TEXTBOOK OF PULMONARY MEDICINE
VOLUME 1

CLINICAL EVALUATION, PHYSIOLOGY, AND INFECTIOUS PATHOLOGIES

Edited by:
Dr. Marie Hyacinth Chiong Tumara

ALLIED
HEALTH
PRESS

Textbook of Pulmonary Medicine Volume 1

Clinical Evaluation, Physiology, and Infectious Pathologies

Dr. Marie Hyacinth Chiong Tumara

Allied Health Press
4164 Lakeshore Road
Burlington ON L7L 1A4
Canada
www.alliedhealthpress.com
Email: orders@arclereducation.com

ISBN: 978-1-77956-812-0

ABOUT THE EDITOR

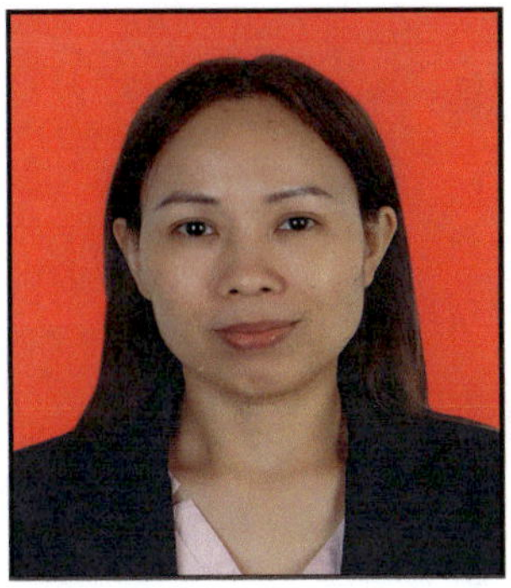

Dr. Marie Hyacinth Chiong Tumara, MD, FPCP, is an Internist with over 16 years of clinical practice and 11 years of government health service. She currently serves as Medical Director and OFW PEME Physician, with expertise in occupational and maritime medicine. A Fellow of the Philippine College of Physicians, she has authored research and medical reports and actively contributes to policy development in hospital and clinical settings. She is presently pursuing her Master's in Health and Hospital Management at Xavier University–Ateneo de Cagayan.

Brief Table of Contents

1. Physical Examination of the Respiratory System 1
2. Growth, Development, and Morphology of the Respiratory Tract 39
3. Normal Respiratory Physiology 75
4. Defense Mechanisms in the Respiratory System 111
5. Diagnostic Methods in Lung Diseases 149
6. Pneumonias, Lung Abscess, and Bronchiectasis 185
7. Tuberculosis 223
8. Infection Due to Nontuberculous Mycobacteria 259
9. Fungal Infections of the Lung and Parasitic Lung Diseases 293
10. Bronchial Asthma 327
11. Chronic Obstructive Pulmonary Diseases 363
12. Respiratory Failure 399

Index 435

Getting Started with This Book

Chapter Openers

A list of Chapter Outline is presented providing a brief Introduction to what will be covered in the chapter.

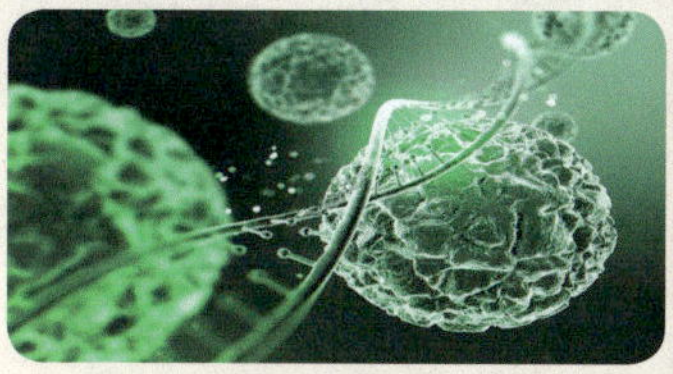

Introduction

Often referred to as the science of life, biology is a broad field of study aimed at comprehending the several kinds of life on Earth, from tiny creatures to sophisticated multicellular entities. Comprising several subfields, including molecular biology, ecology, and evolutionary biology, each of which advances our knowledge of living systems, this field clarifies the mechanisms controlling life events, including development, reproduction, and interaction with the surroundings, which is the central goal of biology. Moreover, biology fills in the void between the natural sciences and medicine by offering a necessary understanding of health, illness, and the interactions between organisms and their environments. Dealing with urgent global issues such as climate change, biodiversity loss, and new diseases depends on an awareness of these complex biological interactions, therefore highlighting the critical part biology plays in modern civilization. Fundamentally, biology explores and tests ideas about the living world using the scientific method. Through methodical observation and experimentation,

LEARNING OBJECTIVES

After studying this chapter, you will be able to:

1. Discuss the scientific method in biology;
2. Explain the cell theory;
3. Discuss the genetics and heredity;
4. Evolution and natural selection;
5. Focus on ecology and ecosystems;
6. Learn about human biology;
7. Evaluate the plant biology;
8. Explain the microbiology;
9. Focus on current trends in biology.

1.1. The Scientific Method in Biology

Learning Outcome

1. Describe the steps of the scientific method;
2. Focus on hypothesis formation;
3. Learn about experimental design.

Learning Outcomes

The beginning of each section of every chapter contains a set of Learning Outcomes that inform students of concepts they should understand. These outcomes help students understand what they should be able to do if they have mastered the material in that section.

Test Your Knowledge

Throughout each chapter, Test Your Knowledge cues you to note which topics have been covered and to self-test your understanding of the material presented.

Test Your Knowledge

1. Explain why correlation does not imply causation in scientific experiments.
2. How does the scientific method help reduce the influence of personal opinions in research?

Chapter Summary

The Summary Section appear at the end of each chapter and summarize main concepts covered throughout the chapter. These points provide key concepts in an engaging and meaningful way.

Summary

The investigation of biological principles highlights the importance of a comprehensive view of life by reflecting the intricate interactions that occur within living systems. The complexity of biology goes beyond individual species or systems, as this essay highlights; it also includes the interactions that mold ecosystems and affect biodiversity. Researchers can conduct in-depth analyses of metabolomic data using sophisticated technologies like MetaboAnalyst, which offer insights into the molecular mechanisms underlying these interactions. As demonstrated by the developments in MetaboAnalyst, for example, the integration of diverse omics data promotes a thorough understanding of metabolic pathways and helps identify important biological markers necessary for research on development and disease (Chong et al., 2018). Additionally, the phenomenon of ecological invasions is a key component of biological research and a vital field of study. The introduction of non-native species into unfamiliar habitats has significant ramifications and calls for multidisciplinary management strategies. Examining the origins and effects of these biological incursions, invasion science has become a crucial field that highlights the need to comprehend ecological dynamics and community interactions. As interest in biological invasions increases, new findings are emerging that put conventional ecological theories and practices to the test. The importance of incorporating various scientific viewpoints is shown by this developing discipline, which also highlights how invasive species shape ecosystems and advances our knowledge of ecological resilience (David et al., 2013). When taken as a whole, these discoveries from invasion science and metabolomics highlight the value of multidisciplinary biology research. Fostering cross-disciplinary collaboration and utilizing technological breakthroughs to improve our comprehension of intricate biological interactions are crucial as we look to the future of biological research. In addition to deepening our understanding of the complexities of life, this method lays the groundwork for tackling urgent environmental issues. Future studies can ensure the continued relevance of biology in a world that is constantly changing by acknowledging the interconnection of biological systems and opening the door to creative solutions that support sustainability and biodiversity conservation. We might imagine a thorough comprehension of life that serves both academia and society at large through ongoing investigation and integration of scientific knowledge.

Knowledge Assessment

The chapter includes material designed to review and reinforce each content. It includes Critical Thinking Questions to help test of your understanding of information presented in the chapter and Short answer Questions to review your understanding of the key concepts presented in the chapter.

Critical Thinking Questions

1. **Who is known as the "Father of Modern Biology"?**
   a. Aristotle
   b. Charles Darwin
   c. Gregor Mendel
   d. Louis Pasteur
2. **What is the basic unit of life?**
   a. Atom
   b. Molecule
   c. Cell
   d. Organism
3. **Which branch of biology studies the interaction of organisms with their environment?**
   a. Genetics
   b. Ecology
   c. Physiology
   d. Botany
4. **Which macromolecule is the main source of energy for living organisms?**
   a. Proteins
   b. Lipids
   c. Carbohydrates
   d. Nucleic acids
5. **DNA is primarily responsible for which function in living organisms?**
   a. Energy production
   b. Protein synthesis
   c. Storing genetic information
   d. Regulating body temperature

Short Answer Questions

1. What is biology, and why is it important to study biology?
2. What are the three main domains of life, and how are they different from one another?
3. Define homeostasis and give an example of how it works in living organisms.
4. What is the cell theory, and why is it fundamental to biology?
5. How do autotrophs and heterotrophs differ in the way they obtain energy?
6. What is the scientific method, and how is it applied in biological research?
7. Discuss how biology helps address global challenges such as climate change, disease, and food security.
8. Explain the levels of biological organization from the smallest unit to the largest. Provide examples at each level.
9. Describe the relationship between structure and function in biology, giving specific examples from cells or organs.
10. How has the discovery of genetics shaped our understanding of inheritance and variation among organisms?

Supplementary Materials

Key Terms: A list of key terms is given for quick reference

KEY TERMS FROM THIS CHAPTER

Annotation enrichment analysis	Biological structure	Cell
Cell theory	Cellular structure	Ecology
Ecosystems	Genetics	Human biology
Microbiology	Natural selection	Organism
Plant biology		

Further Resources: Recommendations for additional readings, websites, and multimedia resources.

References

1. Argelaguet, R., Velten, B., Arnol, D., Dietrich, S., Zenz, T., Marioni, J. C., Buettner, F., et al. (2018). Multi-omics factor analysis—A framework for unsupervised integration of multi-omics data sets. *Molecular Systems Biology, 14*. https://doi.org/10.15252/msb.20178124.
2. Bacher, S., Blackburn, T. M., Essl, F., & Genovesi, P. (2017). *Socio-Economic Impact Classification of Alien Taxa (SEICAT)*. https://core.ac.uk/download/286567949.pdf (accessed on 8th March 2025).
3. Barnett, R., Brace, S., Cucchi, T., & Dobney, K. (2013). *Divergent Evolutionary Processes Associated with Colonization of Offshore Islands*. https://core.ac.uk/download/20664364.pdf (accessed on 8th March 2025).

Detailed Table of Contents

List of Figures — *xv*
Preface — *xxi*

CHAPTER 1

Physical Examination of the Respiratory System — 1

Introduction 1
1.1. Anatomy of the Respiratory System 4
1.1.1. Major Components: Lungs, Trachea, Bronchi 5
1.1.2. Role of the Diaphragm and Intercostal Muscles 6
1.1.3. Upper Vs. Lower Respiratory Tract 7
1.2. Techniques For Physical Examination 8
1.2.1. Inspection: Visual Assessment of the Chest 10
1.2.2. Palpation: Feeling For Abnormalities 11
1.2.3. Auscultation: Listening To Breath Sounds 12
1.3. Common Signs and Symptoms 13
1.3.1. Cough: Types and Significance 14
1.3.2. Shortness of Breath: Causes and Implications 15
1.3.3. Chest Pain: Differential Diagnosis 16
1.4. Diagnostic Tools in Respiratory Examination 18
1.4.1. Spirometry: Measuring Lung Function 18
1.4.2. Peak Flow Meter: Assessing Airflow 19
1.4.3. Imaging Studies: X-Rays and CT Scans 20
1.5. Interpretation of Findings 22
1.5.1. Normal Vs. Abnormal Breath Sounds 22
1.5.2. Identifying Respiratory Distress 23
1.5.3. Correlating Physical Findings With Patient History 24
1.6. Common Respiratory Conditions 26
1.6.1. Asthma: Symptoms and Examination Findings 26
1.6.2. Chronic Obstructive Pulmonary Disease (COPD): Key Indicators 27
1.6.3. Pneumonia: Physical Examination Clues 28
Summary 30
References 33

CHAPTER 2

Growth, Development, and Morphology of the Respiratory Tract — 39

Introduction 39
2.1. Embryonic Development of the Respiratory Tract 43
2.1.1. Formation of the Respiratory Diverticulum 44
2.1.2. Development of the Trachea and Bronchi 45
2.1.3. Role of Genetic Factors in Respiratory Development 45
2.2. Morphological Features of the Respiratory Tract 47
2.2.1. Structure of the Upper Respiratory Tract 48
2.2.2. Anatomy of the Lower Respiratory Tract 49
2.2.3. Histological Differences Across Respiratory Regions 50
2.3. Growth Patterns of the Respiratory Tract 52
2.3.1. Changes During Fetal Development 53

2.3.2. Postnatal Growth and Maturation 54
2.3.3. Factors Influencing Respiratory Growth 55
2.4. Functional Development of the Respiratory System 56
2.4.1. Transition From Fetal To Neonatal Respiration 57
2.4.2. Development of Gas Exchange Capabilities 58
2.4.3. Impact of Environmental Factors On Functional Growth 59
2.5. Pathological Considerations in Respiratory Development 60
2.5.1. Congenital Anomalies of the Respiratory Tract 61
2.5.2. Effects of Prenatal Exposure To Toxins 62
2.5.3. Respiratory Diseases Affecting Growth and Morphology 63
2.6. Comparative Morphology of the Respiratory Tract 64
2.6.1. Differences Between Mammals and Reptiles 65
2.6.2. Adaptations in Avian Respiratory Systems 67
2.6.3. Evolutionary Perspectives On Respiratory Morphology 68
Summary 69
References 72

CHAPTER 3

Normal Respiratory Physiology 75

Introduction 75
3.1. Anatomy of the Respiratory System 78
3.1.1. Major Components of the Respiratory System 79
3.1.2. Structure and Function of the Lungs 80
3.1.3. Role of the Diaphragm and Intercostal Muscles 81
3.2. Mechanics of Breathing 83
3.2.1. Inhalation and Exhalation Processes 83
3.2.2. Role of Pressure Gradients in Respiration 84
3.2.3. Factors Affecting Lung Compliance and Resistance 85
3.3. Gas Exchange 87
3.3.1. Mechanism of Diffusion in Alveoli 88
3.3.2. Role of Hemoglobin in Oxygen Transport 89
3.3.3. Carbon Dioxide Transport and Elimination 90
3.4. Regulation of Breathing 91
3.4.1. Neural Control of Respiration 92
3.4.2. Chemical Regulation Through Blood Gases 93
3.4.3. Reflexes Involved in Respiratory Control 94
3.5. Respiratory Volumes and Capacities 95
3.5.1. Definitions of Tidal Volume, Vital Capacity, And Residual Volume 96
3.5.2 Significance of lung volume measurement 97
3.5.3. Clinical Significance of Altered Respiratory Volumes 98
3.6. Impact of Environmental Factors 99
3.6.1. Effects of Altitude On Respiratory Physiology 100
3.6.2. Influence of Pollutants and Allergens 100
3.6.3. Adaptations To Exercise and Physical Activity 101
Summary 103
References 106

CHAPTER 4

Defense Mechanisms in the Respiratory System 111

Introduction 111
4.1. Anatomy of the Respiratory System 114
4.1.1. Major Components of the Respiratory System 115
4.1.2. Role of the Upper and Lower Respiratory Tracts 116
4.1.3. Interaction With Other Body Systems 117
4.2. Physical Barriers 119
4.2.1. Nasal Hairs and Mucous Membranes 119
4.2.2. Cilia and Their Function in Trapping Particles 120
4.2.3. The Role of the Cough Reflex 121
4.3. Immune Response in the Respiratory System 123
4.3.1. Overview of the Immune Cells Involved 124
4.3.2. Mechanisms of Inflammation in Response To Pathogens 125
4.3.3. Role of Antibodies in Respiratory Defense 126
4.4. Mucociliary Escalator 128
4.4.1. Function of Mucus in Trapping Pathogens 129

4.4.2. Mechanism of Ciliary Movement 130
4.4.3. Importance of the Mucociliary Escalator in Health 131
4.5. Role of Alveolar Macrophages 133
4.5.1. Function and Location of Alveolar Macrophages 133
4.5.2. Mechanism of Pathogen Clearance 134
4.5.3. Interaction With Other Immune Cells 135
4.6. Impact of Environmental Factors 137
4.6.1. Effects of Pollution On Respiratory Defense 137
4.6.2. Influence of Smoking On Defense Mechanisms 139
4.6.3. Role of Allergens in Respiratory Health 140
Summary 142
References 145

CHAPTER 5

Diagnostic Methods in Lung Diseases 149

Introduction 149
5.1. Clinical Evaluation 152
5.1.1. Patient History and Symptom Assessment 153
5.1.2. Physical Examination Techniques 154
5.1.3. Role of Clinical Judgment in Diagnosis 155
5.2. Imaging Techniques 157
5.2.1. Chest X-Rays and Their Diagnostic Value 157
5.2.2. Computed Tomography (CT) Scans 158
5.2.3. Magnetic Resonance Imaging (MRI) Applications 159
5.3. Pulmonary Function Tests (PFTs) 161
5.3.1. Spirometry and Its Significance 162
5.3.2. Diffusion Capacity Testing 162
5.3.3. Bronchodilator Response Assessment 163
5.4. Laboratory Tests 165
5.4.1. Blood Tests For Inflammatory Markers 165
5.4.2. Sputum Analysis and Culture 166
5.4.3. Arterial Blood Gas (ABG) Analysis 167
5.5. Endoscopic Procedures 169
5.5.1. Bronchoscopy and Its Diagnostic Uses 170
5.5.2. Endobronchial Ultrasound (EBUS) 171
5.5.3. Thoracoscopy For Pleural Disease Evaluation 171
5.6. Advanced Diagnostic Techniques 173
5.6.1. Genetic Testing For Hereditary Lung Diseases 173
5.6.2. Biomarkers in Lung Disease Diagnosis 174
5.6.3. Artificial Intelligence in Diagnostic Imaging 176
Summary 177
References 180

CHAPTER 6

Pneumonias, Lung Abscess, and Bronchiectasis 185

Introduction 185
6.1. Types of Pneumonia 189
6.1.1. Community-Acquired Pneumonia (CAP) 190
6.1.2. Hospital-Acquired Pneumonia (Hap) 191
6.1.3. Aspiration Pneumonia 192
6.2. Causes and Risk Factors 193
6.2.1. Infectious Agents (Bacteria, Viruses, Fungi) 194
6.2.2. Environmental Factors (Pollution, Smoking) 195
6.2.3. Underlying Health Conditions (COPD, Immunosuppression) 196
6.3. Symptoms and Diagnosis 198
6.3.1. Common Symptoms of Pneumonia 198
6.3.2. Diagnostic Tests (Chest X-Ray, Sputum Culture) 200
6.3.3. Differentiating Between Pneumonia and Other Conditions 200
6.4. Lung Abscess: Definition and Causes 202
6.4.1. Pathophysiology of Lung Abscess 202
6.4.2. Common Causes (Aspiration, Infections) 203
6.4.3. Risk Factors For Developing Lung Abscess 204
6.5. Symptoms and Treatment of Lung Abscess 206
6.5.1. Clinical Presentation of Lung Abscess 207
6.5.2. Diagnostic Approaches (Ct Scan, Bronchoscopy) 207
6.5.3. Treatment Options (Antibiotics, Surgery) 208
6.6. Bronchiectasis: Overview and Etiology 209
6.6.1. Definition and Pathophysiology of Bronchiectasis 210
6.6.2. Causes (Cystic Fibrosis, Infections) 211

6.6.3. Risk Factors (Genetic, Environmental) 212
Summary **214**
References **217**

CHAPTER 7

Tuberculosis 223

Introduction **223**
7.1. Causes and Transmission **227**
7.1.1. Bacterial Agent: Mycobacterium Tuberculosis 227
7.1.2. Modes of Transmission 228
7.1.3. Risk Factors For Infection 229
7.2. Symptoms and Diagnosis **230**
7.2.1. Common Symptoms of Tuberculosis 231
7.2.2. Diagnostic Tests and Procedures 232
7.2.3. Challenges in Diagnosing Tuberculosis 233
7.3. Treatment Options **234**
7.3.1. Standard Treatment Regimens 235
7.3.2. Drug-Resistant Tuberculosis 236
7.3.3. Importance of Adherence To Treatment 237
7.4. Global Impact **238**
7.4.1. Prevalence of Tuberculosis Worldwide 239
7.4.2. Socioeconomic Factors Influencing Spread 240
7.4.3. Public Health Initiatives and Their Effectiveness 241
7.5. Prevention Strategies **242**
7.5.1. Vaccination Efforts (BCG Vaccine) 243
7.5.2. Screening and Early Detection 244
7.5.3. Education and Awareness Campaigns 245
7.6. Current Research and Developments **246**
7.6.1. Advances in Vaccine Research 247
7.6.2. New Diagnostic Technologies 248
7.6.3. Innovative Treatment Approaches 249
Summary **251**
References **254**

CHAPTER 8

Infection Due to Nontuberculous Mycobacteria 259

Introduction **259**
8.1. Classification of Nontuberculous Mycobacteria **262**
8.1.1. Major Species of Nontuberculous Mycobacteriaand Their Characteristics 263
8.1.2. Environmental Sources of Nontuberculous Mycobacteria 264
8.1.3. Differences Between Nontuberculous Mycobacteriaand ***Mycobacterium Tuberculosis*** ***265***
8.2. Pathogenesis of Nontuberculous Mycobacterial Infections **266**
8.2.1. Mechanisms of Infection and Host Response 267
8.2.2. Risk Factors For NTM Infections 268
8.2.3. Clinical Manifestations of NTM Infections 269
8.3. Diagnosis of Nontuberculous Mycobacterial Infections **270**
8.3.1. Laboratory Techniques For Identification 271
8.3.2. Challenges in Diagnosing nontuberculous mycobacterialnfections 272
8.3.3. Role of Imaging Studies in Diagnosis 273
8.4. Treatment Options For Nontuberculous Mycobacterial Infections **274**
8.4.1. Antibiotic Regimens and Their Effectiveness 275
8.4.2. Duration of Treatment and Patient Adherence 276
8.4.3. Emerging Therapies and Research Directions 277
8.5. Epidemiology of Nontuberculous Mycobacterial Infections **279**
8.5.1. Global Prevalence and Incidence Rates 280
8.5.2. Demographic Factors Influencing Infection Rates 280
8.5.3. Geographic Distribution of NTM Species 281
8.6. Public Health Implications **282**
8.6.1. Impact of NTM Infections On Healthcare Systems 283
8.6.2. Prevention Strategies For At-Risk

Populations 284
8.6.3. Importance of Awareness and Education 285
Summary **287**
References **290**

CHAPTER 9

Fungal Infections of the Lung and Parasitic Lung Diseases **293**

Introduction **293**
9.1. Overview of Fungal Infections **296**
9.1.1. Common Types of Fungal Infections Affecting the Lungs 297
9.1.2. Risk Factors For Developing Fungal Lung Infections 298
9.1.3. Symptoms and Clinical Presentation 299
9.2. Pathophysiology of Fungal Infections **300**
9.2.1. Mechanisms of Fungal Invasion in Lung Tissue 301
9.2.2. Immune Response To Fungal Infections 301
9.2.3. Consequences of Untreated Fungal Infections 302
9.3. Diagnosis of Fungal Lung Infections **304**
9.3.1. Diagnostic Imaging Techniques 305
9.3.2. Laboratory Tests and Cultures 305
9.3.3. Differential Diagnosis 306
9.4. Treatment Options For Fungal Infections **307**
9.4.1. Antifungal Medications 308
9.4.2. Supportive Care and Management Strategies 310
9.4.3. Role of Surgery in Severe Cases 310
9.5. Overview of Parasitic Lung Diseases **312**
9.5.1. Common Parasites That Affect the Lungs 312
9.5.2. Transmission Routes of Parasitic Infections 314
9.5.3. Symptoms and Clinical Presentation 315
9.6. Diagnosis and Treatment of Parasitic Lung Diseases **316**
9.6.1. Diagnostic Methods For Identifying Parasitic Infections 317
9.6.2. Treatment Options and Medications 318
9.6.3. Prevention Strategies For Parasitic Lung Diseases 319
Summary **321**
References **324**

CHAPTER 10

Bronchial Asthma **327**

Introduction **327**
10.1. Causes of Bronchial Asthma **330**
10.1.1. Genetic Factors 331
10.1.2. Environmental Triggers 332
10.1.3. Occupational Exposures 333
10.2. Symptoms of Bronchial Asthma **334**
10.2.1. Shortness of Breath 335
10.2.2. Wheezing 336
10.2.3. Chest Tightness 336
10.3. Diagnosis of Bronchial Asthma **338**
10.3.1. Medical History Assessment 338
10.3.2. Physical Examination 339
10.3.3. Diagnostic Tests (e.g., Spirometry) 340
10.4. Treatment Options For Bronchial Asthma **341**
10.4.1. Medications (e.g., Inhalers) 342
10.4.2. Lifestyle Modifications 343
10.4.3. Allergy Management 344
10.5. Management Strategies For Bronchial Asthma **346**
10.5.1. Asthma Action Plans 346
10.5.2. Monitoring Symptoms 347
10.5.3. Avoiding Triggers 348
10.6. Impact of Bronchial Asthma **350**
10.6.1. Effects On Daily Life 351
10.6.2. Economic Burden 351
10.6.3. Psychological Implications 352
Summary **354**
References **357**

CHAPTER 11

Chronic Obstructive Pulmonary Diseases **363**

Introduction **363**
11.1. Causes of Chronic Obstructive Pulmonary

Diseases 366

11.1.1. Smoking As the Primary Risk Factor 367

11.1.2. Environmental Pollutants and Occupational Hazards 368

11.1.3. Genetic Factors and Alpha-1 Antitrypsin Deficiency 369

11.2. Symptoms and Diagnosis 370

11.2.1. Common Symptoms of COPD 371

11.2.2. Diagnostic Methods Used in Identifying COPD 372

11.2.3. Importance of Early Diagnosis 373

11.3. Pathophysiology of COPD 374

11.3.1. Mechanisms of Airflow Limitation 375

11.3.2. Inflammatory Processes Involved in COPD 375

11.3.3. Impact On Lung Function and Overall Health 376

11.4. Treatment Options 377

11.4.1. Pharmacological Treatments (Bronchodilators, Steroids) 378

11.4.2. Non-Pharmacological Interventions (Pulmonary Rehabilitation) 379

11.4.3. Surgical Options (Lung Volume Reduction Surgery, Transplantation) 380

11.5. Management of COPD 381

11.5.1. Importance of Lifestyle Changes (Smoking Cessation, Exercise) 383

11.5.2. Role of Patient Education and Self-Management 383

11.5.3. Monitoring and Follow-Up Care 384

11.6. Impact of COPD On Quality of Life 385

11.6.1. Physical Limitations and Daily Activities 386

11.6.2. Psychological Effects and Mental Health Considerations 387

11.6.3. Economic Burden and Healthcare Costs 388

Summary 390

References 393

CHAPTER 12

Respiratory Failure 399

Introduction 399

12.1. Types of Respiratory Failure 402

12.1.1. Acute Respiratory Failure 403

12.1.2. Chronic Respiratory Failure 404

12.1.3. Hypoxemic Vs. Hypercapnic Respiratory Failure 405

12.2. Causes of Respiratory Failure 406

12.2.1. Obstructive Lung Diseases 407

12.2.2. Restrictive Lung Diseases 408

12.2.3. Central Nervous System Disorders 409

12.3. Symptoms and Diagnosis 410

12.3.1. Common Symptoms of Respiratory Failure 411

12.3.2. Diagnostic Tests and Procedures 412

12.3.3. Importance of Early Diagnosis 413

12.4. Treatment Options 414

12.4.1. Oxygen Therapy 415

12.4.2. Mechanical Ventilation 416

12.4.3. Pharmacological Interventions 417

12.5. Complications Associated With Respiratory Failure 419

12.5.1. Cardiovascular Complications 419

12.5.2. Infections and Sepsis 421

12.5.3. Long-Term Pulmonary Damage 422

12.6. Prevention Strategies 423

12.6.1. Smoking Cessation Programs 423

12.6.2. Vaccination and Infection Control 424

12.6.3. Management of Chronic Respiratory Conditions 425

Summary 427

References 430

Index 435

LIST OF FIGURES

Figure 1.1. Physical examination of the respiratory system
Figure 1.2. Physical examination
Figure 1.3. Anatomy of the respiratory system
Figure 1.4. Major components of the respiratory system
Figure 1.5. Role of the diaphragm and intercostal muscles
Figure 1.6. Upper vs. lower respiratory tract
Figure 1.7. Techniques for physical examination
Figure 1.8. Visual assessment of the chest
Figure 1.9. Palpation: feeling for abnormalities
Figure 1.9. Auscultating breath sounds
Figure 1.10. Types of cough
Figure 1.11. Causes of shortness of breath
Figure 1.12. Chest pain – differential diagnosis framework
Figure 1.13. Spirometry
Figure 1.14. Peak flow meter
Figure 1.15. Chest X-ray (CXR)
Figure 1.16. Normal vs. abnormal breath sounds
Figure 1.17. Identifying respiratory distress
Figure 1.18. Testing for asthma
Figure 1.19. Chronic obstructive pulmonary disease (COPD): key indicators
Figure 2.1. Growth, development, and morphology of the respiratory tract
Figure 2.2. The respiratory tract
Figure 2.3. Embryonic development of the respiratory tract
Figure 2.6. Formation of the respiratory diverticulum
Figure 2.7. Development of the trachea and bronchi
Figure 2.8. Morphological overview of the human respiratory tract
Figure 2.9. Upper respiratory tract
Figure 2.10. Anatomy of the lower respiratory tract
Figure 2.11. Histological differences across respiratory regions
Figure 2.12. Growth patterns of the respiratory tract

Figure 2.13. Postnatal growth and maturation of the respiratory tract
Figure 2.14. Functional development of the respiratory system
Figure 2.15. Transition from fetal to neonatal respiration
Figure 2.16. Development of gas exchange capabilities
Figure 2.17. Congenital anomalies of the respiratory tract
Figure 2.18. Effects of prenatal exposure to toxins
Figure 2.19. Respiratory tract of the mammals and reptiles
Figure 2.20. Adaptations in avian respiratory systems
Figure 3.1. Physiology of the respiratory system
Figure 3.2. Normal respiratory functions
Figure 3.3. Anatomy of the respiratory system
Figure 3.4. Major components of the respiratory system
Figure 3.5. Structure and function of the lungs
Figure 3.6. Role of the diaphragm and intercostal muscles
Figure 3.7. Mechanics of breathing
Figure 3.8. Inhalation and exhalation processes
Figure 3.9. Role of pressure gradients in respiration
Figure 3.10. Gas exchange
Figure 3.11. Mechanism of diffusion in alveoli
Figure 3.12. Role of hemoglobin in oxygen transport
Figure 3.13. Regulation of breathing
Figure 3.14. Neural control of respiration
Figure 3.14. Reflexes involved in respiratory control
Figure 3.15. Lung volumes and capacities
Figure 4.1. Defense mechanisms of the respiratory system
Figure 4.2. Anatomy df the respiratory system
Figure 4.3. Role of the upper and lower respiratory tracts
Figure 4.4. Respiratory tract interaction with other body systems
Figure 4.5. Nasal mucous is the nose's first line of defence
Figure 4.6. Cilia in lungs
Figure 4.7. The role of the cough reflex
Figure 4.8. Immune response in the respiratory system
Figure 4.9. Mechanisms of inflammation in response to pathogens
Figure 4.9. Role of antibodies in respiratory defense
Figure 4.10. The mucociliary escalator
Figure 4.12. Function of mucus in trapping pathogens

Figure 4.12. Mechanism of ciliary movement
Figure 4.13. Importance of the mucociliary escalator in health
Figure 4.14. Role of alveolar macrophages
Figure 4.15. Function and location of alveolar macrophages
Figure 4.15. Interaction with other immune cells' role in the respiratory system's defense mechanisms
Figure 4.16. Effects of pollution on respiratory defense
Figure 4.17. Tobacco smoke induces and alters immune responses in the lung
Figure 4.18. Role of allergens in respiratory health
Figure 5.1. Diagnostic methods in lung diseases
Figure 5.2. Diagnosing lung diseases
Figure 5.3. Clinical evaluation of lung diseases
Figure 5.4. Patient history and symptom assessment of lung diseases
Figure 5.5. Physical examination techniques for lung diseases
Figure 5.6. Role of clinical judgment in diagnosis
Figure 5.7. Chest X-rays and their diagnostic value
Figure 5.8. Computed tomography (CT) scans
Figure 5.9. Magnetic resonance imaging (MRI)
Figure 5.10. Pulmonary function tests (PFTs)
Figure 5.11. Spirometry
Figure 5.12. Lung diffusion testing
Figure 5.13. Response to bronchodilators in patients with bronchiectasis
Figure 5.14. Inflammatory markers used in blood tests
Figure 5.15. Sputum analysis and culture
Figure 5.16. Arterial blood gas (ABGs) analysis
Figure 5.17. Endoscopy procedure
Figure 5.18. Bronchoscopy and its diagnostic uses
Figure 5.19. Endobronchial ultrasound (EBUS)
Figure 5.20. Genetic testing for hereditary lung diseases
Figure 5.21. Biomarkers in lung disease diagnosis
Figure 6.1. Understanding pneumonia
Figure 6.2. Lung abscess
Figure 6.3. Bronchiectasis
Figure 6.4. Community-acquired pneumonia (CAP)
Figure 6.5. Hospital-acquired pneumonia
Figure 6.6. Aspiration pneumonia
Figure 6.7. Infectious agents

Figure 6.8. Environmental factors
Figure 6.9. Underlying health conditions (COPD, Immunosuppression)
Figure 6.10. Common symptoms of pneumonia
Figure 6.11. Diagnostic tests (Chest X-ray, Sputum Culture) of pneumonia
Figure 6.12. Pathophysiology of lung abscess
Figure 6.13. Infection-associated lung abscess
Figure 6.14. The symptoms of a lung abscess
Figure 6.15. CT scan of lung abscess
Figure 6.16. Overview of bronchiectasis
Figure 6.17. Cystic fibrosis lungs
Figure 7.1. Tuberculosis
Figure 7.2. The historical context of tuberculosis (TB)
Figure 7.3. Bacterial agent: *Mycobacterium tuberculosis*
Figure 7.4. The modes of transmission of tuberculosis (TB)
Figure 7.5. Common symptoms of tuberculosis
Figure 7.6. Challenges in diagnosing tuberculosis
Figure 7.7. Standard treatment regimens for tuberculosis
Figure 7.8. Drug-resistant tuberculosis
Figure 7.9. The global impact of tuberculosis (TB)
Figure 7.10. The spread of tuberculosis (TB)
Figure 7.11. Prevention strategies of tuberculosis (TB)
Figure 7.12. Vaccination efforts (BCG vaccine)
Figure 7.13. Screening and early detection of tuberculosis (TB)
Figure 7.14. Current research and developments of tuberculosis (TB)
Figure 7.15. Advances in vaccine research of tuberculosis (TB)
Figure 7.16. New diagnostic technologies for tuberculosis (TB)
Figure 8.1. Nontuberculous mycobacterial Infections
Figure 8.2. Nontuberculous mycobacteria (NTM)
Figure 8.3. Classification of nontuberculous mycobacteria
Figure 8.4. Major species of Nontuberculous mycobacteria and their characteristics
Figure 8.5. Environmental sources of Nontuberculous mycobacteria
Figure 8.6. Pathogenesis of nontuberculous mycobacterial infections
Figure 8.7. Mechanisms of infection and host response in infection with nontuberculous mycobacteria (NTM)
Figure 8.8. Risk factors for Nontuberculous mycobacteria infections
Figure 8.9. Symptoms of nontuberculous mycobacterial infections
Figure 8.10. Laboratory techniques for identification of nontuberculous mycobacterial infections

Figure 8.11. Role of imaging studies in the diagnosis of nontuberculous mycobacterial infections
Figure 8.12. Treatment options for nontuberculous mycobacterial infections
Figure 8.13. Duration of treatment and patient adherence for nontuberculous mycobacterial infections
Figure 8.14. Epidemiology of nontuberculous mycobacterial infections
Figure 8.15. Demographic factors influencing infection rates
Figure 8.16. Impact of Nontuberculous mycobacteria infections on healthcare systems
Figure 9.1. Fungal infections of the lung and parasitic lung diseases
Figure 9.2. Fungal infections and parasitic diseases
Figure 9.3. Fungal Infections of the lungs
Figure 9.4. Risk factors for developing fungal lung infections
Figure 9.5. Pathophysiology of fungal infections, lung infections
Figure 9.6. Immune response to fungal infections in the lung
Figure 9.7. The consequences of untreated fungal infections in lungs
Figure 9.8. Diagnosis of fungal lung infections
Figure 9.9. Laboratory tests and cultures of fungal lung infections
Figure 9.10. The treatment options for fungal infections of the lung
Figure 9.11. Antifungal medications for lung infections
Figure 9.12. Role of surgery in severe lung infections
Figure 9.13. Parasitic lung diseases
Figure 9.14. Common parasites that affect the lungs
Figure 9.15. Transmission routes of parasitic infections to the lungs
Figure 9.16. Treatment of parasitic lung diseases
Figure 9.17. Diagnostic methods for identifying parasitic infections
Figure 10.1. Bronchial asthma
Figure 10.2. Understanding asthma
Figure 10.3. Causes of bronchial asthma
Figure 10.4. Environmental triggers of bronchial asthma
Figure 10.5. Symptoms of bronchial asthma
Figure 10.6. Shortness of breath
Figure 10.7. Wheezing
Figure 10.8. Chest tightness
Figure 10.9. Diagnosis of bronchial asthma
Figure 10.10. Medical history assessment
Figure 10.11. Diagnostic tests
Figure 10.12. Treatment options for bronchial asthma
Figure 10.13. Medications for bronchial asthma

Figure 10.14. Allergic asthma
Figure 10.15. Asthma action plan
Figure 10.16. Avoiding triggers in bronchial asthma
Figure 10.17. Impact of bronchial asthma
Figure 10.18. The economic burden of bronchial asthma
Figure 11.1. Chronic obstructive pulmonary disease
Figure 11.2. Importance of studying COPD
Figure 11.3. COPD risk factors
Figure 11.4. Genetic factors and alpha-1 antitrypsin deficiency of COPD
Figure 11.5. Symptoms of COPD
Figure 11.6. The importance of early diagnosis in COPD
Figure 11.7. Pathophysiology of COPD
Figure 11.8. Inflammatory processes involved in COPD
Figure 11.9. Pharmacological treatments
Figure 11.10. Non-pharmacological interventions
Figure 11.11. Management of COPD
Figure 11.12. Self-management plan for COPD
Figure 11.13. Impact of COPD on quality of life
Figure 11.14. Psychological effects and mental health considerations of COPD
Figure 12.1. Respiratory failure
Figure 12.2. Woman with respiratory failure, pneumonia, and shortness of breath
Figure 12.3. Acute respiratory failure
Figure 12.4. Hypoxemic respiratory failure
Figure 12.5. The causes of respiratory failure
Figure 12.6. Obstructive lung diseases
Figure 12.7. Restrictive lung diseases
Figure 12.8. Symptoms of respiratory failure
Figure 12.9. Diagnostic tests and procedures for respiratory failure
Figure 12.10. Oxygen therapy
Figure 12.11. Mechanical ventilation
Figure 12.12. Cardiovascular complications with respiratory failure
Figure 12.13. Infections and sepsis with respiratory failure
Figure 12.14. Smoking cessation programs
Figure 12.15. Vaccination and infection control for respiratory failure

PREFACE

Pulmonary medicine is a significant specialty of the field of medical science, focusing on diseases and conditions affecting one of the body's most vital systems—the respiratory system, which is responsible for breathing. Breathing is an involuntary, yet constant, activity, but the illnesses that impede its functioning can be varied, serious, and even life-threatening. From acute infections to chronic inflammatory diseases and structural abnormalities, the specialty demands a thorough understanding of anatomy, physiology, immunology, microbiology, and clinical examination methods. Recognition of subtle signs, establishment of patterns, and response with evidence-based treatment are of utmost value in helping to secure salutary results for patients with respiratory illnesses.

In recent decades, there has been a significant advancement that has transformed the diagnostic and therapeutic landscape of respiratory care. New imaging technology, updated diagnostic criteria, a greater understanding of microbial pathogens, and improved pharmacological and non-pharmacological therapies have all required clinicians to stay current with modern concepts. Pulmonary disease is not just the management of common disorders such as pneumonia and asthma, but also the detection of atypical infections, extrapulmonary manifestations of respiratory diseases, and the impact of comorbidities. A holistic beginning, with the fundamental appreciation of physiology and clinical assessment, remains at the core of accurate diagnosis and effective management.

Textbook of Pulmonary Medicine: Volume 1 has been created to provide a thorough, clinically relevant, and systematically organized foundation in respiratory medicine. It has been penned with a focus on both conceptual clarity and functional usefulness, such that the material finds salience with students at various stages of their professional life. Focused on both practicing clinicians, residents, and medical students, the content represents today's best practices and evidence-based guidelines in a convenient format for use. Priorities have been placed on logical sequence, clear description, explanatory examples, and up-to-date references to make this resource credible and accessible.

Chapter 1 describes physical examination maneuvers and the rationale for examining the respiratory system, prioritizing inspection, palpation, percussion, and auscultation. Clinical significance of each maneuver is described in terms of relating bedside findings to potential underlying pathology. The chapter also focuses on commonly encountered presentations along with how to rule out alternative causes to assist with differential diagnosis.

Chapter 2 deals with developmental biology and morphological organization of the respiratory tract. It describes embryonic development of the airways and lungs, congenital anomalies, and how growth patterns influence respiratory function throughout life. This knowledge of structure forms a basis for understanding both normal function and disease processes.

Chapter 3 provides an overview of normal respiratory physiology. It addresses gas exchange, ventilation, perfusion, lung mechanics, and control of breathing. Basic diagrams and examples effectively convey these concepts with clinical relevance, particularly in relation to understanding abnormal conditions such as respiratory failure and airway obstruction.

Chapter 4 describes the defense mechanisms that ensure the respiratory system from pathogens and toxic materials. Alveolar macrophages, lymphoid tissue, mucociliary clearance mechanism, and systemic immune response are all discussed in detail. To be able to comprehend how infection is prevented or occurs in the case of immunocompromised or structural lung disease patients, these mechanisms have to be clearly understood.

Chapter 5 explains the equipment and techniques used in the diagnosis of lung disease. This includes radiographic imaging, pulmonary function testing, arterial blood gas sampling, bronchoscopy, and microbiological examination. Each method is reviewed in terms of indications, interpretation, limitations, and clinical utility, yielding a comprehensive representation of today's diagnostic capabilities.

Chapter 6 addresses the various types of pneumonia, lung abscess, and bronchiectasis. Infections are classified by etiology—bacterial, viral, or atypical—and then further characterized by risk factors, radiologic findings, clinical presentation, and treatment. Complications management and antibiotic stewardship are also included in the discussion.

Chapter 7 addresses tuberculosis, a significant public health concern in most parts of the world. The chapter includes comprehensive descriptions of primary and secondary tuberculosis, extrapulmonary disease, diagnostic tests such as GeneXpert and imaging, and current treatment regimens. Reference is made to understanding the clinical spectrum of the disease and the importance of coordination with national control programs.

Chapter 8 shifts the emphasis to infection with nontuberculous mycobacteria. These organisms are increasingly recognized more and more as important pathogens, particularly in immunocompromised hosts and in the presence of underlying lung disease. The chapter distinguishes them from tuberculosis and outlines diagnostic subtleties, classification systems, and treatment options.

Chapter 9 describes the fungal and parasitic pneumonias. Aspergillosis, histoplasmosis, and strongyloidiasis are covered under the aspects of clinical presentation, diagnostic technique in the form of serology and culture, and treatment response. Regional epidemiology and host immune status are given added importance while choosing an appropriate evaluation.

Chapter 10 presents bronchial asthma from both clinical and pathophysiologic perspectives. It includes the inflammation of airways, precipitants, reversibility of the obstruction, and diagnostic techniques such as spirometry and peak flow monitoring. Management of acute exacerbation and control measures in the long term, such as pharmacotherapy and lifestyle changes, are elaborated clearly.

Chapter 11 addresses chronic obstructive pulmonary diseases, such as emphysema and chronic bronchitis. The chapter outlines the pathogenesis of airflow limitation, symptom development, management of exacerbation, and rehabilitation. Staging of disease, smoking cessation therapy, and use of inhaled therapies to improve quality of life are particularly emphasized.

Chapter 12 discusses respiratory failure, a potentially life-threatening condition and one that needs to be identified and treated quickly. The chapter discusses types of respiratory failure, etiology, methods of evaluation, including blood gases and imaging, and invasive and noninvasive ventilatory support management techniques. Decision-making in the acute care setting is the primary focus of the chapter, along with guidelines for oxygen therapy and monitoring parameters.

The book is designed for a broad audience within the medical community. Undergraduate students will find the clean underlying information and systematic explanations behind scholarly education. Postgraduate trainees and residents undergoing exams will be able to utilize the sophisticated clinical correlations and evidence-based data. Practicing pulmonologists and internists can use this book as a ready reference to refresh their knowledge on critical areas and make informed decisions regarding patient care. In addition, allied health practitioners like respiratory therapists and nurses will find the material helpful in expanding their understanding of the conditions they encounter in the clinic.

PHYSICAL EXAMINATION OF THE RESPIRATORY SYSTEM

1

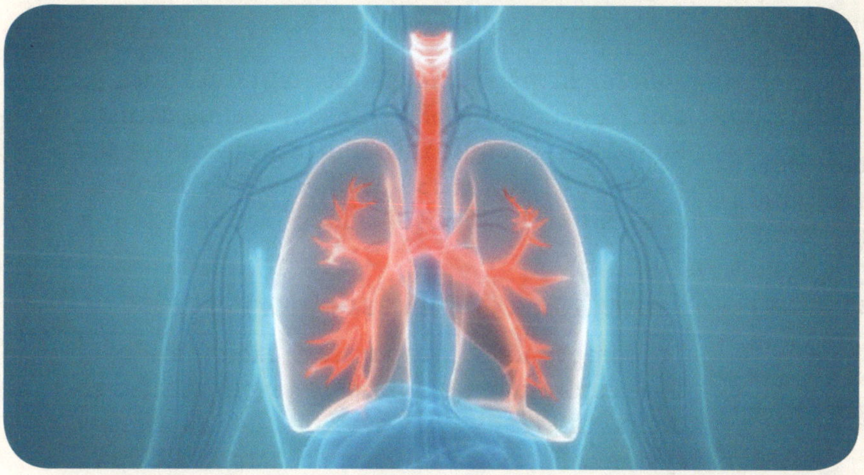

LEARNING OBJECTIVES

After studying this chapter, you will be able to:

1. Discuss the anatomy of the respiratory system
2. List the techniques for physical examination
3. Describe common signs and symptoms
4. Explain diagnostic tools in respiratory examination
5. Focus on the interpretation of findings
6. Explore common respiratory conditions

Introduction

Physical examination of the respiratory system is a crucial component of clinical practice that enhances both diagnostic accuracy and comprehensive patient care. The physical examination is typically a thorough evaluation of respiratory anatomy, function, and pathological dysfunction. The ability of a clinician to provide a practical assessment of respiratory function not only indicates existing respiratory disturbances but may also be a reflection of systemic disturbances potentially resulting from underlying disease processes. Through techniques such as inspection, palpation, percussion, and auscultation, healthcare workers can gather information regarding various conditions that affect airway integrity, lung function, and oxygenation. In addition, a thorough understanding of respiratory physiology enables clinicians to relate clinical findings to potential pathologies, thereby improving the overall efficacy of health interventions and measures. In addition to traditional examination techniques, the development of diagnostic equipment has revolutionized the examination of the respiratory system. Technologies such as spirometry, peak flow meters, and imaging technologies like X-rays and CT scans enhance clinicians' ability to visualize structural and functional disease of the respiratory tract. For example, spirometry provides vital measurements of lung volume and capacity, enabling clinicians to identify obstructive or restrictive pulmonary disorders early. Besides, reconciliation of patient history with examination offers a complete picture of the patients respiratory status, which highlights the multidisciplinary nature of assessments of respiratory systems. As the specialty evolves, ongoing studies continue to reveal new areas for improving diagnostic accuracy and therapeutic outcomes, thereby highlighting the crucial role of detailed respiratory system examinations. Finally, the importance of patient education cannot be emphasized enough in respiratory medicine. Educating patients for their own respiratory disease encourages active participation in their own care.

This involves understanding the need for regular physical inspections, adherence to prescribed therapy, and lifestyle modifications that can aid in maintaining respiratory function. Evidence shows that education interventions can enhance the management of chronic diseases, such as asthma and COPD, by enabling patients to recognize symptoms of exacerbation and seek medical care in a timely manner. Teaching patients about their respiratory system and treatment addresses both the physiological and psychosocial dimensions of care, yielding optimal health benefits. By recognizing the interactive dynamics of education, examination, and intervention, the clinician-patient relationship is ultimately at the center of respiratory health care, which is in alignment with broader objectives of holistic patient-oriented care.

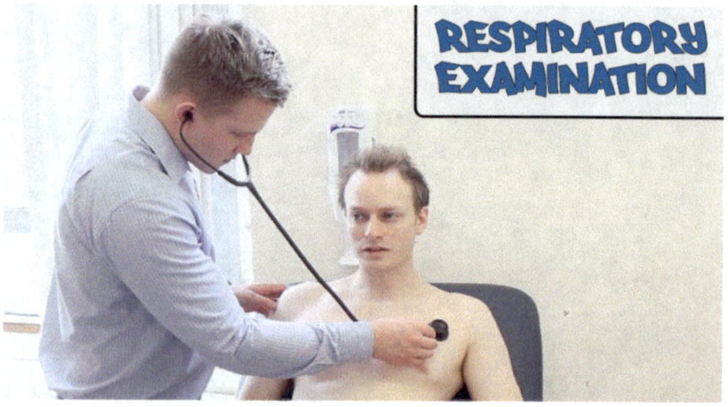

Figure 1.1. Physical examination of the respiratory system.

Source: https://external-content.duckduckgo.com/iu/?u=https%3A%2F%2Fi.ytimg.com%2Fvi%2FGmLvehqi6Yo%2Fmaxresdefault.jpg&f=1&nofb=1&ipt=8837fa1ca39aea53327fc0d07c7046309fc1acf76c4e7fad67d77e55c72d48c9

Definition of the respiratory system

To comprehend the physical examination of the respiratory system, it is essential first to define the respiratory system. The respiratory system refers to the anatomical structures that undertake the process of gas exchange inside the body. The primary components that are included in this process are the nasal cavity, pharynx, larynx, trachea, bronchi, and the lungs, where alveoli assist in the process of oxygen being absorbed into the body and the removal of carbon dioxide. This intricate system serves not only to oxygenate tissues but also to support the function of acid-base balance and maintain temperature during the processes of inhalation and exhalation. As part of the homeostatic process, the respiratory system, if disrupted, can lead to serious health issues, thus further necessitating proper examination techniques for diagnosing respiratory disorders. The effectiveness of the respiratory system depends on its structure and function, with each component given a specific function to allow efficient gas exchange. The upper respiratory system, comprising the nasal passages and sinuses, humidifies and filters air entering the body. The larynx and pharynx serve as tubes that direct air to the trachea. The trachea subsequently bifurcates into the bronchi, which then divide into increasingly smaller bronchioles that lead to alveolar sacs. It is in these microscopic units that the actual gas exchange occurs through thin, moist membranes, where oxygen is absorbed and carbon dioxide is expelled. These are elements to be understood, as they provide a context for the physical examination of the respiratory tract. Practitioners must assess not only the individual structures but also how these intercommunicate to determine conditions that may disrupt the critical process of breathing. Another awareness of the respiratory system involves understanding its physiological components, such as ventilation and perfusion. Ventilation is the mechanical process that allows air to enter and exit the lungs, and perfusion is the blood flow through the pulmonary capillaries surrounding the alveoli. Both are an intrinsic partnership to provide adequate oxygenation to the body and elimination of metabolic waste products. A change in flow in either process will lead to hypoxemia or hypercapnia, exhibited as respiratory distress. The bedside assessment of the respiratory system must therefore encompass measurement of respiratory rate, rhythm, and depth, and auscultation for breath sounds that will help reveal underlying obstructive or infectious pathologies. Familiarity with these definitions and roles underpins comprehensive examination and corresponding interventions in respiratory care, optimizing the efficacy of targeted clinical practice.

Importance of physical examination

The physical examination is a fundamental foundation for assessing respiratory health, enabling clinicians to identify abnormalities that might otherwise go unnoticed. This is followed by a detailed patient history, which will alert the clinician to any underlying conditions, allergies, or previous respiratory diseases. This forms an essential basis for determining the overall well-being of the patient and whether they are at risk for respiratory disease. The following physical examination employs several techniques, including inspection, palpation, percussion, and auscultation. With these, clinicians can detect the occurrence of respiratory pathology, for instance, wheezing, decreased breath sounds, or unusual movement of the chest wall. This initial interaction is typically capable of providing key clues that ultimately direct the diagnostic process to the proper diagnostic imaging or lab tests, which are required for a complete examination. Additionally, a physical assessment of the respiratory system is also helpful for risk assessment and management, particularly in surgical patients. With the aid of modalities like thoracic radiography, clinicians can not only evaluate respiratory disorders but also assess the cardiovascular system, which is essential in anesthesiology planning. Research has found that thoracic radiographs can provide vital information about potential anesthetic risk, especially in animals with already existing respiratory pathologies (Bekta Eş Bilgiç, 2025). The same analysis is similarly crucial in human medicine, as it allows practitioners to stratify patients on physical status and individual risk factors, thus making preoperative assessment more useful. Last, this branch of physical examination reminds us of the value of vigilance in respiratory exams, particularly in patients at higher risk for complications. Additionally, physical examination assessment of health status is of utmost significance to disease prevention across various populations. Diagnosis of demographics and lifestyle from such tests can provide information on broader health trends, especially among young adults. According to evidence, various health determinants, including respiratory system illnesses, are found to be prevalent among medical students, which supports the need for repeated examinations among this age group (Belyaeva et al., 2024). By diagnosing chronically diseased individuals at an early age, preventive measures can be undertaken to avoid the sequelae of chronic respiratory diseases. Prevention is thus essential not only for the immediate clinical outcome but also for promoting improved lifestyles in populations at risk, thereby ensuring public health. The value of the physical exam also extends beyond acute clinical assessment since it can be a turning point in determining public health initiatives and educational programs.

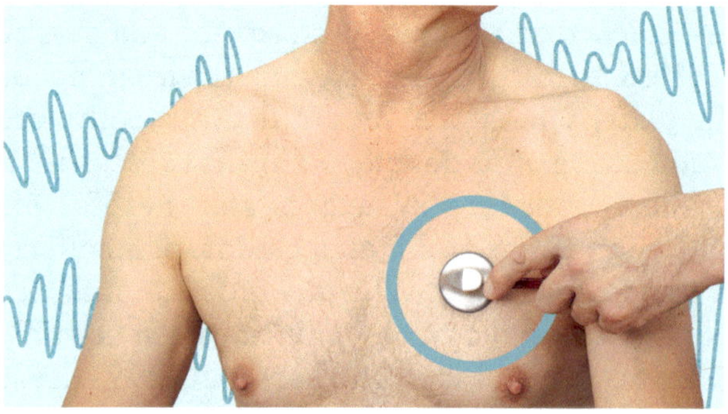

Figure 1.2. Physical examination.

Source: https://cdn-images.ausmed.com/ausmed-articles/20200601_cover_v2.jpg

1.1. Anatomy of the Respiratory System

Learning Outcome

1. Major components: lungs, trachea, bronchi
2. Role of the diaphragm and intercostal muscles
3. Upper vs. lower respiratory tract

The anatomy of the respiratory system is explicitly tailored for gas exchange, a critical function in ensuring the sustenance of life. The system comprises an intricate setup of structures, including the nasal cavity, pharynx, larynx, trachea, bronchi, and lungs. The air inhaled enters the nasal cavity, where it is filtered, warmed, and humidified, and is the initial opening of the respiratory system. Finally, the air passes through the pharynx and larynx, where the epiglottis prevents food from entering the airway during swallowing. The trachea is a cartilaginous tube that divides into the left and right primary bronchi, which extend to the lungs. This division results in the tree-like arrangement of bronchi and bronchioles, which terminate in the alveoli, where gas exchange occurs. It is essential to understand these segments if one is to conduct a comprehensive physical examination of the respiratory system. When inspecting the lungs, it is essential to understand the significance of the alveolar sacs, where oxygen and carbon dioxide exchange with the blood. The alveoli have a thin layer of epithelial cells that allows efficient diffusion of the gases. Surrounding these alveoli are capillaries, creating an immense area for the exchange of oxygen and carbon dioxide during respiration. The physical arrangement of this intricate system can be disrupted by various disease processes, further emphasizing the importance of a thorough physical examination of the respiratory system. Disease processes, such as emphysema, wherein the alveolar walls are weakened, significantly reduce the area for gas exchange. Therefore, an assessment of the respiratory function should not only include a physical check but also an understanding of the underlying anatomy that supports these vital functions. Furthermore, the mechanics of respiration—ventilation—are facilitated by the intercostal muscles and diaphragm, which, through their concerted effort, ventilate the thoracic cavity. During inhalation, the diaphragm descends and the intercostal muscles contract, increasing the volume of the thoracic cavity and sucking in air into the lungs. During exhalation, they relax, decreasing the thoracic volume and expelling air from the lungs. How essential the coordination between these two groups of muscles is can be appreciated by considering what would happen if there were any compromise: it would lead to breathlessness. Physical examination techniques, such as auscultation, can yield abnormal lung sounds indicating the presence of conditions like bronchoconstriction or alveolar flooding of the lungs. Accurate knowledge of respiratory anatomy not only facilitates such techniques but also highlights the significance of various pathologies on respiratory mechanics, guiding physicians in appropriate diagnosis and treatment (Ponikowski et al., 2016; Coté et al., 2019).

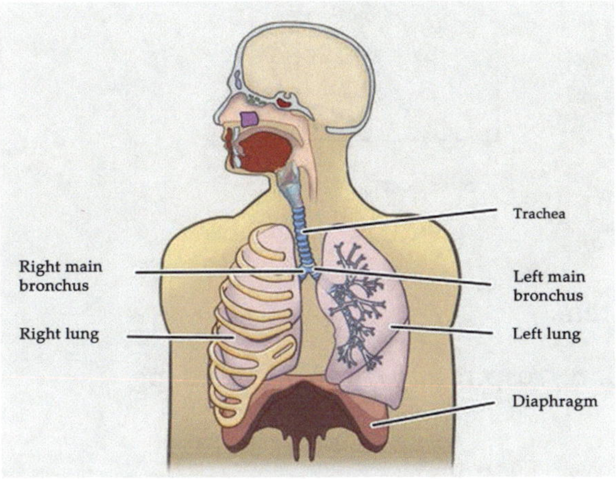

Figure 1.3. Anatomy of the respiratory system.

Source: https://cdn.prod.website-files.com/6320bb946c79f421bd3b702f/6350166d329dc74c5b74cffe_Lower_respiratory_tract.png

1.1.1. Major Components: Lungs, Trachea, Bronchi

The respiratory system is a network with multiple components and is a system that participates in gas exchange. It consists of the lungs, trachea, and bronchi as its principal components. The primary site of oxygen uptake and carbon dioxide expulsion is the lungs, which are composed of lobes and alveoli, where actual gas exchange occurs.

Alveoli are small air sacs that significantly increase the gas exchange area, thereby playing a crucial role in maintaining the efficiency of respiratory function. In addition, the lungs are surrounded by a pleural membrane that enables them to expand and contract during breathing, indicating their dynamic role in the respiratory mechanism. Understanding the structure and function of the lungs is crucial for evaluating respiratory function and diagnosing various pulmonary diseases. The windpipe, also known as the trachea, is a significant air passageway connecting the lungs. Supported structurally by C-shaped cartilaginous rings, the trachea remains open, unobstructing the airway. The trachea extends from the larynx, bifurcating into the left and right bronchi at the carina, an anatomical feature crucial for distributing airflow to the respective lobes of the lungs. The lining of the trachea is also protective, as it captures particles and pathogens and sweeps this mucus up into the throat using cilia. This helps maintain healthy respiratory tracts by preventing them from being infected or clogged, demonstrating the trachea's dual function as a passageway and a protective barrier against respiratory disease.

The bronchi extend from the trachea and play a crucial role in transporting air into the lungs. Once the bronchi enter the lungs, they subdivide further into minute bronchioles, allowing air to flow through to the alveoli where gas exchange occurs. The branching pattern serves to optimize airflow efficiency and penetration through the lung tissue. The bronchi are lined with a mucosal lining identical to that of the trachea, which continues to filter out dirt and humidify the air before it reaches the alveoli. Additionally, their muscular walls allow for the manipulation of airflow and resistance, and thus the bronchi play a crucial role in conditions such as asthma and chronic obstructive pulmonary disease. Knowledge of the anatomy and physiology of the respiratory system's components is essential for conducting a comprehensive physical examination and accurately interpreting pulmonary function tests (Stanojevic et al., 2021).

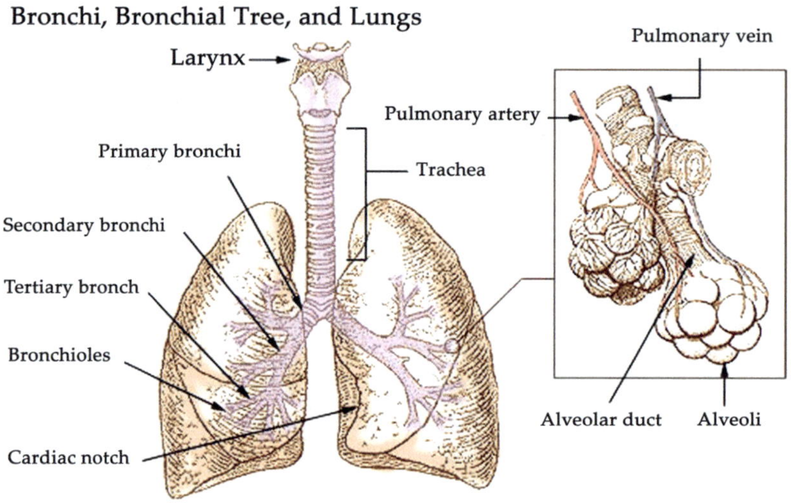

Figure 1.4. Major components of the respiratory system.

Source: https://training.seer.cancer.gov/images/anatomy/respiratory/bronchi_lungs.jpg

1.1.2. Role of the Diaphragm and Intercostal Muscles

The diaphragm and intercostal muscles play essential roles in the mechanism of breathing, effectively influencing respiratory function and efficiency. Below the rib cage lies the primary muscle of respiration, the diaphragm. Contraction during inhalation causes the muscle to be flattened, which widens the thoracic cavity and creates negative pressure for air to enter the lungs. Concomitantly, the external intercostal muscles contract to lift the ribcage and further increase the thoracic volume. Contraction of the two muscle groups simultaneously is essential to ensure adequate air into the lungs and thereby optimal gas exchange. Dysfunction in either of these muscle groups can lead to respiratory inefficiency, highlighting the importance of these muscles in physical examination as well as in clinical assessments of the respiratory system. Inspiratory muscle fatigue has been shown to cause adverse effects on respiratory function, particularly during aerobic exercise that relies heavily on sound breathing mechanics. When the diaphragm and the external intercostals are excessively stressed during strenuous physical labor, the muscles become fatigued and therefore become inefficient in creating the necessary pressures for breathing in. This implies the functional impairments of such muscles and their likely role in overall exercise performance, as evidenced by studies showing that inspiratory muscle fatigue decreases force production and airflow effectiveness. Indeed, the intricate interaction between muscle fatigue and respiratory muscle function is crucial, as it highlights the importance of certain physical examinations in assessing respiratory muscle integrity and endurance, particularly among athletes and patients with chronic respiratory illnesses (Ellis et al., 2024).

Furthermore, engaging in aerobic exercise has been shown to enhance the endurance and strength of the diaphragm and intercostal muscles, resulting in improved respiratory function. Aerobic exercise in the long term leads to physiological adjustments, including increased vital capacity, enhanced alveolar surface area, and improved capillary distribution. Importantly, these adjustments enable enhanced oxygen consumption and delivery at both systemic and cellular levels.

It consequently follows that the more conditioned the respiratory muscles are, the better they will be able to maintain augmented workloads without fatigue. Hence, a comprehensive physical examination of the respiratory system should include consideration of these muscles' function, with a focus on their key role in improving pulmonary efficiency and overall sporting ability (Bekembetova et al., 2024). Such dynamic knowledge will help medical practitioners set up more effective training schedules and therapeutic interventions for those suffering from respiratory complications.

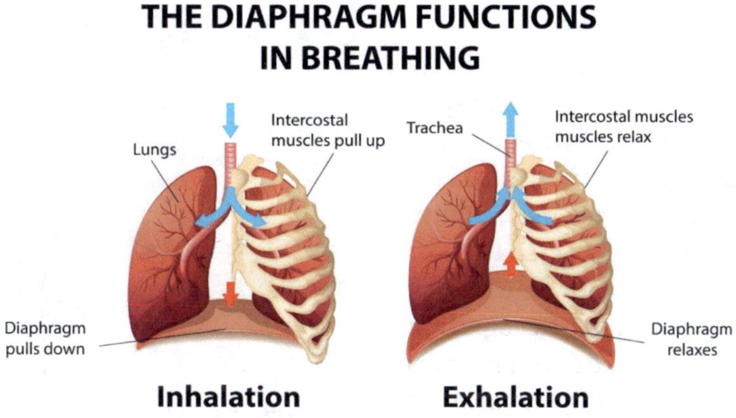

Figure 1.5. Role of the diaphragm and intercostal muscles.

Source: https://blackburnahg.com.au/wp-content/uploads/2023/12/Diaphragm-functions-1024x641.jpg

1.1.3. Upper Vs. Lower Respiratory Tract

During the physical examination of the respiratory system, it is necessary to differentiate between the upper and lower respiratory tracts for accurate diagnosis and treatment of respiratory diseases. The anatomic structures of the upper respiratory tract include the nasal cavity, pharynx, and larynx, and these are primarily responsible for air filtration, warming, and humidification. It is the first defense against airborne pathogens and environmental irritants. Symptoms most often associated with upper respiratory tract infections include nasal congestion, sore throat, and cough, which can significantly impact quality of life and patient comfort. Identification of such symptoms enables health workers to initiate corresponding diagnostic and therapeutic interventions, due to the high prevalence of viral infections in this region, as evidenced by newly emerging respiratory diseases such as those experienced in recent outbreaks (Jin et al., 2020).

Unlike the upper respiratory tract, the lower respiratory tract includes the trachea, bronchi, and lungs. This region is crucial for exchanging gases and must be evaluated critically to identify potential complications of respiratory diseases. Diseases of the lower respiratory tract, such as bronchiolitis and pneumonia, may result in severe respiratory distress and should receive prompt medical care. Symptoms typically include wheezing, tachypnea, and labored work of breathing, which are signs of inflammation or obstruction of the airways. Bronchiolitis, for instance, primarily results from viral infections in infants, which can lead to a range of complications depending on the severity of the condition (Silver et al., 2019). Therefore, a thorough physical examination, including breath sound and respiratory effort evaluation, is essential to differentiate between upper and lower respiratory tract illnesses and ultimately guide treatment. Finally, the treatment of upper and lower respiratory infections differs significantly, which explains the importance of a thorough physical examination.

Upper respiratory tract infections typically resolve on their own and can be managed with symptomatic relief and patient education on hydration and rest. By contrast, diseases affecting the lower respiratory tract may require more intensive therapy, such as oxygenation or bronchodilator therapy, especially in cases of severe obstruction or hypoxemia. Recognition of these variations facilitates healthcare practitioners in individualizing treatment regimens appropriately. For instance, treatment modalities for bronchiolitis vary according to symptom severity, and hence diagnostic specificity becomes a crucial driver of outcomes. Ultimately, recognition of variations between these two tracts maximizes clinical acumen and leads to general improvement in respiratory therapy.

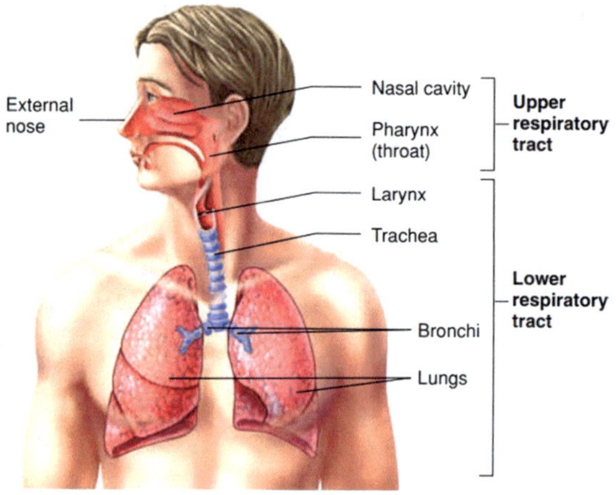

Figure 1.6. Upper vs. lower respiratory tract.

Source: https://img.brainkart.com/article/article-Anatomy-of-the-Respi-jog.jpg

Test Your Knowledge

1. What are the roles of the diaphragm and intercostal muscles?
2. Differentiate upper vs. lower respiratory tract.

1.2. Techniques For Physical Examination

Learning Outcome

1. Inspection: visual assessment of the chest
2. Palpation: feeling for abnormalities
3. Auscultation: listening to breath sounds

The clinical assessment of the respiratory system employs multiple techniques designed to evaluate respiratory well-being and identify any potential disorders. Exhaustive assessment always begins with inspection, which involves observing the patient's respiratory rate, effort, and distress. Visual inspections of the chest wall for symmetry, expansion, and retractions provide practitioners with valuable information about respiratory function. Upon examination, palpation is used to determine tactile fremitus, a method employed to quantify the transmission of vibrations generated by speech through the lung tissue to the chest wall. These vibrations can be abnormal when underlying pathology, such as pleural effusion or consolidation of the lungs, is present, thereby guiding further diagnosis and treatment (Jeny Díaz-Pacheco et al., 2024). Auscultation is another critical physical examination method for the airways, through which physicians can listen to abnormal breath sounds characteristic of diseases of the airway or lung. Clinicians can detect various sounds, such as wheezes, crackles, or rhonchi, through a stethoscope, which can indicate conditions ranging from asthma to pneumonia.

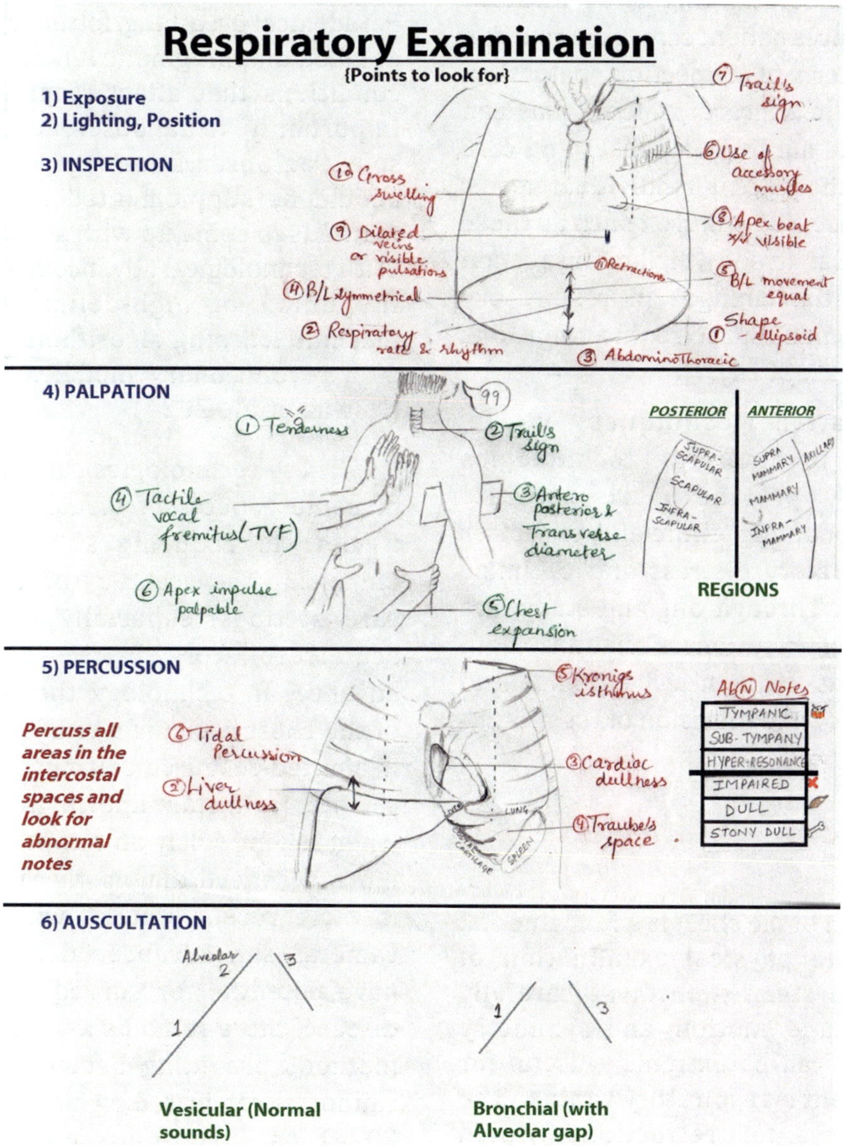

Figure 1.7. Techniques for physical examination.

Source: https://en.wikipedia.org/wiki/Respiratory_examination#/media/File:Respiratory_examn.jpg

It is, however, reliant on the training and experience of the clinicians. New technology, such as airborne ultrasound surface motion cameras (AUSMC), is enabling the possibility of more objective and quantifiable assessments of breath sounds, including vocal fremitus. The technology can potentially make respiratory tests more precise by allowing for high-fidelity recording of lung vibration, ultimately leading to improved diagnostic processes (Wintzenrieth et al., 2024). The use of these testing procedures yields a more complete understanding of respiratory function and enhances patient care. By employing a systematic pattern of inspection, palpation, and auscultation, healthcare professionals can formulate accurate nursing diagnoses and care plans tailored to the patient's individual needs. For instance, in diseased children such as those with spinal muscular atrophy, vigilant inspection can detect essential changes in respiratory patterns that demand precise interventions (Díaz-Pacheco et al., 2024).

As examination techniques evolve, the integration of emerging technologies will increasingly provide more accurate measurements, enabling clinicians to better respond to respiratory distress and optimize patient outcomes. Through ongoing study and innovation, medical practitioners can utilize both traditional methods and high-tech equipment to enhance the efficacy and precision of respiratory system testing.

1.2.1. Inspection: Visual Assessment of the Chest

Visual examination of the chest is a fundamental component of the physical examination of the respiratory system. It involves carefully observing the shape, motion, and symmetry of the chest, and can be extremely useful for assessing a patient's respiratory status. The examiner observes for retractions, which may be a marker of respiratory distress or augmentation of work of breathing. Of special interest are chest shape abnormalities, such as barrel chests. in COPD, that are key indicators of pathophysiology. In addition, the examination is not solely of morphology but must also address the dynamics, such as the breathing pattern and accessory muscle use, both of which can signal complications requiring further testing or intervention (Sang et al., 2025). Visual examination is more than just visual observation, as it leads the clinician to make correlations with likely respiratory illnesses. Paradoxical breathing, for instance, can be a sign of failed diaphragmatic function or neurological conditions that affect respiratory mechanics. Importantly, visual observation should not rely solely on observations made by clinicians, but should be supplemented by other diagnostic methods to come up with an accurate diagnosis. With technological advancements in diagnostics, the union of high-definition imaging and machine learning algorithms is being achieved as a revolutionary modality for the purpose (Nawaz et al., 2024).

These technologies can enable automation of some aspects of visual examination, with a view to reducing subjective biases and enhancing the accuracy of diagnosis in acute care settings, especially in conditions like acute respiratory distress syndrome. Despite advances in technology, the visual assessment of the chest remains a vital clinician skill, even in limited-resource settings. Visual inspection can provide instant information that may be lost when relying solely on computerized systems or more advanced diagnostic machines. As noted in more recent studies, while high-definition cameras and advanced deep-learning models have potential for surveillance of respiratory disease, there remains a vital role for classical methods providing bedside information that cannot be replicated by machines (Nawaz et al., 2024). As such, future practice must focus on a synergistic approach that combines classical visual inspection with new technology to facilitate greater insight into respiratory health and improved patient outcomes across diverse clinical environments.

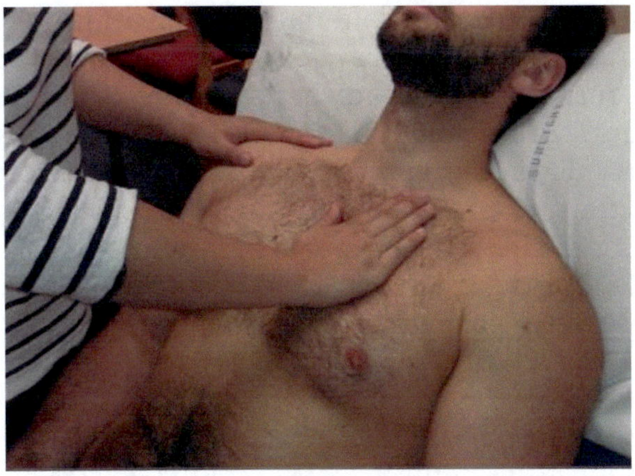

Figure 1.8. Visual assessment of the chest.

Source: https://www.oxfordmedicaleducation.com/wp-content/uploads/2015/08/Untitled13.jpg

1.2.2. Palpation: Feeling For Abnormalities

As part of a comprehensive physical examination of the respiratory tract, palpation is a crucial technique for identifying abnormalities that are not apparent by visual inspection or auscultation. Through stepwise application of pressure on regions of the thorax, clinicians are able to identify for irregularities like asymmetry, tenderness, or pathological masses that would indicate underlying disease.

The clinician typically addresses the intercostal spaces and the anterior and posterior chest wall during palpation. Additionally, palpatory techniques can aid in determining the degree of tactile fremitus, which involves palpating vibrations along the tissue of the lungs during phonation. It differentiates between conditions such as pneumonia, which tends to increase tactile fremitus, and pleural effusion, which decreases it. Apart from this, palpation can also give important information regarding the mechanics of respiration, particularly while assessing for any obstructive or restrictive respiratory disorder. Observation of the chest wall's movement can provide valuable information regarding thoracic expansion and contraction during inspiration and expiration. The clinician will generally observe the symmetry of the chest movements as the asymmetrical expansion suggests underlying conditions like pleural disease or lung consolidation. In addition, irregular respiratory patterns, as uncovered by palpation, can indicate pathophysiologic changes or discomfort in the operation of the lungs. For example, decreased diaphragmatic motion on one side may be a sign of solitary lung disease or diaphragm paralysis, emphasizing the importance of meticulous palpation in providing accurate diagnoses. Lastly, consideration of the skill of palpation is also enhanced by imaging technology advancements that enable more realistic understanding of structures in the thorax.

These be accompanied by the development of new techniques like ultrasound elastography, which allow measurements of tissue stiffness and detection of abnormalities in the lung and surrounding structures without invading the body. Unlike traditional methods that rely on tactile sense, these imaging modalities offer quantitative data on tissue elasticity and can have practical implications in clinical decision-making, particularly in conditions such as fibrosis or tumors. By combining palpation with advanced imaging modalities, clinicians can conduct a comprehensive evaluation of respiratory status, thereby optimizing their diagnostic processes and tailoring treatment plans accordingly. The shifting balance in diagnostic approaches aligns with best practices of today, e.g., as put forth in evidence-based guidelines for the therapy of respiratory illness, thereby validating the irreplaceable role of palpation in the physical examination of the respiratory system.

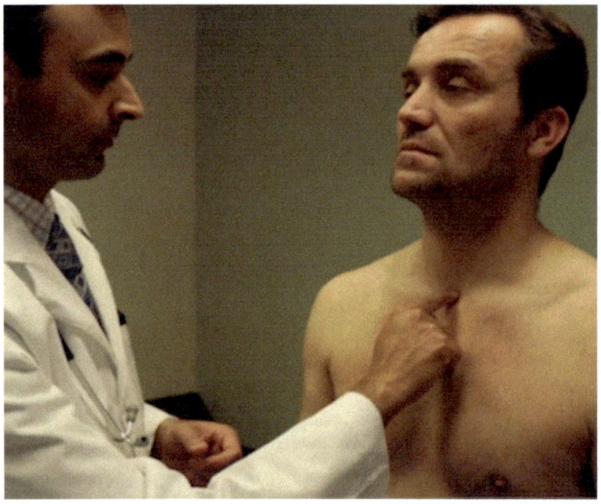

Figure 1.9. Palpation: feeling for abnormalities.

Source: https://www.jove.com/files/media/science-education/science-education-thumbs/10028.jpg

1.2.3. Auscultation: Listening To Breath Sounds

Auscultation is one of the key skills in physical examination of the respiratory system through which breath sounds can be listened to and pulmonary health assessed effectively. It is a technique that involves using a stethoscope to detect abnormal lung sounds indicative of various respiratory disorders. Vesicular, bronchial, or bronchovesicular breath sounds are usually employed to denote normal breath sounds, which reflect air flow dynamics inside the lungs. It is essential for clinicians to be able to distinguish between these sounds as variations such as wheezing, crackles, or stridor can be an indication of conditions such as asthma, pneumonia, or chronic obstructive pulmonary disease (COPD). Detection of such abnormal findings through auscultation early on can enable timely intervention, ultimately contributing to improved patient outcomes and enhancing the quality of care provided in the management of respiratory health. Technical advancements in auscultation have significantly increased its utility in clinical practice. Digital stethoscopes and automated algorithms are now increasingly prevalent, offering improved acoustic analysis and the capability to record and share sounds for further evaluation. Not only do these improvements enhance accuracy in the interpretation of breath sounds, but they also facilitate remote consultation, a crucial function during public health crises such as the COVID-19 pandemic.

Applying telehealth technologies enables practitioners to remotely assess patients' respiratory status with reduced risk of exposure. As respiratory symptoms remain a primary symptom for infectious diseases like COVID-19, adding innovative auscultation technology can streamline diagnostic processes and optimize the utilization of healthcare resources. Healthcare professionals are encouraged to consider the evolving nature of the development in auscultation technology when making treatment decisions and initiating effective care processes. Lastly, good auscultation is not merely the identification of sounds; it entails a complete understanding of the patient's history, clinical presentation, and possibly environmental factors that may affect respiratory function. For instance, individuals residing in environments with high pollution levels often present with distinct, abnormal breath sounds typical of pneumonitis or chronic rhinitis. Similarly, thoughtful attention to social determinants of health, such as access to care and socioeconomic status, is crucial in framing auscultation findings in context. Thus, the ability to combine auscultation results with more comprehensive clinical assessments is critical in delivering tailored care to patients. Proficient auscultation not only guarantees the detection of acute respiratory conditions, but it also promotes preventative interventions addressing longer-lasting conditions in the respiratory tract; therefore, its utmost significance in general respiratory health evaluation and care.

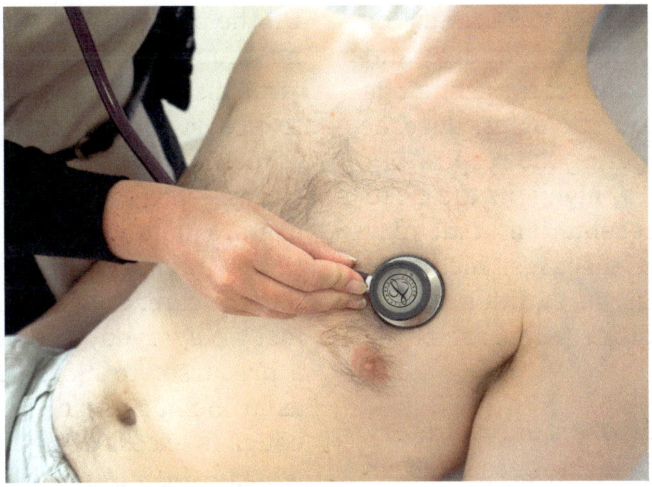

Figure 1.9. Auscultating breath sounds.

Source: https://www.firstaidforfree.com/wp-content/uploads/2017/01/Chest-Auscultation.jpg

Test Your Knowledge

1. How is the visual assessment of the chest done?
2. What is Palpation?

1.3. Common Signs and Symptoms

Learning Outcome

1. Cough: types and significance
2. Shortness of breath: causes and implications
3. Chest pain: differential diagnosis

The respiratory system is often the site of a wide range of manifestations and signs that can indicate a multitude of underlying disorders. Common presentations, such as shortness of breath, cough, and wheezing, are valuable in evaluating respiratory status. Shortness of breath, or dyspnea, can be an acute or chronic complaint and may have several etiologies, including obstructive disorders such as asthma and COPD. The finding of a chronic cough, dry or productive, indicates chronic irritation or inflammation in the airways. Wheezing, characterized by a whistling sound on expiration during inspiration, is a common accompaniment of bronchial constriction and is used to emphasize the need for further diagnostic evaluation, especially when suggestive of broncho-obstructive syndrome (Ibatova S, 2025). An understanding of such typical signs and symptoms forms the basis of effective respiratory exams. Aside from wheezing and cough, clinical manifestations of hypoxemia, such as cyanosis and changes in respiratory rate, usually manifest during the physical examination of the respiratory system. Cyanosis, expressed as a bluish hue of the lips or the extremities, is a sign of insufficient oxygenation of the blood and calls for urgent medical attention. Respiratory rate can also provide information about the presence of a patient's respiratory distress; tachypnea or bradypnea can indicate various respiratory or systemic disease states. Imaging studies and laboratory tests generally support these findings in identifying symptomatic etiologies. Current studies, such as those targeting the respiratory consequences of COVID-19, highlight the need to search for atypical presentations that may be associated with viral diseases, including gastrointestinal symptoms, in addition to the common respiratory findings (Alyousef et al., 2022).

Assessment of physical signs of respiratory distress is also aided by techniques such as auscultation and percussion. On auscultation, the clinician hears the abnormal sounds, which can indicate a variety of conditions—ranging from the presence of fluid in pneumonia to bronchoconstriction, which occurs in asthmatic individuals. Percussion, if performed correctly, will be capable of distinguishing between the normal thoracic resonance and pleural effusion, which is dullness. Furthermore, the recognition of certain patterns, such as tachypnea accompanied by wheezing or crackles, validates the diagnosis of conditions like broncho-obstructive syndrome with prolonged exhalation and respiratory failure (Ibatova, 2025). The multimodal approach reflects the significance of a thorough physical examination, considering both frequent and infrequent signs and symptoms, ultimately culminating in targeted intervention and treatment of respiratory pathologies.

1.3.1. Cough: Types and Significance

Of all the respiratory diseases, the cough is a vital physiological function, and its primary purpose is to eliminate irritants, mucus, and bacteria from the airways. Some types of coughs can be very informative about certain medical conditions. An infectious cough accompanied by sputum production, for instance, typically indicates a bronchial infection, such as pneumonia or chronic obstructive pulmonary disease (COPD). On the other hand, a nonproductive cough with no mucus formation may be a symptom of viral diseases or allergic disorders. According to observation of the nature of cough—acute, chronic, dry, or whether any other symptom is shown—health professionals may continue with a more detailed diagnostic process, in which timely interventions may be strictly required to patient care. Cough has more significance than just an everyday protective function; it can be a precursor to more serious pathologies, such as bronchiectasis or lung carcinoma. Recurrent cough in excess of eight weeks needs aggressive workup because it is an indicator of chronic disease that will accrue unless treated. Secondary symptoms, such as cough (e.g., hemoptysis or dyspnea), also indicate the need for clinical assessment. For instance, patients with chronic cough and weight loss will be at increased risk of malignancies. Furthermore, specific cough characteristics, such as a whooping sound, may be indicative of infections, such as pertussis, and require urgent medical evaluation to prevent the transmission of disease and preserve public health. The evolving understanding of cough as a diagnostic symptom is being put into context in emerging literature with emphasis on the management of viral illnesses like COVID-19. The pandemic has also unveiled how coughing can be an early sign of respiratory distress with viral infection. Cough is usually presented alongside other nonspecific symptoms, such as fever and fatigue, in SARS-CoV-2-infected patients, and thus becomes confusing in the clinical presentation. COVID-19 has been reported to present with a range of cough presentations from mild to severe, accompanied by severe pulmonary infection such as pneumonia. The physical examination of the respiratory system thus includes an accurate evaluation of cough types since the categorization of the cough subtleties would have a great impact on the treatment and clinical management, hence enhancing patient care in an increasingly valued environment that acknowledges cough's critical role in respiratory disease care.

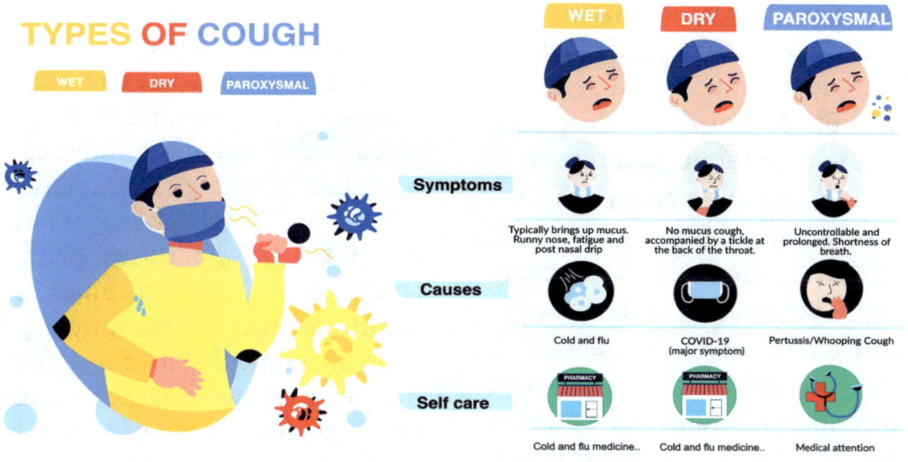

Figure 1.10. Types of cough.

Source: https://www.myhealth1st.com.au/static/assets/images/kEN3842leC3tj5zf3O00o/TYPES%20OF%20COUGH.jpg

1.3.2. Shortness of Breath: Causes and Implications

Breathlessness, also known as dyspnea, is one of the most important signs used in evaluating respiratory function. Numerous etiologies with both respiratory and non-respiratory origins produce it. The most prevalent pulmonary etiology is obstructive diseases, such as asthma and COPD, which lead to restricted airflow and diminished efficiency in gas exchange. Conversely, cardiac disease, e.g., congestive heart failure and arrhythmia, can manifest with respiratory distress due to fluid overload and perfusion. Other diseases, such as pneumonia, can significantly impair lung function, which can actually exacerbate breathlessness. To ensure proper management of these etiologies, it is essential to understand their causes. Although patterns such as in Humbert et al., (2022) stress individualized treatment regimens, it is crucial that clinicians determine the causality of dyspnea as a preliminary step to direct precise interventions.

Shortness of breath crosses clinical presentations and has far-reaching implications that overflow into noteworthy alterations in quality of life in the patients. Dyspnea patients will commonly find that activities of daily living become more strenuous, followed by subsequent self-limited mobility, social withdrawal, and heightened anxiety regarding their state of health. Such an additive effect not only affects physical function but also can cause mental distress and a vicious cycle of declining health function. For health professionals, the consciousness of both psychosocial factors and respiratory symptoms is essential. The integration of interventions targeting both the physical and emotional aspects of dyspnea is most likely to improve patient care overall. Besides, recent research underscores the importance of using physical examination techniques to establish the scope and likely etiology of dyspnea and thus initiate early and proper therapy, as is called for by various clinical practice guidelines, for example, guidelines in Rosen et al., (2018). In conclusion, evaluating breathlessness requires a comprehensive consideration of its multifaceted etiology, as well as its primary impact on patient well-being. Physicians are required to use rigorous testing methods to determine the causative diseases of dyspnea, enabling the formulation of optimal treatment regimens. Systemic treatment of both respiratory and extrapulmonary diseases underlying this symptom, quality of care can be significantly enhanced by medical interventions. Furthermore, by recognizing the broader impacts of dyspnea on a patient's life, care is valued, as it must be multidisciplinary. While we try to optimize interventions and optimize outcomes in dyspneic patients, combining recent recommendations and experienced guidance in Humbert et al. (2022) and Rosen et al. (2018) once again present clinicians with valuable tools to deal with the complex clinical phenomenon.

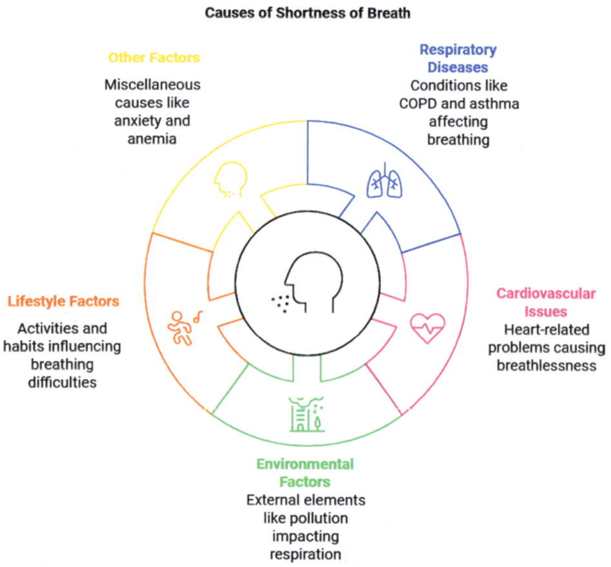

Figure 1.11. Causes of shortness of breath.

Source: https://avicennacardiology.com/wp-content/uploads/2024/10/shortness-of-breath.png

1.3.3. Chest Pain: Differential Diagnosis

Chest pain is a significant diagnostic challenge, especially in respiratory system examination, since a heterogeneous array of clinical conditions may cause it. A range of differential diagnoses includes not only common respiratory illnesses like pneumonia or pleuritis but also more life-threatening illnesses like pulmonary embolism and lung cancer. Associated symptoms of pain in the chest may often narrow down the potential diagnoses, with characteristics (dull, sharp, or stabbing) of pain, onset, duration, and accompanying features being used in clinical decision-making. Sharp pain provoked by deep breathing, for instance, may presage pleuritic disorders, whereas repeated dull pain may indicate the presence of an underlying malignancy. Therefore, a thorough physical examination, along with a detailed patient history, is essential for establishing the causes of chest pain, with life-threatening causes being prioritized. Appreciation of the high priority of pulmonary embolism in the differential diagnosis of chest pain is essential for the correct management of patients. This condition classically presents with acute onset chest pain and is characterised by the signs and symptoms of dyspnea and tachycardia, indicative of its acute presentation. Adaptation of current guidelines to practice is key to improving diagnostic accuracy. Recent updates recommend that clinicians become increasingly aware of the signs and symptoms of pulmonary embolism on presentation, especially in high-risk groups. As highlighted in the guidelines mentioned in Konstantinides et al., (2019), appropriate utilization of diagnostic tools like D-dimer testing and imaging studies can be incredibly beneficial and result in timely interventions. Therefore, detection of this condition during chest pain evaluation can greatly enhance outcomes in patients.

The significance of merging proven guidelines with clinical acumen cannot be overstated, particularly regarding the nuanced evaluation of chest pain. The ESC guidelines emphasize that healthcare professionals need to balance their interpretations with the latest evidence and recommendations, thereby adopting a balanced approach to diagnosis. As indicated in Adler et al., (2015), the guidelines do not relinquish the clinician's personal responsibility to make a decision but enhance the process that they follow. Adequate diagnosis of chest pain requires practitioners to consider not just the functioning of the respiratory system but also interactions with cardiac disease and musculoskeletal illness. Such an integrated assessment strategy not only helps determine the underlying pathology but also does justice to the ethical obligation to provide comprehensive patient care, thereby upholding trust and strengthening the therapeutic relationship between clinician and patient.

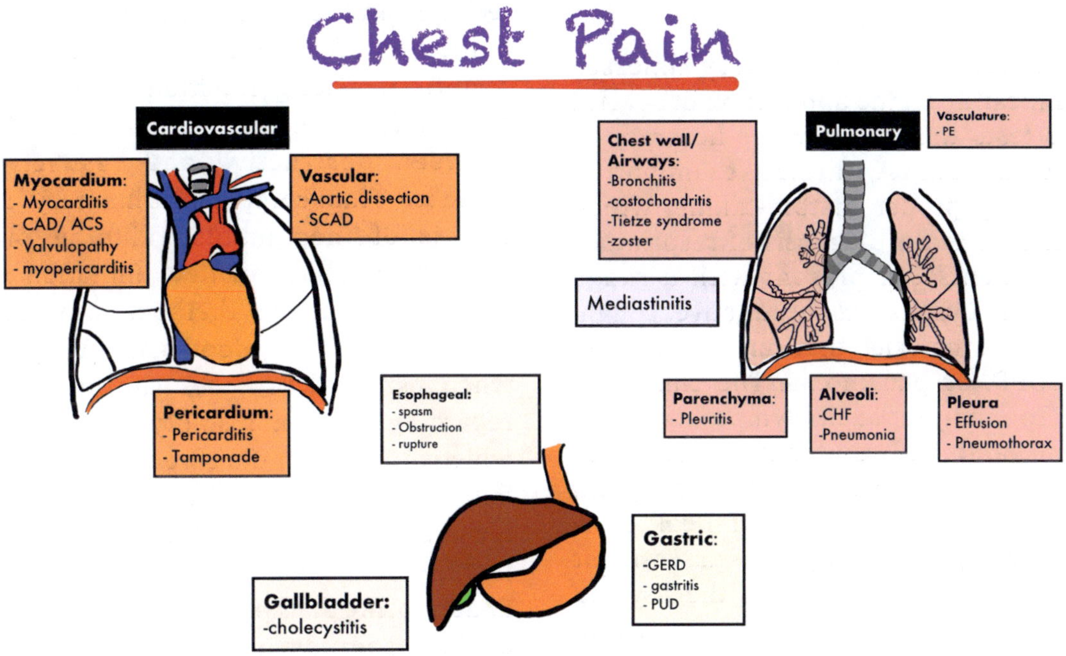

Figure 1.12. Chest pain – differential diagnosis framework.

Source: https://img.grepmed.com/uploads/9911/differential-original.jpeg

Test Your Knowledge

1. What is a cough, and explain the types of cough?
2. What are the causes of shortness of breath?

1.4. Diagnostic Tools in Respiratory Examination

Learning Outcome

1. Spirometry: measuring lung function
2. Peak flow meter: assessing airflow
3. Imaging studies: X-rays and CT scans

Effective assessment of respiratory illnesses relies significantly on the application of several diagnostic tests that enhance the accuracy of clinical evaluations. A physical examination is preceded by proper history-taking, which remains crucial in the diagnosis of respiratory illnesses. Patients can present with a range of signs from dyspnea to productive cough, representing pathologies that can be linked to asthma, COPD, or pneumonia. The clinician's capacity to analyze such symptoms is of paramount value and commonly necessitates the assistance of other diagnostic equipment. For instance, the application of peak flow meters can complement objective assessment of lung function, particularly in the asthma patient, allowing for early intervention and management. Additionally, technologies such as pulse oximetry enable the quick determination of oxygen saturation levels, providing insight into the extent of respiratory compromise, especially during emergent conditions. In addition to these screening devices, more advanced diagnostic procedures are necessary to carry out a complete evaluation. Auscultation remains a significant part of the respiratory examination, with the clinician listening for pathologic lung sounds, such as wheezing or crackles, that may indicate pathology in the airways or alveoli. Percussion will also reveal the condition of the underlying lung parenchyma and differentiate between fluid accumulation or consolidation. Notably, recent advancements in imaging technologies have significantly contributed to the diagnosis of respiratory conditions. Chest X-rays and computed tomography (CT) scans are essential diagnostic tools in making precise diagnoses of complex thoracic diseases, including tumors and interstitial lung diseases, therefore allowing health professionals to formulate specific treatments based on accurate diagnoses.

The integration of diagnostic technology in respiratory examination has kept up with technological advances, increasing the clinician's ability to offer optimal care. For example, quantitative lung function measurement by spirometry is helpful in the discrimination between obstructive and restrictive lung disease. This complex pulmonary function test is of inestimable value in providing information about air flow limitation and lung volume, and affects therapeutic management. Similarly, arterial blood gas (ABG) analysis, when instituted, provides valuable information regarding a patient's ability to exchange gases, which is crucial in the care of acute respiratory failure. The diagnosis of disorders through these techniques aligns with the demand for timely interventions that improve patient outcomes, underscoring their pivotal role in physical exams of the respiratory system (Evans et al., 2021; Cruz-Jentoft et al., 2018).

1.4.1. Spirometry: Measuring Lung Function

Spirometry is a key component in measuring lung function and provides valuable information about a patient's respiratory status. It is a non-invasive test that measures crucial variables such as Forced Vital Capacity (FVC) and Forced Expiratory Volume in one second (FEV1). Spirometry assists medical practitioners in calculating how much air the patient can inhale and exhale, enabling them to diagnose a variety of respiratory diseases, including asthma and COPD. Measurements derived from spirometry not only impact clinical diagnosis but also enable the monitoring of disease progression and the efficacy of treatment. Awareness of these measurements allows clinicians to tailor intervention measures to effectively achieve improved patient outcomes in the management of respiratory diseases. Measurements derived through spirometry help differentiate between restrictive and obstructive lung disease. For instance, a reduced FEV1/FVC ratio, reflecting airflow obstruction, can imply the existence of asthma or COPD and is treated accordingly. Both FEV1 and FVC are reduced in restrictive lung diseases; therefore, further evaluation of lung volumes and capacities is necessary. The use of spirometry together with other pulmonary function tests enables clinicians to define lung health more clearly. For example, studies demonstrate that mountain populations exhibit phenomenal adjustments in lung function during chronic hypoxia, with significant disparities in lung volumes and capacities compared to their low-altitude counterparts (Fatima S[1] et al., 2024). Such data best explains why spirometric results need to be interpreted in broader physiological and environmental contexts. In addition to measuring baseline lung function, spirometry is a critical component of ongoing monitoring in patients with pre-existing respiratory disease and is increasingly significant in specialist groups. Studies have reported that variables such as age, sex, and overall health conditions significantly influence lung function test results. For instance, women with rheumatoid arthritis-related interstitial lung disease possess typical pulmonary measurements corresponding to their clinical status, demonstrating the nuanced applications of spirometry in different patient groups (de Deucher et al., 2023). Through the use of spirometry not only for diagnosis but also for ongoing monitoring, medical personnel can institute timely interventions that significantly improve patient quality of life. With the inclusion of spirometry in routine physical examinations, the comprehensive administration of respiratory health gains an invaluable foundation, ultimately benefiting efforts to minimize the impact of lung disease.

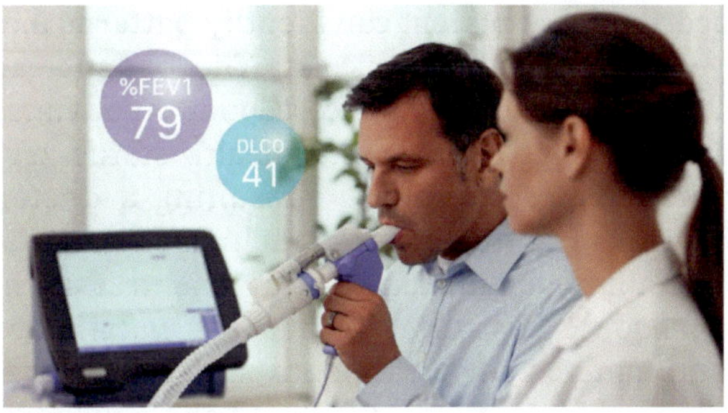

Figure 1.13. Spirometry.

Source: https://cdn.nddmed.com/posts/spirometer-test-1080x720.webp

1.4.2. Peak Flow Meter: Assessing Airflow

A peak flow meter is a valuable instrument applied to measure airflow within the respiratory system, particularly among asthma and chronic respiratory disorder patients. The instrument is handheld and measures the fastest rate of exhalation, providing crucial information about lung performance in a patient. Specialists employ the device to monitor airway obstruction and treatment outcomes over a period of time. As one blows across the peak flow meter's mouthpiece, the peak expiratory flow rate (PEFR) is measured, which indicates a shift in airway reactivity and airflow. The monitoring of such values enables clinicians to make adjustments in interventions, adjust medications, and tailor patient management. Such dynamic management is especially crucial in patients whose airflow varies due to environmental stimuli or drug effects, thus underscoring the utility of peak flow meters in dynamic respiratory diagnosis and treatment. Peak flow metering is used for measurement; it is a valuable technique in patient education and self-management of respiratory disease. Patients are typically requested to perform peak flows daily, which encourages independence and increased awareness of respiratory disease. Through symptom diary and PEFR recording, the patient can identify patterns and precipitants of their disease. The patient can interpret such readings to respond in advance to any change in his or her health status, e.g., switching medication or consulting a doctor. The self-monitoring approach used here is particularly significant during the treatment of chronic diseases because it maximizes compliance with treatments and encourages informed decision-making based on knowledge. Thus, incorporating peak flow meter monitoring into the patient's plans can guarantee improved respiratory symptom control as well as quality of life. Utilization of peak flow meters is also emphasized in the field of study and clinical practice that researches respiratory mechanics and muscle function. Recent advancements in methods have provided the underpinnings for greater precision in understanding how respiratory muscles operate under varying conditions, such as exercise and acute stress.

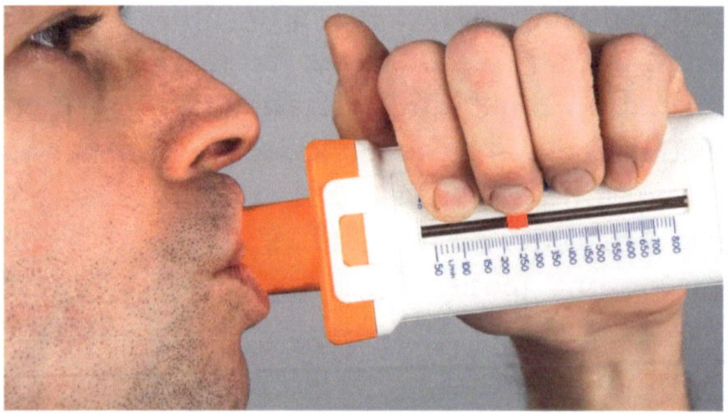

Figure 1.14. Peak flow meter.

Source: https://i0.wp.com/images-prod.healthline.com/hlcmsresource/images/topic_centers/Asthma/1296x728_Peak_Expiratory_Flow_Rate.jpg?w=1155&h=1528

This type of study highlights the complex relationship between airflow measurement and respiratory muscular performance, suggesting that instruments like the peak flow meter can detect significant changes in response to treatment or therapeutic assessment. By examining the sensitivity of peak expiratory flow in relation to other assessments of respiratory function, clinicians are better equipped to accurately measure the efficacy of treatment and prevent complications. By doing so, the value of peak flow meters is strengthened in practice, and the need for continuing work on the subject of respiratory physiology and patient management is reinforced (Laveneziana et al., 2019). Accordingly, the peak flow meter is both a diagnostic tool and an instrument for acquiring knowledge of respiratory health.

1.4.3. Imaging Studies: X-Rays and CT Scans

Imaging procedures are a part of the physical examination of the respiratory system, and especially the diagnosis of many diseases of pulmonary pathology. X-rays and computed tomography (CT) scans are the most commonly used modalities, and each provides unique advantages in imaging lung architecture and disease. X-rays are a quick way in which the lungs can be screened, and findings of abnormalities like pneumonia, masses in the lung, or pleural effusion can be identified. However, their relatively low sensitivity can lead to false negatives or missed diagnoses of early diseases. Due to these factors, chest CT scans have gained increasing attention as they offer higher resolution and can produce cross-sectional images of the lungs, providing detailed information about the presence of interstitial lung diseases or complications of infections, such as those associated with COVID-19 (Humbert et al., 2022). Additionally, CT scans are becoming increasingly important in the new dynamic of respiratory diseases. They enable a detailed examination of lung disease that cannot be identified with regular X-rays. For instance, during the COVID-19 pandemic, rapid and reliable imaging studies played a key role in diagnosing and treating patients with extreme respiratory disease. A CT scan will reveal ground-glass opacities, consolidations, and bilateral and peripheral patterns of lung involvement, all of which are classic for COVID-19 pneumonia (Guarracino et al., 2020).

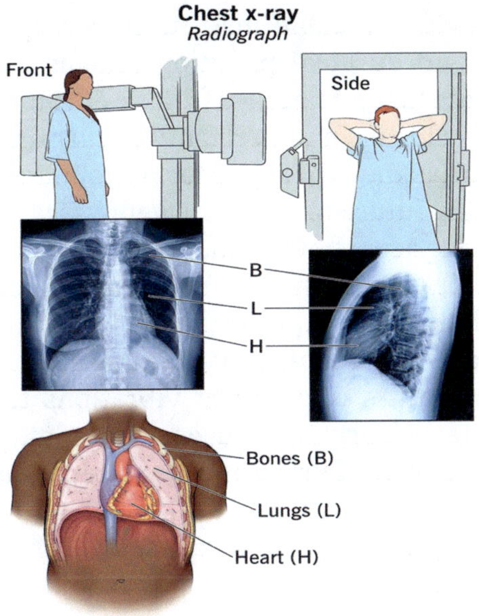

Figure 1.15. Chest X-ray (CXR).

Source: https://my.clevelandclinic.org/-/scassets/images/org/health/articles/10228-chest-x-ray

Accurate imaging enables the medical team to accurately estimate the severity of pneumonia and tailor management accordingly, thereby becoming an integral part of the management protocols for patients with respiratory failure. Lastly, the synergism between X-rays and CT scans underscores their complementary nature in comprehensive lung evaluation. While X-rays will hopefully guide the clinician on the initial assessment, CT scans provide the subtle degree of detail needed to establish a diagnosis or guide therapeutic intervention. In practice, this equates to one patient with a respiratory illness potentially receiving an initial X-ray, which, if diagnostic, would result in further investigation being conducted immediately using CT scanning. The use of both imaging techniques optimizes diagnostic accuracy, critical to informed treatment protocols. Lastly, imaging studies complement the physical assessment of the respiratory system through diagnostic resolution, enabling the successful treatment of multiple pulmonary disease processes (Humbert et al., 2022).

Test Your Knowledge

1. What are the different tests used to measure the lung function in spirometry?
2. What are X-rays and CT scans?

1.5. Interpretation of Findings

Learning Outcome

1. Normal vs. abnormal breath sounds
2. Identifying respiratory distress
3. Correlating physical findings with patient history

The clinical interpretation of physical examination findings in the respiratory system plays a crucial role in diagnosing respiratory disorders. Through the use of instruments such as palpation, a doctor assesses tactile fremitus, a measure of the conduction of vibrations produced by vocalizations through the lung tissue. Traditional techniques heavily rely on the doctor's subjective measurement, which can introduce variability into the measurement results. However, tools such as the airborne ultrasound surface motion camera (AUSMC) provide an objective, quantitative estimate of such vibrations, thereby improving the validity of the findings. Through more reproducible vocal fremitus mapping, not only is subjective judgment eliminated, but also a more nuanced interpretation of thoracic well-being in diverse groups can be obtained, as seen through large-scale data collection in health screening among volunteers. The use of the technology seeps into improved diagnostic roles in the clinical setting (Wintzenrieth et al., 2024). Additionally, interpretation of results from respiratory examination entails consideration of the potential for surgical procedures. Tracheostomy and thoracotomy are procedures where a proper understanding of physical examination findings is required to make informed surgical intervention decisions. In veterinary surgeons, careful examination and evaluation of nasal air flow, thoracic structure symmetry, and palpation of the affected anatomical structures is essential before any surgical intervention. These tests guide clinicians in evaluating potential complications, prognosis, and operability, which in turn informs post-operative care and recovery in patients. A close examination of findings from such tests necessitates improved surgical practices, as effective and precise evaluations can provide valuable insights into respiratory health and surgical planning (Dugassa et al., 2020). Evaluating findings from respiratory tests not only aids us in understanding current states but also has the capacity to form a foundation for predicting future respiratory wellness issues. By integrating acoustic examination techniques, such as auscultation, with more modern technologies, practitioners can gain a complete understanding of a patient's respiratory function. Knowing the correlation of aberrant vibrations to most probable underlying causes makes diagnosis more accurate. Furthermore, as technological progress leads to further seeking of meticulous data analysis, caregivers can design predictive models that can identify vulnerabilities and facilitate more effective preventative medicine in respiratory therapy. Thus, interpretation of results becomes an essential factor in respiratory disease management, allowing for timely intervention and, potentially, prevention of undiagnosed cases-related morbidity (Dugassa et al., 2020; Wintzenrieth et al., 2024).

1.5.1. Normal Vs. Abnormal Breath Sounds

Assessment of breath sounds is a crucial part of the physical examination of the respiratory system and is extremely useful in monitoring underlying respiratory pathology. Normal breath sounds, in accordance with their clarity and homogeneity, vary in each thoracic area. Bronchial sounds, typically heard over the trachea, are higher-pitched and of briefer duration during expiration than during inspiration, for instance. By contrast, vesicular breath sounds, which are typical over the lung fields, are lower in pitch, less loud, and longer on inspiration than on expiration. These are characteristic of everyday sounds and indicate unimpeded passage of air through the tracheobronchial tree and the lung parenchyma, a reflection of flawless respiratory function. Proper distinction of these normal sounds is essential because any deviation from the normal can lead to early detection of potential respiratory pathologies. In contrast to normal breath sounds, abnormal breath sounds can indicate severe medical conditions and need further investigation. These adventitious sounds, such as wheezes, crackles, and rhonchi, are alterations in airflow and potential blockages within the airways. Wheezing, for instance, typically implies constricted airways, most often accompanied by asthma or COPD. Crackles, or rales, can be indicative of fluid in the alveoli, most commonly encountered in the context of pneumonia or congestive heart failure. Rhonchi, being rumbling and low-pitched in nature, typically signify mucus within the large airways. These sounds are significant for clinicians to recognize since they can guide diagnostic procedures and treatment regimens for a variety of pulmonary pathologies. Bedside evaluation of breath sounds, therefore, emphasizes the integration of findings of auscultation with clinical and physiological backgrounds. Pathologic breath sounds do not occur independently; they are instead frequently a feature accompanying a patient's history, physical examination, and even radiographic findings. An instance is a patient with crackles presenting with respiratory failure and hypoxemia, and hence necessitating prompt therapeutic intervention for the underlying pathology. Methods such as respiratory function scoring systems and systematic approaches to interpreting breath sounds are vital for healthcare professionals. An increased understanding of normal and abnormal breath sounds enables more thorough respiratory assessments, facilitating improved patient care and management. As science evolves, as it does with the development of novel diagnostic biomarkers for lung illnesses, the significance of fine physical examination techniques will remain critical to practice.

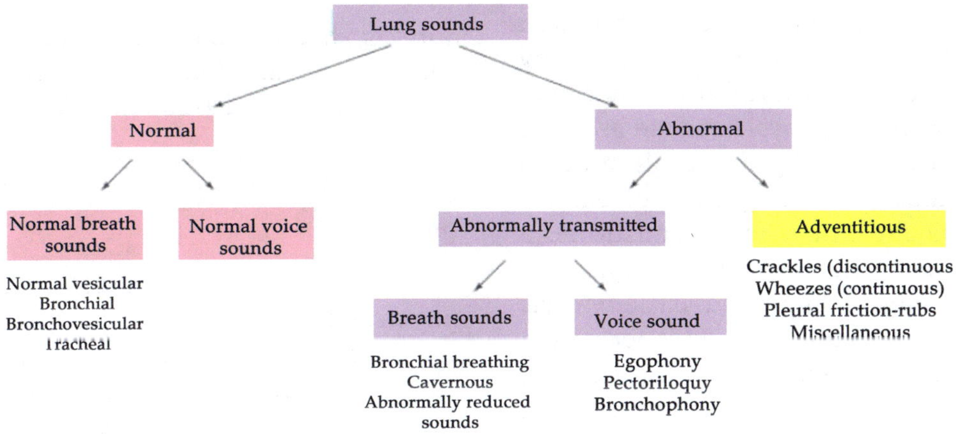

Figure 1.16. Normal vs. abnormal breath sounds.

Source: https://ars.els-cdn.com/content/image/3-s2.0-B0123708796003550-gr2.jpg

1.5.2. Identifying Respiratory Distress

Recognition of respiratory distress is an essential component of the respiratory system physical examination and involves sensitive awareness of clinical presentation and underlying physiology. Presentation of respiratory distress often manifests through observable behaviors and physiological patterns, such as increased respiratory rate, effortful breathing, or the use of accessory muscles during respiration. Clinicians must have the ability to recognize these signs because any delay in recognizing these signs will compound the patient's illness. Healthcare providers must also consider the context in which these symptoms occur, as underlying medical conditions—such as asthma or COPD—will significantly impact how respiratory distress manifests. By total history along with physical examination findings, it is possible to have a more accurate estimation of the severity and potential etiology of the distress, ultimately deciding on appropriate intervention. Additionally, biomarkers have been identified that enhance the detection of respiratory distress. For instance, studies have determined the significance of siglec-9 expression in patients with acute respiratory distress syndrome (ARDS) as a diagnostic marker (Liu et al., 2025). High plasma concentrations of this biomarker are highly correlated with ARDS severity and emphasize its clinical relevance in evaluation. Identification of such biomarkers is an essential for clinicians because it would not only assist in measuring the extent of the condition but may also result in targeted therapeutic interventions. Furthermore, by combining these biomarkers with traditional examination techniques, physicians can promote early intervention, thereby greatly improving patient outcomes. This integration of clinical findings and biochemical markers constitutes a multi-modal diagnostic paradigm to respiratory distress, resulting in improved patient care. Involvement of technological advancements, such as imaging tests and innovative drug delivery systems, also influences the identification and management of respiratory distress. For example, recent therapy employing mannosylated lipid nanoparticles to enhance the delivery of therapeutic molecules, such as miR-146a, to alveolar macrophages has been reported to alleviate lung injury in mechanical ventilation significantly (Fei et al., 2023). This approach not only treats acute physiological discomfort but also targets the underlying inflammatory processes causing the condition. Therefore, by combining new technologies with intensive physical examination techniques, one not only accurately diagnoses respiratory distress but also opens up new avenues for beneficial intervention. Continual improvement in the diagnosis and treatment of respiratory conditions underpins the necessity of continuous education in the clinical environment, enabling healthcare providers to stay abreast of best practice management.

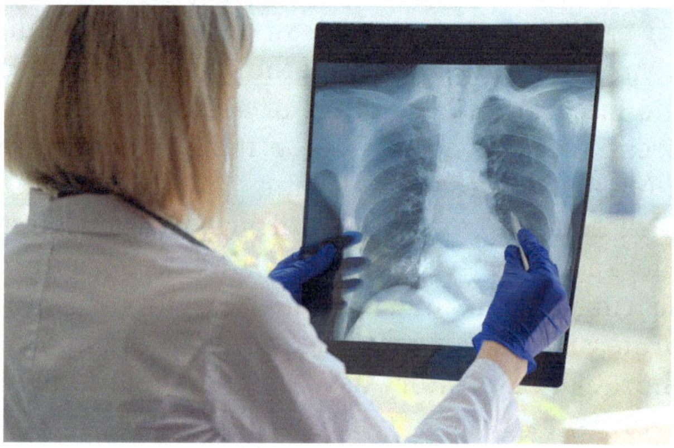

Figure 1.17. Identifying respiratory distress.

Source: https://medicare.wedelo.co.uk/wp-content/uploads/2022/08/respiratory-distress-syndrome-covid-19-1024x677.jpg

1.5.3. Correlating Physical Findings With Patient History

In the context of respiratory tests, matching physical findings with a patient's history is crucial to achieving an effective diagnosis. The comprehensive aspect of patient history—spanning from past illnesses to environmental and familial conditions—enables the inclusion of critical context that informs clinicians about potential underlying pathologies, which is critical. For instance, a chronic cough patient can manifest with various physical findings that vary from wheezing or diminished breath sounds, and can bear a history of asthma or chronic obstructive pulmonary disease (COPD). Such correlations not only aid in the identification of underlying respiratory issues but also guide clinicians in establishing an overall image of the patient's health, highlighting the importance of comprehensive questioning on history taking (Bone et al., 2024).

Besides, the integration of physical examination findings with patient history enhances clinical decision-making and results in the management of respiratory ailments. While physical exam results, such as lung auscultation overtones, may provide early indicators of ventilatory function, they are of greater significance when considered in the context of chronological data. A physician assessing a patient with a smoking history and chronic respiratory infection, for example, will consider abnormal breath sounds more menacingly than one who is assessing a non-smoker with an acute upper respiratory illness. This amalgamation of information significantly enhances diagnostic confidence by excluding benign conditions from potentially severe diseases, thereby reducing the risk of misdiagnosis (Fukuzawa et al., 2023).

Lastly, technological innovations such as artificial intelligence underscore the ongoing value of a thorough patient history, complemented by the addition of physical findings. Recent studies have reported that AI systems can utilize patient histories to enhance diagnostic accuracy, demonstrating that medical history plays a vital role in achieving a very high percentage of correct diagnoses. The addition of results from physical examinations and laboratory findings further enhances diagnostic accuracy (Fukuzawa et al., 2023). This double treatment benefits not only a more enriching diagnostic process but also justifies the clinician's role in integrating different data in addressing respiratory ailments. In this regard, underscoring this connection enables a comprehensive approach toward understanding patient conditions, which ultimately informs more effective treatment regimens.

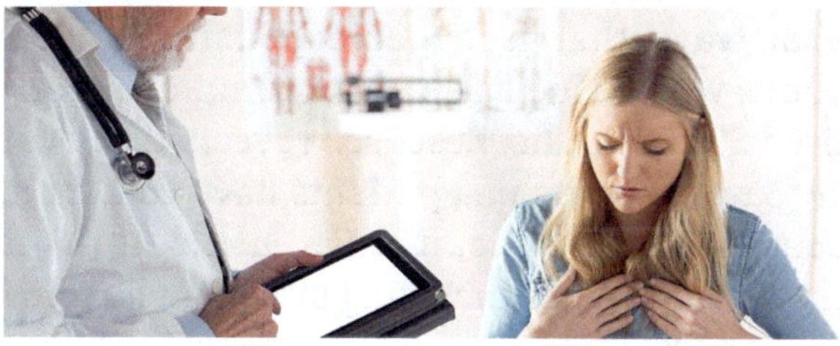

Source: https://www.hopkinsmedicine.org/-/media/images/health/1_-conditions/stomach-and-gut/woman-experiencing-gerd-hero.jpg?h=500&iar=0&mh=500&mw=1300&w=1297&hash=C2DDB6E072844F9D7406D9ED319DE485

Test Your Knowledge

1. What is normal vs. abnormal breath sounds?
2. How to identify respiratory distress?

1.6. Common Respiratory Conditions

Learning Outcome

1. Asthma: symptoms and examination findings
2. Chronic obstructive pulmonary disease (COPD): key indicators
3. Pneumonia: physical examination clues

The common respiratory illnesses have a significant impact on public health, with asthma and chronic obstructive pulmonary disease (COPD) being among the most prominent ones. Asthma, an inflammatory condition of the airways that is hyperresponsive, affects millions worldwide and is quite common among United States adults. Research reveals that over half (61.6%) of asthma patients have comorbid diseases, whose healthcare utilization is considerably higher, including overnight hospital stays where utilization is a staggering 21.6% with comorbidities versus only 7.4% without (Hanna A Frank et al., 2024). This is evidence of the intricate relationship between asthma control and the existence of other health issues, which presents the need for adequate physical examination to be capable of assessing asthma's impact and the comorbidities that worsen it. Chronic obstructive pulmonary disease is another common and disabling respiratory ailment that is characterized by airflow limitation and persistent respiratory symptoms. COPD most often leads to serious complications like pulmonary bullae that are capable of deteriorating lung function and significantly impacting patients' quality of life. It is also challenging to treat pulmonary bullae since the standard surgical intervention, bullectomy, is also risky with threats like postoperative complications as well as high recurrence rates (Zhu et al., 2024). New interventional respiratory techniques are proving to be of great promise as an alternative for patients who cannot undergo surgery due to compromised lung function or other disease. With practitioners eyeing the entire spectrum of respiratory pathology, a skilled physical examination comes in handy in guiding appropriate intervention and overall management for COPD patients.

Physical examination is useful in diagnosing and managing common respiratory illnesses. A thorough evaluation not only assesses lung function and airway reactivity but also screens for signs of comorbid diseases that may complicate these disorders. It is the responsibility of clinicians to apply auscultation tests to identify irregularities in the sounds produced by the lungs that indicate pathology, along with the incorporation of the patient's medical history, particularly smoking or occupational exposure. Such a comprehensive evaluation can inform interventions targeting primary respiratory diseases, as well as their associated comorbidities. By focusing on extensive assessment, health professionals can significantly reduce the rate of emergency admissions and improve the overall management of respiratory wellness, ultimately leading to better patient outcomes in managing chronic conditions such as asthma and COPD.

1.6.1. Asthma: Symptoms and Examination Findings

The clinical presentation of asthma is best defined as a range of respiratory symptoms that often include wheezing, dyspnea, chest tightness, and a persistent cough, mainly nocturnal or morning. Wheezing, the most recognizable sound of asthma, is produced by turbulent airflow through narrowed airways, which creates a high-pitched musical quality. These symptoms are episodic in nature and can be triggered by a variety of precipitating factors such as allergens, respiratory infections, exercise, and environmental agents. In the process of establishing a physical examination, these symptoms can be reinforced by objective measurements such as peak expiratory flow rate (PEFR), which can demonstrate variability in airflow limitation. Clinicians must examine the frequency and pattern of these signs to analyze the severity of asthma and the need for individualized management strategies (Vogelmeier et al., 2017). Some physical examination findings may also offer further information on the presence of asthma. Bilateral wheezing on lung auscultation indicates bronchial hyperreactivity and airway obstruction. With severe illness, there may be decreased air movement and a prolonged expiratory phase, reflecting severe airflow limitation. The use of accessory muscles in the patient may also be observed as a compensatory response to respiratory distress, reflecting the severity of the case. The presence of atopic signs, such as eczema or allergic rhinitis, may also be prevalent in patients with asthma, relating the condition to basic allergic responses. The clinician's perception of these physical findings is essential in creating a comprehensive picture of the patient's respiratory status and guiding management (Butt et al., 2017). A thorough history is as important as a physical examination in asthma evaluation. Clinicians may query the onset, duration, frequency, and precipitating factors of symptoms to understand the patient's individual asthma phenotype. Identifying related comorbidities, such as allergic rhinitis or gastroesophageal reflux disease, can aid in developing a comprehensive treatment plan. History of medications, including adherence to inhaled corticosteroids and use of relievers, is also essential to evaluate asthma control, and patient education on inhaler technique should not be overlooked. With the integration of clinical presentation from both history and examination, clinicians are better able to classify the severity and category of asthma, thus ultimately informing maximized management and better outcomes for patients (Vogelmeier et al., 2017).

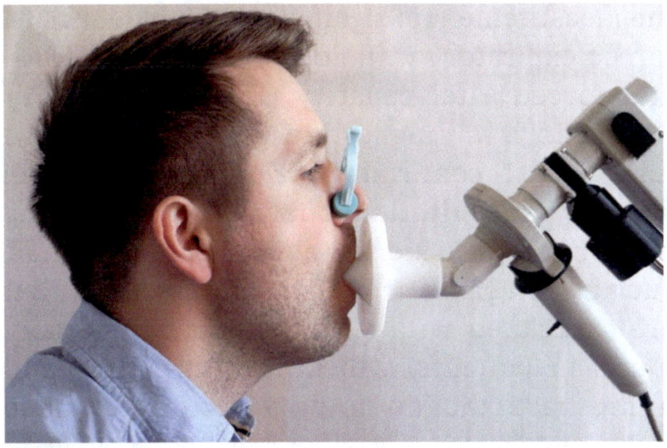

Figure 1.18. Testing for asthma.

Source: https://www.health.com/thmb/4juk1a8AgIMFvptXGpu_Qk6O-Ho=/2121x0/filters:no_upscale():max_bytes(150000):strip_icc()/GettyImages-937846468-118d4a5614ec4a7991cdb488863cbeb5.jpg

1.6.2. Chronic Obstructive Pulmonary Disease (COPD): Key Indicators

Chronic obstructive pulmonary disease (COPD) is characterized by chronic airflow limitation, which is most frequently caused by exposure to noxious gases or particles, such as tobacco smoke. The primary symptoms of COPD are excessive smoking history, dyspnea, repeated respiratory infections, and impaired exercise tolerance. During physical examination, a clinician can observe increased respiratory rate, accessory muscle utilization on expiration, and digital clubbing. Their identification is key to differentiating COPD from other respiratory diseases. Moreover, clinical guidelines in practice emphasize the importance of prompt diagnosis and management to retard the condition and improve the patient's quality of life. The detection of these key indicators ensures early intervention, which is vital when incorporated into an entire respiratory assessment (Humbert et al., 2022). Physical evaluation of suspected COPD patients must include spirometry, with the measurement of significant variables such as forced expiratory volume in one second (FEV1) and forced vital capacity (FVC). Low FEV1/FVC ratio is a diagnostic sign for obstructive lung disease, confirming the existence of COPD. Further, auscultation analysis of breathing patterns can also identify abnormal lung sounds, such as wheezing or prolonged expiration, that are associated with airflow limitation, usually found in patients with COPD. Physicians and nurses are taught how to recognize these signs and symptoms effectively, as they form the basis for primary differential diagnosis. Emphasizing these parameters during a physical examination can lead to a more precise diagnosis and, consequently, better treatment plans that are tailored to the patient's individual clinical presentation and overall health status (Vogelmeier et al., 2017).

Treatment for COPD also entails a wide understanding of comorbidities that usually accompany the disease, such as cardiovascular disorders and anxiety. Identifying the interrelationship between all these comorbidities and COPD is essential during the physical examination. The clinician must attentively look out for manifestations of chronic diseases that complicate respiratory conditions, as this has significant implications for treatment strategies and the prognosis of the patient. These interventions, such as smoking cessation, pulmonary rehabilitation, and drug therapy, must also be optimally coordinated with the overall plan of a patient since they contribute to the reduction of both respiratory and systemic complications associated with COPD. Such integrated management of major indicators ensures that patients receive comprehensive care, which enhances the long-term prognosis and quality of life among COPD patients (Humbert et al., 2022).

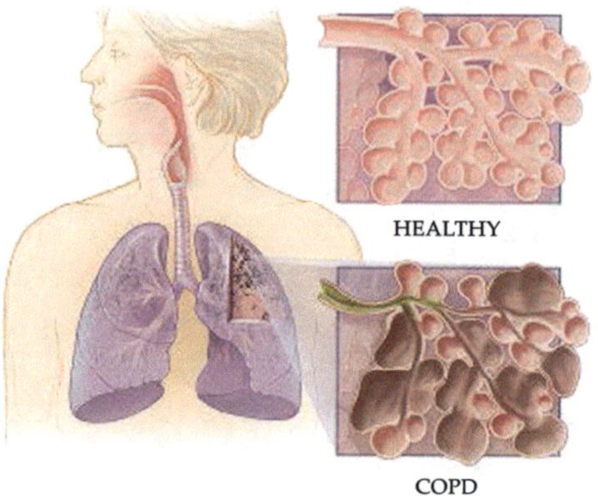

Figure 1.19. Chronic obstructive pulmonary disease (COPD): key indicators.

Source: https://upload.wikimedia.org/wikipedia/commons/5/59/COPD_versus_healthy_lung.jpg

1.6.3. Pneumonia: Physical Examination Clues

A physical examination of the patient suspected of having pneumonia involves a series of systematic checks that can be of significant assistance in determining the presence and severity of the disease. The examination begins with the inspection of the patient's general appearance, vital signs, and respiratory effort. Tachypnea, or an increased respiratory rate, is a significant finding on physical examination that can indicate respiratory distress. Additionally, the clinician should check for a crackle or rale on auscultation, as rattling breath sounds may indicate fluid in the alveoli. In addition, the finding of diminished breath sounds or appreciable dullness to percussion can indicate a pleural effusion that is related to the pneumonia, necessitating further evaluation and treatment. Identification of these physical findings can help facilitate a quick diagnosis and enhance patient outcomes. Throughout the examination, clinicians also use percussion and palpation techniques to detect abnormalities in lung function. Percussion is utilized to distinguish areas of consolidation from normal lung tissue, as the presence of dullness will indicate underlying pneumonia, while normal lung is characterized by resonance. Palpation may indicate tactile fremitus alterations; increased fremitus is observed over areas of consolidation, while reduced fremitus can indicate effusion or other obstructions. In addition, inspection of the patient's color and overall circulation may imply systemic disease or hypoxia due to pneumonia. Early recognition of such a possible subtle yet significant physical examination finding plays important and essential role in the management direction of acute pneumonia, which may include antibiotics and supportive therapy targeted to the patient's unique situation. Detailed physical exam findings can also illustrate the underlying etiology of pneumonia and is essential in guiding treatment. For instance, in cases where aspiration is suspected to be the cause of pneumonia, focal findings on exam, such as fetid breath or the presence of a unilateral wheeze due to obstructed airways, may be found by the physician. Certain populations, such as the elderly or patients with comorbidities, may have a non-typical presentation, with less extreme examination findings. Moreover, knowledge of the circumstances of such physical findings directs the clinician's selection of diagnostic imaging or laboratory testing. Thus, effective physical examination skills remain an essential component in the early diagnosis of pneumonia with prompt intervention and monitoring for potential complications, such as respiratory failure or sepsis, particularly in vulnerable patient populations, as highlighted in discussion of mental health implications during the COVID-19 pandemic (Salari et al., 2020) and increased need for the early diagnosis of pulmonary disorders such as pulmonary fibrosis (Lederer et al., 2018).

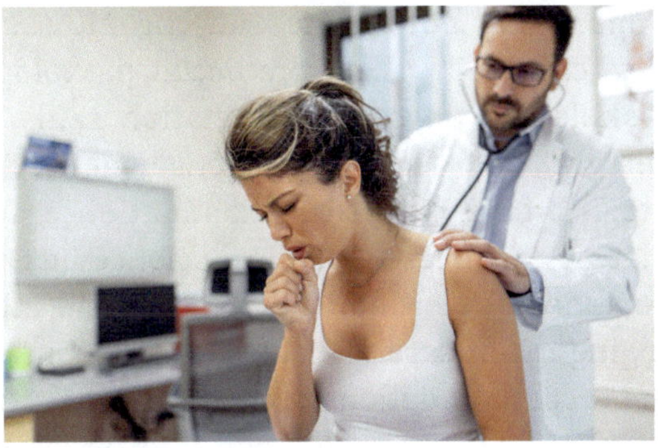

Source: https://hospitalvozandes.com/wp-content/uploads/2023/11/Foto-Neumonia-BLOG-HVQ-scaled.jpg

Test Your Knowledge

1. What are the symptoms of asthma?
2. What are the key indicators of chronic obstructive pulmonary disease (COPD)?

SUMMARY

A walk-through of the physical examination of the respiratory system is essential to consider the multifaceted function that this assessment can play in diagnosing and managing respiratory diseases. The process is carried out systematically, dependent on observation, palpation, percussion, and auscultation to outline the actual health condition of the lungs and airways. Widespread physical examination techniques not only enable recognition of common pathologies but also provide avenues to instant interventions, directly influencing the patient's outcomes. Additionally, whenever new healthcare breakthroughs occur, the inclusion of imaging modalities in the diagnostic process increases the diagnostic capacity to address the challenges faced by respiratory diseases today.

The benefits of a comprehensive respiratory examination far exceed those of initial evaluations. With the current global health emergencies, most notably the COVID-19 pandemic, there has been an increased appreciation for the utility of this clinical skill in identifying potential complications and managing both acute and chronic respiratory issues. Careful evaluation of the respiratory system can avert risks from occult pathologies, directing healthcare professionals to remain alert and skilled in physical examination skills. Actually, physical examination is a significant aspect of integral care for patients, ensuring not only accurate diagnosis but also optimal therapeutic strategies. Lastly, physical examination practices on the respiratory system should catch up with the latest advances in medical science and technology. The findings of all research emphasize the importance of continuing education and modification of examination practices to keep pace with changing healthcare scenarios. In this context, the development of comprehensive guidelines, such as the recommendations for respiratory rehabilitation that consider both physical and psychological aspects, is crucial. To this end, the psychological well-being of patients must not be overlooked, as evidenced by studies that indicate the psychological impacts of respiratory diseases during crisis situations, such as the COVID-19 pandemic (Salari et al., 2020; Zhao et al., 2020). Such considerations are crucial to creating an integrated care approach that emphasizes both physical and mental health, thereby enriching the quality of life for patients.

Physical examination of the respiratory system in clinical medicine plays a critical role in the diagnosis and the monitoring of pulmonary function. Some important factors to consider are a systematic process of inspection, palpation, percussion, and auscultation. These techniques collectively reveal important information about lung function and disease. Visual observation, for instance, can detect respiratory distress such as cyanosis or the use of accessory muscles. Moreover, palpation is also capable of identifying deviations, such as chest wall tenderness or asymmetry, whereas percussion allows clinicians to determine if lung fields are resonant or dull, thereby suggesting subdiagnoses like pleural effusion or consolidation. A sound appreciation of the maneuvers forms the basis of an entire evaluation of respiratory wellness and guides subsequent medical care. Another significant focus of the physical examination is the detection of abnormal breath sounds via auscultation. Detection of wheezes, crackles, or silent areas during the process can alert clinicians to specific pulmonary illnesses, ranging from asthma to pneumonia or COPD. Pathologic breath sounds are a critical diagnostic clue, prompting further investigation and management measures. The nuances of such sounds, particularly their timing in the respiratory cycle and their location within the patients entire clinical context, enhance a physician's ability to build an accurate diagnosis. An appreciation of the clinical relevance of such observations is crucial, as it can significantly impact treatment pathways and patient outcomes in respiratory therapy. In addition, the interaction between physical examination findings and broader epidemiological data cannot be overstated. For example, the importance of examination is not only in the direct clinical setting but also determines public health surveillance, particularly where there are epidemic respiratory diseases instigated by environmental causes. The COVID-19 pandemic has highlighted the importance of the link between regular physical examinations and the basis for tracking disease spread and initiating public health interventions (Hale et al., 2021). Moreover, the identification of underlying comorbidities through respiratory tests enables the development of thorough management strategies, as diseases like COPD require multidisciplinary interventions that account for additional health issues (Vogelmeier et al., 2017). Hence, incorporation of test findings with cumulative data enhances clinical understanding and public health interventions.

KEY TERMS FROM THIS CHAPTER

- Inspection
- Percussion
- Respiratory rate
- Tactile fremitus
- Cyanosis
- Use of accessory muscles
- Barrel chest
- Hyperresonance
- Vesicular breath sounds
- Wheezes
- Palpation
- Auscultation
- Chest expansion
- Tracheal deviation
- Clubbing
- Intercostal retractions
- Pectus excavatum
- Dullness (on percussion)
- Bronchial breath sounds
- Crackles (rales)

CRITICAL THINKING QUESTIONS

1. During chest percussion, which of the following findings is most consistent with pleural effusion?

a. Hyperresonance
b. Dullness to percussion
c. Tympany
d. Resonance

2. Which of the following is the correct sequence for physical examination of the respiratory system?

a. Percussion → Inspection → Palpation → Auscultation
b. Inspection → Palpation → Percussion → Auscultation
c. Palpation → Inspection → Auscultation → Percussion
d. Auscultation → Percussion → Palpation → Inspection

3. What type of breath sound is normally heard over the trachea?

a. Vesicular
b. Bronchial
c. Bronchovesicular
d. Adventitious

4. Which of the following adventitious breath sounds is most likely to be heard in a patient with bronchial asthma?

a. Crackles
b. Stridor
c. Wheezing
d. Pleural rub

5. Tactile fremitus is decreased in which of the following conditions?

a. Lung consolidation
b. Pulmonary edema
c. Pleural effusion
d. Lobar pneumonia

Short Answer Questions

1. What are the four main components of the physical examination of the respiratory system?
2. What does dullness to percussion over the lungs suggest?
3. What chest shape abnormality is commonly seen in chronic obstructive pulmonary disease (COPD)?
4. Which condition is indicated by decreased tactile fremitus and dullness to percussion?
5. What does increased tactile fremitus suggest?
6. What kind of percussion note is expected over a normal lung field?
7. Which breath sounds are normally heard over most peripheral lung areas?

Answer to Critical Thinking Questions

1. (b) 2. (b) 3. (b) 4. (c) 5. (c)

REFERENCES

1. Adler, Y., Charron, P., Imazio, M., Badano, L., Barón-Esquivias, G., Bogaert, J., Brucato, A., Gueret, P., Klingel, K., Lionis, C., Maisch, B., Mayosi, B., Pavie, A., Ristić, A. D., Tenas, M. S., Seferovic, P., Swedberg, K., Tomkowski, W., Achenbach, S., . . . Nesukay, E. (2015). 2015 ESC Guidelines for the diagnosis and management of pericardial diseases. *European Heart Journal, 36*(42), 2921–2964. https://doi.org/10.1093/eurheartj/ehv318Akyol, M. U., Alden, T. D., Amartino, H., Ashworth, S., et al. (2019). Recommendations for the management of MPS VI: Systematic evidence- and consensus-based guidance. https://core.ac.uk/download/323074857.pdf (accessed on 16th June 2025).

2. Alyousef, I. A., Alsaileek, Z. A., Alabdulsalam, M. A., Almohanna, M. A., Alshaqhaa, N. A., Alqahtani, M. M., Al Alyany, A. A., et al. (2022). Mesenteric panniculitis and COVID-19: A rare association. *Cureus, 14.* https://www.semanticscholar.org/paper/0b5999b0c095cb2917ebd308c5be531f1259c0aa (accessed on 16th June 2025).

3. Baumgartner, H., De Backer, J., Babu-Narayan, S. V., Budts, W., Chessa, M., Diller, G. P., Lung, B., et al. (2020). 2020 ESC guidelines for the management of adult congenital heart disease. *European Heart Journal, 42*, 563–645. https://doi.org/10.1093/eurheartj/ehaa554 (accessed on 16th June 2025).

4. Bekembetova, R., Konakbayev, B., & Mazhenov, S. (2024). Dynamics of maximum oxygen consumption under extreme physical exertion in ski racers. *Теория и методика физической культуры.* https://www.semanticscholar.org/paper/8f0bd486d3610a17771e926a839d3aebb89ae0d0 (accessed on 16th June 2025).

5. Belyaeva, Y., & Shemetova, G. (2024). Assessment of socio-hygienic factors affecting health and morbidity among university students. *Social Aspects of Population Health.* https://www.semanticscholar.org/paper/be655515443d1056264bd3f45aef4b2424834e3e (accessed on 16th June 2025).

6. Bilgiç, E. B. (2025). Anesthetic risk analysis with routine preoperative thoracic radiography in dogs and cats. *Revista Científica de la Facultad de Ciencias Veterinarias.* https://www.semanticscholar.org/paper/d8c27eb9e43311303569a26a5b880505ed43cb3f (accessed on 16th June 2025).

7. Bone, H., & Diamond-Fox, S. (2024). Assessment and examination of the respiratory system. *British Journal of Nursing, 33*(13), 606–611. https://www.semanticscholar.org/paper/ac9ffca6d0ec2ef8d0a1ec640d0bc85ba4afae4f (accessed on 16th June 2025).

8. Butt, N. M., Lambert, J., Ali, S., Beer, P., Cross, N. C. P., Duncombe, A., Ewing, J., et al. (2017). Guideline for the investigation and management of eosinophilia. *British Journal of Hematology, 176*, 553–572. https://doi.org/10.1111/bjh.14488 (accessed on 16th June 2025).

9. Clark, T. A., Cohn, A. C., Farley, M. M., Hall, A. J., et al. (2016). Meningococcal disease in patients with human immunodeficiency virus infection: A review of cases reported through active surveillance in the United States, 2000–2008. https://core.ac.uk/download/323082103.pdf (accessed on 16th June 2025).

10. Coté, C. J., & Wilson, S. (2019). Guidelines for monitoring and management of pediatric patients before, during, and after sedation for diagnostic and therapeutic procedures. *Pediatrics, 143.* https://doi.org/10.1542/peds.2019-1000 (accessed on 16th June 2025).

11. Cruz-Jentoft, A. J., Bahat, G., Bauer, J. M., Boirie, Y., Bruyère, O., Cederholm, T., Cooper, C., et al. (2018). Sarcopenia: Revised European consensus on definition and diagnosis. *Age and Ageing, 48*, 16–31. https://doi.org/10.1093/ageing/afy169 (accessed on 16th June 2025).

12. Deucher, R. A. O., Reis, L. F. F., Papathanasiou, J., Azevedo, B. L. P. A., Oliveira, J. G. M., Silva, M. M., Sales, R. C., et al. (2023). Estimating cardiopulmonary fitness with a new sampling technology in patients with rheumatoid arthritis-associated interstitial lung disease. *Physiotherapy Research International: The Journal for Researchers and Clinicians in Physical Therapy.* https://www.semanticscholar.org/paper/ca1e0fdd100f1e01ff2dcf632e31b1a4595583d1 (accessed on 16th June 2025).

13. Díaz-Pacheco, J., & Cabanillas-Chávez, M. T. (2024). Nursing process applied to a preschooler with spinal muscular atrophy and chronic respiratory failure. *Multidisciplinary (Montevideo).* https://www.semanticscholar.org/paper/c7ca40f0b8c183ae2f05dbcc22702cd2bdbb2825 (accessed on 16th June 2025).

14. Ding, X., Clifton, D. A., Ji, N., Lovell, N. H., Bonato, P., Chen, W., Yu, X., et al. (2020). Wearable sensing and telehealth technology with potential applications in the coronavirus pandemic. *IEEE Reviews in Biomedical Engineering, 14*, 48–70. https://doi.org/10.1109/rbme.2020.2992838 (accessed on 16th June 2025).

15. Dugassa, J., & Wirtu, A. (2020). Review on surgical affections of respiratory system and thoracic cavity in dogs. *Volume, 2*, 39. https://www.semanticscholar.org/paper/0d25ea0ae051d5877b566f48dc59bf950b554b0a (accessed on 16th June 2025).

16. Ellis, M., & Faghy, M. (2024). The role of inspiratory muscle fatigue and its impact on strength and respiratory function. *Graduate Journal of Sports Science, Coaching, Management, & Rehabilitation.* https://www.semanticscholar.org/paper/1482cfacb2e0609effba9e1af66018268f618fba (accessed on 16th June 2025).

17. Evans, L., Rhodes, A., Alhazzani, W., Antonelli, M., Coopersmith, C. M., French, C., Machado, F. R., et al. (2021). Surviving Sepsis Campaign: International guidelines for management of sepsis and septic shock 2021. *Critical Care Medicine, 49*, e1063–e1143. https://doi.org/10.1097/ccm.0000000000005337 (accessed on 16th June 2025).

18. Fatima, S., Ijaz, S., Asadullah, S., Arslan, I., Mohammed, M., Ali, K., Sultan, P., et al. (2024). Comparative anatomy of the respiratory systems in high altitude vs. low altitude populations. *Journal of Health and Rehabilitation Research.* https://www.semanticscholar.org/paper/11154b0e8b9df3b2102faf65279cee038e7cc6d5 (accessed on 16th June 2025).

19. Fei, Q., Shalosky, E., Barnes, R., Shukla, V., Xu, S., Ballinger, M., Farkas, L., et al. (2023). Macrophage-targeted lipid nanoparticle delivery of microRNA-146a to mitigate hemorrhagic shock-induced acute respiratory distress syndrome. *ACS Nano.* https://www.semanticscholar.org/paper/e56a78b0e8713f4b4da4351a92809fcb00c30416 (accessed on 16th June 2025).

20. Frank, H. A., & Karim, M. E. (2024). Physical comorbidity is associated with overnight hospitalization in U.S. adults with asthma: An assessment of the 2005–2018 National Health and Nutrition Examination Surveys. *Journal of Asthma, 62*, 155–166. https://www.semanticscholar.org/paper/7f88e6939e2b8d1589e5d03da2e833faa232bf44 (accessed on 16th June 2025).

21. Fukuzawa, F., Yanagita, Y., Yokokawa, D., Uchida, S., Yamashita, S., Li, Y., Shikino, K., et al. (2023). Importance of patient history in artificial intelligence–assisted medical diagnosis: Comparison study. *JMIR Medical Education, 10.* https://www.semanticscholar.org/paper/11

c680ffdd149d551b35737329a0b9bca6c589c3 (accessed on 16th June 2025).

22. Guarracino, F., Vetrugno, L., Forfori, F., Corradi, F., Orso, D., Bertini, P., Ortalda, A., et al. (2020). Lung, heart, vascular, and diaphragm ultrasound examination of COVID-19 patients: A comprehensive approach. *Journal of Cardiothoracic and Vascular Anesthesia, 35*, 1866–1874. https://doi.org/10.1053/j.jvca.2020.06.013 (accessed on 16th June 2025).

23. Gyawali, B., Ramakrishna, K., & Dhamoon, A. S. (2019). Sepsis: The evolution in definition, pathophysiology, and management. *SAGE Open Medicine, 7.* https://doi.org/10.1177/2050312119835043 (accessed on 16th June 2025).

24. Hale, T., Angrist, N., Goldszmidt, R., Kira, B., Petherick, A., Phillips, T., Webster, S., et al. (2021). A global panel database of pandemic policies (Oxford COVID-19 Government Response Tracker). *Nature Human Behavior, 5*, 529–538. https://doi.org/10.1038/s41562-021-01079-8 (accessed on 16th June 2025).

25. Humbert, M., Kovács, G., Hoeper, M. M., Badagliacca, R., Berger, R. M. F., Brida, M., Carlsen, J., et al. (2022). 2022 ESC/ERS guidelines for the diagnosis and treatment of pulmonary hypertension. *European Respiratory Journal, 61*, 2200879–2200879. https://doi.org/10.1183/13993003.00879-2022 (accessed on 16th June 2025).

26. Ibatova, S. (2025). Bronchial obstruction syndrome in young children: Clinical features, diagnosis and treatment. *Medical Science of Uzbekistan.* https://www.semanticscholar.org/paper/c9865ee38e9ddbd9264eea72569c0008b7022f63 (accessed on 16th June 2025).

27. Jin, Y., Cai, L., Cheng, Z., Cheng, H., Deng, T., Fan, Y., Fang, C., et al. (2020). A rapid advice guideline for the diagnosis and treatment of 2019 novel coronavirus (2019-nCoV) infected pneumonia (standard version). *Military Medical Research, 7.* https://doi.org/10.1186/s40779-020-0233-6 (accessed on 16th June 2025).

28. Kalyan, B. G. P., & Kumar, L. (2022). 3D printing: Applications in tissue engineering, medical devices, and drug delivery. *AAPS PharmSciTech, 23.* https://doi.org/10.1208/s12249-022-02242-8 (accessed on 16th June 2025).

29. Konstam, M. A., Kiernan, M. S., Bernstein, D., Bozkurt, B., Jacob, M., Kapur, N. K., Kociol, R. D., et al. (2018). Evaluation and management of right-sided heart failure: A scientific statement from the American Heart Association. *Circulation, 137.* https://doi.org/10.1161/cir.0000000000000560 (accessed on 16th June 2025).

30. Konstantinides, S., Meyer, G., Becattini, C., Bueno, H., Geersing, G. J., Harjola, V. P., Huisman, M. V., et al. (2019). 2019 ESC guidelines for the diagnosis and management of acute pulmonary embolism developed in collaboration with the European Respiratory Society (ERS). *European Respiratory Journal, 54*, 1901647–1901647. https://doi.org/10.1183/13993003.01647-2019 (accessed on 16th June 2025).

31. Laveneziana, P., Pereira de Albuquerque, A. L., Aliverti, A., Babb, T. G., Barreiro, E., Dres, M., Dubé, B. P., et al. (2019). ERS statement on respiratory muscle testing at rest and during exercise. *European Respiratory Journal, 53*, 1801214–1801214. https://doi.org/10.1183/13993003.01214-2018 (accessed on 16th June 2025).

32. Lederer, D. J., & Martínez, F. J. (2018). Idiopathic pulmonary fibrosis. *New England Journal of Medicine, 378*, 1811–1823. https://doi.org/10.1056/nejmra1705751 (accessed on 16th June 2025).

33. Liu, X. G., Lu, Z. H., Cai, Y. C., Yang, Z., Sun, X. W., Zhu, J., & Su, X. (2025). [Preliminary study on the role of siglec-9 expression in peripheral blood of acute respiratory distress syndrome patients]. *Zhonghua Jie He He Hu Xi Za Zhi = Zhonghua Jiehe He Huxi Zazhi = Chinese Journal of Tuberculosis and Respiratory Diseases, 48*(2), 123–129. https://www.semanticscholar.org/paper/4c600b39d6f2bf0fc34bdeccdd112d2c1768ca43 (accessed on 16th June 2025).

34. Morice, A. H., Millqvist, E., Biekšienė, K., Birring, S. S., Dicpinigaitis, P. V., Domingo, C., Hilton Boon, M., et al. (2019). ERS guidelines on the diagnosis and treatment of chronic cough in adults and children. *European Respiratory Journal, 55*, 1901136–1901136. https://doi.org/10.1183/13993003.01136-2019 (accessed on 16th June 2025).

35. Nawaz, W., Jouvet, P., & Noumeir, R. (2024). Automated detection of acute respiratory distress using temporal visual information. *IEEE Access, 12*, 142071–142082. https://www.semanticscholar.org/paper/52fa053ea3ce0ce02c2add27a8a56991e384c0aa (accessed on 16th June 2025).

36. Panti, A. (2018). Norme per gli autori. *Ricerche di Psicologia.* https://www.semanticscholar.org/paper/a31a6d3f2d3640a017a2e8f8c117a8baa2329301 (accessed on 16th June 2025).

37. Papa, S. M., Brundin, P., Fung, V. S. C., Kang, U. J., Burn, D. J., Colosimo, C., Chiang, H. L., et al. (2020). Impact of the COVID-19 pandemic on Parkinson's disease and movement disorders. *Movement Disorders, 35*, 711–715. https://doi.org/10.1002/mds.28067 (accessed on 16th June 2025).

38. Ponikowski, P., Voors, A. A., Anker, S. D., Bueno, H., Cleland, J. G. F., Coats, A. J. S., Falk, V., et al. (2016). 2016 ESC guidelines for the diagnosis and treatment of acute and chronic heart failure. *European Heart Journal, 37*, 2129–2200. https://doi.org/10.1093/eurheartj/ehw128 (accessed on 16th June 2025).

39. Rosen, R., Vandenplas, Y., Singendonk, M., Cabana, M. D., DiLorenzo, C., Gottrand, F., Gupta, S. K., et al. (2018). Pediatric gastroesophageal reflux clinical practice guidelines. *Journal of Pediatric Gastroenterology and Nutrition, 66*, 516–554. https://doi.org/10.1097/mpg.0000000000001889 (accessed on 16th June 2025).

40. Ross, D. S., Burch, H. B., Cooper, D. S., Greenlee, M. C., Laurberg, P., Maia, A. L., Rivkees, S. A., ct al. (2016). 2016 American Thyroid Association guidelines for diagnosis and management of hyperthyroidism and other causes of thyrotoxicosis. *Thyroid, 26*, 1343–1421. https://doi.org/10.1089/thy.2016.0229 (accessed on 16th June 2025).

41. Salari, N., Hosseinian-Far, A., Jalali, R., Vaisi-Raygani, A., Rasoulpoor, S., Mohammadi, M., Rasoulpoor, S., et al. (2020). Prevalence of stress, anxiety, depression among the general population during the COVID-19 pandemic: A systematic review and meta-analysis. *Globalization and Health, 16.* https://doi.org/10.1186/s12992-020-00589-w (accessed on 16th June 2025).

42. Sang, B., Wen, H., Junek, G., Neveu, W., Di Francesco, L., Romberg, J., & Ayazi, F. (2025). A MEMS seismometer respiratory monitor for work of breathing assessment and adventitious lung sounds detection via deep learning. *Scientific Reports, 15.* https://www.semanticscholar.org/paper/b22bdf957f8d1f0ae1f9889aa8705e6863aafbae (accessed on 16th June 2025).

43. Sigrist, R., Liau, J., El Kaffas, A., Chammas, M. C., & Willmann, J. K. (2017). Ultrasound elastography: Review of techniques and clinical applications. *Theragnostic, 7*, 1303–1329. https://doi.org/10.7150/thno.18650 (accessed on 16th June 2025).

44. Silver, A. H., & Nazif, J. (2019). Bronchiolitis. *Pediatrics in Review, 40*, 568–576. https://doi.org/10.1542/pir.2018-0260 (accessed on 16th June 2025).

45. Slathia, D. S. (2012). Effects of yogic practices on different organs of an athlete. *Paripex Indian Journal of Research, 3*, 216–218. https://www.semanticscholar.org/paper/01c8002e4a1090740500caabaf0d65cc2d945b2e (accessed on 16th June 2025).

46. Stanojevic, S., Kaminsky, D. A., Miller, M. R., Thompson, B., Aliverti, A., Barjaktarević, I., Cooper, B., et al. (2021). ERS/ATS technical standard on interpretive strategies for routine lung function tests. *European Respiratory Journal, 60*, 2101499–2101499. https://doi.org/10.1183/13993003.01499-2021 (accessed on 16th June 2025).

47. Vogelmeier, C., Criner, G. J., Martínez, F. J., Anzueto, A., Barnes, P. J., Bourbeau, J., Celli, B. R., et al. (2017). Global strategy for the diagnosis, management, and prevention of chronic obstructive lung disease: 2017 report. GOLD executive summary. *American Journal of Respiratory and Critical Care Medicine, 195*, 557–582. https://doi.org/10.1164/rccm.201701-0218pp (accessed on 16th June 2025).

48. Wintzenrieth, F., Couade, M., Lehanneur, F., Laveneziana, P., Niérat, M., Verger, N., Fink, M., et al. (2024). Airborne ultrasound for the contactless mapping of surface thoracic vibrations during human vocalizations: A pilot study. *AIP Advances.* https://www.semanticscholar.org/paper/de059aee29129a0976a3dd0afa34e84d350b4f40 (accessed on 16th June 2025).

49. Zhao, L., Xie, Y. X., & Wang, C. (2020). Recommendations for respiratory rehabilitation in adults with coronavirus disease 2019. *Chinese Medical Journal, 133*, 1595–1602. https://doi.org/10.1097/cm9.0000000000000848 (accessed on 16th June 2025).

50. Zhu, J., Yin, W., Xiao, Y., Yuan, M. L., Ni, F., & Hu, Y. (2024). [Application of interventional respiratory techniques in the treatment of pulmonary bullae: An update]. *Zhonghua Jie He He Hu Xi Za Zhi = Zhonghua Jiehe He Huxi Zazhi = Chinese Journal of Tuberculosis and Respiratory Diseases, 47*(3), 259–264. https://www.semanticscholar.org/paper/b8e06e70b50ab2534c093f4983c43a460834d5d1 (accessed on 16th June 2025).

GROWTH, DEVELOPMENT, AND MORPHOLOGY OF THE RESPIRATORY TRACT

2

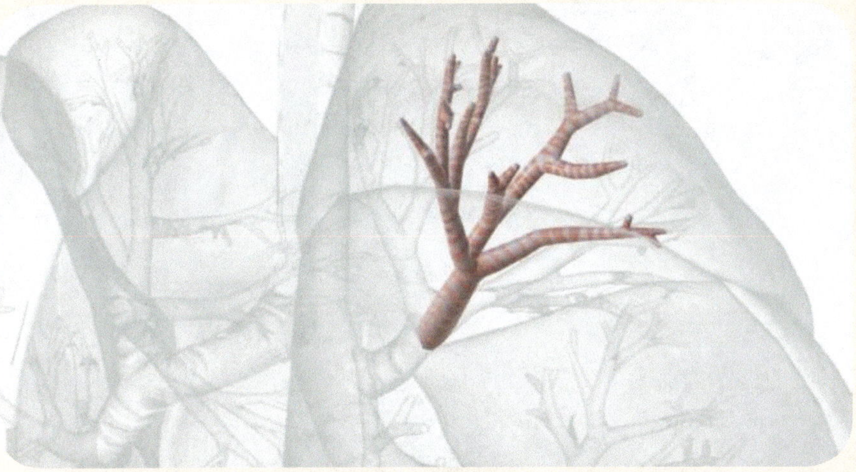

LEARNING OBJECTIVES

After studying this chapter, you will be able to:

1. Explore the embryonic development of the respiratory tract
2. Explain morphological features of the respiratory tract
3. List the growth patterns of the respiratory tract
4. Describe the functional development of the respiratory system
5. Focus on the pathological considerations in respiratory development
6. Discuss the comparative morphology of the respiratory tract

Introduction

The respiratory system is a fundamental aspect of life that participates in the exchange of gases as well as plays a variety of metabolic and immunologic roles. The system develops and matures over a long period, particularly during prenatal and neonatal life, adapting to the organism's requirements from a uterine to an independent respiratory regime. The morphology of the respiratory tract varies radically through such stages, producing structures from the nasal passages to the lung alveoli. Knowledge of the intricacies of such developmental processes is important not only for understanding normal respiratory function, but also for recognizing possible associated pathological conditions affecting breathing and lung health in later life. A detailed examination of the ontogeny of the respiratory tract reveals the intricate interplay of genetic, environmental, and endogenous factors that can influence its morphology and function. During embryogenesis, the development of the respiratory tract is intricately regulated by various signaling pathways that govern the formation of critical structures, such as the trachea and bronchi. The function of epithelial-mesenchymal interactions, through which these structures form appropriately, indicates the contribution of both genetic and environmental processes to the development of the respiratory tract. Disruptions of this window of development could potentially result in congenital defects that impair lung function. Such examination of these lines of development enables researchers to track the source of many respiratory diseases, connecting embryologic disturbances to clinical symptoms. Furthermore, with the growing body of knowledge regarding respiratory tract morphology, the importance of factors such as the mother's health, exposure to outdoor pollutants, and even nutritional intake in influencing in utero and postpartum lung growth is established, emphasizing the need for extensive studies in this regard.

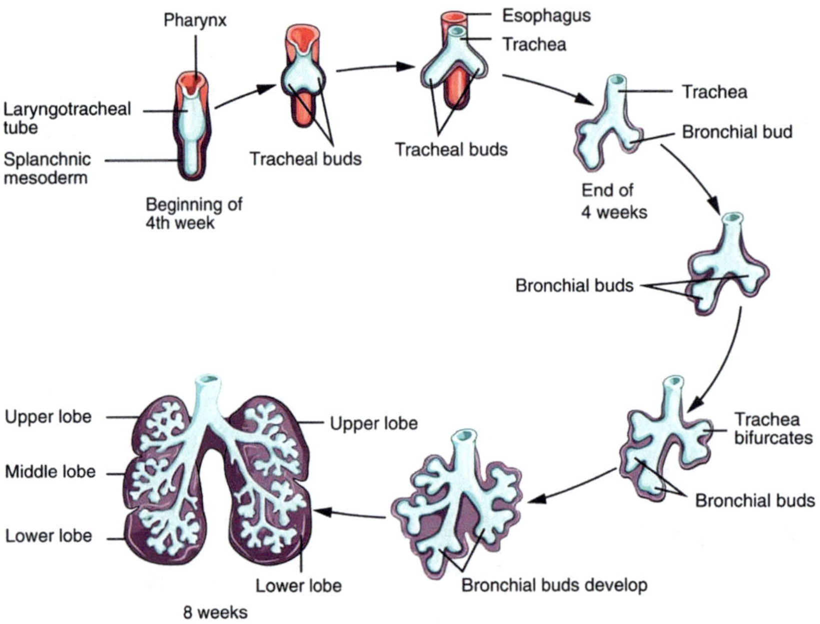

Figure 2.1. Growth, development, and morphology of the respiratory tract.

Source: https://teachmeanatomy.info/wp-content/uploads/Development-of-the-Lower-Respiratory-System-Respiratory-Diverticulum-1024x778.jpg

The integration of data on growth, development, and morphology of the respiratory tract is rapidly gaining relevance in modern medical research. Most of the recent research has been focused on understanding the microbiome and respiratory health, with an emphasis on the potential impact on lung development and lung function. For instance, microbial exposure in early life may have a long-term effect on immune maturation as well as respiratory health, promoting resilience to common respiratory disease. Alongside this, research is growing on the impacts of microplastics and environmental toxins on lung function, emphasizing the need to examine morphological changes in conjunction with ecological exposures (Ragusa et al., 2020). Of interest to investigate are also the influences of the microbiota-gut-brain axis on respiratory conditions, as new evidence has linked gut health to systemic outcomes that could impact respiratory disease (Cryan et al., 2019). Overall, the multidimensional approach to the investigation of respiratory tract growth, development, and morphology is the key to unlocking complex relationships required for developing a therapeutic approach.

Definition of the respiratory tract

The respiratory tract is an important anatomical route that is responsible for the process of exchanging gases between the outside environment and the circulatory system. The respiratory tract is primarily divided into the upper and lower respiratory tracts, and both are extremely important but different in their functions as regards respiration and gas exchange. The nasal passage, pharynx, and larynx are upper respiratory structures that provide for early air inhalation processes and filtration. These structures also humidify and warm air being inhaled, hence protecting the lower respiratory tract's vulnerable tissues. The lower respiratory tract comprises the trachea, bronchi, bronchioles, and alveoli, where essential gas exchange processes occur. This duality is an expression of the sophisticated respiratory system morphology and functional differentiation, each of which alone ensures successful respiration.

Morphogenesis of the respiratory system starts early in embryogenesis and extends into late childhood and is an essential factor in respiratory health. During early development, the respiratory system originates as a respiratory diverticulum from the foregut and subsequently develops into the trachea and its branching bronchi. As the embryo develops, these become more peripheral bronchioles and alveoli necessary for proper gas exchange. Naturally, the infant's respiratory system is a bit immature at birth, with more and more alveoli developing after birth to keep up with the rising metabolic needs. Ideal pulmonary function is dependent on gradual maturation; defective alveolar growth can lead to respiratory distress. Modern research also emphasizes the importance of multiple environmental exposures and factors during the developmental stage, with a critical need for comprehensive understanding of respiratory morphology and development.

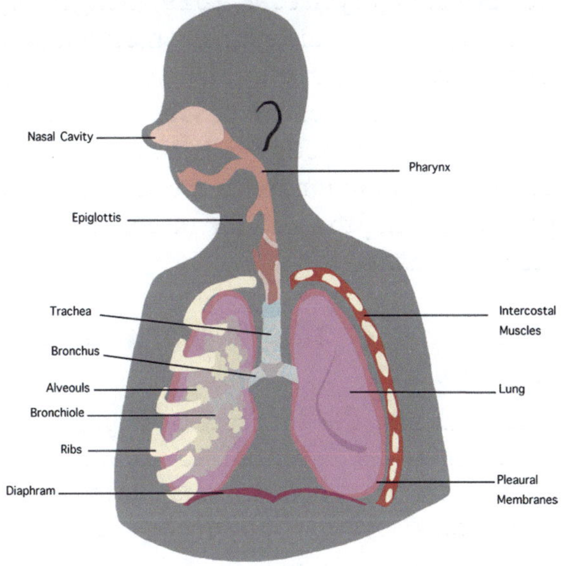

Figure 2.2. The respiratory tract.

Source: https://library.fiveable.me/_next/image?url=https%3A%2F%2Fstorage.googleapis.com%2Fstatic.prod.fiveable.me%2Fsearch-images%252F%2522Upper_and_Lower_Respiratory_Tract_anatomy_diagram_showing_structures_and_functions_in_human_respiratory_system%2522-Respiratory_System.png&w=750&q=75

The definition of the respiratory airway is not restricted to standard anatomical definitions but also encompasses physiological and environmental interactions that facilitate homeostasis. Composition of the respiratory tract microbiota also has a critical role as a protective system for avoiding invading pathogens, but regulating the immune response and the overall state of respiratory health. These microbes are able to affect the development of the respiratory tract because various factors, like mode of delivery and early antibiotic exposure, may impact the composition of the microbiota. More evidence has been accumulating to suggest that the health of the respiratory microbiome may influence other human body systems, including the gut-brain axis and the interconnectivity of body systems (Cryan et al., 2019; Alengebawy et al., 2021). An interdisciplinary methodology in the research of the respiratory tract is therefore needed, one that encompasses its structural development, functional mechanisms, and ecological interactions with the rest of the body systems, paving the way for future therapeutic interventions.

Importance of studying growth and development

Understanding the intricacies of growth and development is essential to examining the respiratory tract's form and function. The respiratory system undergoes significant changes from embryonic development through adulthood, making the study of these alterations crucial to medical practitioners and researchers. An understanding of respiratory tract development can aid in identifying congenital abnormalities or developmental disorders that may be detrimental to respiratory function. For instance, developmental malformations at crucial stages of development can lead to conditions such as bronchopulmonary dysplasia or pulmonary hypoplasia.

Investigating such development processes not only improves early diagnosis but also facilitates potential interventions and preventive measures. Such knowledge enables the achievement of enhanced clinical outcomes and improved therapeutic measures in the management of respiratory diseases, ultimately contributing to better patient care and quality of life (Colavita et al., 2020). Additionally, studies on the relationship between development, growth, and the environment are crucial for a better understanding of pulmonary disease. Maternal health, exposure to harmful substances, and diet have been found to affect the development of the respiratory system. Evidence supports that early exposure to toxic chemicals can yield irreversible outcomes on lung anatomy and function, rendering a person susceptible to diseases like asthma and Chronic Obstructive Pulmonary Disease (COPD) later in life. Studies focusing on these themes emphasize the importance of a healthy pregnancy and early childhood years, as well as the potential for prevention in early life to mitigate the long-term health impacts of respiratory disease. By carefully examining these variables, better public health education programs and policies can be designed to promote respiratory well-being (Cryan et al., 2019).

Finally, the study of development and growth of the respiratory tract can lead to the production of innovations in the practice of medicine. As researchers begin to explore the developmental biology of respiratory organs, novel stem cell-based therapies, regenerative medicine modalities, and innovative surgical procedures can be developed. For example, understanding the mechanisms that regulate lung maturity can lead to improved methods for treating premature infants with underdeveloped lungs.

Furthermore, the application of precision medicine, such as tailoring treatments to individual patterns of growth, is becoming increasingly advanced as our understanding of growth and anatomical change improves. In this case, enhanced knowledge of respiratory development not only informs clinical practice but also stimulates innovation in biomedical research, underscoring the necessity for continuous research in this field (Colavita et al., 2020).

2.1. Embryonic Development of the Respiratory Tract

Learning Outcome

1. Formation of the respiratory diverticulum
2. Development of the trachea and bronchi
3. Role of genetic factors in respiratory development

Embryonic development of the respiratory tract is a complex process that starts early during gestation, an essential time in the overall growth and morphology of the respiratory tract. It typically begins in the fourth week of gestation, when the respiratory diverticulum emerges from the ventral wall of the foregut, a crucial event in the transition from foregut to respiratory structures. This diverticulum undergoes series of branching processes, giving rise to the trachea and primary bronchi, which serve as templates for organizing the overall plan of the respiratory system. The growth and differentiation of various cell types at this stage form the basis for air conduction and the complex alveolar structures involved in gas exchange. Understanding these early stages is crucial because any disruption here will lead to congenital anomalies that will cause serious respiratory issues after birth. With the advancement in development, lung branching morphogenesis further demonstrates the complexity of respiratory tract development. By week seven, the terminal bronchial branches bifurcate into secondary bronchi, which correlates with the development of lung lobes. It is during this stage that mesenchymal interactions play a crucial role in guiding epithelial fate and the progression of lung maturation. Cellular signaling mechanisms, including those mediated by fibroblast growth factor and vascular endothelial growth factor, play a crucial role in this process, guiding cell proliferation and differentiation within the developing lung tissue. Refining these structures is crucial for maintaining a functional respiratory capacity at birth, highlighting the importance of both environmental and genetic influences on fetal growth.

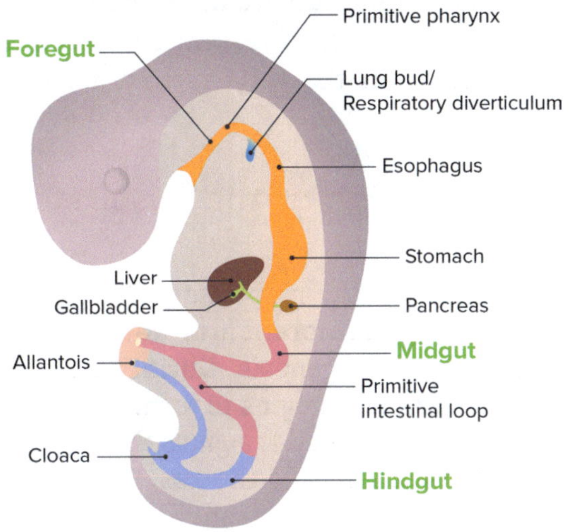

Figure 2.3. Embryonic development of the respiratory tract.

Source: https://cdn.lecturio.com/assets/Embryonic-development-of-the-gut-tube_NEW.png

Additionally, the interaction between cellular signaling and extracellular matrix components lays the foundation for subsequent lung performance and resilience to respiratory illnesses. Importantly, understanding the embryonic development of the respiratory tract also forms the foundation for later therapeutic approaches and the prevention of respiratory diseases. Developments in molecular cartography, as presented in Mén et al., (2015), also enlighten us about tissue-specific proteomes which play a role in lung development and may have implications of targeted therapy for congenital respiratory disease. Observations from such studies can help determine how specific proteins interact during critical developmental phases, ultimately affecting lung morphology and function. Furthermore, research on the influences on embryonic growth, such as maternal condition and environmental exposure, underscores the complexity of respiratory system development. These studies can uncover possible early interventions for individuals at risk so that the first components of respiratory health are safeguarded from the very earliest formative phases.

2.1.1. Formation of the Respiratory Diverticulum

The formation of the respiratory diverticulum is a critical developmental landmark in respiratory embryogenesis. During the fourth week of gestation, it begins to form as a ventral outpouch of the foregut. It signals the beginning of the differentiation of the respiratory tract from that of the gastrointestinal tract. As this diverticulum elongates, it gives rise to the trachea and the primary bronchi, which are essential in forming the pulmonary airways. The critical nature of the developmental process underscores the importance of proper regulatory pathways, specifically signaling and gene expression patterns, that direct the growth and branching morphogenesis of the respiratory system. Identifying this developmental pathway provides insight into congenital anomalies that may develop from disturbances in the process and require intensive inquiry into the underlying mechanisms. During its maturation, the respiratory diverticulum is exposed to a cascade of morphological changes permitting the development of the respiratory tract's architecture. The initial phases of differentiation involve the formation of differentiated epithelial cell types, i.e., ciliated and secretory cells, which are the basis for the functional characteristics of the adult respiratory epithelium. At this point, interaction between epithelial and mesenchymal tissue assumes significance as mesenchymal signals are implicated in the control of proliferation and differentiation of epithelial cells. The branching morphogenesis, occurring coincidentally with the extension of the diverticula, is a necessity for the development of the complex tree-like morphology that characterizes lungs. Such elaborate processes indicate the dynamic interplay between growth and development in the formation of respiratory tract morphology and highlight how alterations may lead to teratogenic developmental disorders, additionally demanding extensive research in this area. The later development of the diversifying respiratory diverticulum is characterized by lung bud differentiation and the initial formation of alveoli. As further growth of the terminal bronchi of the bronchial tree proceeds, the alveolar epithelium emerges as a development from a simple cuboidal to a more specialized one constituted by type I and type II alveolar cells.

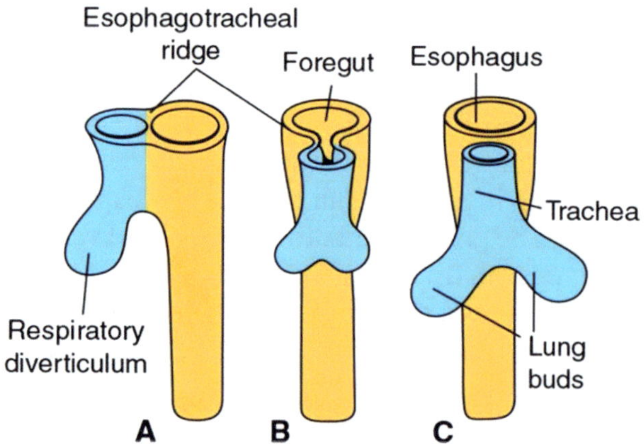

Figure 2.6. Formation of the respiratory diverticulum.

Source: https://encrypted-tbn0.gstatic.com/images?q=tbn:ANd9GcRFybnuj0FqU1oIcHNPXEtslZ1Mj9KQrap1DA&s

This development is crucial in pulmonary function because alveolar cells carry out gas exchange and produce surfactants. Proper development of the respiratory diverticulum not only matters for developing a working lung anatomy but also for correctly placing the lungs so they can meet the respiratory demands of the developing organism. Disruptions during this advanced maturation period can lead to respiratory distress syndromes, highlighting the importance of understanding the development and morphology of the respiratory tract in both health and disease (Adler et al., 2014; Hickling et al., 2015).

2.1.2. Development of the Trachea and Bronchi

Development of the trachea and bronchi is a critical component of tracing the process and morphology of the respiratory tree. Originating from the embryonic foregut, the tracheobronchial tree undergoes a series of distinctive morphological changes during early fetal development, typically beginning between the fourth week of gestation. The development is controlled by intricate signal pathways that dictate the differentiation of progenitor cells into the trachea and bronchi. It begins with the formation of the tracheal diverticulum, which subsequently divides to form the right and left main bronchi. Reciprocal proper formation of these structures is important as any disruption could lead to congenital defects such as tracheoesophageal fistula or bronchial agenesis, both of which have significant clinical implications as they compromise airway patency and lung function.

As the trachea and bronchi develop, they acquire specific histological features that are of crucial significance for respiratory function. The lining epithelium in the airways is differentiated into specific cell types like ciliated cells, goblet cells, and basal cells which all contribute to respiratory maintenance and health. Among these, the ciliated cells are vital as they possess motile cilia, which remove mucus and debris from the airway. Mucociliary clearance is paramount in maintaining a sterile lung condition, thereby preventing infections and other lung diseases. The function of ciliated cells in airway functioning highlights the importance of understanding their developmental processes and the significance of structural defects in disorders such as primary ciliary dyskinesia, as these defects can hinder the critical clearance process (Tilley et al., 2014).

The postnatal environment also influences the maturation of the trachea and bronchi, with several factors affecting development, including air exposure and respiratory pathogens. With the growth of the individual from fetal to neonatal respiration, the architecture of the bronchi and trachea adapts to the higher demands of respiration outside the uterus. Maturation can be influenced by mechanisms such as mechanical stretching during breathing and environmental stimuli, which enhance the remodeling and repair of the epithelium. The exploration of the tracheobronchial epithelium's cellular and molecular mechanisms of adaptation reveals the dynamic nature of the tracheobronchial epithelium throughout postnatal life, as well as its sensitivity to external stimuli. Understanding such balanced growth and adaptation of the bronchi and trachea to such stimuli may hold a clue to respiratory developmental disorders and future treatment (Bustamante-Marin et al., 2016).

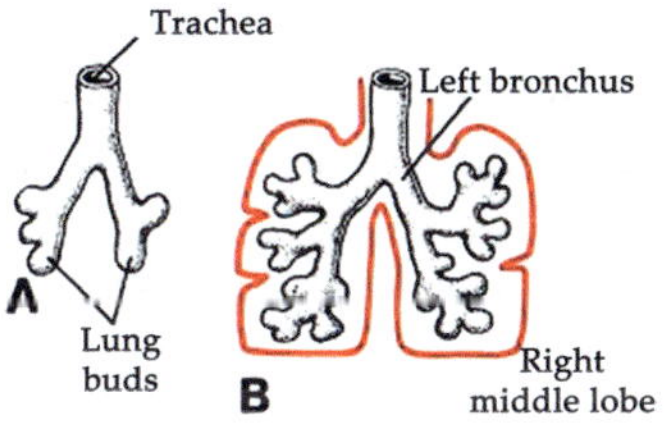

Figure 2.7. Development of the trachea and bronchi.

Source: https://encrypted-tbn0.gstatic.com/images?q=tbn:ANd9GcQCGAH5taeg5JmEieCtjz8gvdaU5t06o9hOJw&s

2.1.3. Role of Genetic Factors in Respiratory Development

Genetic factors play a central role in the respiratory development of the human individual, establishing the structural and functional characteristics of the respiratory tract throughout embryonic development and into adulthood. Genetic variation is a key factor in the morphogenesis of the lung, influencing major processes such as branching morphogenesis, epithelial cell differentiation, and pulmonary vasculature development. Critical. Genes such as fibroblast growth factors and homeobox genes control the development of airways and alveoli. Deviations from these gene pathways can cause numerous respiratory pathologies, which suggests the crucial role of preserving genetic integrity in ensuring respiratory homeostasis. Understanding these genetic factors not only enriches our insight into normal respiratory development but also facilitates the identification of potential genetic susceptibility to respiratory disease, which is equally applicable in considering insight into complex traits and diseases such as asthma and chronic obstructive pulmonary disease. The interaction between environmental factors and genetic predisposition further contributes to the complexity of the dynamics that affect respiratory development. For instance, genetic susceptibility to certain airborne pollutants may increase the risk of getting chronic respiratory disease. Indeed, exposure to microplastics and other contaminants may interfere with the normal growth of lungs, with possible long-term health consequences. Studies have shown that microplastics can be detected in the human body, including in human placentas, indicating the impact of environmental exposures on prenatal respiratory health (Ragusa et al., 2020). Therefore, genetic factors do not work in isolation, but there is an interaction between them and environmental factors to influence respiratory outcomes. Such synergy highlights the need for an integrative research strategy in respiratory health research, considering both genetic and environmental factors in disease susceptibility. In addition, the genetic organization of the respiratory system has far-reaching implications in the description of disease processes, as illustrated by the instance of viral infections of the respiratory system, such as COVID-19. Studies have shown that certain genetic backgrounds may lead to variable levels of susceptibility to respiratory infections, such as those caused by SARS-CoV-2. The presence of genetic variability in the angiotensin-converting enzyme 2 (ACE2), a viral receptor, indicates the contribution of genetic susceptibility to disease severity and susceptibility (Guo et al., 2020). This interaction of genetic factors and lung development highlights the complexity of respiratory disease, where both acquired and inherited genetics intersect. Thus, investigation of the genetic mechanisms of lung development is essential in the formulation of our knowledge of developmental biology and respiratory disease pathogenesis, and in making specific therapeutic measures possible.

Test Your Knowledge

1. What is the development of the trachea and bronchi?
2. What are the role of genetic factors in respiratory development?

2.2. Morphological Features of the Respiratory Tract

Learning Outcome

1. Structure of the upper respiratory tract
2. Anatomy of the lower respiratory tract
3. Histological differences across respiratory regions

The respiratory tract has a highly intricate architecture that changes considerably during development and, in turn, affects both function and efficiency. The initial separation of the tract into the upper and lower tracts has different physiological functions. The upper respiratory tract, the nasal cavity, and the pharynx are lined with a specialized epithelium that consists of ciliated as well as mucus-secreting cells.

This unique morphology enables the trapping of particulates and pathogens, protecting the lower respiratory tract. As development proceeds, changes in airway dimensions and cellular content occur, reflecting the increasing respiratory demands. The lower respiratory system, comprising the trachea, bronchi, and alveoli, features a distinct morphological configuration characterized by smooth muscle layers and an increasing number of alveolar sacs for efficient gas exchange.

These findings underscore the importance of respiratory functional changes in morphology throughout growth and development. Further examination confirms that the microscopic structure of the respiratory tract is paramount to its immunological responses. The presence of specialized cells within the respiratory epithelium forms the basis for sensing and responding to environmental insults, including allergens and pathogens. Interestingly, the respiratory system is also supplied with an extensive vascular bed and infiltrating immune cells, allowing for a rapid response to inhalants. The characteristic histological axis enables the mucociliary clearance mechanism to operate, where mucus captures inhaled particles and pathogens, and cilia move them towards the oropharynx for expulsion. And, as studies demonstrate, alterations in the structure of these tissues can have a profound impact on respiratory health and disease susceptibility. Disruptions of homeostasis in the respiratory tracts due to environmental stressors, as suggested by recent research, can lead to pathological conditions that highlight the interconnection between the morphology and function of the respiratory apparatus (Ragusa et al., 2020).

Furthermore, the understanding of the developmental morphology of the respiratory tracts extends to more universal physiological conditions, such as those involving the microbiota. New evidence has put the microbiota-gut-brain axis in the forefront in the control of homeostasis, and its implications extend to respiratory health. The content of the gut microbiota is shown to influence and modulate respiratory system immune responses, exhibiting a multifaceted interplay of relations surpassing reductionist anatomical issues (Cryan et al., 2019).

The interconnection between the respiratory tract's morphology and the microbiome underscores the importance of a comprehensive understanding of respiratory health, particularly in relation to growth and development. Understanding these interactions can inform therapy in respiratory disease and promote general well-being throughout life by highlighting the contribution of morphological features in regulating these complex biological processes.

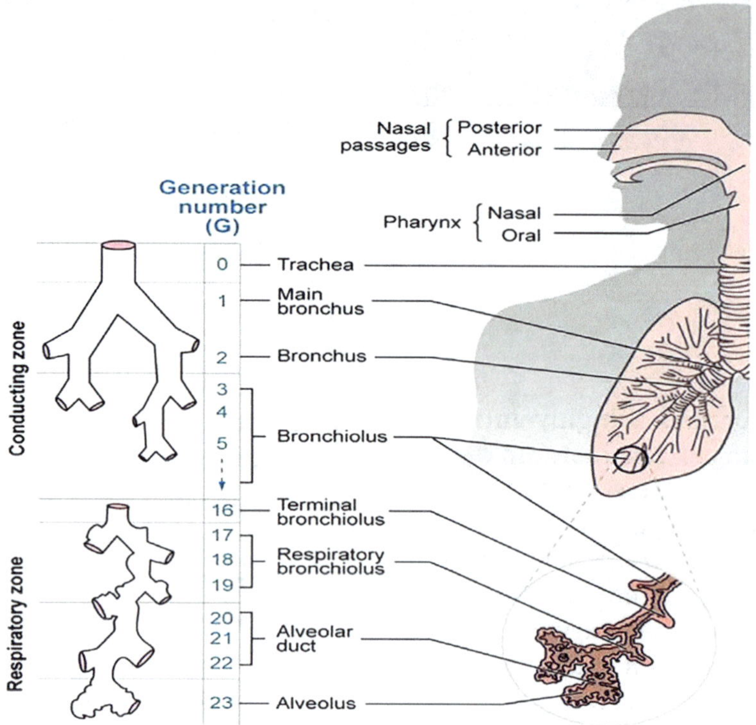

Figure 2.8. Morphological overview of the human respiratory tract.

Source: https://external-content.duckduckgo.com/iu/?u=https%3A%2F%2Fwww.researchgate.net%2Fpublication%2F367099248%2Ffigure%2Ffig1%2FAS%3A11431281113926002%401674145652502%2FMorphological-overview-of-the-human-respiratory-tract-14_Q320.jpg&f=1&nofb=1&ipt=8836ed27ffe228a1c3814fadd6868a1db15a1cc9432deac02218d2653529b7a9

2.2.1. Structure of the Upper Respiratory Tract

The upper respiratory tract is the first pathway for air to penetrate the body and is responsible for numerous physiological functions. In terms of structure, it consists of the nasal cavity, paranasal sinuses, pharynx, and larynx, each of which functions uniquely in respiratory function. The nasal cavity, lined with ciliated epithelial cells and mucus-secreting glands, enables the filtration, humidification, and warming of the air. This structure not only protects the lower respiratory tract from external contaminants and pathogens but also facilitates olfaction, illustrating the multifunctional nature of this tract. The intricate structure of the upper respiratory tract highlights its role in maintaining respiratory health and optimizing the efficiency of gas exchange throughout the entire respiratory system. In order, the pharynx, which connects the nasal cavity to the larynx and esophagus, is also divided into nasopharynx, oropharynx, and laryngopharynx. There is space for each segment to hold different functions, like airway passage, and as a drainage area for the sinuses and Eustachian tubes. The oropharynx and laryngopharynx also play an important role in supporting both respiration and digestion, a complexity that highlights the evolutionary adaptation of the human respiratory tract. The anatomy of the larynx that houses the vocal cords is not only critical for sound production but also for protecting the trachea from food aspiration. Such interplay between structure and function is critical in the upper respiratory tract contribution to overall respiratory health and function. Furthermore, upper respiratory tract diseases can have a significant impact on growth and development, particularly in children. Structural anomalies, such as adenoid hypertrophy (AH), may be responsible for obstructing the airway and manifesting as impairments in craniofacial development and respiratory function (Li et al., 2022). These obstructions tend to cause chronic mouth breathing, which can alter facial morphology and adversely affect growth patterns. Indeed, children with chronic obstruction may present with nasal airway resistance, reduced nasopharyngeal volume, and even impaired sleep quality due to flow limitation (Li et al., 2022). Thus, understanding the normal anatomy of the upper respiratory tract and what goes wrong if it is not normal is of paramount importance in curing not only the immediate health conditions but also long-term developmental impacts on the individuals.

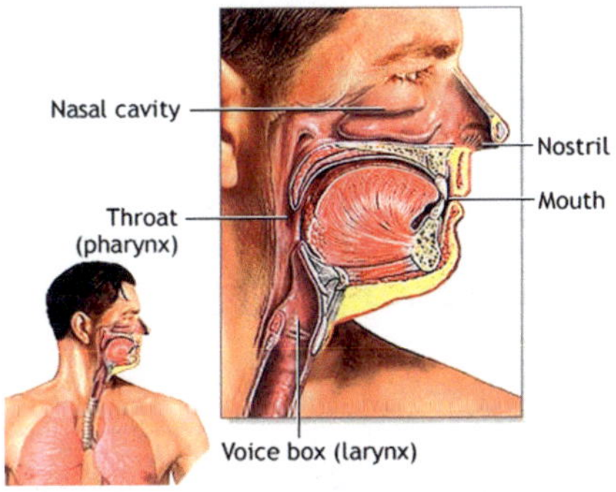

Figure 2.9. Upper respiratory tract.

Source: https://medlineplus.gov/ency/images/ency/fullsize/19378.jpg

2.2.2. Anatomy of the Lower Respiratory Tract

Lower respiratory tract anatomy is crucial to understanding its role in the growth, development, and morphology of the respiratory system. The trachea, bronchi, bronchioles, and alveoli comprise this part of the respiratory system, which facilitates airway conduction and gas exchange. The trachea, cushioned by C-shaped cartilaginous rings, bifurcates into the main bronchi, each of which passes into the corresponding lung. The structure of these airways is evolutionarily suited to permit the streamlined flow of air while protecting against pathogens and irritants. Notably, the branching bronchi and bronchiole network greatly increases the surface area to be utilized to effect gas exchange, allowing for maximal oxygenation and carbon dioxide removal as respiratory demands change, particularly with exercise or disease conditions like COVID-19 that significantly involve the respiratory system (Baumgartner et al., 2020). As development progresses from embryonic to adult life, the lower respiratory tract undergoes significant morphological development, thereby maximizing its function. Indeed, during the pseudoglandular stage, the respiratory system is essentially a simple airway. As pregnancy advances through canalicular and saccular development, alveolar structures begin to form and the epithelial lining becomes specialized. This intricate interplay between cell and tissue maturation is augmented by the expansion of capillary networks, which form the boundary between the blood and the alveolar airspace. This type I/type II alveolar cell differentiation is critical; type II cells synthesize surfactant, thus lowering surface tension and making respiratory efficiency possible. Such developmental milestones play a critical role in preparing the lungs for gas exchange at birth and are adversely affected by pregnancy conditions, leading to chronic respiratory complications (Baumgartner et al., 2020).

Moreover, the anatomical nuances of the lower respiratory passages play a key part in rendering it susceptible to infectious conditions, like viral infections, including SARS-CoV-2. The availability of specific receptors, namely angiotensin-converting enzyme 2 (ACE2), on lung epithelial cells enables the virus to enter and subsequently disrupt cells. This is what contributes to the respiratory distress and pneumonia clinical presentations, thereby highlighting the significance of understanding the anatomy and physiology of tracts in clinical practice. The complexity of the lower airway shows not only how we breathe but also how inherent structural features dictate respiratory disease and health. As more research is conducted, the emphasis on the development and morphology of such structures will become increasingly essential for designing preventive and therapeutic measures aimed at respiratory disease (Guo et al., 2020).

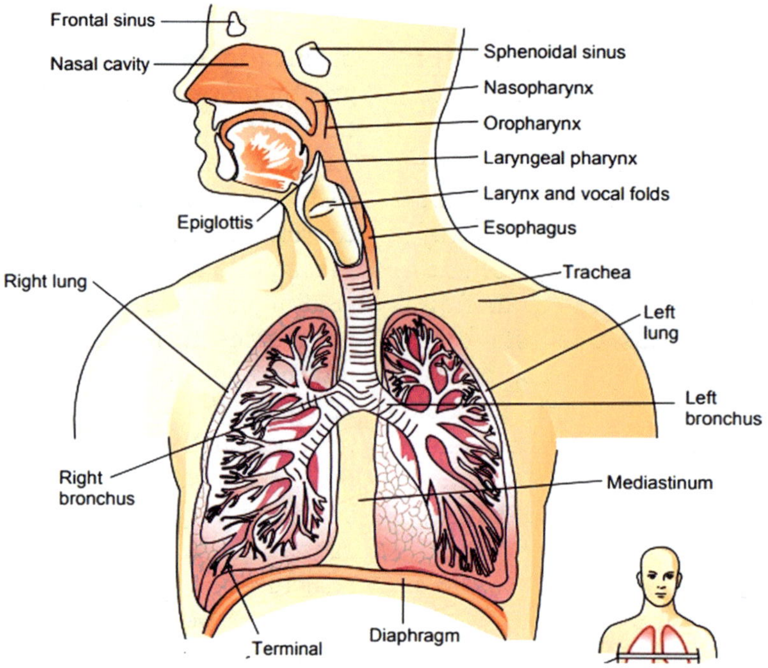

Figure 2.10. Anatomy of the lower respiratory tract.

Source: https://img.brainkart.com/article/article-Anatomy-of-the-Lower-nBb.jpg

2.2.3. Histological Differences Across Respiratory Regions

The respiratory tract is composed of various regions, each with characteristic histological features that are essential for its specific functions. The nasal cavity is the first defense mechanism against airborne particles and pathogens, wherein the epithelium is typically composed of ciliated pseudostratified columnar cells dispersed with goblet cells. These goblet cells also produce mucus, which traps particles and provides a moist environment required for effective gas exchange. The presence of olfactory epithelium in certain areas continues to underscore the sensory function of the nasal cavity, illustrating histological adaptation that supports both respiratory and sensory functions. Understanding these histological characteristics is the foundation for recognizing pathological conditions that may arise in this context (Habib et al., 2015). Moving further down the respiratory tract, the histological morphology of the trachea and bronchi differs markedly from that of the nasal passage. Here, the epithelium gives way to a more advanced type, maintaining its ciliated pseudostratified columnar tissue while supplementing it with smooth muscle and cartilage to support airflow and maintain structural integrity. The submucosal glands also occur here, secreting mucus to trap additional particles caught by inhalation. The architecture of this region is essential to adequate mucociliary clearance, a key defense against infection in the lungs. Histological analysis of the tracheobronchial tree reveals that these adaptations are critical in environments with high exposure to particulate matter, thereby impacting respiratory health and susceptibility to disease (Priori et al., 2015).

Further down in the respiratory system, the alveolar regions exhibit a striking contrast in histological arrangement compared to the previous segments. The alveolar sac is lined by simple squamous epithelium, which facilitates the efficient exchange of gases between alveoli and pulmonary capillaries. Type II alveolar cells, which produce surfactants, are crucial in reducing surface tension and preventing the collapse of alveoli during the respiratory cycle. Such a minimalist structure mimics the functional demands of the alveoli, which primarily exist to ensure the efficiency of gas exchange rather than pathogen filtration or particle trapping. The specific histological adaptations of the different respiratory regions reflect pressures on the respiratory apparatus through evolution, highlighting the need for specialized morphology to serve various functional needs along the tract (Habib et al., 2015).

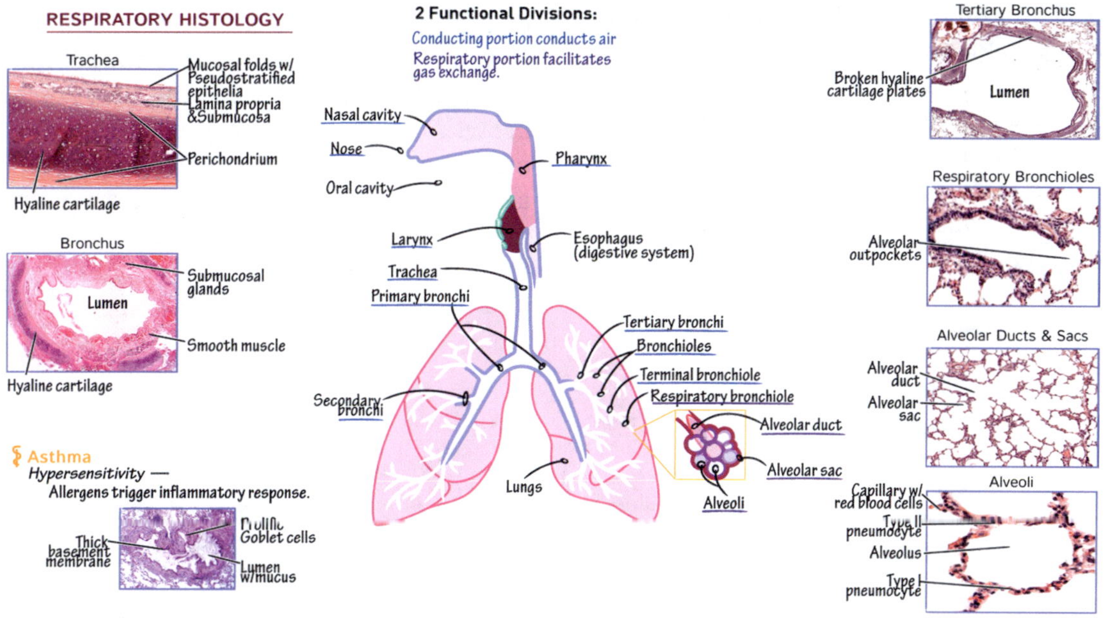

Figure 2.11. Histological differences across respiratory regions.

Source: https://d1j63owfs0b5j3.cloudfront.net/tutorial/finalImage/1385-1480370270586.png

Test Your Knowledge

1. Illustrate the Structure of the upper respiratory tract
2. What are the histological differences across respiratory regions?

2.3. Growth Patterns of the Respiratory Tract

Learning Outcome

1. Changes during fetal development
2. Postnatal growth and maturation
3. Factors influencing respiratory growth

Respiratory tract development is a process that involves multiple steps and is influenced by genetic, environmental, and physiologic factors. The respiratory system undergoes qualitative alterations during embryogenesis with the initiation of lung bud formation from the foregut. The buds grow and differentiate into conducting airways and alveoli. Noteworthy is that the branching morphogenesis of the respiratory epithelium is controlled by numerous signaling molecules, including fibroblast growth factors and vascular endothelial growth factor, which affect the growth and development of the airway walls. Moreover, external stimuli from maternal smoking or pollutants can exert a negative impact on the proper direction of growth, potentially leading to chronic respiratory diseases in the future. An evident understanding of these patterns of growth is thus crucial for early intervention in strategies to improve respiratory health among children and adults. From embryonic development, postnatal growth patterns in the respiratory system have some uncharacteristic features. Infancy is a period of rapid growth, during which the alveolar zone increases in size and the airways remodel. According to recent studies, development in the early years is crucial in shaping lung function and capacity, with the first years of life being a period of maximum exposure to environmental insults. The ongoing structural development of alveolar surfaces and airway epithelium in childhood and adolescence is concomitant with changes in metabolic demands and exercise. The growth of the respiratory tract is reflected not only in the expansion of the lungs' volume but also in the adaptation of conducting airways to meet the greater airflow needs.

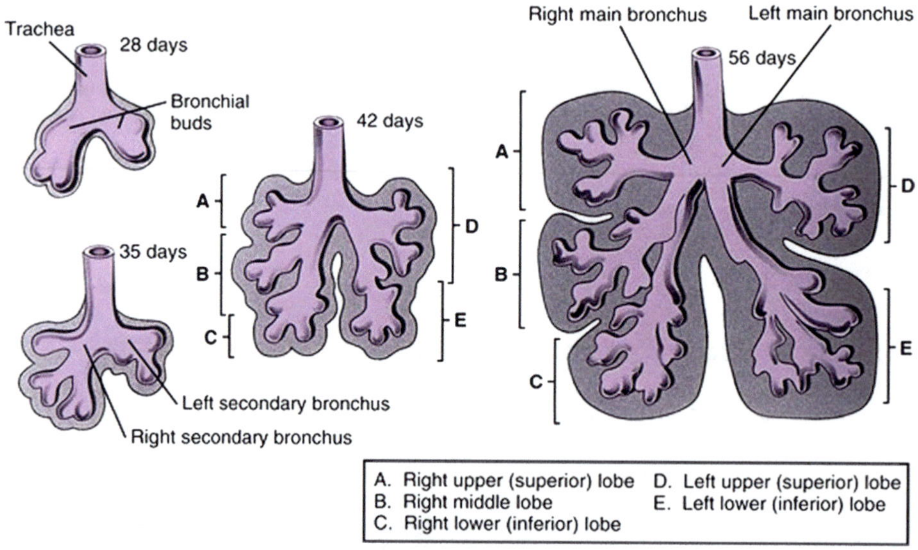

Figure 2.12. Growth patterns of the respiratory tract.

Source: https://radiologykey.com/wp-content/uploads/2015/12/B9780323081764000483_f048-002-9780323081764.jpg

These developmental landmarks are crucial to recognize in understanding periods of susceptibility to respiratory disease, thereby informing clinical practice and population health interventions targeting lung health. The interaction between genetic predispositions and the environment keeps affecting the growth patterns of the respiratory tract throughout life. It is interesting that the pathogenesis of respiratory diseases, such as asthma or COPD, may often be attributed to initial development periods during which abnormal growth patterns may have developed. For instance, the adverse effects of particulate matter or allergens during sensitive developmental periods can lead to chronic alterations in respiratory function. Furthermore, recent research emphasizes the role of pregnant mothers' health, including exposure to infectious agents, potentially exerting long-lasting effects on the lung development of the offspring. Knowledge of the interaction between these factors not only helps in the depiction of growth trends but also emphasizes the necessity of specific interventions to prevent risks related to adverse respiratory health outcomes, highlighting continued challenges in the prevention and management of respiratory disease throughout the life cycle (Jeevanandam et al., 2018; Guo et al., 2020).

2.3.1. Changes During Fetal Development

Embryonic development is a complex and intricate process that includes sequential formation of various organ systems, chief among them the respiratory tract. To begin with, during the embryonic phase, respiratory tract development starts with the formation of laryngeal and tracheobronchial structures. As development of the embryo progresses, a series of branching morphogenesis processes occurs that leads to the formation of the bronchial tree. This is an extremely sensitive phase to external influences, such as environmental toxins that can disrupt the normal growth of respiratory tissues. The effects of toxicants exposed at this time are profound, and they may result in malformations or functional deficits in the respiratory system in adulthood, showing the intricate relationship between developmental biology and the environment, as discussed when reference is given to heavy metals and pesticides in Alengebawy et al. (2021). As fetal growth proceeds into the second trimester, the respiratory system becomes increasingly specialized and mature. Now, the primary airways have been established by the lungs and intricate alveolar structures are starting to develop. Respiratory epithelium differentiation is a key component of this process, which involves specific cellular responses to intrinsic developmental cues as well as extrinsic environmental stimuli. Notably, environmental exposures to toxicants such as lead, which are stored in the ecological environment due to their chemical and physical characteristics, are of special interest to normal respiratory development and function, as seen in Wani et al., (2015). The complexity of these developmental stages also underscores the need to continue researching the ways in which early-life exposures reorganize respiratory structure and function to achieve long-term health consequences. The final stages of fetal lung development in the late third trimester are crucial in preparing the fetus for independent breathing at birth. During this period, type II alveolar cells mature and produce surfactant, a critical substance that reduces surface tension in the lungs, enabling effective gas exchange at birth. However, conditions such as preterm birth can cease this vital developmental milestone and result in conditions such as neonatal respiratory distress syndrome. Preterm birth could furthermore increase the vulnerability of the infant to disease in later years due to the impact of foreign toxins, as the study of environmental toxicants in Alengebawy et al. (2021) identifies. It is essential to acknowledge these changes in the fetus both for the purpose of giving improved neonatal care and to design interventions to counteract the effects of environmental hazards on respiratory function to usher in healthier generations.

2.3.2. Postnatal Growth and Maturation

Postnatal life is a period of crucial growth and maturation of the respiratory system, characterized by significant anatomical and functional changes. Shortly after birth, the lungs undergo a sequence of changes that prepare them for the imperative role of gas exchange. Beginning with lung tissue inflation, the alveoli increase in number and surface area, thereby enabling the maximal absorption of oxygen and removal of carbon dioxide. It is a time when the airway epithelium matures from a developmentally primitive state to a mature, complex structure. This postnatal growth is controlled by the intricate interplay of environmental and genetic influences, emphasizing the significance of understanding respiratory health outcomes within the framework of early life development. Hence, it is necessary to investigate the multiple factors involved in this rapid process of maturation, as they significantly impact respiratory health throughout a person's entire lifespan. Since the respiratory tract continues to develop postnatally, the coordination of the diverse microbial communities is the most crucial element in the establishment and maintenance of lung homeostasis. Recent research highlights the importance of specific microorganisms that colonize lower airways, which are capable of having a direct impact on lung development and functioning. For instance, studies have revealed the existence of specific protective bacteria, such as Paenibacillus odorifer, that are associated with protection against lung carcinogenesis through the generation of metabolites, including acetic acid. All such microbiological interactions underscore the importance of understanding the role of respiratory microbiomes during periods of growth.

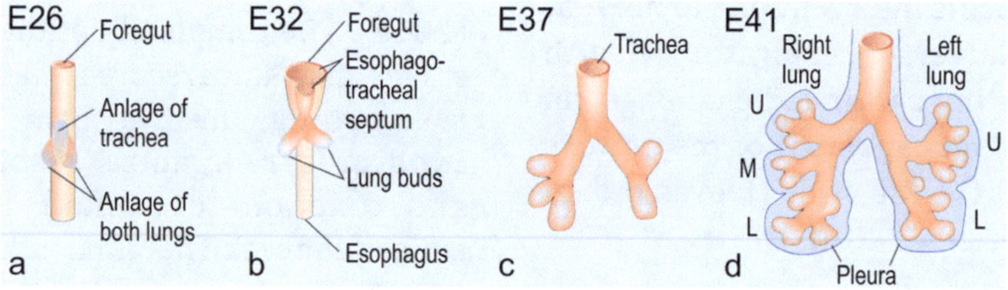

Figure 2.13. Postnatal growth and maturation of the respiratory tract.

Source: https://static.cambridge.org/binary/version/id/urn:cambridge.org:id:binary:20170202072500913-0032:9781139680349:07209fig7_2.png?pub-status=live

The interaction of the respiratory microbiome with the maturation of the lungs thus highlights how alterations in microbial balance could potentially lead to adverse health outcomes. On this basis, further studies of such processes in postnatal life have the potential to enhance lung health and prevent respiratory disease in adulthood. In investigating postnatal respiratory system morphology, the necessity of understanding growth patterns becomes clear in order to recognize developmental abnormalities. The study using animal models, including the mouse model, gives important information concerning normal respiratory development, from which researchers can distinguish between regular anatomical features and those modified by disease. A comprehensive understanding of the respiratory tract's developmental timeline is necessary for accurate evaluation of respiratory health. This stance is supported by methods that yield high-resolution visual accounts of respiratory anatomy at stages of development. These tools are gold-standard resources for investigators because they confirm chronological age and morphological integrity in research on development. Emphasizing the necessity of thorough studies on postnatal development and morphology is critical because it ultimately decides on clinical ways of diagnosing and treating respiratory diseases among human beings (Chen et al., 2024; Parslow et al., 2024).

2.3.3. Factors Influencing Respiratory Growth

The intricate development of the air passage is significantly influenced by genetic, environmental, and physiological forces that act in combination during development. During embryogenesis, specific genes guide the airway epithelial branching morphogenesis, resulting in a competent and complex respiratory organ. Gene signals are of utmost significance in shaping the anatomy of the lung, influencing the configuration of airways and alveoli. Environmental considerations, such as maternal health and exposure to toxins, also introduce complexity to this pattern of development. Specifically, maternal smoking or exposure to contaminants has adverse effects on fetal lung development with resultant long-term respiratory implications.

These interactions serve to demonstrate the subtle interplay between environmental stimuli and hereditary determinants in the patterning of respiratory growth during critical intervals of opportunity. Compounding the complexity of respiratory growth are postnatal factors, such as nutrition and exposure to disease agents. Imbalance in diet during early childhood years can have far-reaching effects on lung development and lung function. For instance, the loss of essential vitamins and minerals can impair respiratory tract integrity, making the respiratory system more susceptible to infection. Additionally, the postnatal presentation of environmental stimuli, such as infectious agents or allergens, can modify airway responsiveness and exacerbate respiratory disorders like asthma. The reciprocal interaction between immune system development and respiratory tract anatomy is of interest, since acute infection may induce alterations in airway architecture that can perpetuate chronic respiratory conditions. This presentation of risk factors highlights the multifaceted nature of respiratory development and the various ways in which health during infancy and early childhood can impact long-term respiratory outcomes. Current research emphasizes the role of modern-day environmental adversity, specifically exposure to microplastics and infection, in respiratory growth.

Microplastics, which have polluted ecosystems and food chains, are being introduced as a probable respiratory health risk factor. There is evidence that microplastics can permeate human tissues, and their exposure at critical stages of development may trigger inflammatory responses in the respiratory system (Ragusa et al., 2020). Moreover, the emergence of respiratory viruses, particularly SARS-CoV-2, has prompted an investigation into how viral infections affect lung development and function (Guo et al., 2020). The ability of such pathogens to cause robust immune responses can impact lung morphology and growth patterns over the long term, especially in susceptible groups. Ultimately, insight into the interaction of environmental exposures, viral impacts, and nutrition is crucial for promoting optimal respiratory development and addressing existing health disparities in populations.

Test Your Knowledge

1. What are the changes during fetal development?
2. What is postnatal growth and maturation?

2.4. Functional Development of the Respiratory System

Learning Outcome

1. Transition from fetal to neonatal respiration
2. Development of gas exchange capabilities
3. Impact of environmental factors on functional growth

The functional development of the respiratory system is a complex process that progresses through several stages, with a key breakthrough driven by both environmental and genetic factors. During embryonic development, the respiratory system originates from the foregut and matures into the trachea and bronchial airways, which branch out. This early differentiation is critical as it establishes the architecture for gas exchange in life after birth. With the development of the fetus, development of alveoli and pulmonary vasculature is necessary, allowing eventual transition to placental to pulmonary respiration. Not only are anatomical changes a mark of this transition, but also significant physiological adjustments, such as the production of surfactant, which lowers alveolar surface tension. The presence and function of such structures are essential for successful gas exchange in the neonate, underscoring the intricate relationship between morphology and function in the development of the respiratory system. Postnatal respiratory system maturation involves enhancement of its structures to enable increased lung capacity and efficiency. In early infancy, alveolar surface area rises exponentially, allowing for more oxygenation and the removal of carbon dioxide. This continues through early childhood, with respiratory rate, lung volumes, and the respiratory system overall remodeling to support the metabolic demands of a growing body. Additionally, several external factors, including environmental toxins and pathogens, can influence respiratory development during this period of heightened susceptibility. There is evidence to suggest that exposure to adverse environmental conditions may delay functional development, potentially leading to respiratory issues throughout life. Therefore, understanding such mechanisms is crucial for facilitating respiratory health during infancy and preventing risks associated with compromised development, thereby highlighting the role of environmental and genetic interactions at this stage of development. Interaction between the respiratory tract and microbiome also requires attention for such functional development. Recent research has suggested that the gut microbiota can influence lung function and development through the microbiota-gut-brain axis, with microbial metabolites affecting physiological responses in various organ systems. As the microbiome develops during early life, it influences the immune system, possibly determining inflammatory reactions of the respiratory tract. This conversation takes on special significance because it points to the role of healthy microbiota in asthma and other respiratory conditions. The impact of these associations is not yet fully understood, with a need for further research on targeted interventions that could potentially leverage the benefits of a healthy microbiota for improved respiratory outcomes. These observations not only increase our understanding of respiratory function but also reveal potential avenues for therapeutic intervention towards optimizing respiratory health across the life course.

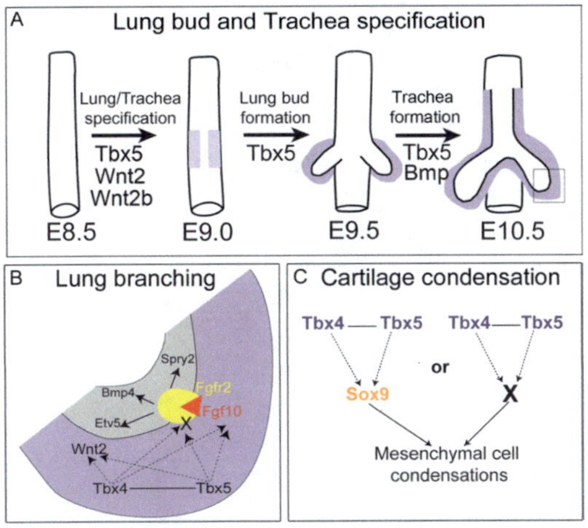

Figure 2.14. Functional development of the respiratory system.

Source: https://embryology.med.unsw.edu.au/embryology/images/thumb/7/77/Mouse_respiratory_Tbx4_and_Tbx5.jpg/400px-Mouse_respiratory_Tbx4_and_Tbx5.jpg

2.4.1. Transition From Fetal To Neonatal Respiration

The transition from fetal to neonatal respiration is a period of great importance in which an infant's respiratory system undergoes a radical transformation in its physiological function. In fetal life, the fetus depends on placental perfusion and maternal respiration for gas exchange, which occurs within the placenta and not through the lungs. The highly vascularized fetal lung environment primarily serves as a conduit for respiratory structure development and maturation, rather than for gas exchange. This unique adaptation allows the fetus to exist in comparatively hypoxic environments, as opposed to the requirement for direct air in the postnatal condition. By birth time, the baby is then forced to adapt rapidly to life outside the uterus, with independent breathing being a prerequisite for survival. This transition involves significant anatomical and physiological remodeling, essentially transforming the body's manner of obtaining oxygen and expelling carbon dioxide, which sets the stage for neonatal life. During the initiation of breathing, several structural adjustments of the respiratory tract are initiated. The lungs become aerated for the first time, triggering different biochemical reactions that enable the immediate oxygenation of the blood. The transformation also results in the closure of fetal shunts, including the ductus arteriosus and the foramen ovale, which minimizes shunting across the lungs. The adaptation enhances the effectiveness of gas exchange and accommodates the newborns' metabolic needs. Second, the formation of functional residual capacity means that the lungs are set for adequate ventilation. With inhalation through the newborn, pulmonary surfactant, which is secreted within the alveoli, reduces surface tension, preventing alveolar collapse and promoting lung compliance. As a result, these anatomical and physiological adaptations create an environment conducive to effective neonatal breathing, enhancing robust oxygenation and carbon dioxide removal, which are crucial to survival through the initial several seconds after birth. The immune role of the lung also becomes more prominent at this transition. Since it is now the primary organ of gas exchange and is brought directly into contact with the outside world, the structure of the lungs is most important to its numerous functions, one of which is protection against pathogens. The presence of both innate and adaptive immune cells makes this immune response possible, one that is made possible by the lungs' exposure to air-borne pathogens and foreign particles. The transition to neonatal circulation also affects the immune function of the lungs, particularly as the infant is exposed to a wide range of environmental stimuli, including allergens and potential infections. Notably, the differences in the immune response—specifically regarding the nature of pathogens encountered—impact the vulnerability to illnesses such as pneumonia and acute respiratory distress syndrome among neonates. An understanding of these mechanisms is an essential one since they underscore the importance of respiratory tract growth, development, and morphology in determining an effective and adaptive respiratory function that promotes lifelong health against the backdrop of fluctuating environmental conditions (Tan et al., 2019; Kumar, 2020).

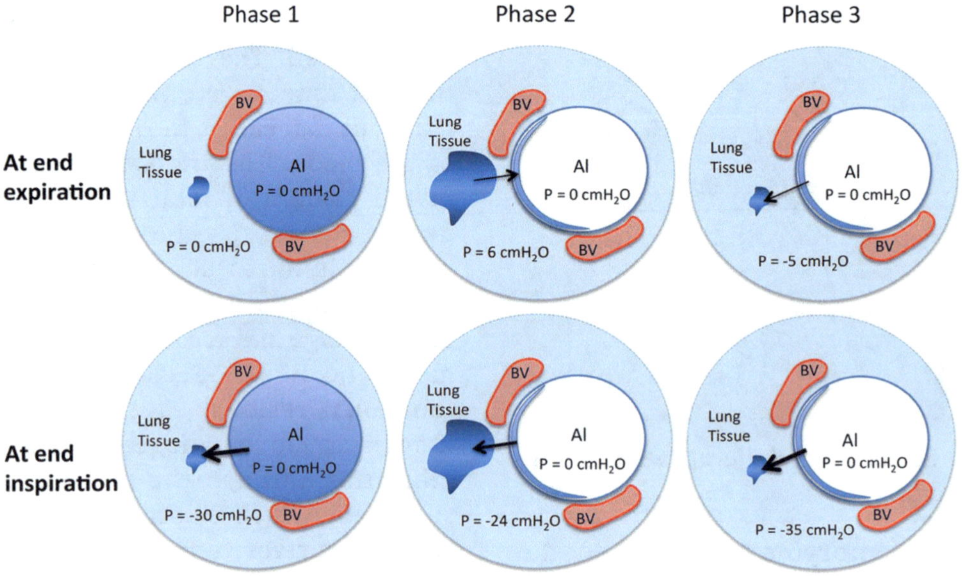

Figure 2.15. Transition from fetal to neonatal respiration.

Source: https://fn.bmj.com/content/fetalneonatal/101/3/F266/F1.large.jpg

2.4.2. Development of Gas Exchange Capabilities

The formation of gas exchange is a part of the total morphological and growth process of the respiratory system. During early embryogenesis, respiratory structures begin to form, establishing the groundwork for effective gas exchange. Pulmonary development includes the differentiation of epithelial cells, which will form alveoli lining and permit oxygen to be absorbed while allowing carbon dioxide to be eliminated. Alveolar sacs result from bronchiole branching, significantly increasing the surface area for gas exchange. Such complexity is essential to the efficient respiratory process since the increased surface area allows more diffusion of gases. An appreciation of these stages of development illuminates the complex mechanisms of respiratory health and disease, which mirror the manner in which structural malformations can lead to compromised respiratory function in adulthood, underscoring the importance of early developmental milestones in lung function. During later developmental stages, the mechanism of surfactant production lies at the heart of refining gas exchange ability. Surfactant, a complex blend of lipids and proteins, reduces the surface tension within alveoli, preventing collapse and providing stability during breathing cycles. The initiation of surfactant synthesis is a critical milestone in the respiratory system, typically occurring between the 24th and 28th week of gestation. This development is crucial not only for facilitating gas exchange but also for the lungs' readiness for independent function upon birth. Inadequate surfactant synthesis can lead to conditions such as neonatal respiratory distress syndrome (NRDS), highlighting the susceptibility of developmental processes necessary for optimal respiratory well-being. Furthermore, ongoing research into surfactant biology holds promise for therapeutic interventions that enhance gas exchange in compromised neonatal lungs, underscoring the importance of this critical period in respiratory development. Besides structural and biochemical transformations, gas exchange abilities also involve the maturity of vascular networks associated with the lungs. The pulmonary capillary bed undergoes an enormous expansion, providing adequate blood for gas exchange. The expansion is such that oxygen-depleted blood can properly be supplied with oxygen and simultaneously facilitate carbon dioxide removal. There should be interaction between the developing circulatory and respiratory systems since interference will lead to inefficient gas exchange with subsequent clinical implications. Environmental agents, such as pathogens and pollutants, to which the lungs are exposed after birth can further stress the delicate balance of gas exchange. Understanding these complex interactions emphasizes the importance of continued research in respiratory medicine to clarify the way various variables affect lung development and function, as these discoveries hold long-term implications for respiratory health during the entire life span.

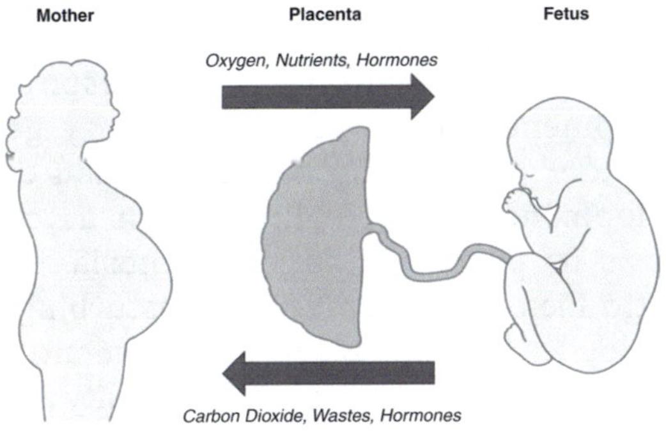

Figure 2.16. Development of gas exchange capabilities.

Source: https://static.cambridge.org/binary/version/id/urn:cambridge.org:id:binary:20200413035534776-0236:9781108163705:19480fig5_1.png?pub-status=live

2.4.3. Impact of Environmental Factors On Functional Growth

The function of environmental determinants in functional development is a critical aspect of respiratory tract development, particularly during the initial stages of life. Various components, such as the quality of air, exposure to pollutants, and nutritional status, may significantly influence the respiratory environment. For example, components such as heavy metals, including cadmium and lead, in conjunction with pesticide exposure, have been shown to cause harm to lung development and function. They can cause oxidative stress and inflammation, which are detrimental to cellular processes governing the growth and resistance of respiratory tissues (Alengebawy et al., 2021). Consequently, these harmful effects can not only be viewed as compromised lung function in childhood but also have late-life implications in respiratory health, thus elevating the significance of how environmental agents can interfere with developmental events in the respiratory tract. Also, ecological stressor impacts vary with exposure timing and duration, and this highlights the idea of a critical window during respiratory development. The developmental stage early in life, which is highly susceptible to disruption by external pollutants, is characterized by excessive proliferation and cell differentiation. Studies have found that exposure to environmental toxins and particulate air pollution at this stage can alter the morphology and structure of the respiratory tract, leading to long-term health impacts. Gut-brain axis studies have also emerged, demonstrating that microbial well-being is associated with respiratory outcomes. The communication between environmental factors and gut microbiota can then influence systemic inflammatory reactions, linking poor quality environment with abnormal respiratory development both indirectly and directly (Cryan et al., 2019). This multi-level interaction highlights the networks that need to be examined in order to understand the complexity of respiratory development fully. The implications of these results extend to individual health, as population-level assessments of environmental impacts are also crucial for informing public health policy. Sustained exposure to environmental pollution in urban settings has been linked to higher rates of respiratory disease in populations, underscoring the need for effective legislation to mitigate environmental toxicity. Furthermore, education systems that foster awareness of the interconnections between environmental health and respiratory well-being have the potential to spark community action towards improved air quality. By understanding the harmful effects of pollutants and toxicants on functional development, stakeholders can prioritize prevention and intervention programs that support respiratory health in various socioeconomic contexts. Thus, dealing with the issue of the influence of the environment on respiratory tract development is not only a scientific problem but also a part of public health policy aimed at making future generations healthier.

Test Your Knowledge

1. How do gas exchange capabilities develop?
2. What is the impact of environmental factors on functional growth?

2.5. Pathological Considerations in Respiratory Development

Learning Outcome

1. Congenital anomalies of the respiratory tract
2. Effects of prenatal exposure to toxins
3. Respiratory diseases affecting growth and morphology

The complex respiratory developmental process is vulnerable to several pathological conditions that can significantly impair normal growth and function. Tracheoesophageal fistula and congenital diaphragmatic hernia are examples of this critical hindrance to development. These malformations interfere with the anatomic alignment of the respiratory tract and may result in severe respiratory distress at birth. In addition, exposure to environmental toxins such as tobacco smoke and air pollution during the critical periods of lung development can cause respiratory disease in adulthood. These pathological considerations must be taken into account by health professionals, as timely diagnosis and treatment can optimize respiratory outcomes and reduce the long-term consequences of such developmental challenges. In addition to congenital conditions, more evidence is emerging that implicates genetic factors in respiratory development. Mutations in regulatory genes can hinder proper lung maturation and cause developmental abnormalities, such as cystic fibrosis or primary ciliary dyskinesia. These genetic factors, in addition to disturbing the pathologies of respiratory development, also cause significant morbidity and mortality among children. The incorporation of genetic screening into clinical practice can enhance early diagnosis and provide targeted therapeutic interventions. Furthermore, the utilization of lengthy guidelines highlights the necessity of treating such pathological regions during a child's growth stage, so that all healthcare professionals are aware of identifying and treating congenital and genetic disorders (Humbert et al., 2022). Lastly, an overall understanding of the pathophysiologic mechanisms of respiratory development can aid in preventive interventions that minimize risk factors for abnormal lung growth. Interventions such as counseling expectant women on avoiding teratogenic agents during pregnancy are crucial in minimizing the occurrence of congenital defects. Further studies on the effects of prenatal and postnatal environmental exposures are also critical for providing evidence-based standards for practitioners. The ESC has emphasized that healthcare professionals need to remain vigilant and responsive to the evolving landscape of respiratory health standards, incorporating them into practice to enhance patient care (Pelliccia et al., 2020). Such an inclusive approach to education and addressing pathological considerations in the context of respiratory development ultimately aims for better health futures for generations to come.

2.5.1. Congenital Anomalies of the Respiratory Tract

Congenital respiratory tract anomalies are significant birth defects that happen during embryogenesis and influence the development of the lungs and airways. They are classified into structural malformations, such as tracheoesophageal fistula and congenital diaphragmatic hernia, and functional impairments that undermine respiratory efficiency. The embryonic mechanisms that influence these anomalies are complex and result from genetic mutations and environmental factors during critical phases of fetal development. Congenital anomalies can lead to severe respiratory distress at the time of birth, which could demand immediate medical intervention. It is essential to understand the morphological development of the respiratory tract, as it forms the basis for understanding how deviations from normal development can lead to malformations and, consequently, impact neonatal outcomes and long-term respiratory function. Congenital respiratory anomalies have been reported to be rare by most studies, yet their impact can be severe. For instance, congenital diaphragmatic hernia occurs in approximately 1 in 2,200 live births and can be accompanied by profound pulmonary hypoplasia or underdevelopment of lung tissue. This necessitates intensive prenatal screening and management during neonatal period to avoid complications. Other malformations, including bronchogenic cysts or lung agenesis, are also connected with various degrees of respiratory impairment and require individual therapeutic strategies depending on the individual patient's requirements. Their medical management is multidisciplinary in nature, incorporating pediatric surgery, neonatology, and reconstructive therapies, and giving emphasis to the importance of early detection and treatment in achieving a good prognosis in infants with such conditions. Aside from the direct clinical utility of congenital respiratory tract anomalies, there is the reality that such anomalies manifest significant concerns about lung development and respiratory wellness in general.

The combination of environmental exposures and genetic vulnerabilities in utero, such as maternal infection or smoking, can have a lasting effect on the form and function of the respiratory system. Furthermore, health professionals are faced with the task of integrating guidelines and evidence-based practice into clinical decision-making to optimize outcomes. Therefore, although congenital respiratory anomalies initially present as localized problems, they often exhibit systemic pathologies affecting respiratory function and require ongoing investigation and education within pediatric respiratory medicine. Recognizing the sophisticated nature of the anomalies, particularly in light of the guidelines established by health authorities, is crucial for delivering optimal patient care (Baumgartner et al., 2020; Pelliccia et al., 2020).

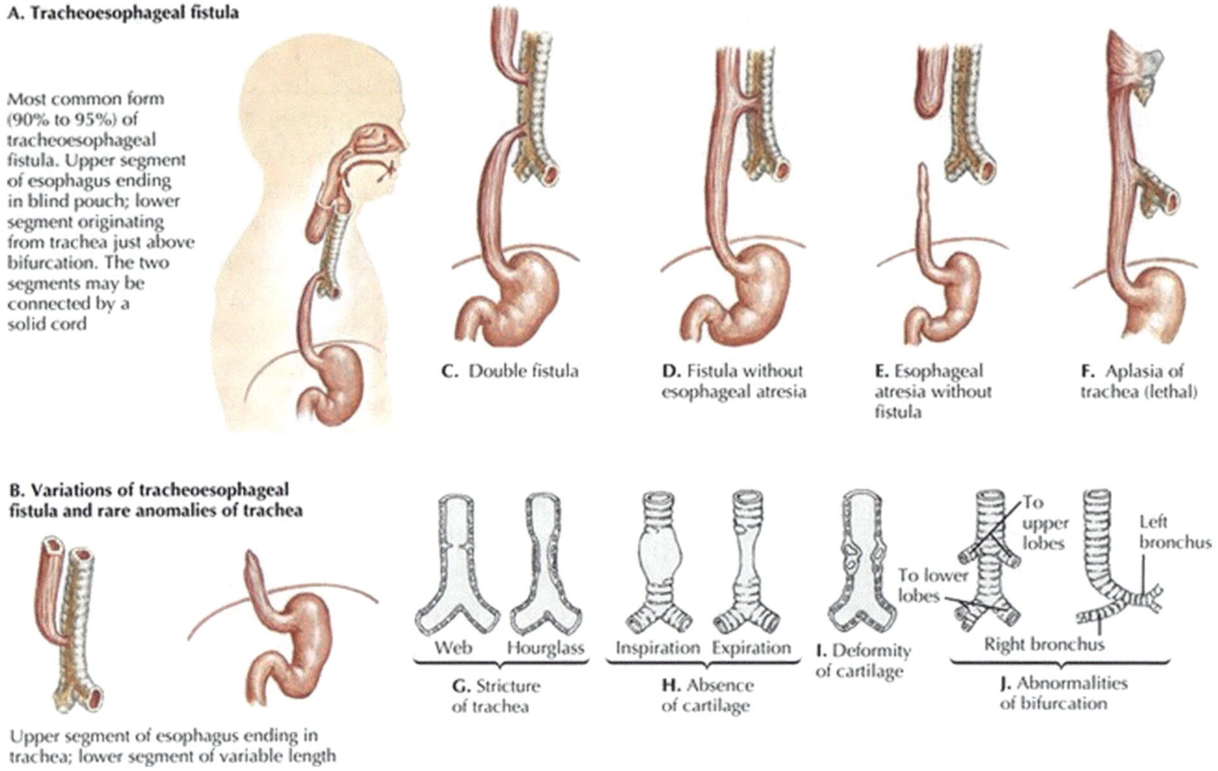

Figure 2.17. Congenital anomalies of the respiratory tract.

Source: https://obgynkey.com/wp-content/uploads/2016/06/B9781437711554000390_f039-001-9781437711554.jpg

2.5.2. Effects of Prenatal Exposure To Toxins

The toxic implications of prenatal toxin exposure, particularly environmental toxins, have garnered more attention in recent decades due to their impacts on respiratory tract morphogenesis and fetal development. Research indicates that toxins such as heavy metals, air pollutants, and microplastics can cause aberrant morphogenesis of the respiratory system. For instance, delicate particulate matter (PM2.5) exposure has been associated with alterations in infant lung architecture and function that manifest as asthma and chronic bronchial hyperreactivity. Also, maternal microplastic exposure, which is increasingly widespread in different ecosystems, is potentially toxic to developing fetuses. These small particles can translocate biological barriers, leading to systemic exposure with negative impacts on fetal development, respiratory tract morphology, and ultimately, long-term respiratory health (Osman et al., 2023).

At the same time, the effect of toxins on the maternal microbiome has become significant to study in prenatal health. The microbiome in the gut is a key factor in the metabolism of xenobiotic exposure while pregnant and can, subsequently, influence fetal development. Environmental toxins can potentially induce dysbiosis, altering microbial composition and its function in metabolizing nutrients and drugs. The alteration has the potential to enhance xenobiotics' toxicity or impair the effectiveness of treatment interventions, further complicating respiratory health outcomes in infants.

Evidence suggests that alterations in maternal microbiota, following toxin exposure, can even affect the ontogeny of the offspring's immune system, leading to increased vulnerability to respiratory infections and allergic disorders (Clarke et al., 2019).

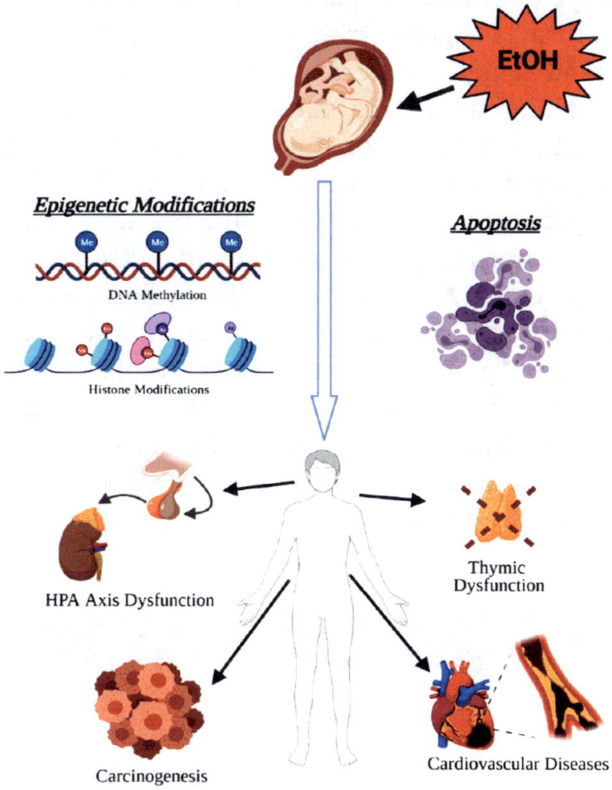

Figure 2.18. Effects of prenatal exposure to toxins.

Source: https://www.mdpi.com/ijms/ijms-22-08785/article_deploy/html/images/ijms-22-08785-g003.png

A profound understanding of this is essential to avert deleterious consequences after prenatal exposure to toxins. Moreover, the timing and duration of exposure to prenatal toxins are crucial determinants of their effects on respiratory development. Susceptibility periods vary with each other and are particularly vulnerable in some of the trimesters due to the accelerated fetal organ development. Exposure during the first trimester, for example, during the development of the respiratory system, may cause more pronounced morphological deformities than that at subsequent periods. Additionally, concomitant exposures to multiple toxins have synergistic actions that contribute to the intricacy during lung development. A multifactorial risk such as this highlights the need for public health intervention in pollution mitigation and maternal education. Preventing exposure to environmental toxins is not only likely to protect maternal health but also ensure generations to do not endure respiratory diseases, a significant step in maintaining public health in general (Osman et al., 2023).

2.5.3. Respiratory Diseases Affecting Growth and Morphology

The growth and morphology of the respiratory tract are also significantly influenced by the onset of various respiratory diseases, which can impose permanent structural and functional alterations. For instance, exposure to particulate matter, particularly PM2.5, has been reported to impair immune function in the respiratory tract, leading to increased susceptibility to microbial infections that can exacerbate diseases like asthma or chronic obstructive pulmonary disease. These disorders not only manifest with inflammatory responses but also induce morphological changes in the airways and lung parenchyma, which ultimately impair the normal respiratory process. As highlighted in recent research, the interaction of PM2.5 with the respiratory immune system reveals the complexity of microbial pathogenesis and how environmental factors can negatively impact respiratory health, further necessitating ongoing investigation of appropriate interventions and actions to avert adverse outcomes of such exposures (Ma et al., 2024).

Another significant characteristic of respiratory disease is its role in the developmental course of the respiratory tract. The pathogens, such as Bordetella spp., which include B. pertussis and B. bronchiseptica, are universal causative agents that can influence the growth and morphological integrity of airway structures. Their potential to infect, coupled with their ability to modulate immunity, highlights their impact on respiratory health, particularly in vulnerable populations such as children. Empirical data indicate that these infections can lead to chronic pulmonary pathology, characterized by abnormal airway responsiveness and compromised lung mechanics, with a direct impact on growth and development. It is thus imperative to understand the pathogenesis mechanisms of Bordetella and its interaction with host factors since this determines potential targets of therapy that could alleviate the burden of such respiratory illnesses (First et al., 2023). Moreover, the relationship between malnutrition and pulmonary disease also bears consideration in development and growth. Acute respiratory infection, for instance, can exacerbate malnutrition, stunting growth, and morphological development of the respiratory system as a whole. Malnutrition is known to exacerbate respiratory disease as well, creating a cycle in which impaired respiratory function in turn damages nutritional status. Children also stand at high risk because stunted development and lung damage may have long-term effects on health and respiratory function. The latter point highlights the importance of integrated health approaches that address both the treatment of respiratory infections and nutritional supplementation to achieve the highest results for growth and respiratory morphology in affected patients. Thus, future studies must identify these associations intending to establish holistic interventions that will counteract the detrimental effect of respiratory diseases on growth and development in all populations.

Test Your Knowledge

1. What are the congenital anomalies of the respiratory tract?
2. What are the effects of prenatal exposure to toxins?

2.6. Comparative Morphology of the Respiratory Tract

Learning Outcome

1. Differences between mammals and reptiles
2. Adaptations in avian respiratory systems
3. Evolutionary perspectives on respiratory morphology

The comparative anatomy of the respiratory tract across various species demonstrates extreme adaptations that maximize survival in diverse environmental situations. These morphological differences are paramount, as they enable effective gas exchange and serve essential functions in thermoregulation, filtration, and sound production. For example, in aquatic animals such as fish, gills are adaptive features that maximize oxygen uptake from water, illustrating the contrast between evolutionary forces and those of land-dwelling vertebrates, which rely on lungs. The structural intricacy in such breathing apparatuses is similarly observed by comparing the patterns of lung branching and lung area in mammals, which evolved to optimize gas exchange through increased alveolar surface area. This comparative approach emphasizes how various evolutionary forces have shaped respiratory function, leading to specialized adaptations that enhance each species' capacity to meet metabolic demands and survive in their environment. Developmentally, the respiratory tract undergoes intricate morphogenetic processes that are essential for its successful function throughout a lifetime. The embryonic stage is critical as the formation of the tracheobronchial tree is sequential and influenced by genetic, environmental, and nutritional factors. For instance, disruptions at this developmental stage can lead to congenital malformations that affect respiratory efficiency and overall health (Habib et al., 2015). Additionally, during the development of organisms from infancy to maturity, the respiratory tract undergoes persistent structural and functional alterations, reflecting changes in metabolic requirements. The capacity to easily regulate airflow and gas exchange becomes increasingly significant as the organism's demands increase, suggesting the importance of morphogenetic mechanisms in forming a functional respiratory apparatus capable of sustaining life. Furthermore, comparative morphology of the respiratory tract enables an understanding of the evolutionary pathways taken by various species. Mechanisms such as the mammalian evolution of alveoli versus the more primitive air sacs of reptiles illustrate how respiratory systems evolve to meet the demands of aerobic respiration in various environments. In addition, birds' respiratory physiology, characterized by a single air sac system for unidirectional air flow, reveals an excellent adaptation for the optimal efficiency of oxygen extraction (Cryan et al., 2019). Understanding such evolutionary differences not only educates evolutionary biology but also adds to the medical sciences, particularly in the evolution of interventions and treatments for respiratory diseases. The transfer of morphological knowledge across species allows for a framework for improvement in respiratory health and disease research, supporting innovations in treatment that draw on successful adaptive mechanisms in the natural world.

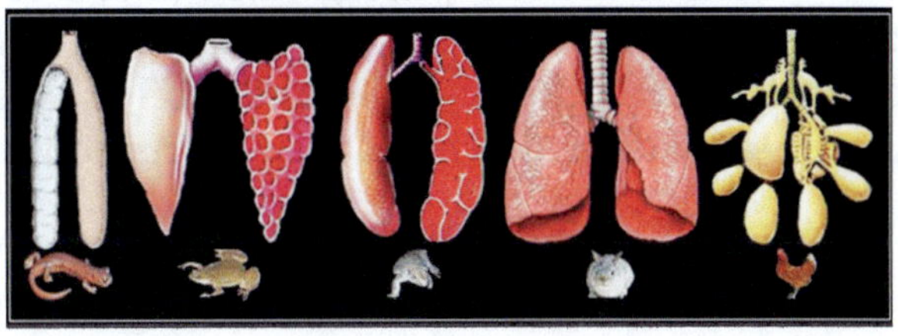

Source: https://www.researchgate.net/profile/Maina-John/publication/287595560/figure/fig1/AS:314862539427840@1452080487518/The-different-morphologies-of-lungs-Notes-Left-to-right-lungs-of-a-urodele-amphibian.png

2.6.1. Differences Between Mammals and Reptiles

The split between mammals and reptiles encompasses several of the most significant physiological differences, most notably in the respiratory system. The well-developed and efficient respiratory system of mammals consists of alveoli, which have a large surface area across which gas exchange can occur. The physical structure enables more efficient oxygen uptake and carbon dioxide expulsion, which are necessary to sustain their high metabolic demands. In contrast to that, reptiles have a more basic lung morphology, typically involving a chain of connected air sacs and fewer, less effective areas of gas exchange. The simple respiratory morphology mirrors the broader metabolic demands of mammals, which require an uninterrupted and higher oxygen supply than reptiles, who, due to their ectothermic lifestyle, can support less effective respiratory systems and economy-saving mechanisms. Furthermore, the development of mammalian and reptilian respiratory tracts differs due to distinct embryological processes. In mammals, the respiratory system is derived from the endoderm and undergoes a complex pattern of branching morphogenesis to establish the well-organized lung structure, which is necessary for their active lifestyle. Their development is highly regulated by neuroendocrine mechanisms such as the hypothalamic-pituitary-thyroid axis, which governs the production of thyroid hormones that are necessary for normal lung development. This is in contrast to reptiles, which have a less complex development of ribosomal organs, fewer branching points, and a simpler lung pattern. This divergence in growth and development patterns reflects the evolutionary differentiation of these groups and the manner in which their respiratory systems are adapted to meet their corresponding ecological and metabolic needs (Paul et al., 2022).

Additionally, the thermoregulatory divergence between mammals and reptiles also helps explain their respiratory adaptations. Endothermic (warm-blooded) mammals have a constant metabolic cost to maintain their body temperature, which necessitates an efficient respiratory system to supply the energy needed to sustain this type of living. Birds and mammals possess mechanisms such as non-shivering thermogenesis (NST), which is facilitated by various anatomical organs, reflecting the evolutionary forces that have developed their adaptations (Grigg et al., 2021). Conversely, reptiles, being ectotherms (cold-blooded), are dependent on environmental heat and have a lower basal metabolism, leading to a lesser oxygen requirement. This environmental context determines the path and shape of their respiratory systems because reptiles have adapted to their environments with less focus on the efficiency of gas exchange, unlike mammals. Thus, the similarities between reptiles and mammals indicate an interesting convergence of ecology, physiology, and evolution in shaping their shared respiratory processes.

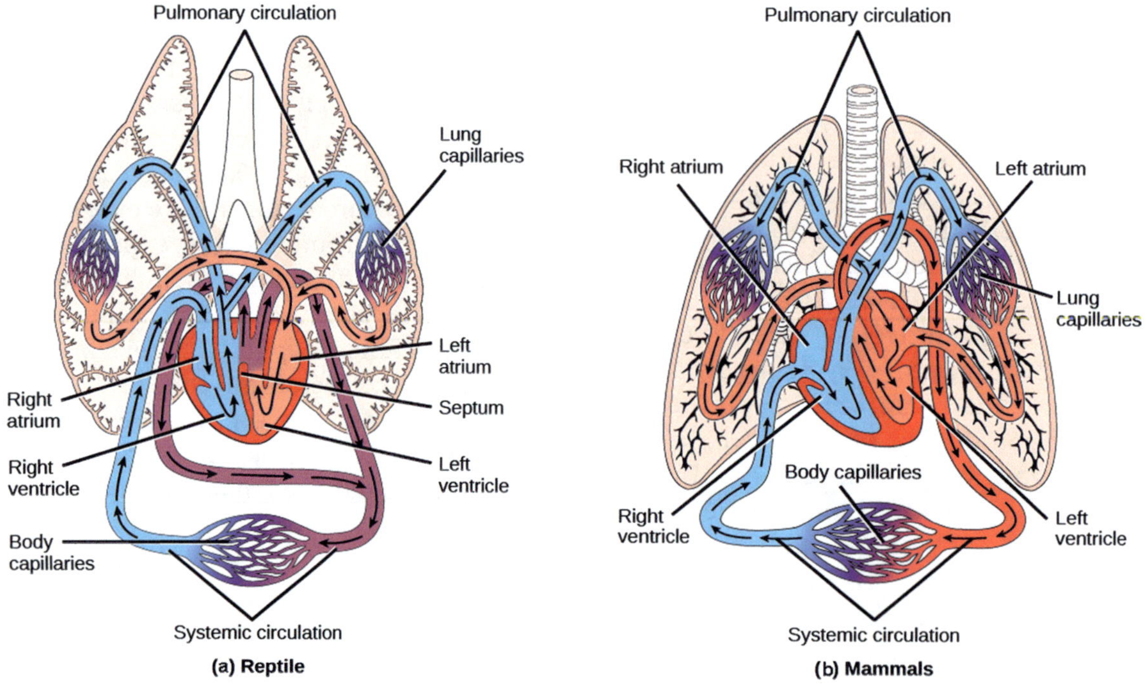

Figure 2.19. Respiratory tract of the mammals and reptiles.

Source: https://rotel.pressbooks.pub/app/uploads/sites/78/2024/08/ReptilesMammals-circulatory-systems.jpeg

2.6.2. Adaptations in Avian Respiratory Systems

The respiratory processes observed among bird species highlight their remarkable evolutionary history, particularly in terms of meeting the demands of flight and altitudinal environments. Birds possess an atypical respiratory system consisting of rigid lungs complemented by a vast air sac network. This structural arrangement is significant, as it optimizes the efficiency of gas exchange during inspiration and expiration, a crucial function given the high metabolic rate associated with flight. The distinctive structure of the avian lung — securely anchored to the ribcage and vertebrae — facilitates maximum operation under varying pressures encountered at varying altitudes. These shifts reflect a significant divergence with respiratory approaches of terrestrial vertebrates, providing a complex interrelationship between anatomy and selective pressures that has granted birds unparalleled respiratory efficiency across a broad spectrum of habitats (Maina et al., 2025). The bird respiratory system's high efficiency can be largely attributed to numerous specific morphometric characteristics. The bird lungs are characterized by a fragile blood-gas barrier that has a low resistance but high oxygen diffusion into the blood. The barrier provides ample respiratory surface area, along with plenty of pulmonary capillaries that allow effective gas exchange at high rates. Of particular interest is how the allometric thinning of the blood-gas barrier is indicative of a systematic optimization towards gas exchange across a broad range of body size. In addition, the significant correlation between respiratory surface density and body mass suggests the evolutionary refinement of the respiratory tissues in birds, which highlights how these adaptations contribute to enhancing their capacity to survive and function in ecological niches where oxygen concentrations fluctuate (Maina, 2025).

Also, the continuous and unidirectional movement of air along the respiratory tract of birds is a critical adaptation that differentiates birds from other classes of air-breathing vertebrates. This is achieved through coordinated movements of the air sacs, ensuring an uninterrupted flow of oxygenated air through the lungs. This dynamic system minimizes the mixing of fresh and spent air to an absolute degree, allowing for maximum oxygen extraction at each stage of respiration. Secondly, the specific arrangement of gas exchange tissue approximates countercurrent and crosscurrent designs, optimizing respiratory efficiency during both the uptake and expulsion of air. These modifications not only highlight the evolutionary advances in bird respiratory physiology but also emphasize the functional importance of these structural patterns in various habitats, fulfilling essential roles in meeting the high bird life requirements (Maina, 2025).

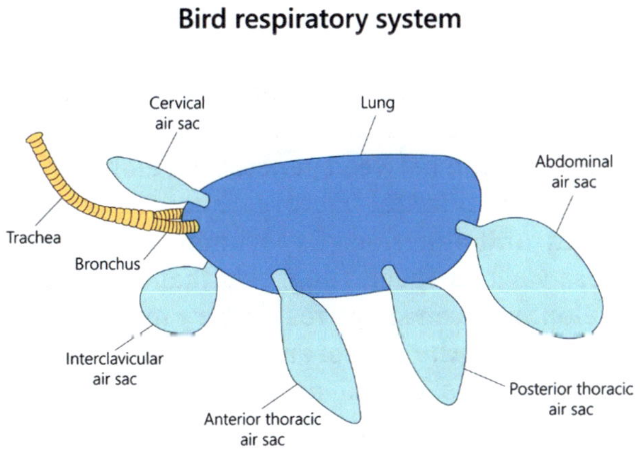

Figure 2.20. Adaptations in avian respiratory systems.

Source: https://images.birdfact.com/production/bird-respiratory-system_2024-02-14-213540_hpwh.jpg?w=1200&h=900&q=80&auto=format&fit=crop&dm=1707946543&s=61548670f14ea796198f4ae997621b5d

2.6.3. Evolutionary Perspectives On Respiratory Morphology

The evolution of respiratory morphology is a fascinating subplot to the greater tale of biological adaptation. There is a tremendous diversity of respiratory systems among different species that have evolved to meet their unique environmental needs and physiological requirements. The development of advanced lung morphology in terrestrial vertebrates, for instance, is a critical evolutionary step from gill morphology in aquatic life. These developments highlight the significance of respiratory efficiency and the efficacy of gas exchange across various environments. These morphological transitions have enabled the occupation of varied environments by optimizing oxygen uptake in a manner congruent with the metabolic requirements of the organisms. Furthermore, the development of respiratory systems demonstrates the integration of environment and physiology, serving as an indication of evolutionary forces that have molded life forms over millennia in response to adapting to their niches. Morphological growth in the respiratory system is often influenced by the interaction between genetic, developmental, and environmental factors that can impact growth and function. Experimental evidence across various species suggests that embryonic development can shape respiratory morphology, specifically the differentiation of various lung elements or gill arches. Differentiation not only represents a demonstration of biological complexity but also responds to the evolutionary adaptability of respiratory systems to environmental changes. For instance, air-breathing animals may have a more complex branching of their bronchial trees to achieve a maximum surface area for gas exchange on land. Aquatic animals, on the other hand, exhibit a range of morphological adaptations, such as the flattened shapes in gills, to attain maximal extraction of oxygen from water. Such factors account for how evolutionary pressures have influenced respiratory morphology among various taxa. The interaction between respiratory anatomy and environmental pressure extends beyond basic anatomical characteristics; it essentially influences an organism's survival and reproductive fitness. Alterations in respiratory systems tend to express an adaptation to ecological stress, such as fluctuations in oxygen tension, temperature, and habitat type. For instance, certain amphibians possess highly developed cutaneous respiration, which allows them to survive in low-oxygen environments. Conversely, intense selection pressure in high-altitude species has given rise to adaptations that enhance oxygen acquisition by way of specialized lung morphology and hemoglobin variants with improved oxygen-affinity binding. These examples illustrate that respiratory morphology evolves as a dynamic evolutionary response to the outside world, and hence it is imperative that evolutionary perspectives on the subject be taken into account. Lastly, a consideration of these evolutionary paths presents keen insights into the diversities and complexities of life's respiratory adaptations to developmental, growth, and respiratory tract morphological roles in general.

Test Your Knowledge

1. What are the differences between mammals and reptiles?
2. What are the evolutionary perspectives on respiratory morphology?

SUMMARY

The intricate processes in the growth, development, and morphology of the respiratory system underscore its indispensable role in human health. Aside from facilitating the exchange of gases necessary for homeostasis, the system also serves as an environmental barrier against infectious agents. The interplay between genetic, environmental, and biological factors during embryogenesis is a major contributor to the efficient functioning of the respiratory tract. An understanding of these mechanisms may help in developing more effective clinical approaches to treating respiratory diseases and achieving better patient outcomes. Future research must investigate the developmental plasticity of the respiratory system and the mechanisms by which environmental exposures affect its morphology and function throughout a lifespan in greater detail. In particular, studies on how such exposures, such as microplastics and viral infections, would affect respiratory health are essential (Ragusa et al., 2020; Colavita et al., 2020). In addition, the morphology of the respiratory tract is not entirely a result of its anatomical structure but is also largely influenced by environmental determinants. Imaging techniques and histological techniques have provided insights into how the individual architecture of the respiratory tract alters and develops in reaction to varying ecological stresses. One such example is how pollutants affect ciliated epithelial cells, a marker of how environmental stresses can alter the respiratory system's architecture and lead to potential pathologies. Additional research would be required to establish the adaptive mechanisms through which the respiratory tissues adapt to persistent stressors. Such research is crucial in designing preventive and therapeutic interventions against disease development due to intrinsic malformations and extrinsic injuries, thereby ensuring lung resistance and optimal respiratory function well into adulthood (Ragusa et al., 2020; Colavita et al., 2020).

Lastly, the dynamics between developmental biology and environmental influences characterize the architecture of the respiratory system, which is critical in maintaining respiratory health throughout an individual's lifetime. Maintenance of respiratory morphology during various stages of development assures proper functioning of lungs and optimal gas exchange. Future research in this field would be well-advised to examine how early formative stages of life provide the foundation for respiratory well-being and disease susceptibility. An understanding of such developmental trajectories would help healthcare providers design efficient intervention strategies for individuals susceptible to respiratory diseases due to genetic predisposition or environmental stimuli. Lastly, integrating respiratory morphology understanding and clinical practice will enhance the management of respiratory diseases and lead to improved health outcomes for the target populations (Ragusa et al., 2020; Colavita et al., 2020).

The development, growth, and morphology of the respiratory tract are critical aspects of human physiology, encompassing various structural and functional modifications from embryonic life to adulthood. During the embryonic period, airway and pulmonary structures develop in number through a process of branching morphogenesis, providing a foundation for respiratory functions. Respiratory epithelium differentiates through a tightly regulated process, where specific signaling pathways determine the formation of distinct cell types, such as ciliated epithelial and goblet cells. These cellular products are essential for airway patency and mucociliary clearance, which protects the respiratory tract from infections and other inhaled toxicants. Understanding these processes clearly provides vital data regarding congenital disease and anomalies that can arise as a consequence of uneven development, which affects respiratory well-being later in life.

Nutrition in the developmental phase of the respiratory system cannot be overstated, particularly for immune system integrity. As implied by research, proper intake of nutrients is essential in the development of the respiratory system and the body's immune defense against respiratory infections. For instance, food components such as vitamins C and D, along with certain antioxidants, have been found to enhance immune responses and, therefore, protect against respiratory pathogens. Micronutrient deficiencies can increase susceptibility to infection, emphasizing the importance of a balanced diet throughout critical developmental periods. This relationship between nutrition and respiratory health takes on special significance when assessing public health interventions and approaches aimed at achieving optimized outcomes in vulnerable populations, such as children and the elderly, who are at a higher risk of nutritional deficiency. In the development of the respiratory tract, environmental influence and morphology interact with rising relevance. Pollution, cigarette smoke, and allergens are among the environmental factors that significantly impact the growth and functional maturity of the respiratory system. Scientific research has demonstrated that early exposure to environmental stressors may have long-lasting effects, some of which include susceptibility to chronic respiratory diseases like asthma and chronic obstructive pulmonary disease (COPD). This highlights the importance of creating protective factors and healthy environments in early childhood. In addition, the role of the gut microbiota in modulating immune responses, as illustrated by its impact on the respiratory tract, also suggests that the microbiota-gut-brain axis may potentially lead to novel therapeutic strategies for improving respiratory function. Increasing recognition of these intricate interactions will be necessary to advancing our understanding of respiratory development and to developing interdisciplinary approaches to improving respiratory health across the lifespan.

KEY TERMS FROM THIS CHAPTER

- Embryonic stage
- Canalicular stage
- Alveolar stage
- Lung bud
- Bronchial tree
- Secondary bronchi
- Alveoli
- Type I pneumocytes
- Cilia
- Respiratory epithelium
- Pseudoglandular stage
- Saccular stage
- Branching morphogenesis
- Tracheoesophageal septum
- Primary bronchi
- Tertiary bronchi
- Surfactant production
- Type II pneumocytes
- Goblet cells
- Pleura

CRITICAL THINKING QUESTIONS

1. **Which embryonic structure gives rise to the respiratory tract?**
   a. Mesonephric duct
   b. Endoderm of the foregut
   c. Neural crest
   d. Paraxial mesoderm
2. **At what gestational age do alveoli begin to form?**
   a. 8 weeks
   b. 16 weeks
   c. 24 weeks
   d. 36 weeks
3. **What is the function of surfactant in the fetal lung?**
   a. Inhibits lung development
   b. Increases airway resistance
   c. Reduces surface tension in alveoli
   d. Promotes bronchoconstriction
4. **Which of the following structures is not part of the conducting zone of the respiratory system?**
   a. Trachea
   b. Bronchi
   c. Terminal bronchioles
   d. Alveolar sac
5. **Postnatal lung development continues up to approximately what age?**
   a. 6 months
   b. 2 years
   c. 8 years
   d. 20 years

Short Answer Questions

1. What is the function of pulmonary surfactant, and when does it typically begin to be produced in fetal lungs?
2. Name the stages of lung development in chronological order.
3. Which lung development stage is characterized by formation of terminal sacs (primitive alveoli)?
4. What separates the trachea and esophagus during embryonic development?
5. How many lobes does the right lung have compared to the left lung?

Answer to Critical Thinking Questions

1. (b) 2. (c) 3. (c) 4. (d) 5. (d)

REFERENCES

1. Adler, D., & Liu, R. (2014). Duplication cysts: Diagnosis, management, and the role of endoscopic ultrasound. *Endoscopic Ultrasound, 3*(3), 152. https://doi.org/10.4103/2303-9027.138783Alengebawy, A., Abdelkhalek, S. T., Qureshi, S. R., & Wang, M. Q. (2021). Heavy metals and pesticides toxicity in agricultural soil and plants: Ecological risks and human health implications. *Toxics, 9*, 42–42. https://doi.org/10.3390/toxics9030042 (accessed on 16th June 2025).
2. Baumgartner, H., De Backer, J., Babu-Narayan, S. V., Budts, W., Chessa, M., Diller, G. P., Lung, B., et al. (2020). 2020 ESC guidelines for the management of adult congenital heart disease. *European Heart Journal, 42*, 563–645. https://doi.org/10.1093/eurheartj/ehaa554 (accessed on 16th June 2025).
3. Bustamante-Marin, X. M., & Ostrowski, L. E. (2016). Cilia and mucociliary clearance. *Cold Spring Harbor Perspectives in Biology, 9*, a028241–a028241. https://doi.org/10.1101/cshperspect.a028241 (accessed on 16th June 2025).
4. Chen, X., Qiu, D., Wang, Y., Ju, Q., Zhao, C. L., Zhang, Y. S., Wang, M., et al. (2024). Acetate-producing bacterium *Paenibacillus odorifer* hampers lung cancer growth in lower respiratory tract: An *in vitro* study. *Microbiology Spectrum, 12.* https://www.semanticscholar.org/paper/2da8248ecf2193d5866ac6a49aedebb1cc484ba2 (accessed on 16th June 2025).
5. Clarke, G., Sandhu, K. V., Griffin, B. T., Dinan, T. G., Cryan, J. F., & Hyland, N. P. (2019). Gut reactions: Breaking down xenobiotic–microbiome interactions. *Pharmacological Reviews, 71*, 198–224. https://doi.org/10.1124/pr.118.015768 (accessed on 16th June 2025).
6. Colavita, F., Lapa, D., Carletti, F., Lalle, E., Bordi, L., Marsella, P., Nicastri, E., et al. (2020). SARS-CoV-2 isolation from ocular secretions of a patient with COVID-19 in Italy with prolonged viral RNA detection. *Annals of Internal Medicine, 173*, 242–243. https://doi.org/10.7326/m20-1176 (accessed on 16th June 2025).
7. Cryan, J. F., O'Riordan, K. J., Cowan, C. S. M., Sandhu, K. V., Bastiaanssen, T. F. S., Boehme, M., Codagnone, M. G., et al. (2019). The microbiota-gut-brain axis. *Physiological Reviews, 99*, 1877–2013. https://doi.org/10.1152/physrev.00018.2018 (accessed on 16th June 2025).
8. First, N. J., Pedreira-Lopez, J., San-Silvestre, M. R. F., Parrish, K., Lu, X., & Gestal, M. C. (2023). *Bordetella* spp. utilizes the type 3 secretion system to manipulate the VIP/VPAC2 signaling and promote colonization and persistence of the three classical *Bordetella* in the lower respiratory tract. *Frontiers in Cellular and Infection Microbiology, 13.* https://www.semanticscholar.org/paper/8731188e1ea2efa95cc9e9e9cefb64f81800b842 (accessed on 16th June 2025).
9. Flerlage, T., Boyd, D. F., Meliopoulos, V., Thomas, P. G., & Schultz-Cherry, S. (2021). Influenza virus and SARS-CoV-2: Pathogenesis and host responses in the respiratory tract. *Nature Reviews Microbiology, 19*, 425–441. https://doi.org/10.1038/s41579-021-00542-7 (accessed on 16th June 2025).
10. Grigg, G. C., Nowack, J., Bicudo, J. E. P. W., Bal, N. C., Woodward, H. N., & Seymour, R. S. (2021). Whole-body endothermy: Ancient, homologous and widespread among the ancestors of mammals, birds and crocodylians. *Biological Reviews/Biological Reviews of the Cambridge Philosophical Society, 97*, 766–801. https://doi.org/10.1111/brv.12822 (accessed on 16th June 2025).

11. Guo, Y. R., Cao, Q. D., Hong, Z. S., Tan, Y. Y., Chen, S. D., Jin, H. J., Tan, K. S., et al. (2020). The origin, transmission and clinical therapies on coronavirus disease 2019 (COVID-19) outbreak–An update on the status. *Military Medical Research, 7.* https://doi.org/10.1186/s40779-020-00240-0 (accessed on 16th June 2025).
12. Habib, G., Lancellotti, P., Antunes, M. J., Bongiorni, M. G., Casalta, J. P., Del Zotti, F., Dulgheru, R., et al. (2015). 2015 ESC guidelines for the management of infective endocarditis. *European Heart Journal, 36*, 3075–3128. https://doi.org/10.1093/eurheartj/ehv319 (accessed on 16th June 2025).
13. Hickling, D., Sun, T. T., & Wu, X. R. (2015). Anatomy and physiology of the urinary tract: Relation to host defense and microbial infection. *Microbiology Spectrum, 3.* https://doi.org/10.1128/microbiolspec.uti-0016-2012 (accessed on 16th June 2025).
14. Humbert, M., Kovács, G., Hoeper, M. M., Badagliacca, R., Berger, R. M. F., Brida, M., Carlsen, J., et al. (2022). 2022 ESC/ERS guidelines for the diagnosis and treatment of pulmonary hypertension. *European Respiratory Journal, 61*, 2200879–2200879. https://doi.org/10.1183/13993003.00879-2022 (accessed on 16th June 2025).
15. Iddir, M., Brito, A., Dingeo, G., Sosa, S., Samouda, H., La Frano, M. R., & Bohn, T. (2020). Strengthening the immune system and reducing inflammation and oxidative stress through diet and nutrition: Considerations during the COVID-19 crisis. *Nutrients, 12*, 1562–1562. https://doi.org/10.3390/nu12061562 (accessed on 16th June 2025).
16. Jeevanandam, J., Barhoum, A., Chan, Y. S., Dufresne, A., & Danquah, M. K. (2018). Review on nanoparticles and nanostructured materials: History, sources, toxicity and regulations. *Beilstein Journal of Nanotechnology, 9*, 1050–1074. https://doi.org/10.3762/bjnano.9.98 (accessed on 16th June 2025).
17. Kumar, V. (2020). Pulmonary innate immune response determines the outcome of inflammation during pneumonia and sepsis-associated acute lung injury. *Frontiers in Immunology, 11.* https://doi.org/10.3389/fimmu.2020.01722 (accessed on 16th June 2025).
18. Landrigan, P. J., Stegeman, J. J., Fleming, L. E., Allemand, D., Anderson, D. M., Backer, L. C., Brücker-Davis, F., et al. (2020). Human health and ocean pollution. *Annals of Global Health, 86*, 151–151. https://doi.org/10.5334/aogh.2831 (accessed on 16th June 2025).
19. Lee, Y., Berríos-Vázquez, G., Maes, R. K., Kiupel, M., Desmarets, L., Nauwynck, H., & Soboll Hussey, G. (2023). Development of immortalized feline respiratory epithelial cells in an air-liquid-interface culture system for feline herpesvirus-1 study. *Virus Research, 326*, 199063–199063. https://doi.org/10.1016/j.virusres.2023.199063 (accessed on 16th June 2025).
20. Li, H., Wang, H., Hao, H., An, H., & Geng, H. (2022). Influences of airway obstruction caused by adenoid hypertrophy on growth and development of craniomaxillofacial structure and respiratory function in children. *Computational and Mathematical Methods in Medicine, 2022*, 1–7. https://doi.org/10.1155/2022/5096406 (accessed on 16th June 2025).
21. Ma, J., Chiu, Y. F., Kao, C. C., Chuang, C. N., Chen, C. Y., Lai, C. H., & Kuo, M. L. (2024). Fine particulate matter manipulates immune response to exacerbate microbial pathogenesis in the respiratory tract. *European Respiratory Review, 33.* https://www.semanticscholar.org/paper/bbf820b87221213424fb451776caad80c7c9460d (accessed on 16th June 2025).
22. Maina, J. (2025). Structure and function of the avian respiratory system. *Philosophical*

Transactions B, 380. https://www.semanticscholar.org/paper/68e6328c3494ff742768d1a01f70c630e5b39031 (accessed on 16th June 2025).

23. Maina, J., & Schachner, E. R. (2025). Biology of the avian respiratory system: Development, evolutionary morphology, function and clinical considerations. *Philosophical Transactions of the Royal Society B: Biological Sciences, 380.* https://www.semanticscholar.org/paper/ab28719510c0ea0117f35be88d6e761b88b44336 (accessed on 16th June 2025).
24. Nobile, C. J., & Johnson, A. D. (2015). *Candida albicans* biofilms and human disease. *Annual Review of Microbiology, 69*, 71–92. https://doi.org/10.1146/annurev-micro-091014-104330 (accessed on 16th June 2025).
25. Osman, A. I., Hosny, M., Eltaweil, A. S., Omar, S., Elgarahy, A. M., Farghali, M., Yap, P. S., et al. (2023). Microplastic sources, formation, toxicity and remediation: A review. *Environmental Chemistry Letters, 21*, 2129–2169. https://doi.org/10.1007/s10311-023-01593-3 (accessed on 16th June 2025).
26. Parslow, V. R., Elmore, S. A., Cochran, R. Z., Bolon, B., Mahler, B., Sabio, D., & Lubeck, B. A. (2024). Histology atlas of the developing mouse respiratory system from prenatal day 9.0 through postnatal day 30. *Toxicologic Pathology, 52*, 153–227. https://www.semanticscholar.org/paper/35dabd419767bf9e112f3fe172d8a0b52a2f3754 (accessed on 16th June 2025).
27. Paul, B., Sterner, Z. R., Buchholz, D. R., Shi, Y. B., & Sachs, L. M. (2022). Thyroid and corticosteroid signaling in amphibian metamorphosis. *Cells, 11*, 1595–1595. https://doi.org/10.3390/cells11101595 (accessed on 16th June 2025).
28. Pelliccia, A., Sharma, S., Gati, S., Bäck, M., Börjesson, M., Caselli, S., Collet, J. P., et al. (2020). 2020 ESC guidelines on sports cardiology and exercise in patients with cardiovascular disease. *European Heart Journal, 42*, 17–96. https://doi.org/10.1093/eurheartj/ehaa605 (accessed on 16th June 2025).
29. Priori, S. G., Blomström-Lundqvist, C., Mazzanti, A., Blom, N., Borggrefe, M., Camm, A. J., Elliott, P., et al. (2015). 2015 ESC guidelines for the management of patients with ventricular arrhythmias and the prevention of sudden cardiac death. *European Heart Journal, 36*, 2793–2867. https://doi.org/10.1093/eurheartj/ehv316 (accessed on 16th June 2025).
30. Ragusa, A., Svelato, A., Santacroce, C., Catalano, P., Notarstefano, V., Carnevali, O., Papa, F., et al. (2020). Plasticity: First evidence of microplastics in human placenta. *Environment International, 146*, 106274–106274. https://doi.org/10.1016/j.envint.2020.106274 (accessed on 16th June 2025).
31. Tan, C., & Lewandowski, A. J. (2019). The transitional heart: From early embryonic and fetal development to neonatal life. *Fetal Diagnosis and Therapy, 47*, 373–386. https://doi.org/10.1159/000501906 (accessed on 16th June 2025).
32. Tilley, A. E., Walters, M. S., Shaykhiev, R., & Crystal, R. G. (2014). Cilia dysfunction in lung disease. *Annual Review of Physiology, 77*, 379–406. https://doi.org/10.1146/annurev-physiol-021014-071931 (accessed on 16th June 2025).
33. Uhlén, M., Fagerberg, L., Hallström, B. M., Lindskog, C., Oksvold, P., Mardinoğlu, A., Sivertsson, Å., et al. (2015). Tissue-based map of the human proteome. *Science, 347.* https://doi.org/10.1126/science.1260419 (accessed on 16th June 2025).
34. Wani, A. L., Ara, A., & Usmani, J. A. (2015). Lead toxicity: A review. *Interdisciplinary Toxicology, 8*, 55–64. https://doi.org/10.1515/intox-2015-0009 (accessed on 16th June 2025).

NORMAL RESPIRATORY PHYSIOLOGY

3

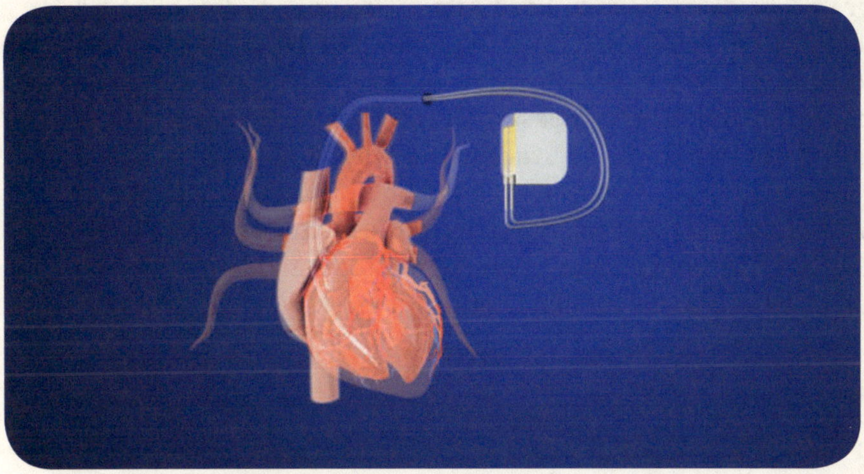

LEARNING OBJECTIVES

After studying this chapter, you will be able to:

1. Discuss the anatomy of the respiratory system
2. Explore the mechanics of breathing
3. Define gas exchange
4. Focus on the regulation of breathing
5. Explain respiratory volumes and capacities
6. List the impact of environmental factors

Introduction

The initial section of this chapter serves as a background by introducing the key mechanisms and processes of the respiratory system. This crucial system facilitates gas exchange, sending oxygen into the body and removing carbon dioxide effectively. Identification of these processes not only accounts for the central role of respiration in maintaining homeostasis but also sheds light on the clinical aspects of respiratory disease. With the integration of current research, such as the recent inclusion of exercise pulmonary hypertension (exPH) into the main guidelines, awareness of how physiological changes impact respiratory function during exercise has heightened. This context provides a foundation for evaluating the normal physiology of the respiratory system and illustrates how deviations from expected physiology can predict pathological states, ultimately affecting patient outcomes and mortality rates in various populations (Zeder et al., 2024).

Throughout this essay, the complexity of respiratory mechanics will be revealed, thereby offering a deeper understanding of the forces at work in breathing. Not only does the respiratory system work in conjunction with the cardiovascular system, but it also adapts to variations in stimuli and environmental conditions. Anomalies, such as exercise-induced alterations in pulmonary hemodynamics, illustrate the intricate interdependence of respiratory physiology and overall health. By examining components such as lung volumes, capacities, and driving forces for ventilation, we can understand how normal physiology provides a template against which respiratory pathologies are quantified. This platform aligns substantially with the argument that having complete knowledge of normal respiratory function is essential for timely disease detection, thereby connecting physiology to applied health consequences (Gadadhar et al., 2021). To put it in a nutshell, the introduction lays out the entire process of an integrated study of Normal Respiratory Physiology, emphasizing its application in both disease and health. This essay aims to bridge the gap between practical application and theoretical knowledge, elucidating why knowledge of respiratory mechanics enhances our treatment and prevention methods for respiratory diseases. Through a focus on both the fundamentals of the field and recent advances within it, the study of healthy lung function seeks not only to account for why the lungs are healthy but also to highlight the broader significance of respiratory health to overall health. With emerging research methods and a better understanding of the disease manifestations, the interplay between respiratory physiology and other health outcomes becomes more evident, indicating the need for additional research (Gadadhar et al., 2021; Zeder et al., 2024).

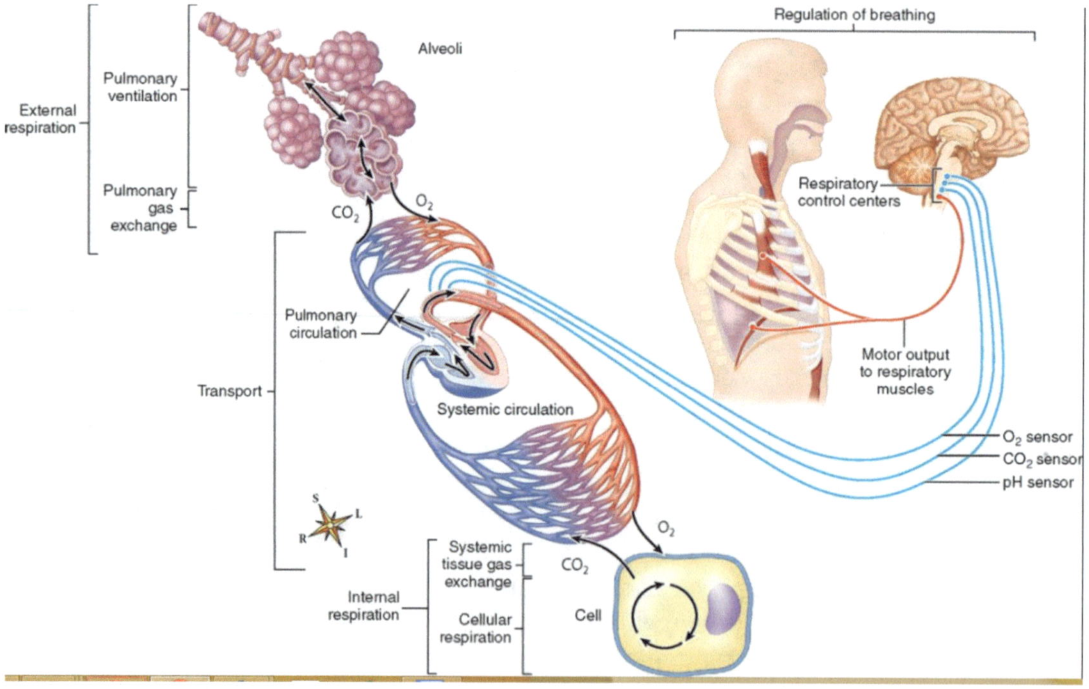

Figure 3.1. Physiology of the respiratory system.

Source: https://basicmedicalkey.com/wp-content/uploads/2016/05/F500402f27-01-9780323096003.jpg

Definition of respiratory physiology

Respiratory physiology can be described as the science of the biochemical and mechanical processes involved in gas exchange between an organism and its external environment. The study of respiratory physiology not only focuses on the physical movement of air in and out of the lungs, but also on the molecular movement that allows for gas exchange at the level of the alveoli. It is essential to understand the mechanisms involved, as they enable the delivery of oxygen to tissues and the elimination of carbon dioxide, a byproduct of cellular metabolism. It is essential to appreciate how respiratory physiology informs us about various pathophysiological states, thereby guiding clinical practice and treatment plans. The present research in this subject also encompasses broad areas of human physiology, illuminating how the function of the respiratory system impacts and is in turn impacted by other systems, thereby illustrating the integrated functional nature of bodily functions. Respiratory physiology also entails examining how the mechanics of ventilation contribute to maintaining homeostasis within the body. An essential aspect of this regulation is mediated by chemoreceptors that respond to changes in blood gases and pH levels, causing alterations in breathing depth and rate. As an example, when there is an increase in carbon dioxide concentration, chemoreceptors cause an increase in ventilation to eliminate excess CO_2, demonstrating a feedback mechanism essential for acid-base balance maintenance. Additionally, other variables such as physical activity and environmental conditions affect respiratory function, necessitating dynamic control of ventilatory variables. This interplay illustrates the sophistication of respiratory physiology as it operates in real-time, adapting to physiological requirements while facilitating efficient gas exchange. The study of respiratory physiology, thus, not only adds to what is understood about respiratory mechanisms but also to an understanding of the importance of respiratory health to overall well-being. Finally, respiratory physiology knowledge encompasses the understanding of the impact of respiratory pathology on overall health status. Various diseases, such as chronic obstructive pulmonary disease (COPD) and asthma, disrupt normal respiratory processes, making this physiological component necessary to learn. With an understanding of the pathogenesis of such diseases and their impact on gas exchange and lung mechanics, medical professionals can develop effective methods for diagnosis, management, and rehabilitation. Recent research into respiratory physiology also examines how lifestyle factors, such as smoking or air pollution, result in alterations in lung function and respiratory well-being. Recent research has highlighted the gut-lung axis and its relevance to respiratory disease, revealing compelling correlations between the respiratory system and the overall health of the body. Hence, the field of respiratory physiology broadens from being an abstraction of physiological processes to a comprehensive understanding of how such processes form the core of disease and health and that this eventually directs clinical approaches as well as health interventions.

Importance of understanding normal respiratory function

Understanding normal respiratory function helps establish deviations, which may indicate underlying health issues. The respiratory system is an intricate network of organs designed to facilitate gas exchange, primarily through the intake of oxygen and the removal of carbon dioxide. The intricate process begins with breathing in air that travels via the nasal passages, pharynx, and larynx and ends up in the lungs, where oxygen is absorbed into the bloodstream. When doctors understand the complexity of this physiologic process, they are better equipped to diagnose and treat respiratory diseases. Given the role the respiratory system plays in overall well-being, understanding its normal function facilitates the early identification of conditions that would otherwise result in severe complications, thereby underscoring the importance of comprehensive respiratory physiology instruction. The health significance of the respiratory system extends beyond the patient to public and societal scales, affecting public health policy and economic realities. As an instance, chronic lower respiratory disease has been quoted to be the third most frequent cause of death in the United States, emphasizing the significance of these diseases in the population at large (Miller et al., 2017). It facilitates clinicians and researchers planning preventive measures, therapy, and educational interventions to reduce morbidity and mortality from respiratory disorders. Moreover, insights derived from research on respiratory physiology can enhance the quality of life and life expectancy of affected populations, thereby constituting a keystone element of modern healthcare practice. Thus, focusing on normal respiratory function lays a foundation for promoting respiratory health and effective intervention strategies. Second, familiarity with normal respiratory physiology aids in the development of new treatment practices and enhances existing practice in respiratory care. Research using models with highly accurate human-like respiratory physiology has provided valuable insights into disease pathogenesis and the effects of environmental determinants on lung conditions (Miller et al., 2017). For example, clarifying how allergens and pollutants inhaled interact with respiratory architecture has the promise of unveiling new therapeutic targets. In addition, knowledge of normal function is crucial in vaccine development and evaluation, which are essential for managing respiratory infections. This ongoing research reaffirms the importance of respiratory physiology in developing effective remedies and policies that focus on the respiratory system. As knowledge is developed, the ability to translate findings into improved patient outcomes increases, making a comprehensive understanding of normal respiratory function imperative.

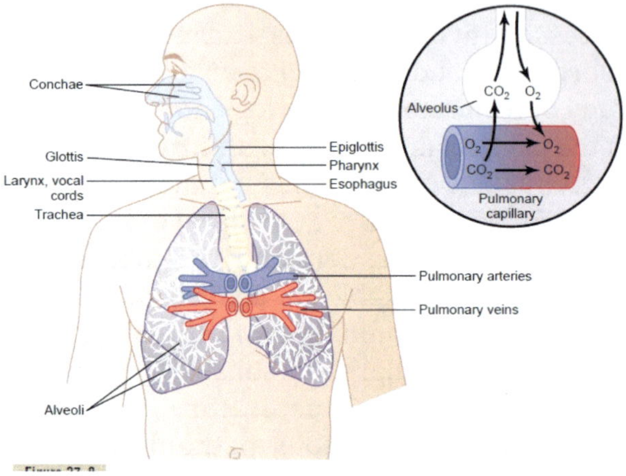

Figure 3.2. Normal respiratory functions.

Source: https://img.brainkart.com/imagebk20/vdwiTvx.jpg

3.1. Anatomy of the Respiratory System

Learning Outcome

1. Major components of the respiratory system
2. Structure and function of the lungs
3. Role of the diaphragm and intercostal muscles

The respiratory system is anatomically very organized, with a lot of structures that play the most critical roles in gas exchange. From the upper airway, air flows through the nasal passages where it is filtered, humidified, and warmed. The nasal cavity has mucous membranes covered in ciliated epithelial cells that filter and remove particulate matter and pathogens, thereby representing a first line of defense. Air then proceeds through the pharynx and larynx and into the trachea, which bifurcates into the left and right bronchi, branching out into the lungs. This passage not only provides a means by which air can travel, but also protects the lower respiratory tract from invading pathogens, demonstrating the two-in-one nature that exists within and throughout the anatomy of the respiratory system. As such, an understanding of these structures is crucial to comprehending the complexities of normal respiratory pathophysiology and physiology in respiratory diseases. The lungs themselves are made up of a highly specialized architecture that optimizes the process of gas exchange. The bronchi subdivide into increasingly smaller bronchioles throughout the lungs, eventually terminating in the alveoli, which are microscopically small air sacs where the critical exchange of carbon dioxide and oxygen occurs. The walls of the alveoli are thin, fragile, and allow efficient gas diffusion with the help of an enormous surface area that has a grape-like cluster structure. Capillaries are present around the alveoli to provide oxygen from the inhaled air and pass it directly into the blood, transporting carbon dioxide in the opposite direction to be expelled during exhalation. This precise organization emphasizes the respiratory system's evolutionary adaptation to best function, illustrating how form follows function at every level of the anatomy, which ultimately results in the maintenance of homeostasis throughout the body. Pathological diseases, such as Chronic Obstructive Pulmonary Disease (COPD), exemplify why this anatomy is so crucial in maintaining respiratory health. In COPD, characterized by progressive airflow limitation, airway and lung parenchymal structural integrity is disrupted, affecting their efficacy in performing their functions. Changes in airway resistance and lung elastance are associated with respiratory mechanics, as revealed by fluctuations in forced expiratory volume (FEV) and lung volumes (Beris et al., 2022). The relationship between anatomy and physiological response becomes crucial in understanding the systemic consequences of such diseases, especially during periods of sustained hypoxia. Hence, learning the anatomy of the respiratory system is not merely a classroom exercise; it provides valuable insights into the comprehension of disease processes, aiding in the development of specific therapeutic strategies aimed at restoring normal respiratory physiology (Miller et al., 2017).

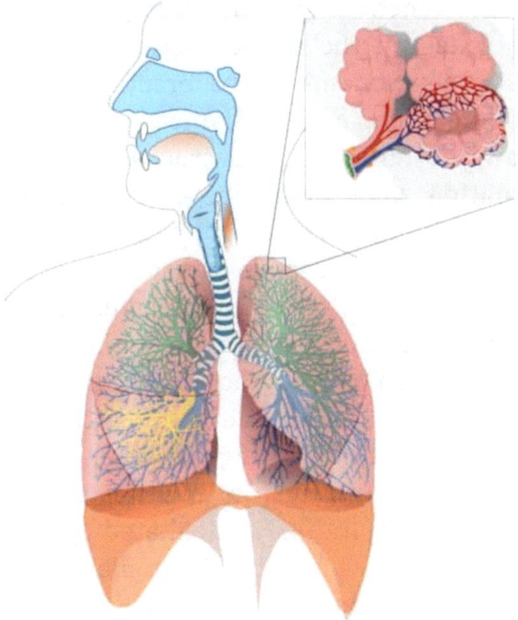

Figure 3.3. Anatomy of the respiratory system.

Source: https://teachmeanatomy.info/wp-content/uploads/The-Bronchial-Tree.jpg

3.1.1. Major Components of the Respiratory System

The main components of the respiratory system all work together to facilitate the exchange of life-giving gases. Air from the nose and mouth moves through the trachea and splits into bronchi, which then branch into minute bronchioles, ultimately reaching the alveoli, where gas exchange occurs. The alveoli are tiny air spaces that provide a large surface area for the diffusion of oxygen and carbon dioxide through the walls of the alveoli and the capillaries. The design is highly efficient, as the alveolar walls are extremely thin, reducing the distance traveled by the gases. Furthermore, the vast alveolar population of the lungs considerably enhances the surface area for gas exchange, and consequently provides adequate oxygen transport to the blood to meet the body's requirements under various activities, including exercise and rest.

The functioning of the respiratory system also relies on the supporting structures and muscle components of the breathing process. The diaphragm, a dome-shaped muscle located below the lungs, plays a crucial role in both inhalation and exhalation. As the diaphragm contracts, it increases the volume of the thoracic cavity, causing a negative pressure that attracts air into the lungs. The intercostal muscles, which are between the ribs, assist in the inflation and deflation of the thoracic cavity during that process as well. This concerted action maintains optimum lung function, allowing efficient gas exchange. In addition, the entire process of respiration is facilitated by various reflex mechanisms that help maintain the airways and promote efficient airflow, thereby maintaining the integrity of gas exchange in the face of environmental adversity. Additionally, the respiratory system exhibits excellent adaptations that enable various physiological states, particularly in high-altitude environments where oxygen is scarce. Most notably, birds have evolved specialized respiratory systems that enable them to thrive in hypoxic environments. As explained in research, birds perform adaptations along their pulmonary and circulatory systems to optimize oxygen uptake at a minimum cost of energy on flight, particularly in migratory patterns at high altitudes (Altshuler et al., 2006). These types of adaptations are representative of the plasticity of respiratory systems and illustrate how environmental demands affect physiological adaptation. Additionally, age brings about structural and physiological alterations that may affect lung function, including reduced elasticity and changes in airways, which can increase the incidence of conditions such as COPD (Ebejer et al., 1999). The reader should be able to value the complexities of the elements of the respiratory system and the way they function in maintaining normal physiology by understanding these parameters.

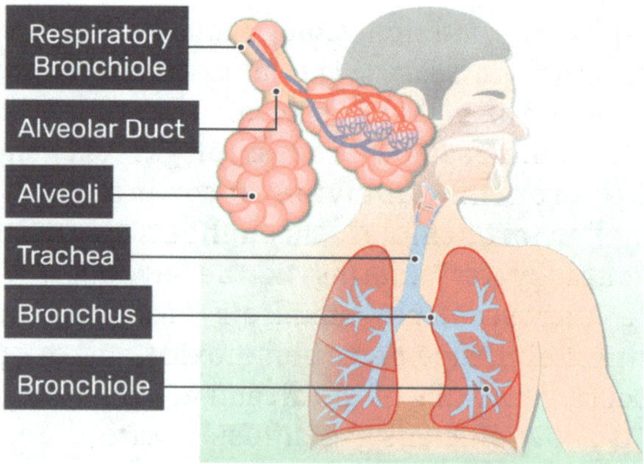

Figure 3.4. Major components of the respiratory system.

Source: https://www.getbodysmart.com/wp-content/uploads/2017/09/Respiratory-lower-tract-1024x732.png

3.1.2. Structure and Function of the Lungs

Lungs are the primary organs of the respiratory system that facilitate gas exchange, a vital process required for survival. They are anatomically divided into lobes, with three for the right lung and two lobes for the left lung, consistent with the location of the heart. The asymmetrical arrangement not only accommodates space for the placement of the hearts but also enables efficient surface area for gas exchange. The alveoli, tiny air, are the primary locations for oxygen and carbon dioxide exchange. Surrounding each alveolus is a close network of capillaries, which form a suitable mechanism for gases to be diffused through. This remarkable structure highlights the lungs' role in maintaining homeostasis, absorbing oxygen required for metabolic reactions and removing carbon dioxide, a byproduct of these reactions, thereby regulating the body's acid-base balance and supporting cellular respiration. An integrated cooperation of various physiological mechanisms regulates the functioning of the lungs. Ventilation, or the movement of air into and out of the lungs, occurs through inhalation and exhalation, a process primarily initiated by the diaphragm and intercostal muscles. During inhalation, the diaphragm relaxes, expanding the thoracic cavity and reducing intrapulmonary pressure, allowing air to enter the lungs. During exhalation, these muscles relax, and elastic recoil of the lung tissue assists in expelling air. This dynamic process is also facilitated by surfactant, a substance that reduces alveolar surface tension, preventing the alveoli from collapsing and facilitating effective gas exchange. Understanding such a function is essential because it highlights the subtle balance required for effective pulmonary function and how this relies on overall respiratory health within the context of normal respiratory physiology. Current advances in imaging techniques have significantly enhanced our understanding of the functional and structural properties of the lungs. For instance, the application of micro-computed tomography (micro-CT) enables researchers to visualize the arteries' architectures in great detail and obtain valuable information about their distensibility and mechanics. Such techniques have played a crucial role in studying diseases such as chronic hypoxia-induced pulmonary hypertension, where the pulmonary vasculature undergoes structural alterations. Through high-resolution imaging and subsequent evaluation, researchers can quantify changes in the mechanical properties of pulmonary vessels, thereby gaining useful information regarding the effect of pathologies on lung structure and function. The integration of imaging technology within the discipline of respiratory physiology not only broadens the area of pulmonary disease mechanics but also facilitates focused therapeutic interventions for lung disease, thereby enhancing the role of structure in function in the respiratory system (Dawson et al., 2000; Dawson et al., 2004).

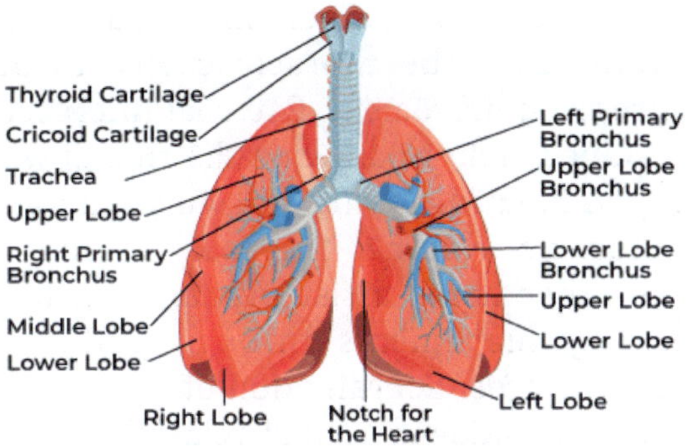

Figure 3.5. Structure and function of the lungs.

Source: https://media.geeksforgeeks.org/wp-content/uploads/20240221123034/Human-Lung.png

3.1.3. Role of the Diaphragm and Intercostal Muscles

Within the context of regular respiratory physiology, the diaphragm and intercostal muscles are the main facilitators of respiration. The diaphragm, a dome-shaped muscle located at the bottom of the thoracic cavity, contracts during inhalation, generating a negative pressure within the thoracic cavity that draws air into the lungs. Neural signals primarily drive this contraction, making efficient neuromechanical coupling essential for maximizing respiratory ability. The relationship between the activity of the diaphragm and intrathoracic pressure dynamics is of utmost significance; as the diaphragm descends, it not only expands the thoracic volume but also augments the mechanical advantage of the respiratory apparatus to deliver greater tidal volume and to enable effective gas exchange. The understanding of this relationship brings out the diaphragm's central role in maintaining healthy respiratory mechanics, particularly in pathologic conditions where neuromuscular functioning is compromised. In addition to the diaphragm, the intercostal muscles play a crucial role in breathing, particularly during forced breathing exercises. These are the muscles that lie between your ribs and assist in expanding and decreasing the volume of the thoracic cavity through synchronized movement. External intercostals, for instance, help in drawing the ribs upwards during inhalation, which in turn increases the thoracic volume. Internal intercostals, on the other hand, assist primarily in forced expiratory movements through pulling the ribs downwards. Coordination of these muscle groups is essential; in normal, relaxed breathing, a synergistic pattern exists, maximizing flow and pressure control within the lungs. Research has examined the interaction between invasive and non-invasive measures of this muscle activity, emphasizing the need to understand function in evaluating respiratory mechanics in both the healthy and compromised lungs (Petrocelli et al., 2019; Jané Campos et al., 2018). In addition, the measurement of inspiratory muscle function, including the intercostal muscles and the diaphragm, has advanced with the development of both invasive and non-invasive techniques. Invasive techniques, such as crural diaphragm electromyography and transdiaphragmatic pressure measurement, remain the gold standard for measuring respiration-induced muscle activity. Non-invasive techniques, such as mechanomyography and surface electromyography, are newly introduced alternatives to invasive measurement methods for assessing muscle function with minimal risks. Recent findings have demonstrated solid correlations between these non-invasive measures and traditional gold standards, and their clinical application has been emphasized (Jané Campos et al., 2018; Petrocelli et al., 2019). These developments in the quantification of respiratory muscle dynamics underscore the complex nature of these muscle groups in lung activity and their importance in explaining and treating most respiratory diseases.

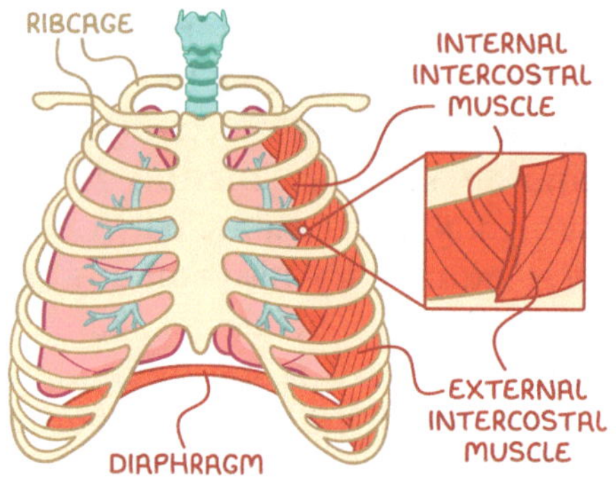

Figure 3.6. Role of the diaphragm and intercostal muscles.

Source: https://s3.eu-west-2.amazonaws.com/elements.cognitoedu.org/0b53e062-d17e-4b62-b88e-5513f94c3b3a/ribcage-muscles-ventilation-diagram.png

Test Your Knowledge

1. What are the major components of the respiratory system?

What are the roles of the diaphragm and intercostal muscles?

3.2. Mechanics of Breathing

Learning Outcome

1. Inhalation and exhalation processes
2. Role of pressure gradients in respiration
3. Factors affecting lung compliance and resistance

The mechanics of breathing are a precise interaction between numerous structures of the respiratory system, the most important of which are the lungs, chest wall, and diaphragm. The diaphragm is the primary muscle of respiration, contracting to create a negative pressure in the thoracic cavity and allowing air to enter the lungs. Chest wall compliance, or its ability to stretch and accommodate changes in lung volume, is crucial to this process. Chest wall compliance changes can substantially influence the effectiveness of inhalation and exhalation. To illustrate, in extremely severe conditions, such as in very preterm infants, decreased chest wall stiffness can impair the development of sufficient intrathoracic pressure for adequate ventilation and lead to severe respiratory impairment (Brandes et al., 2018). Availability of lung ventilation models enabled researchers to describe the dynamics of respiratory mechanics better. Through a continuum poroelastic model, these models simulate the interaction between the airway tree and lung parenchyma, providing useful insights into the response of lung tissue under varying physiological conditions. Through numerical simulation, scientists can observe how airway constriction, reduction in tissue elasticity, and other mechanisms affect ventilation efficiency and the distribution of alveolar pressure. These models are crucial in understanding the mechanics of healthy lung function as well as diseased states such as chronic obstructive pulmonary disease and pulmonary fibrosis. The capability to model these interactions enables us to gain a better understanding of respiratory mechanics, which facilitates more effective diagnostic and therapeutic interventions (Berger et al., 2015).

Furthermore, understanding breathing mechanics is crucial in developing non-invasive respiratory support for vulnerable populations, such as preterm infants. These difficulties emphasize the importance of characterizing chest wall mechanics as well as overall respiratory system dynamics. New modeling methods enable researchers to investigate how interventions, such as continuous positive airway pressure (CPAP), can help maintain lung volume while also enhancing pulmonary function in the setting of increased chest wall compliance. By incorporating parameters such as laryngeal braking into these models, scientists can predict the impact of interventions on breathing efficiency and tissue health. Therefore, this research not only contributes to theoretical knowledge but also gains immense clinical importance in the treatment of respiratory ailments in vulnerable populations (Brandes et al., 2018).

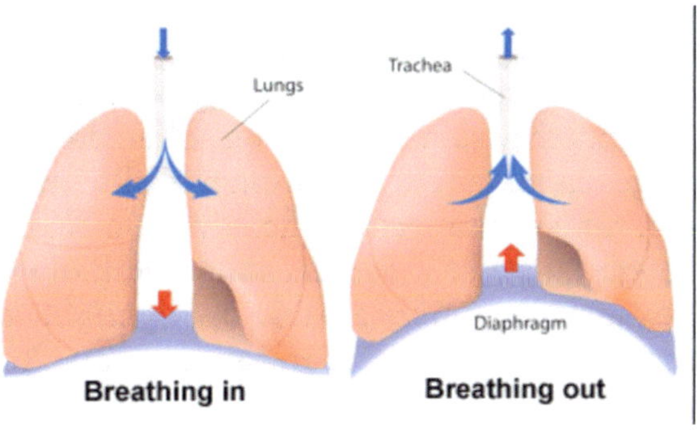

Figure 3.7. Mechanics of breathing.

Source: https://teachpe.com/images/anatomy-physiology/breathing-mechanics356.jpg

3.2.1. Inhalation and Exhalation Processes

Inhalation and exhalation are crucial components of the complex physiology of the normal respiratory process. Active is inhalation, or inspiration, where the diaphragm tightens and intercostal muscles cause the thoracic cavity to move outward, decreasing intrathoracic pressure. The pressure gradient enables air in the environment to flow into the lungs and fill alveoli with oxygen-rich air for gas exchange. The efficiency of this process largely depends on factors such as airway resistance and lung compliance, as increased resistance or decreased compliance may impede airflow (Lancmanová et al., 2024). Understanding inhalation mechanics in the diagnosis of respiratory disorders, as well as for optimal oxygen delivery in clinical settings, is thus crucial, and the importance of maintaining proper respiratory function for optimal health becomes apparent. Exhalation, or expiration, can be separated into active and passive phases. During passive expiration, the intercostal muscles and diaphragm relax, allowing the lungs to recoil automatically due to their elastic properties. This results in increased intrathoracic pressure, which pushes air containing carbon dioxide out of the lungs. Active exhalation involves muscular effort, typically during vigorous exercise, through abdominal and internal intercostal muscles that push air out. The physiology of exhalation highlights the respiratory system's sensitivity to changes in metabolic requirements, illustrating the organism's capacity to achieve homeostasis through successful gas exchange. Pathologies of exhalation, such as COPD, highlight the importance of an understanding of these mechanisms for intact respiratory function and management of respiratory conditions (Bosma et al., 2023). Breakthroughs in computational simulations of airflow dynamics in recent years have provided significant contributions to the knowledge on inhalation and exhalation dynamics. Computational simulations using the Reynolds-Averaged Navier-Stokes equations have been successful in simulating turbulent airflow in the human upper airways, resulting in a major improvement in respiratory mechanics during normal breathing (Lancmanová et al., 2024). Such investigations prioritize the precise imitation of physiological situations to expand the understanding of airflow behavior, which is critical to the development of successful treatments for respiratory diseases. The simulations not only enable the determination of complex interactions between airflow patterns and respiratory physiology but also create a platform for future investigations into more intricate parameters, such as time-dependent effects and nonuniform flow rates. By further studying these processes, clinical practices can be enhanced, ultimately improving patient outcomes and quality of life in patients with respiratory complications.

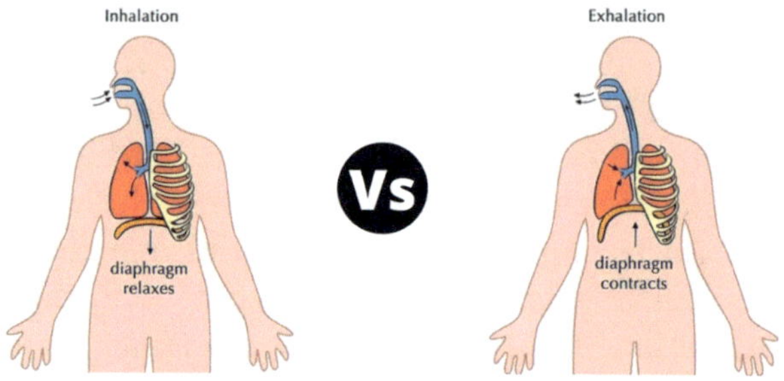

Figure 3.8. Inhalation and exhalation processes.

Source: https://biologynotesonline.com/wp-content/uploads/2022/01/Inhalation-vs-Exhalation-scaled-1.jpg

3.2.2. Role of Pressure Gradients in Respiration

The respiratory process is greatly dependent on the complex dynamics of pressure gradients that allow air to enter and exit the lungs. During inhalation, intrathoracic pressure decreases as the diaphragm and intercostal muscles contract, establishing a pressure gradient between atmospheric pressure and the pressure within the thoracic cavity. This pressure gradient allows air to flow from an area of higher pressure (the atmosphere) to an area of lower pressure (the lungs). This understanding helps shed light on the underlying mechanisms of ventilation, as alterations in pressure have a significant impact on lung inflation and the overall economy of gas exchange. Therefore, understanding pressure gradients is fundamental to comprehending the broader aspects of pulmonary physiology, i.e., how other factors affect respiratory mechanics. Exhalation, on the other hand, induces a shift in mechanics and reversal of pressure gradients. Relaxed diaphragm and intercostals raise intrathoracic pressure and push air out of the lungs back into the environment. Understanding these pressure forces is significant for research conditions such as obstructive lung disease, which can annihilate normal pressure gradients and interfere with airflow. For cases where airway resistance is high, such as in asthma or Chronic Obstructive Pulmonary Disease (COPD), the lungs can struggle to generate suitable pressure gradients for effective exhalation. This disruption is adequate to decrease the effectiveness of carbon dioxide removal from the blood, demonstrating the significance that pressure gradients play in maximizing respiratory function and overall body homeostasis. The physiological reaction to external stimuli, such as water immersion, also demonstrates the significance of pressure gradients in respiration. For example, research has shown that immersion can alter intrathoracic pressure and, in turn, impact respiratory mechanics, thereby supporting the notion that external pressure conditions profoundly affect intrapulmonary pressure dynamics (Dorchak et al.). Furthermore, the interaction of cardiovascular systems with the respiratory process is also under non-periodic flow phenomena because arterial pressures can vary due to various physiological changes further underlining the complexity of pressure gradient effects in respiratory processes (Figueroa et al., 2010). This awareness underscores the necessity of considering the knowledge of pressure gradients in various physiological contexts to gain a more comprehensive understanding of normal respiratory physiology and its abnormalities.

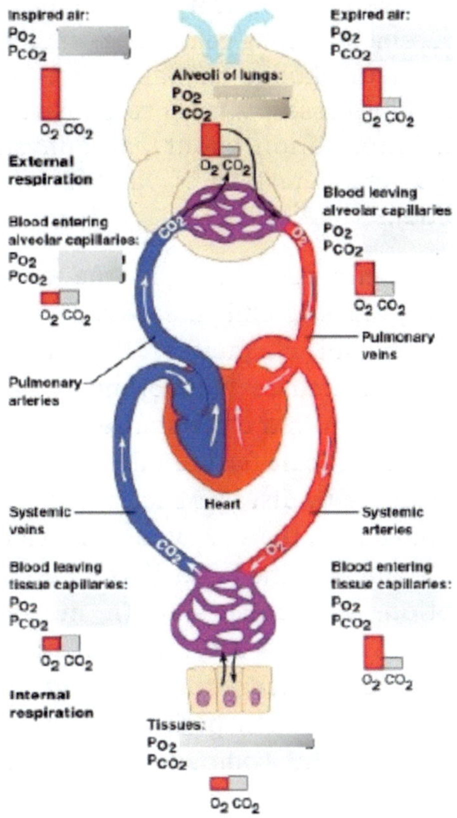

Figure 3.9. Role of pressure gradients in respiration.

Source: https://o.quizlet.com/CYtuJAmLVEEsRl7upXBhDQ_b.png

3.2.3. Factors Affecting Lung Compliance and Resistance

Lung compliance, the ability of the lung to expand and relax, is measured by numerous physiological and pathological conditions. A primary one is surfactant secretion, which lowers surface tension at the alveolar level, allowing the lung to inflate more easily. Conditions such as neonatal respiratory distress syndrome may result from surfactant deficiency with resultant decreased lung compliance. Moreover, the elastic properties of lung tissue, which are influenced by age and disease, also play a significant role. For instance, pulmonary fibrosis leads to stiffening of lung tissue, further decreasing compliance and altering respiratory mechanics. In the measurement of lung compliance, methods such as the methacholine challenge test (MCT) are employed to assess airway responsiveness and reveal information about pathophysiological changes characteristic of various respiratory conditions (N/A, 2024).

Systemic resistance in the respiratory pathway is instead measured by airway diameter and elasticity. When the airway diameter decreases with bronchoconstriction or inflammation, the resistance increases, and it is more difficult for the air to flow. This can be illustrated by diseases such as asthma, where inflammation of the airways and hyperreactivity cause significant increases in resistance. Mucus secretion, bronchial smooth muscle tone, and airway edema are also causative factors for this resistance. Moreover, the fact that collateral ventilation pathways exist provides insight into the compensatory mechanisms of the lung when there is obstruction. These pathways can maintain gas exchange during regional occlusion of the airway, thus reducing the cumulative impact of increased resistance (Delaunois, 1989). How each of these factors interacts to affect airway resistance is essential in effectively treating most respiratory illnesses. Compliance and resistance are interrelated in normal respiratory physiology; changes in one can significantly affect the other. For example, increased resistance can lead to more substantial inspiratory efforts, which may raise compliance of the lungs, but high demand can render respiratory muscles fatigued after some time. Such balance is critical during exercise, where increased ventilation demand requires efficient lung mechanics. Disorders affecting only one mechanism, such as restrictive lung disease, may produce abnormal dynamics in both compliance and resistance. As the body responds to maintain homeostasis, it is essential to understand how these two factors interact to diagnose and treat respiratory diseases effectively. The interaction between lung compliance and resistance also highlights the complexity of respiratory physiology in both disease and health, demonstrating that more than one factor needs to be considered when conducting a clinical assessment (N/A, 2024).

Test Your Knowledge

1. Discuss inhalation and exhalation processes.
2. What are the factors affecting lung compliance and resistance?

3.3. Gas Exchange

Learning Outcome

1. Mechanism of diffusion in alveoli
2. Role of hemoglobin in oxygen transport
3. Carbon dioxide transport and elimination

In everyday respiratory physiology, gas exchange plays a primary role in the homeostasis of the human body. It occurs predominantly in the alveoli, where oxygen in the inspired air is transferred into the blood, and carbon dioxide, a waste product of metabolism, moves in the opposite direction. Gas exchange effectiveness is governed by several factors, including the surface area available for diffusion and gas concentration gradients. These must be preserved, and one example is that the partial pressure of oxygen must be higher in alveolar air than in venous blood to permit its uptake. Furthermore, effective gas exchange is essential for supplying tissues with sufficient oxygen, supporting cellular metabolism, and maintaining blood pH levels by eliminating carbon dioxide.

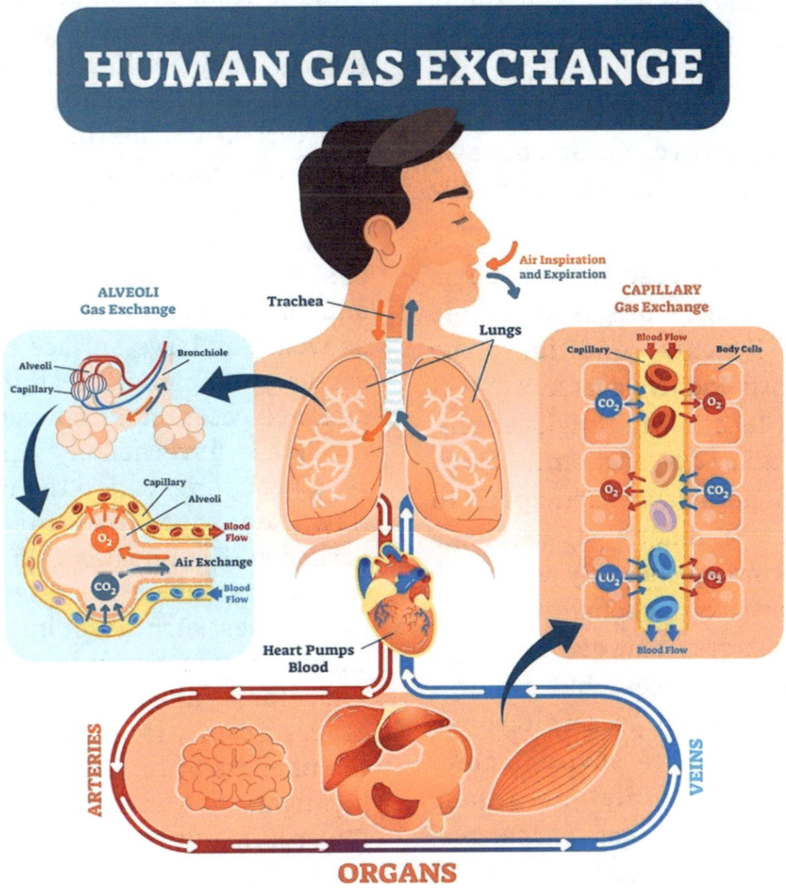

Figure 3.10. Gas exchange.

Source: https://www.mrgscience.com/uploads/2/0/7/9/20796234/published/content-human-gas-exchange-system-vector-illustration-oxygen-travel-from-lungs-to-heart-to-all-body-cells-and-back-to-lungs-as-CO_2-948356058-962x1094-1.jpeg?1679074098

The mechanical role of respiration is also equally important in facilitating efficient gas exchange. The mechanism includes inhalation that lowers intrathoracic pressure, raising venous return to the heart, and maximizing cardiac output to enable efficient gas exchange. A delicate balance has been observed in the respiratory pump, where a controlled intrathoracic pressure gradient, ideally less than −10 cmH2O, provides maximal cardiovascular performance while minimizing unwanted hemodynamic effects from excessive variations in intrathoracic pressure, as evidenced by recent literature. The coordination of respiratory mechanics and cardiovascular physiology underscores the necessity of an integrated system of these organs for overall respiratory health. Physiological processes that control gas exchange not only facilitate respiration but also highlight the interdependence of different bodily functions.

In addition, the body's reaction to hypoxia underscores the flexibility of gas exchange processes. During hypoxic conditions, the upregulation of hypoxia-inducible factors (HIFs) is to control immune function and angiogenesis, thereby maintaining tissue oxygenation. Research suggests that such pathways participate in inflammatory processes, linking gas exchange to broader systemic consequences. By regulating gene expression during oxygen homeostasis, the HIF pathway demonstrates that gas exchange is not merely a physical process, but rather a highly advanced biochemical process through which the body can adapt to environmental variations. Having such intricate interactions provides understanding for gas exchanges' crucial role in normal respiratory physiology, ensuring ongoing oxygen delivery at rest and during exercise, and thus its significance beyond just basic breathing (Watts et al., 2018; Convertino, 2019).

3.3.1. Mechanism of Diffusion in Alveoli

Alveolar diffusion is necessary for gas exchange to occur, a vital component of normal respiratory physiology. Alveoli, the tiny air bubbles of the lungs, are specially constructed to optimize this function, with a vast amount of surface area and a thin membrane between the blood and air. Oxygen, when it enters the alveoli during inhalation, moves through the alveolar membrane into the blood of the capillaries, where it becomes bound to the hemoglobin in red blood cells. Carbon dioxide, the waste byproduct of metabolic functions, is a gas that diffuses from the blood into the alveoli to be exhaled. This gas exchange is primarily achieved through simple diffusion, with the influence of differences in the partial pressures of oxygen and carbon dioxide between alveolar air and capillary blood illustrating the principles of passive transport in biological systems. Furthermore, diffusion is affected by the level of surface area, the thickness of the membrane, and the concentration gradients of the gases as well. The large surface area of the alveolar capillary complex and its thin walls decrease the distance gases must diffuse. This relationship is further governed by ventilation-perfusion (V/Q) coupling, where the ratio of air to blood flow rates optimizes the efficiency of gas exchange. The imbalance in V/Q ratios actually causes inefficient gas exchange, as observed in diseases such as pulmonary embolism or chronic obstructive pulmonary disease (COPD). Therefore, understanding the diffusional processes in the alveoli not only illustrates the fineness of respiratory physiology but also highlights the importance of these processes towards maintaining the body's homeostasis. Revolutionary research being conducted is further clarifying our understanding of the mechanics of gas exchange in the alveoli, utilizing mathematical models to measure variables that affect diffusion. For instance, recent work demonstrates that determinants such as respiratory patterns and the composition of soluble gases in exhaled breath influence the gas exchange values obtained. A model, for instance, relates end-tidal breath concentrations to systemic blood levels of volatile organic compounds (VOCs), extending beyond classical models like the Farhi equation, and highlights the physiological complexities of alveolar gas exchange. Current findings indicate that gas exchange across the airways is primarily responsible for concentration changes in the breath during varying levels of activity, thereby underscoring the significance of the alveolar microclimate in respiratory physiology. We are also capable of learning more about such factors and their application in disease and health management, particularly in the detection and treatment of respiratory disease (Amann et al., 2010, 2011).

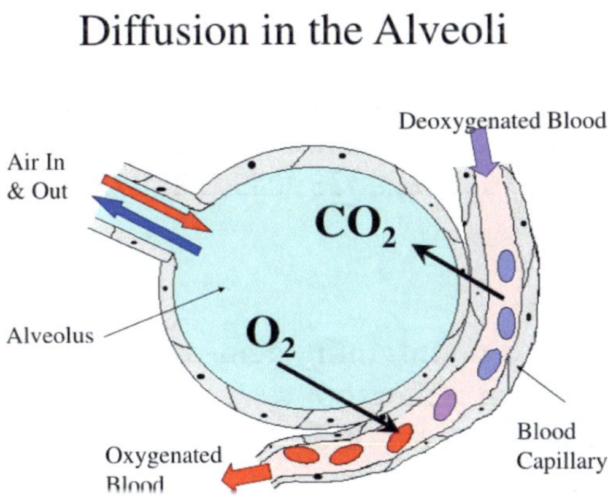

Figure 3.11. Mechanism of diffusion in alveoli.

Source: https://external-content.duckduckgo.com/iu/?u=https%3A%2F%2Fimage2.slideserve.com%2F3869286%2Fdiffusion-in-the-alveoli-n.jpg&f=1&nofb=1&ipt=5ea1d9b95b385e7fe45c340c62fc71f6f0d3940137073e5665e4e7dd09bc0144

3.3.2. Role of Hemoglobin in Oxygen Transport

The role of hemoglobin in oxygen transport is a fundamental aspect of normal respiratory physiology, as it is the primary protein responsible for the delivery of oxygen from the lungs to tissues. Hemoglobin, within red blood cells, sequesters oxygen molecules at higher partial pressures within the lungs, where oxygen is in abundance. It is achieved through a process known as cooperative binding; each oxygen molecule binds to hemoglobin, enhancing the affinity of hemoglobin for further oxygen molecules. This allows not only for the maximal uptake of oxygen but also for the sufficient provision of oxygen to meet the metabolic demands of various tissues. The efficiency of this oxygen delivery system is one of the most crucial parameters in maintaining cellular homeostasis, particularly in organs that require high oxygen tensions, such as the heart and brain. Moreover, hemoglobin's affinity for oxygen is significantly influenced by various physiological states, including pH level, temperature, and carbon dioxide levels. For instance, during highly active metabolism, storage of carbon dioxide and lactic acid in the blood causes a decrease in pH, an effect known as the Bohr effect. This results in a decreased hemoglobin affinity for oxygen, leading to increased oxygen release in metabolically active tissues. Furthermore, elevated temperatures, typically associated with increased metabolic rates, increase oxygen unloading from hemoglobin. These adaptive processes reflect the intricate interaction between hemoglobin's function and the organism's needs, illustrating the essential role of hemoglobin in successfully adapting to the organism's metabolic status. In pathologic conditions such as hypertension, however, the importance of hemoglobin's role in oxygen delivery is even more emphasized. It has been found that conditions such as essential hypertension alter microcirculation processes, hence affecting tissue oxygen consumption. One study prominently demonstrated that spontaneously hypertensive rats possessed a higher maximum rate of oxygen consumption (VO_2) compared to normotensive rats, which indicated an impairment of normal hemoglobin oxygen delivery-mitochondrial function coupling. Such observations point to the fact that the oxygen transport regulatory mechanisms, like hemoglobin's binding properties, need to be viewed within the broad physiological context, in which factors such as acid-base status and microcirculatory sufficiency get intertwined with tissue oxygenation (White et al.; Shah et al., 2017).

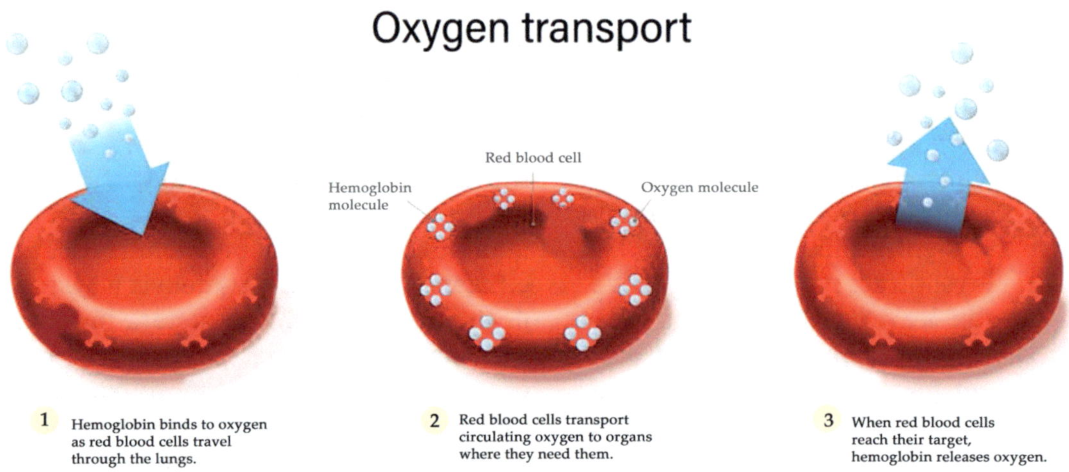

Figure 3.12. Role of hemoglobin in oxygen transport.

Source: https://external-content.duckduckgo.com/iu/?u=https%3A%2F%2Fas1.ftcdn.net%2Fv2%2Fjpg%2F05%2F65%2F82%2F50%2F1000_F_565825079_olkI9gqwD8oldmi04m7i6kQGGEvhj3My.jpg&f=1&nofb=1&ipt=ec82d9bf383b3a6f68259a0d5e491b7ed576e89eaab239ca58521b7374442d89

3.3.3. Carbon Dioxide Transport and Elimination

Transport and removal of carbon dioxide (CO_2) are crucial to maintaining acid-base balance and normal respiratory physiology. After carbon dioxide is formed as a metabolic waste product during cellular respiration, it is diffused from the tissues into the blood. Most of CO_2 (approximately 70%) is carried in the form of bicarbonate ions (HCO3-) generated by an enzymatic reaction catalyzed by carbonic anhydrase. This process not only facilitates efficient transport but also helps buffer blood pH, allowing the body to remain in a state of homeostasis. The excess CO_2 is either physically dissolved in plasma or bound to hemoglobin, facilitating efficient CO_2 delivery to the lungs for exhalation. This intricate system highlights the fundamental interdependence between metabolism, gas exchange, and respiratory function in order to maintain physiological equilibrium within the human body. Once CO_2 has passed through pulmonary capillaries, it diffuses into the alveoli, where body removal through exhalation occurs. It is necessary since the alveolar air and blood concentration gradient results in diffusion of CO_2 out of the bloodstream. The process is enhanced by the large alveolar surface area, as well as the thin alveolar-capillary membrane barrier, which minimizes the diffusion distance. Additionally, a suitable ventilation-perfusion ratio is necessary to facilitate effective gas exchange. Airway resistance and lung compliance can affect the ratio, potentially leading to ventilatory complications. In explaining the conditions that impair elimination of CO_2, the dynamics involved must be appreciated, and how they may undermine homeostasis and result in a range of physiological disturbances. Apart from its role in respiratory physiology, transport and removal of CO_2 are also crucial for systemic physiology. CO_2 concentration has a direct effect on the pH of blood, and thus any defect in its transport and removal is a critical aspect of the prevention of acid-base imbalance. Defects in CO_2 transport and removal may lead to respiratory acidosis or alkalosis, abnormalities resulting from defective respiratory or metabolic derangements, respectively. Consistently, the body can compensate with processes like changing the rate and depth of breathing to offset such imbalances. Moreover, recent evidence also suggests that CO2's interaction with reactive species implicates CO2 levels in influencing tissue responses to oxidative stress, further highlighting its intricacy in normal physiology (cite29, cite30). This complex relationship underscores the importance of effective CO2 control in maintaining respiratory health and preventing disease.

Test Your Knowledge

1. Explore the mechanism of diffusion in alveoli.
2. What is the role of hemoglobin in oxygen transport?

3.4. Regulation of Breathing

Learning Outcome

1. Neural control of respiration
2. Chemical regulation through blood gases
3. Reflexes involved in respiratory control

The regulation of breathing is a complex and dynamic function critical to the support of homeostasis within the body. The physiological process involved in this is under the control of the central nervous system, which regulates respiratory rhythms through a group of neurons in the brainstem. These neurons respond to various stimuli, such as changes in blood carbon dioxide and oxygen levels, allowing breathing patterns to adjust and accommodate the body's metabolic demands. During physical exertion, for example, the rate and depth of breathing are increased to supply more oxygen and remove more carbon dioxide. It is essential to understand the intricacies of these neural control mechanisms, as alterations could lead to respiratory disease, which in turn impacts overall health and wellness. Therefore, a thorough understanding of these control mechanisms is crucial for studying normal respiratory physiology. In addition to neural control, breathing is also regulated by various biochemical variables that govern respiratory function. The peripheral and central chemoreceptors are interconnected to detect variations in blood gases, particularly carbon dioxide and pH levels. When there is a rise in the concentration of carbon dioxide or a decrease in pH, these chemoreceptors send signals to the brain's respiratory centers, which cause an elevation in the respiratory rate. This response is essential not only for ensuring adequate gas exchange but also for the prevention of respiratory acidosis and maintenance of acid-base balance in the body. Moreover, recent research emphasizes the significance of intracellular mechanisms, including mitochondrial respiratory pathways, in modulating the impact of respiration on cardiac rhythm and blood pressure regulation at various stages of respiration. These observations highlight the interrelationship between respiratory physiology and other physiological functions, as well as their contribution to health disorders, including breathing diseases and stress-related conditions (Barnes et al., 2014). Moreover, the participation of the neurotransmitter systems, particularly serotonin, in playing a central role in controlling respiration is also elucidated. The role of serotonin is best demonstrated in disorders such as Rett syndrome, where deficiencies in serotonergic function may result in severe autonomic perturbations, manifesting as irregular patterns of breathing and hyperventilation or apneic spells (Abdala et al., 2014). Such perturbations reinforce the necessity of studying neurotransmitter dynamics in modulating regular respiratory activity. Novel therapeutic strategies targeting elevated serotonergic activity, particularly the utilization of biased agonists, hold promise for alleviating respiratory distress and enhancing overall respiratory well-being. This new perspective on the interconnectivity between neurotransmission and respiration broadens the scope of what is known about mechanisms that govern normal respiratory physiology, ushering in new forms of therapy for respiratory dysfunction as well as related disorders.

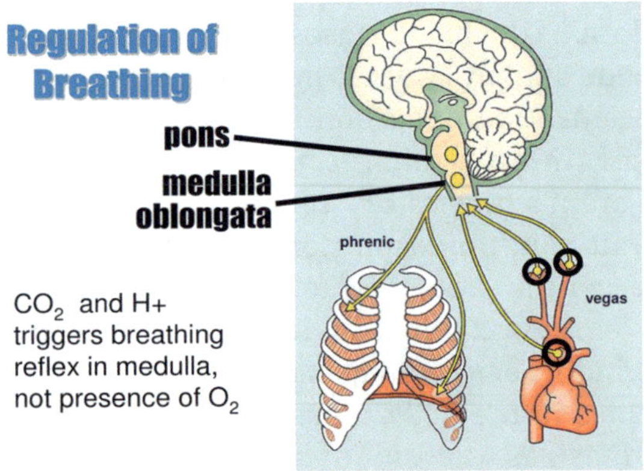

Figure 3.13. Regulation of breathing.

Source: https://external-content.duckduckgo.com/iu/?u=https%3A%2F%2Fimage1.slideserve.com%2F1779231%2Fregulation-of-breathing-l.jpg&f=1&nofb=1&ipt=f4768960c8b843cc0847a2cef7fc041cebd0726b082c24eeb3d153fb8c10ce99

3.4.1. Neural Control of Respiration

The neural regulation of respiration is an intricate process involving more than one interconnected network within the central nervous system. The brainstem houses central centers that play a fundamental role in regulating the rhythmic pattern of breathing, including medulla oblongata and pons. The ventral respiratory column (VRC), comprising the preBötzinger complex, is a localized area that generates respiratory rhythms within the medulla. These neuronal populations coordinate the muscular contractions required for inhalation and exhalation through diverse motoneuron outputs. Peripheral receptor feedback, such as from chemoreceptors, also adjusts respiratory patterns based on the levels of oxygen and carbon dioxide in blood to provide homeostasis during dynamic exercise, such as rest or exercise. Such an integrated mechanism is a model of the neural basis of normal respiratory physiology under which the body is able to adapt to varying demands of the external environment. Neural control pathway disruptions are capable of inducing severe respiratory distress, underscoring the importance of understanding these pathways. Diseases such as Late-Onset Pompe Disease (LOPD) illustrate how genetic mutations affect neuronal function, resulting in suboptimal airway clearance and respiratory deficiency. Fulleren et al. (2013) and DeRuisseau et al. (2009) describe how in LOPD, the accumulation of glycogen in the neural milieu is liable for inducing dysfunction within the neurons in the medulla, thereby decreasing inspiratory neuron activity. The interaction among respiratory motoneurons is thus disrupted, leading to inefficient coughing responses as well as impaired lung ventilation. The implications of such studies present significant questions about the neuropathophysiological mechanisms liable for inducing respiratory insufficiencies. Understanding these dysfunctions can provide insight into targeted therapeutic interventions for the management of respiratory-related illnesses. In addition, the role of endogenous opioids in respiration adds another layer of complexity to neural control. Opioid-induced respiratory depression (OIRD) provides a prime example of how exogenous substances can alter the standard respiratory drive significantly. Research in the activity of mu-opioid receptors (MORs) in the VRC has shown that activation can lead to a significant decline in respiratory volume and rate, primarily under conditions of overdose. Penk+ neuron experiments in the preBötzinger complex shed light on the key role of enkephalin in maintaining respiratory stability. Pharmacological modulation studies indicate that, while enkephalinergic signaling is a part of respiratory rhythm, it's not via direct MOR routes but via glutamatergic pathways. The comprehension of the highly intricate interaction of opioids within the respiratory neural circuits guides not only clinical effects for treatment of overdose but also indicates possible targets for therapeutic intervention in the prevention of OIRD and thereby enhancement of respiratory performance during pathological conditions.

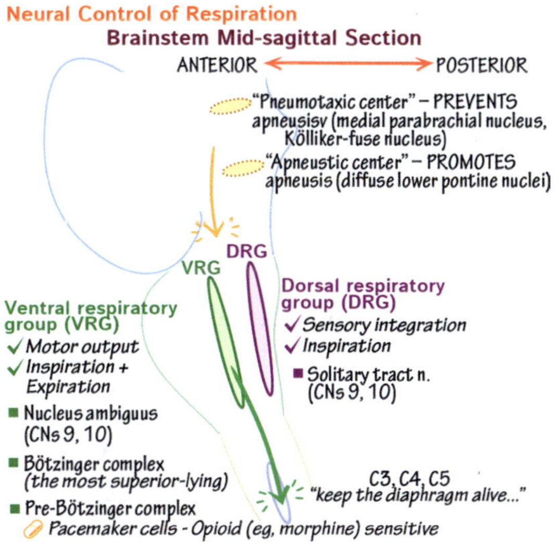

Figure 3.14. Neural control of respiration.

Source: https://d1j63owfs0b5j3.cloudfront.net/term/images/neural-control-of-respiration-5643.png

3.4.2. Chemical Regulation Through Blood Gases

The delicate balance of blood gases plays a crucial role in the chemical control of respiration, thereby serving as the interface between metabolic function and respiratory function. Concentrations of oxygen (O_2) and carbon dioxide (CO_2) regulate depth and rate of ventilation through several mechanisms. When cellular metabolism increases, such as during exercise, CO2 production also increases, resulting in a decrease in blood pH. This acid-base change is detected by chemoreceptors, primarily the carotid and aortic bodies, which cause an increase in respiratory rate to eliminate CO2 and normalize acid-base balance. This interaction shows how the body gains homeostasis and dynamically responds to metabolic requirements, delivering adequate oxygenation and removal of waste in accordance with usual respiratory physiology principles. The respiratory response to alterations in blood gases involves peripheral and central chemoreceptors that transmit signals to the central nervous system to initiate corresponding respiratory responses. Medulla oblongata central chemoreceptors are stimulated by input almost exclusively due to CO_2 change and resultant pH modification in cerebrospinal fluid. Peripheral chemoreceptors respond almost entirely to changes in arterial O_2 levels, with an augmented response when the partial pressure of oxygen (PaO_2) falls below a certain level. Integrated activity produced as a result modulates ventilation in proportion to metabolic requirements, thereby ensuring the efficient exchange of gases across the alveoli. These intricate mechanisms of regulation validate the function of chemical signaling in maintaining respiratory competence across a range of physiological states and activity levels, thereby ensuring cellular function and overall health in a constantly changing world. Understanding the regulation of breathing by blood gases further justifies the benefits of exercise and physical training for enhancing respiratory efficiency. Regular exercise enhances ventilatory capacity by strengthening cardiovascular health, which may maximize gas exchange and augment the delivery of oxygen to tissues. When exercising, the body's metabolic demands increase, resulting in elevated CO2 production and a subsequent decrease in blood pH. Based on current studies, the cerebral cortex plays a central role in response to physical exercise by modifying the cardiorespiratory function, demonstrating the integration of the respiratory system with neuromuscular functions (Svitlana Tymchik et al., 2021). Consequently, subjects who exercise regularly exhibit improved hypoxic responses and tolerance to high levels of CO2, illustrating the significant impact of exercise on regulating respiratory physiology and homeostasis through alterations in metabolic conditions (Kelly, 2004).

3.4.3. Reflexes Involved in Respiratory Control

Control of respiratory function ultimately relies on an accurate interplay of reflexes, which yields homeostasis within the respiratory system. Central to this is automatic respiratory control, which operates via neural loops that act as feedback systems. The loops respond to a range of stimuli, adjusting the rate and depth of respiration to meet the body's oxygen needs, much like a thermostat regulates temperature. However, beyond automaticity, reflexes also respond to behavior and emotion, demonstrating the fine control between voluntary and involuntary actions. Research indicates that specific neurons, those expressing Tac1 in the lateral parabrachial nucleus, play a crucial role in this state-dependent modulation, allowing for significant deviations from homeostatic breathing rhythms under certain conditions (Arthurs et al., 2024). Reflex mechanisms are especially evident in the regulation of muscles of the upper airway, which is vital to ensure unhindered airflow when breathing. Control of the upper airway by neural mechanisms comprises complex control with multiple reflex arcs acting in response to pressure, stretch, and chemical stimulus in the blood. Importantly, pulmonary receptors provide input on lung inflation and airway resistance that initiates reflexes to correct for optimal breathing efficiency. In addition to this, chemoreceptor reflexes also respond to changes in carbon dioxide and oxygen levels in the blood, initiating vital adjustments in the depth and rate of breathing to maintain arterial gas homeostasis. The influence of baroreceptors is also equally vital, as they control airflow to prevent potential collapsibility of the upper airway under changing physiological states, such as sleep and wakefulness (Horner, 2012). Such knowledge is not merely of theoretical interest, as it has profound implications for respiratory clinical disease.

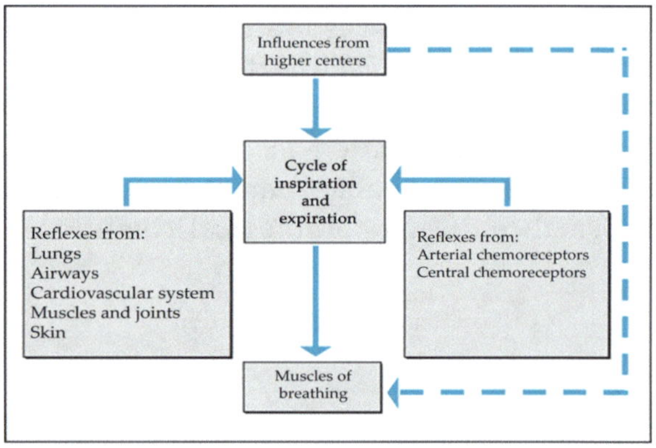

Figure 3.14. Reflexes involved in respiratory control.

Source: https://basicmedicalkey.com/wp-content/uploads/2016/06/m_levi8_c009f001.png

For instance, the disruption of these neural control mechanisms can be responsible for pathologies such as obstructive sleep apnea, where, the tone of the airway muscles is lost, leading to massive functional disabilities. Furthermore, substances such as alcohol, sedatives, and opioids also modify neural control of the upper airway to exacerbate collapsibility-related abnormalities and respiratory function. By studying the interaction of reflexes in normal respiratory physiology, science can define therapeutic targets that enhance respiratory stability and address the origins of respiratory disorders, resulting in improved patient outcomes and an increase in our understanding of respiratory health (Horner, 2012).

Test Your Knowledge

1. What is neural control of respiration?
2. What are the chemical regulations that occur through blood gases?

3.5. Respiratory Volumes and Capacities

Learning Outcome

1. Definitions of tidal volume, vital capacity, and residual volume
2. Importance of measuring lung volumes
3. Clinical significance of altered respiratory volumes

The concept of respiratory volumes and capacities is significant in considering normal respiratory physiology, as the values reflect the adequacy of the respiratory system. Various sections of lung volumes include tidal volume, inspiratory reserve volume, expiratory reserve volume, and residual volume, each of which carries a unique function in facilitating effective gas exchange. Tidal volume refers to the amount of air breathed in and out during spontaneous breathing. In contrast, inspiratory and expiratory reserve volumes refer to the extra air that can be inhaled and exhaled over tidal volume. Total lung capacity encompasses all the volumes and is highly significant in assessing overall respiratory status. Changes in these volumes can indicate pathological conditions or physiological adaptations, for example, during pregnancy, when an ever increasing uterus shifts physiological adaptations. For instance, during pregnancy, the uterus alters the diaphragmatic position, consequently diminishing lung volumes and capacities over time (Bhambhi et al., 2021).

The relationship between different lung volumes is particularly significant in clinical assessment, as it aids in the diagnosis of pulmonary disease. For instance, the forced expiratory volume in one second (FEV1) to forced vital capacity (FVC) ratio is a critical measure in determining whether a lung pattern is obstructive or restrictive. In obstructive lung function, including asthma or Chronic Obstructive Pulmonary Disease (COPD), FEV1 will usually decrease relative to FVC, indicating constricted airways that obstruct airflow. Conversely, restrictive lung diseases have reduced total lung capacities and volumes, but a normal FEV1/FVC ratio is otherwise observed. The distinction is of significant importance to clinicians to formulate accurate interventions and care plans. By examining these values, caregivers can monitor trends over time, guiding interventions to improve lung function and quality of life in affected patients (Mannino, 2021). Furthermore, the implications of respiratory volumes are not limited to clinical diagnosis but also have a significant impact on physical functioning and well-being. Proper lung capacity is crucial for sports performance because it directly influences the uptake of oxygen and the removal of carbon dioxide during physical activity. Trained athletes usually undergo training exercises that aim for the development of strength for the respiratory muscle and its efficiency, such as the Respiratory Muscle Stretch Gymnastic (RMSG). Such exercise has been found to enhance lung volumes and capacity, particularly among groups such as pregnant women, where physiological adjustments necessitate effective respiratory adjustments (Bhambhi et al., 2021). Understanding the dynamics of respiratory volume not only educates clinical practice but also widens our appreciation of the intricate interdependency between respiratory health and overall body fitness. Therefore, ongoing observation and study of such parameters remain of critical concern to health workers and those seeking to optimize their respiratory function.

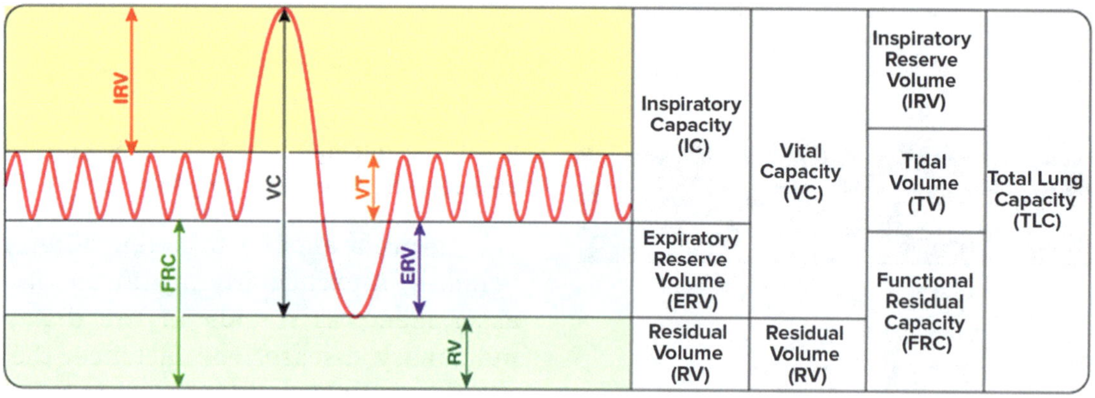

Figure 3.15. Lung volumes and capacities.

Source: https://cdn1.byjus.com/wp-content/uploads/2019/04/Lung-Volumes-and-Lung-Capacity2.png

3.5.1. Definitions of Tidal Volume, Vital Capacity, And Residual Volume

Lung volume division is essential for interpreting normal respiratory physiology, and tidal volume, vital capacity, and residual volume are crucial parameters in assessing pulmonary function. Tidal volume (TV) is the amount of air inhaled or exhaled during a resting, unforced breath. In healthy adults, the volume is usually between 500 and 600 mL per breath. This measure is significant as it measures an individual's effort and efficiency in respiration while exchanging gases. Tidal volume measurement further provides information regarding the physiological response under stressful situations, such as examinations, as supported by studies that have tested physiological indices among students subjected to significant anxiety and stressors that influence respiratory function (Suleimenova et al., 2024). Understanding tidal volume is an important essential in diagnosing and managing varied respiratory conditions, as deviations from standard measurements may indicate underlying pathophysiologic mechanisms. Vital capacity (VC) refers to the maximum amount of air that can be forcibly exhaled after maximal inspiration and comprises tidal volume, inspiratory reserve volume, and expiratory reserve volume. The parameter is essential in evaluating pulmonary function and overall respiratory status. Normal vital capacity is a predictor of function for various conditions, enabling clinicians to quantify lung mechanics and distinguish between restrictive and obstructive disease. Because dimensions like body composition and physical fitness levels can have a significant influence on vital capacity, the measurement is typically adjusted in the clinical setting to accommodate variation between patients (Nardo MD et al., 2019). Thus, an understanding of vital capacity would aid in our management of conditions like acute respiratory distress syndrome, as it requires attention to the fine balance between lung volumes and respiratory mechanics necessary for effective clinical management. Residual volume (RV) is the volume of air remaining in the lungs during maximum exhalation and is a crucial component in assessing lung function. Under resting conditions, this volume is approximately 1,200 mL in normal adults and is crucial for maintaining alveolar inflation stability and facilitating gas exchange during the respiratory cycle. Residual volume not only serves to avoid the complete collapse of alveoli but also acts as an air reservoir, and pulmonary ventilation is improved during subsequent breaths. Significantly, dramatic alterations in residual volume can indicate many pathologies, such as chronic obstructive pulmonary disease (COPD) or restrictive lung diseases, with compromised residual air dynamics (Suleimenova et al., 2024). Awareness of the relationship between tidal volume, vital capacity, and residual volume allows healthcare professionals to assess respiratory health better and develop specific treatment modalities for patients with compromised ventilation.

3.5.2 Significance of lung volume measurement

Lung volume measurement is significant for the study of respiratory physiology and the diagnosis of many pulmonary diseases. Lung volume quantification refers to the functional ability of the respiratory system, allowing medical practitioners to assess the presence and severity of conditions such as chronic obstructive pulmonary disease (COPD), restrictive lung disease, and asthma. Through the measurement of parameters such as tidal volume, vital capacity, and residual volume, clinicians can identify abnormalities in lung function that may uncover hidden pathologies. Quantitative measurement forms the basis of respiratory care, guiding therapy and disease surveillance. Furthermore, measuring lung volume can aid in assessing patient response to therapy, optimizing management strategies, and improving patient outcomes. In situations like acute respiratory failure, the relevance of lung volume measurement is yet more increased. The exacerbation of COPD and acute respiratory distress syndrome (ARDS) necessitates precise measurements of lung function to direct the application of therapies such as noninvasive mechanical ventilation (NIV) (Rochwerg et al., 2017). NIV is now a necessary intervention for the treatment of respiratory failure, particularly in patients with evidence of abnormal lung volumes due to disease states. An understanding of these measurements allows clinicians to tailor ventilation parameters for the prevention of ventilator-induced lung injury while ensuring adequate gas exchange. Accurate measurement of lung volumes can further be utilized to establish patient needs for supportive therapy and weaning strategies, ultimately translating to enhanced patient safety and outcome. Additionally, measuring lung volumes helps establish the risk of complications from respiratory interventions. In ventilated patients, large tidal volumes can lead to ventilator-associated lung injury, a key concern that necessitates careful monitoring of lung compliance and volume (Brochard et al., 2016). Through observation of lung volumes, healthcare providers can implement lung-protective measures and adjust ventilatory settings to prevent injury due to excessive transpulmonary pressure swings. This represents aggressive management of the respiratory system, highlighting the cardinal application of lung volume measurement in both diagnosis and the dynamic regulation of therapeutic interventions. Thus, continuous monitoring of lung volumes is a crucial component of effective respiratory management, leading to overall improvements in patient outcomes across various clinical conditions.

3.5.3. Clinical Significance of Altered Respiratory Volumes

The clinical significance of altered respiratory volumes can be vast, particularly in defining how deviations from normal physiology may reflect underlying medical conditions. In evaluating patients in the clinical environment, measurements such as tidal volume, vital capacity, and residual volume are essential in the diagnosis of lung disease. For instance, reduced vital capacity can point towards restrictive lung disease, while increased residual volume can be a sign of obstructive disease. These respiratory volume changes not only give us insight into the mechanics of ventilation but also relate to cardiovascular effects. Research has shown that compromised respiratory volumes can enhance cardiovascular risk, particularly among populations at risk of conditions such as preterm birth, where interrupted development can result in long-term dysfunction in respiratory and cardiac function. This interdependence emphasizes the need for comprehensive assessments to manage the pulmonary and systemic effects of altered respiratory volume in clinical practice (Lewandowski, 2019). In patients with chronic anemia, respiratory compensation is particularly significant because it illustrates the interdependence of cardiac and pulmonary function. With decreased hemoglobin, the body compensates by increased cardiac output and ventilation rates, and this results in a modification of respiratory volume. This adaptive process involves the augmentation of respiratory minute volume and a reduction in vital capacity, with possible exertional dyspnea and other symptoms of respiratory distress. These compensatory mechanisms, although transiently effective, may over time become a strain on both the respiratory and cardiovascular systems, making clinical observation of respiratory volumes in such patients worthwhile. Understanding these dynamics can guide clinical interventions to be performed in a timely manner, thereby treating anemia and its pulmonary impact, and enhancing overall health outcomes for patients affected (Blumgart et al., 1948). Longitudinal studies that track shifts in respiratory capacity across different populations reveal notable patterns that merit attention from clinicians. For instance, preterm infants' alterations in lung function may lead to extreme physiological changes when adapting to life outside the womb. Preterm youths and young adults may have elevated left and right ventricular volumes due to adaptive changes following defective respiratory mechanics. This highlights a critical time for monitoring respiratory and cardiac health, as early interventions can help avoid future complications. Evidence indicates that thorough management of the changes is able to reduce the cardiovascular disease in adulthood. The relationship between respiratory function and cardiovascular disease points towards the importance of rigorous patient evaluation. Medical professionals should therefore continuously monitor individuals with altered respiratory volumes to address potential health risks ahead of time and improve overall quality of life (Lewandowski, 2019).

Test Your Knowledge

1. Give definitions of tidal volume, vital capacity, and residual volume.
2. What are the important advantages of measuring lung volumes?

3.6. Impact of Environmental Factors

Learning Outcome

1. Effects of altitude on respiratory physiology
2. Influence of pollutants and allergens
3. Adaptations to exercise and physical activity

The interaction between environmental factors plays a significant role in normal respiratory physiology, impacting lung function and overall well-being. Other environmental conditions, such as air quality, altitude, and exposure to allergens, can create alterations in respiratory mechanics and the efficiency of gas exchange. For instance, airborne contaminants such as particulate matter, ozone, and nitrogen dioxide can trigger inflammatory reactions, thereby impairing lung function. Prolonged exposure to such agents has been associated with increased risk of getting respiratory illnesses like asthma and chronic obstructive pulmonary disease (COPD). Research confirms that children who grow up in cities with poorer air quality have lower lung function scores compared to those in cleaner cities, indicating that environmental factors play a significant role in respiratory health from an early age. Notably, health disparities observed among populations exposed to various environmental conditions underscore the need for a more nuanced understanding of how factors interact with genetic predispositions and other social determinants of health. Moreover, socio-economic status has an intrinsic association with environmental exposures that affect respiratory physiology. Individuals with lower socio-economic status are likely to reside in areas with higher pollution and fewer healthcare facilities, thereby aggravating the health risks associated with poor air quality. These disparities can perpetuate a cycle of health disparities where at-risk populations have increased rates of respiratory illness compared to richer counterparts. Furthermore, specific work environments expose workers to harmful respiratory agents, such as chemical toxins and dust, which further exacerbate health disparities. Working to address these environmental factors, policies can be developed to minimize exposure and maximize public health benefits. Interestingly, ongoing research investigates the complex relationships between environmental quality, socioeconomic status, and respiratory illness, aiming to develop more effective interventions that promote healthier communities. Parallel to this is the physiological response to environmental stressors, which underscores the need for targeted public health interventions aimed at optimizing lung health. Evidence of the mechanism of environmental action, such as hypoxia signal transduction pathways, suggests that environmental factors exert an effect on immune responses and inflammatory mechanisms in the lungs. For instance, hypoxic stimuli are capable of activating specific transcription factors that determine the severity of lung inflammation, as observed in various pathological conditions. The interaction between environmental effects and these cell pathways of signaling underscores the requirement for integrated healthcare approaches that are attentive to both environmental and physiological inputs in lung health. An increased understanding of how environmental exposures and genetic susceptibilities contribute to respiratory physiology can lead to more effective prevention and therapeutic outcomes for respiratory diseases, ultimately resulting in a healthier population. The urgency to prioritize causes of the environment is brought to the fore by a study indicating that tailored interventions have the potential to significantly improve lung function and reduce the prevalence of respiratory disorders in such populations, as evidenced in congruent health disparities literature (Watts et al., 2018; Bhakta et al., 2021).

3.6.1. Effects of Altitude On Respiratory Physiology

As altitude increases, the environment around organisms in the environment becomes drastically altered, particularly in terms of respiratory physiology. The most critical change is in oxygen availability. At high altitudes, the partial pressure of oxygen decreases significantly, and in extreme cases, it can be as low as 26% of sea-level conditions. This hypoxic condition poses a challenge to migratory animals or those residing in such areas, as it hinders oxygen diffusion into the blood during inhalation. Organisms then need to adapt their respiratory organ to provide adequate oxygenation to accommodate metabolic requirements. For example, various species have physiological mechanisms that enhance lung efficiency and increase the oxygen-carrying capacity of their blood, allowing them to sustain low oxygen levels while maintaining normal respiratory functions that sustain life, as demonstrated in avian and mammalian species. Furthermore, the decrease in air density with rising altitude affects respiratory mechanics and total physiological function. Lower air density results in variations in drag and lift across different modes of locomotion, particularly for birds. While reduced drag is beneficial to forward flight, the requirement for higher lift during hovering becomes more pronounced, necessitating higher power from aerodynamic structures like wings. Studies have observed that birds, such as hummingbirds, show morphological adaptations to resist such hypodense air. Their body-weight-scaled wing amplitudes are greater, and their amplitude of wingbeat increases with high-altitude hovering. Hummingbirds can maintain consistent power requirements at varying altitudes through these specializations, evidencing the refined interaction of altitude and respiratory physiology, and the refinement of adaptations for survival at high altitude, characteristic of ordinary respiratory physiological function. Interestingly, exposure to hypoxia for a sustained period not only affects respiratory function but also imposes a metabolic burden at the cellular level. Hypoxic conditions are found to be accompanied by deranged cardiac energetics and dysregulated mitochondrial function, with principal effects on complex I respiration and increased oxidative stress due to increased levels of reactive oxygen species. The changes are ultimately capable of inhibiting the total production of energy in the tissues. However, nutritional therapy, such as nitrate supplementation, has been shown to reverse several of the damaging effects of hypoxia on cardiac physiology. By enhancing mitochondrial function and maintaining increased blood supply, dietary nitrate reestablishes equilibrium between oxidants and antioxidants. This is to appreciate the role of altitudes in impacting the respiratory physiology and the general metabolic processes essential for the support of normal physiological function against conditions of stress prevalent in high-altitude settings, and the potentiality for dietary mechanisms reversing such physiological disadvantages, most particularly in human and other mammals with varying conditions for the environment, as demonstrated in several experimental research studies (Altshuler et al., 2006; Murray et al., 2014).

3.6.2. Influence of Pollutants and Allergens

Respiratory physiology is highly specialized for filtering and exchanging gases, but the introduction of pollutants and allergens can have an unfavorable impact on this normal physiology. Environmental pollutants, such as particulate matter, volatile organic compounds, and gases including ozone, can lead to oxidative stress, resulting in an unfavorable impact on lung function. This kind of stress results from the lack of balance between reactive oxygen species and the ability of the body to detoxify these toxic endproducts. Sustained exposure to such pro-oxidant factors, as supplied by M-Rad et al., (2020), not only deteriorates the lung's structure but also compromises its functional integrity to the extent of repeatedly inducing inflammatory reactions. Over time, these inflammatory responses predispose subjects to asthma, chronic obstructive pulmonary disease (COPD), and other respiratory disorders that diminish quality of life and increase healthcare costs. Allergens like pollen, mold spores, and pet dander also pose some of the most significant challenges to respiratory wellness. When they gain access to the airways, they trigger an immune response, leading to wheezing, inflammation, and shortness of breath. The airway hypersensitivity in individuals with allergies exposes them to these allergens more frequently, leading to increased inflammatory responses. Notably, the phenomenon is also associated with oxidative stress since the body's response to allergens will result in reactive oxygen species that ultimately cause damage to lung tissues. The synergism of allergens and pollutants will increase respiratory diseases, and this results in an aggravating effect on treatment and management. The interaction of these environmental factors and respiratory physiology highlights the importance of protection against exposure to maintain lung health. Moreover, the nutritional status of an individual plays a crucial role in modulating the effects of allergens and pollutants on the respiratory tract. A poor supply of key nutrients, such as vitamins E and C, can weaken antioxidant defense and increase the risk of respiratory disease. These anti-inflammatory vitamins provide protective benefits against oxidative damage induced by allergens and pollutants. According to (Iddir et al., 2020), a balanced diet rich in antioxidants can build the immune system and minimize the adverse effects of environmental stressors. Some nutrients also influence gene expression that controls inflammation, signaling pathways, and the body's response to oxidative stress. Thus, having an appropriate diet becomes essential for individuals exposed to substantial quantities of airborne allergens and pollutants, confirming the connection between diet and respiratory status.

3.6.3. Adaptations To Exercise and Physical Activity

The human body undergoes significant physiological adaptations in response to regular exercise and physical conditioning, particularly in terms of respiratory function. Adaptations are crucial in enhancing athletic performance and overall health. The body's involvement in activities such as endurance training causes the respiratory system to become more effective, which improves aerobic capacity. Augmented pulmonary ventilation provides for more efficient oxygenation and carbon dioxide removal, hence boosting the overall efficiency of the cardiovascular system. Furthermore, structural and functional alterations within the lungs, such as increased alveolar surface area, facilitate enhanced gas exchange, which is crucial during intense activity. These physiological adaptations are , essential not just for the athlete but for healthy, optimal function in the wider population as well. Mitochondrial biogenesis plays a significant role in the body's adaptation to regular endurance exercise. With increased exercise intensity, there is a linear increase in the oxidative capacity of skeletal muscle, driven by a greater number and greater efficiency of mitochondria. Such adaptation enables the body to utilize fat as a primary energy source during sub-maximal exercise, with a reduced reliance on glycogen stores. The improved mitochondrial function translates into enhanced endurance performance, expressed through improved oxygen consumption (VO_2max) values that are critical measures of cardiorespiratory fitness. Such adaptation comes about from specific biochemical stimuli triggered by physical exertion, reaffirming the importance of continuous training. While endurance training has numerous benefits for mitochondrial adaptation, it is equally important to examine various training modalities that can further enhance these effects, thereby maximizing overall physical performance (Acheson et al., 2015). Aside from endurance training, high-intensity interval training (HIIT) has been shown to induce significant physiological changes comparable to those of traditional endurance training. Evidence from recent research indicates that sprint interval training (SIT) is a reliable method for enhancing aerobic capacity and various physiological variables, including resting heart rate and blood pressure. These adaptations may lead to increased physical work capacity, contributing to improved overall health and enhanced performance measures. For instance, simultaneous SIT with endurance training can trigger further desirable changes in metabolic health, particularly regarding cholesterol levels and glucose metabolism. Such convergence of different training modalities provides the potential to optimize exercise prescriptions for individuals seeking health benefits over brief periods of time. In the long run, a customized approach to physical activity, such as varied training modalities, can help sustain a robust cardiorespiratory system and improve long-term health benefits (Hurst et al., 2014).

Test Your Knowledge

1. What are the effects of altitude on respiratory physiology?
2. What are the adaptations to exercise and physical activity?

SUMMARY

The complexities of healthy respiratory physiology underscore the fine-tuned balance required to maintain homeostasis in the human body. The respiratory system, however, is not a closed system; instead, it is synchronized with heterogeneous physiological processes to ensure effective gas exchange, blood pH control, and compensation for metabolic demands. The rhythmical production of respiratory patterns, primarily regulated by the pre-Bötzinger complex, was discovered to be remarkably resilient. Evidence indicates that even with widespread destruction of the preBötzinger complex, compensatory mechanisms occur, highlighting the importance of neural plasticity in maintaining respiratory function. This plasticity becomes essential where respiratory control is compromised, as evidenced by research that identifies alterations in breathing patterns in pathological conditions (Bonis et al., 2009). Furthermore, the role of vascular endothelial growth factor (VEGF) in respiratory physiology is evidence of the connection between respiratory health and systemic inflammatory reactions. Acute respiratory distress syndrome (ARDS) illustrates well how the function of the respiratory system can be impaired by inflammatory processes that alter critical regulatory variables such as bioactive VEGF. The detection of soluble VEGF receptor-1 (sVEGFR-1) in ARDS patients indicates an exquisitely regulated modulatory system that can suppress the effect of VEGF during stress. This information not only enhances our knowledge of respiratory physiology but may also direct therapeutic interventions aimed at reversing dermal function in disease (Armstrong et al., 2005). The insight gained by examining normal respiratory physiology identifies avenues for future research, most importantly, the discovery of interventions that are able to reduce the impact of respiratory disease. Research currently underway into the flexibility of the respiratory network and the influence of biochemical modulators can lead to improved clinical outcomes. Because respiratory physiology has such a profound interplay with the general health of the body, it is necessary to continue to increase our understanding of both healthy and diseased states. From unraveling these complexities in the future, research will drive the advancement of novel therapies that enhance respiratory function and overall health, once again underlining the significance of the respiratory system in maintaining not just breath, but life.

When examining normal respiratory physiology, several key points are noteworthy in terms of the intricate mechanisms of the respiratory system. One such point is ventilation, which enables effective gas exchange. Ventilation is the physical act of breathing, as the diaphragm and intercostal muscles must function together. Ventilation is required to introduce oxygen into the lungs and expel carbon dioxide. This mechanism keeps the body's metabolic needs in good condition. Ventilation is controlled by various factors, including neural mechanisms and chemical feedback systems, which respond to changes in the levels of carbon dioxide and oxygen in the blood. Understanding these dynamics thus explains why the respiratory system is so impressive in responding to physiological needs and environmental changes. Additionally, the development of imaging modalities has enabled more detailed investigation into pulmonary physiology, allowing for the acquisition of formerly inaccessible information about lung function. For example, the importance of gating during lung imaging to prevent motion artifacts has been highlighted. In many cases, live imaging of the lungs must be synchronized with the ventilatory cycle to obtain an accurate representation. The technological challenges posed by high ventilation rates, particularly in small animal models, have prompted the development of new strategies, such as post-acquisition gating, where computer algorithms are applied to analyze ventilatory phases efficiently. This measure enhances both qualitative and quantitative evaluations in pulmonary research, facilitating improved understanding of normal respiratory performance and driving advancements in clinical implementation as well as research methodology (Dawson et al., 2004). Additionally, ongoing research using animal models is evaluating respiratory physiology in relation to translational medicine. Research in dystrophic mice, for example, generates a significant amount of information regarding muscular and respiratory function, as their pathophysiology parallels that of human conditions like Duchenne muscular dystrophy (DMD). The D2/mdx mouse model novel is unique through its genetic features that are expected to emulate the severity of symptoms experienced by DMD patients. Research through these models enables the testing of therapeutic effectiveness and disease modifiers, thereby bridging the gap in respiratory science. By integrating data on both respiratory capabilities and general physiological characteristics of these models, researchers can enhance their understanding of healthy respiratory mechanics and disease, ultimately guiding future therapy (Aartsma-Rus et al., 2018).

KEY TERMS FROM THIS CHAPTER

Ventilation	Perfusion
Diffusion	Tidal volume
Inspiratory reserve volume	Expiratory reserve volume
Residual volume	Total lung capacity
Vital capacity	Functional residual capacity
Alveolar ventilation	Partial pressure of oxygen (PaO2)
Partial pressure of carbon dioxide (PaCO2)	Hemoglobin
Oxyhemoglobin dissociation curve	Respiratory rate
Minute ventilation	Pulmonary surfactant
Hypoxic drive	Chemoreceptors

CRITICAL THINKING QUESTIONS

1. **What is the primary muscle responsible for quiet inspiration?**
   a. External intercostals
   b. Diaphragm
   c. Internal intercostals
   d. Sternocleidomastoid
2. **Which of the following best describes the partial pressure of oxygen (PaO_2) in arterial blood under normal conditions?**
   a. 40 mmHg
   b. 75 mmHg
   c. 100 mmHg
   d. 150 mmHg
3. **Which of the following lung volumes cannot be measured by simple spirometry?**
   a. Tidal volume
   b. Vital capacity
   c. Residual volume
   d. Inspiratory reserve volume
4. **The majority of oxygen in the blood is transported in which form?**
   a. Dissolved in plasma
   b. Bound to hemoglobin
   c. As bicarbonate ions
   d. Bound to myoglobin
5. **Which receptor type primarily detects changes in arterial CO_2 levels to regulate breathing?**
   a. Peripheral chemoreceptors
   b. Central chemoreceptors
   c. Mechanoreceptors
   d. Baroreceptors

Short Answer Questions

1. What is the primary muscle responsible for inspiration?
2. Define tidal volume and give its approximate normal value in an adult.
3. What is the normal partial pressure of oxygen (PaO_2) in arterial blood?
4. Explain the role of surfactant in lung function.
5. What is the difference between ventilation and perfusion in the respiratory system?

Answer to Critical Thinking Questions

1. (b) 2. (c) 3. (c) 4. (b) 5. (b)

REFERENCES

1. Gordish-Dressman, H., Willmann, R., Pazze, L. D., Kreibich, A., Van Putten, M., Heydemann, A., Bogdanik, L., Lutz, C., Davies, K., Demonbreun, A. R., Duan, D., Elsey, D., Fukada, S., Girgenrath, M., Gonzalez, J. P., Grounds, M. D., Nichols, A., Partridge, T., Passini, M., . . . Aartsma-Rus, A. (2018). "Of Mice and Measures": a project to improve how we advance Duchenne muscular dystrophy therapies to the clinic. *Journal of Neuromuscular Diseases, 5*(4), 407–417. https://doi.org/10.3233/jnd-180324Abdala, A. P., Bissonnette, J., & Newman-Tancredi, A. (2014). Pinpointing brainstem mechanisms responsible for autonomic dysfunction in Rett syndrome: Therapeutic perspectives for 5-HT1A agonists. https://core.ac.uk/download/29027032.pdf (accessed on 16th June 2025).
2. Acheson, A., Munters, A., Alexander, J., Andersen, B., Atherton, R., Baar, K., et al. (2015). Utilizing small nutrient compounds as enhancers of exercise-induced mitochondrial biogenesis. https://core.ac.uk/download/323068533.pdf (accessed on 16th June 2025).
3. Altshuler, D. L., & Dudley, R. (2006). The physiology and biomechanics of avian flight at high altitude. https://core.ac.uk/download/4887664.pdf (accessed on 16th June 2025).
4. Amann, A., Hinterhuber, H., Hartmann, K., King, J., Koc, H., et al. (2011). A modeling-based evaluation of isothermal rebreathing for breath gas analyses of highly soluble volatile organic compounds. http://arxiv.org/abs/1105.0864 (accessed on 16th June 2025).
5. Amann, A., Lumb, A. B., Schrikker, A. C., Mörk, A. K., Amann, A., et al. (2010). A mathematical model for breath gas analysis of volatile organic compounds with special emphasis on acetone. http://arxiv.org/abs/1003.4475 (accessed on 16th June 2025).
6. Armstrong, L., McAuley, D. F., Millar, A., Perkins, G. D., et al. (2005). Regulation of vascular endothelial growth factor bioactivity in patients with acute lung injury. https://core.ac.uk/download/12436.pdf (accessed on 16th June 2025).
7. Arthurs, J., Bush, N., Reilly, E., Guan, S., & Baertsch, N. (2024). Conditional activity of parabrachial Tac1 neurons turns on rapid breathing. *Physiology.* https://www.semanticscholar.org/paper/46961d4f273ea1012eb1f5f5a8f521d431280c28 (accessed on 16th June 2025).
8. Azzalini, D., Rebollo, I., & Tallon-Baudry, C. (2019). Visceral signals shape brain dynamics and cognition. *Trends in Cognitive Sciences, 23*, 488–509. https://doi.org/10.1016/j.tics.2019.03.007 (accessed on 16th June 2025).
9. Barnes, V. A., Crawford, M. W., Harden, K., Ravinder, R., et al. (2014). Widespread depolarization during expiration: A source of respiratory drive? https://core.ac.uk/download/131210052.pdf (accessed on 16th June 2025).
10. Berger, L., Bordas, R., Burrowes, K., Grau, V., et al. (2015). A pyroclastic model coupled to a fluid network with applications in lung modelling. http://arxiv.org/abs/1411.1491 (accessed on 16th June 2025).
11. Beris, A. N., Chalant, A., Chen, L., Gee, A., et al. (2022). A systems engineering approach to modeling and analysis of chronic obstructive pulmonary disease (COPD). http://arxiv.org/abs/2212.13207 (accessed on 16th June 2025).
12. Bhakta, N. R., Kaminsky, D. A., Bime, C., Thakur, N., Hall, G. L., McCormack, M. C., & Stanojevic, S. (2021). Addressing race in pulmonary function testing by aligning intent and evidence

with practice and perception. *CHEST Journal, 161*, 288–297. https://doi.org/10.1016/j.chest.2021.08.053 (accessed on 16th June 2025).

13. Bhambhi, K., & Rathod, P. V. (2021). The effect of respiratory muscle stretches gymnastic (RMSG) on pulmonary function test among pregnant ladies: An experimental study. *International Journal of Science and Research (IJSR).* https://www.semanticscholar.org/paper/b99ad213c16ec5559c6cb35597d5333487744af6 (accessed on 16th June 2025).
14. Blumgart, H. L., & Altschule, M. (1948). Clinical significance of cardiac and respiratory adjustments in chronic anemia. *Blood, 3*(4), 329–348. https://www.semanticscholar.org/paper/07e16d9baf81aa9d54cb02e93f755387ea0808e1 (accessed on 16th June 2025).
15. Bonis, J. M., Davis, S. E., Forster, H., Kiner, S., et al. (2009). Normal breathing pattern and arterial blood gases in awake and sleeping goats after near total destruction of the presumed pre-Bötzinger complex and the surrounding region. https://core.ac.uk/download/213078626.pdf (accessed on 16th June 2025).
16. Bosma, K., Martin, C. M., Burns, K., Mancebo Cortés, J., Suarez Montero, J., Skrobik, Y., Thorpe, K., et al. (2023). Study protocol for a randomized controlled trial of proportional assist ventilation for minimizing the duration of mechanical ventilation: The PROMIZING study. *Trials, 24.* https://www.semanticscholar.org/paper/599c5564a17f05f88dd2478fd2ad5863bfe4864c (accessed on 16th June 2025).
17. Brandes, M., Fix, L. E., Khoury, J., Linkous, M. T., et al. (2018). Theoretical open-loop model of respiratory mechanics in the extremely preterm infant. https://core.ac.uk/download/232207327.pdf (accessed on 16th June 2025).
18. Breijyeh, Z., & Karaman, R. (2020). Comprehensive review on Alzheimer's disease: Causes and treatment. *Molecules, 25*, 5789–5789. https://doi.org/10.3390/molecules25245789 (accessed on 16th June 2025).
19. Brochard, L., Slutsky, A. S., & Pesenti, A. (2016). Mechanical ventilation to minimize progression of lung injury in acute respiratory failure. *American Journal of Respiratory and Critical Care Medicine, 195*, 438–442. https://doi.org/10.1164/rccm.201605-1081cp (accessed on 16th June 2025).
20. Campos, J., Jolley, J., Lozano, M., Moxham, J., et al. (2018). Surface mechanomyography and electromyography provide non invasive indices of inspiratory muscle force and activation in healthy subjects. https://core.ac.uk/download/187265990.pdf (accessed on 16th June 2025).
21. Chang, S.-W., & Lee, H.-C. (2019). Vitamin D and health–The missing vitamin in humans. *Pediatrics & Neonatology, 60*, 237–244. https://doi.org/10.1016/j.pedneo.2019.04.007 (accessed on 16th June 2025).
22. Convertino, V. A. (2019). Mechanisms of inspiration that modulate cardiovascular control: The other side of breathing. *Journal of Applied Physiology, 127*, 1187–1196. https://doi.org/10.1152/japplphysiol.00050.2019 (accessed on 16th June 2025).
23. Crozier, K., & Gruneberg, F. (2015). Delayed cord clamping in the compromised baby. https://core.ac.uk/download/41993077.pdf (accessed on 16th June 2025).
24. Dawson, C. A., Haworth, S. T., Hu, J., Molthen, R., et al. (2004). Post-acquisition small-animal respiratory gated imaging using micro cone-beam CT. https://core.ac.uk/download/213084633.pdf (accessed on 16th June 2025).

25. Dawson, C. A., Haworth, S. T., Johnson, R. H., Karau, K., et al. (2000). Micro-CT image-derived metrics quantify arterial wall distensibility reduction in a rat model of pulmonary hypertension. https://core.ac.uk/download/213083603.pdf (accessed on 16th June 2025).

26. Delaunois, L. (1989). Anatomy and physiology of collateral respiratory pathways. *The European Respiratory Journal, 2*(9), 893–904. https://www.semanticscholar.org/paper/b4e197f74122a395371cf6135bad9f49ccfe4b6d (accessed on 16th June 2025).

27. Di Meo, S., Reed, T. T., Venditti, P., & Víctor, V. M. (2016). Role of ROS and RNS sources in physiological and pathological conditions. *Oxidative Medicine and Cellular Longevity, 2016.* https://doi.org/10.1155/2016/1245049 (accessed on 16th June 2025).

28. Di Nardo, M., & Grasso, S. (2019). Should we set tidal volume in children using the driving pressure? *Pediatric Critical Care Medicine.* https://www.semanticscholar.org/paper/fd85865072abfc09f046d8a87e9c0e139dc5d297 (accessed on 16th June 2025).

29. Dorchak, K. J., Greenleaf, J. E., Kollias, J., Vanderveer, D., et al. (2025). Physiologic responses to water immersion in man: A compendium of research. https://core.ac.uk/download/pdf/42884411.pdf (accessed on 16th June 2025).

30. Ebejer, M. J., & Lesauskaite, V. (1999). Age-related changes in the respiratory system. https://core.ac.uk/download/46601782.pdf (accessed on 16th June 2025).

31. Figueroa, C. A., Jansen, K. E., Taylor, C. A., & Vignon-Clementel, I. E., et al. (2010). Outflow boundary conditions for 3D simulations of non-periodic blood flow and pressure fields in deformable arteries. https://core.ac.uk/download/47107935.pdf (accessed on 16th June 2025).

32. Gadadhar, S., Alvarez Viar, G., Hansen, J. N., Gong, A., Kostarev, A., Ialy-Radio, C., Leboucher, S., et al. (2021). Tubulin glycation controls axonemal dynein activity, flagellar beat, and male fertility. *Science, 371.* https://www.semanticscholar.org/paper/40afb086720e6bf1aad25073 3db4e901ffa4b0ef (accessed on 16th June 2025).

33. Horner, R. (2012). Neural control of the upper airway: Integrative physiological mechanisms and relevance for sleep disordered breathing. *Comprehensive Physiology, 2*(1), 479–535. https://www.semanticscholar.org/paper/a14e20ca5eb088e05de4fb1504d40cc1e42da014 (accessed on 16th June 2025).

34. Hurst, R. A. (2014). The effects and differences of sprint interval training, endurance training and the training types combined on physiological parameters and exercise performance. https://core.ac.uk/download/29841767.pdf (accessed on 16th June 2025).

35. Iddir, M., Brito, A., Dingeo, G., Sosa, S., Samouda, H., La Frano, M. R., & Bohn, T. (2020). Strengthening the immune system and reducing inflammation and oxidative stress through diet and nutrition: Considerations during the COVID-19 crisis. *Nutrients, 12*, 1562–1562. https://doi.org/10.3390/nu12061562 (accessed on 16th June 2025).

36. Kelly, L. (2004). *Essentials of Human Physiology for Pharmacy.* https://www.semanticscholar.org/paper/4219f4edcfbeb281dc54006ce947a2795fbfb510 (accessed on 16th June 2025).

37. Lancmanová, A., & Bodnár, T. (2024). Numerical study of the steady airflow in the human respiratory system during inhaling and exhaling. *Topical Problems of Fluid Mechanics 2024.* https://www.semanticscholar.org/paper/7e54b70f6acea6f4c86bcaa214bdc131879bba91 (accessed on 16th June 2025).

38. Lewandowski, A. (2019). The preterm heart: A unique cardiomyopathy? *Pediatric Research, 85*, 738–739. https://www.semanticscholar.org/paper/e3df9f3bf940deaafc69d1133d243ff4463d6d72 (accessed on 16th June 2025).

39. Loginov, G., Arthurs, J., Atkinson, W., Reilly, E., & Baertsch, N. (2024). Unraveling the role of enkephalin signaling in respiratory control. *Physiology.* https://www.semanticscholar.org/paper/6e8a97d5da76d72d9a5e4f8677d038702cb47bee (accessed on 16th June 2025).

40. Mannino, D. (2021). Insights into the spectrum of chronic lower respiratory disease: Low lung function is still bad. *American Journal of Respiratory and Critical Care Medicine, 204*, 873–874. https://www.semanticscholar.org/paper/9246152cc71c3b89905ccf7e6b674ede40c5f7d3 (accessed on 16th June 2025).

41. Miller, L., Pinkerton, K., Royer, C., Schelegle, E., et al. (2017). Nonhuman primate models of respiratory disease: Past, present, and future. https://core.ac.uk/download/323069778.pdf (accessed on 16th June 2025).

42. Murray, A. J., Cowburn, A. S., Fernandez, B. O., Branco-Price, C., West, J. A., Griffin, J. L., Heather, L. C., et al. (2014). Dietary nitrate increases arginine availability and protects mitochondrial complex I and energetics in the hypoxic rat heart. https://core.ac.uk/download/29473739.pdf (accessed on 16th June 2025).

43. Olsen, W., Smith, B., Pitts, T., Napoli, N., & Bolser, D. C. (2024). Respiration and cough in Pompe disease: Results from a neuromechanical computational model of the respiratory control system. *Physiology.* https://www.semanticscholar.org/paper/f98980a4217a3d519fe94980e2914f12431ce7e1 (accessed on 16th June 2025).

44. Petrocelli, L. C. E., Campos, J., Jolley, J., Lozano García, M., et al. (2019). Noninvasive assessment of inspiratory muscle neuromechanical coupling during inspiratory threshold loading. https://core.ac.uk/download/294829794.pdf (accessed on 16th June 2025).

45. Pulmonary Function and Clinical Respiratory Physiology Committee of Chinese Association of Chest Physicians, Chinese Thoracic Society, & Pulmonary Function Group of Respiratory Branch of Chinese Geriatric Society. (2024). [Standard technical specifications for methacholine chloride (Methacholine) bronchial challenge test (2023)]. *Zhonghua Jie He He Hu Xi Za Zhi = Zhonghua Jiehe He Huxi Zazhi = Chinese Journal of Tuberculosis and Respiratory Diseases, 47*(2), 101–119. https://doi.org/10.3760/cma.j.cn112147-20231019-00247 (accessed on 16th June 2025).

46. Rochwerg, B., Brochard, L., Elliott, M., Hess, D., Hill, N. S., Nava, S., Navalesi, P., et al. (2017). Official ERS/ATS clinical practice guidelines: Noninvasive ventilation for acute respiratory failure. *European Respiratory Journal, 50*, 1602426–1602426. https://doi.org/10.1183/13993003.02426-2016 (accessed on 16th June 2025).

47. Shah, H. (2017). PO_2 dependence of oxygen consumption in skeletal muscle of hypertensive and normotensive rats. https://core.ac.uk/download/84613284.pdf (accessed on 16th June 2025).

48. Sharifi-Rad, M., Kumar, N. V. A., Zucca, P., Varoni, E. M., Dini, L., Panzarini, E., Rajković, J., et al. (2020). Lifestyle, oxidative stress, and antioxidants: Back and forth in the pathophysiology of chronic diseases. *Frontiers in Physiology, 11.* https://doi.org/10.3389/fphys.2020.00694 (accessed on 16th June 2025).

49. Suleimenova, A. E., Tatayeva, R. K., Isaeva, N. B., & Nurzhankyzy, A. (2024). Influence of exam stress on the level of anxiety and respiratory indicators of the body of students with different somatotypes. *Bulletin of the L.N. Gumilyov Eurasian National University. Bioscience Series.* https://www.semanticscholar.org/paper/38092efc73666f90f880fde69db1a3768ea75e5e (accessed on 16th June 2025).

50. Watts, E., & Walmsley, S. R. (2018). Inflammation and hypoxia: HIF and PHD isoform selectivity. *Trends in Molecular Medicine, 25*, 33–46. https://doi.org/10.1016/j.molmed.2018.10.006 (accessed on 16th June 2025).

51. White, R. J. (2025). Acid-base homeostasis in the human system. https://core.ac.uk/download/pdf/42869639.pdf (accessed on 16th June 2025).

52. Zeder, K., Douschan, P., Foris, V., Sassmann, T., Maron, B. A., Olschewski, H., & Kovacs, G. (2024). The prognostic relevance of exercise pulmonary hypertension in cardiac and pulmonary diseases. *Current Opinion in Pulmonary Medicine, 30*, 451–458. https://www.semanticscholar.org/paper/78ed9896ef277c785f0106299e8d50fd1f1a6316 (accessed on 16th June 2025).

53. Tymchik, S., Bryksin, O., & Omelyanchuk, E. (2021). Influence of different types of loads on the cardiovascular and muscular systems in the process of physical education classes in the department of athletic gymnastics. https://www.semanticscholar.org/paper/5704d51c5152cd6b59af3495cb84e4bff9e6b77d (accessed on 16th June 2025).

DEFENSE MECHANISMS IN THE RESPIRATORY SYSTEM

4

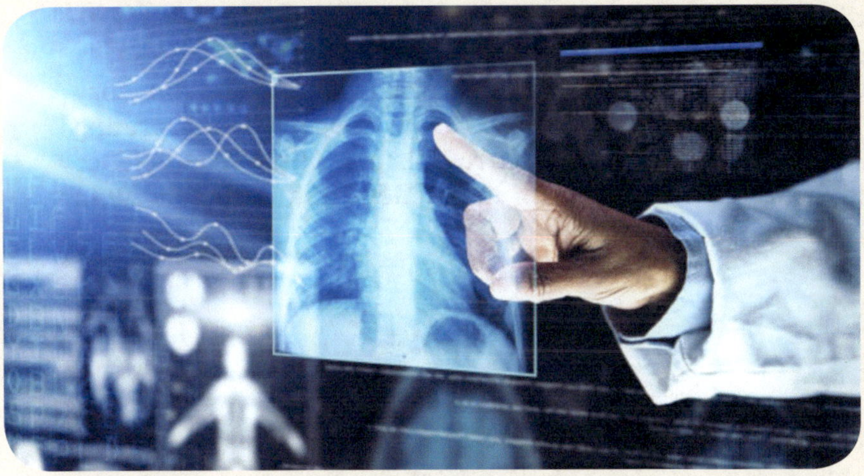

Introduction

Understanding the complexities of the respiratory system is an essential part of learning about the many defense mechanisms that protect the body from invasion by pathogens and toxins in the environment. Respiratory airways are not just conduits for oxygenation but also a frontline defence mechanism against inhaled microbe and toxin particles. Since the lungs are constantly exposed to pathogenic organisms, the body has evolved subtle immune mechanisms to counter infections and inflammation that may arise. Such defense mechanisms range from mechanical barriers such as mucosal surfaces and the ciliary escalator to sophisticated immunity with specialized cells and proteins. An appreciation of the significance of such processes is central to the design of effective therapeutic strategies to enhance respiratory health. Of primary concern to the defence mechanisms of the respiratory system is the bronchus-associated lymphoid tissue (BALT), an essential organ in coordinating immune responses to aerial pathogens. BALT

LEARNING OBJECTIVES

After studying this chapter, you will be able to:

1. Illustrate the anatomy of the respiratory system
2. Describe physical barriers
3. Explore immune response in the respiratory system
4. Explain the mucociliary escalator
5. Define the role of alveolar macrophages
6. Identify the impact of environmental factors

is located in areas where the primary bronchus branches into secondary bronchi and is of crucial significance for the aetiology of the immune response in birds, as documented in the literature. Interestingly, the BALT organs form quite early in life, indicating their crucial role in developing an effective immune response. According to research, the organized pattern of BALT, including both B and T cell areas, favors synergistic activity against infiltrating pathogens. Appreciation of the complex interactions in BALT enhances the understanding of the respiratory system's capacity to develop an effective defence against infections, highlighting its functional characteristics in pulmonary homeostasis. Furthermore, the microbiota inhabiting the respiratory tract plays an important role in the body's global defense mechanisms, a notion better understood in recent immunological research. These resident microorganisms not only exist in harmony with the host, but actually modulate immune functions, conferring immunity against potential pathogens. The principle of "co-immunity" proposes that the host immune system and its microbials collaborate to resist infection, where the latter can suppress the activity of pathogens without necessarily eliminating them. By containing and controlling pathogenic microorganisms, the respiratory microbiota fosters the host's ability to deal effectively with respiratory infections. Interpreting the role of BALT and resident microbiota in the respiratory tract reveals a multi-layered defence mechanism, which documents the complexity of host-pathogen interactions and ultimately with respect to the necessity of further research within the field.

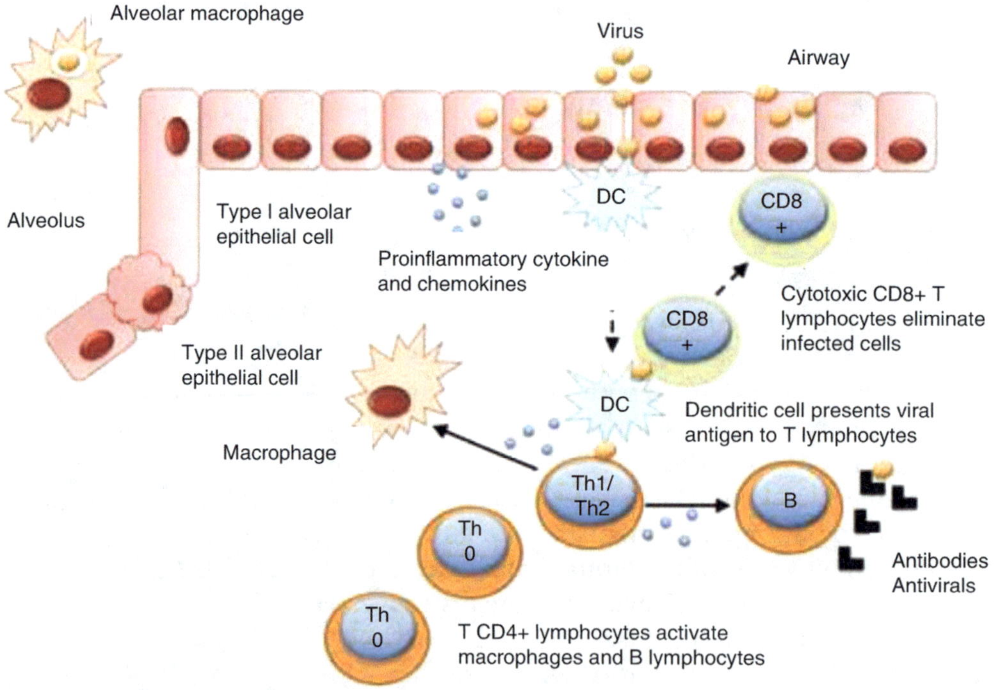

Figure 4.1. Defense mechanisms of the respiratory system.

Source: https://thoracickey.com/wp-content/uploads/2020/11/441522_1_En_6_Fig1_HTML.png

Definition of the respiratory system

The respiratory system is an intricate organization of organs and structures that facilitate gas exchange, essential to sustaining life. Composed nearly entirely of the lungs, trachea, bronchi, and diaphragm, the system is responsible for introducing oxygen into the circulatory system while simultaneously eliminating carbon dioxide, a waste product of metabolism. The intricate organization of the respiratory system maximizes surface area for gas exchange, particularly in alveoli, tiny air spaces of the lungs, where diffusion of oxygen and carbon dioxide occurs. Besides, the respiratory system is not autonomic but dynamically interacts with other physiological systems, such as the circulatory system, to maximize homeostasis. As we explore the defense mechanisms inherent in the respiratory system, it becomes clear that these mechanisms are essential to maintaining a healthy respiratory system, defending against external organisms and environmental irritants.

Central to the definition of the respiratory system is the presence of an array of defense mechanisms, which protect the body against deadly invaders. The initial barrier is mechanical and consists of mucous membranes and cilia lining the respiratory system, which screen out and eliminate foreign particles and microorganisms. Resident microbiota also play a significant role in facilitating immunity; they not only occupy niches but also assist in resistance against pathogens, thus showing the interdependency of microbiomes and the immune system. As noted, protective microbes can exert an impact beyond their niche, interrupting the entry, establishment, growth, and spread of disease-causing microorganisms (Abt et al., 2017). This indicates the co-immunity premise, where both the host's immune defense and its microbiota collaborate to enhance resistance to respiratory disease, contemplating the respiratory system's protective aspect. Progress in medical strategies, including immunization against respiratory pathogens, also illustrates the importance of the respiratory system in public health. The case in point is the seasonal influenza vaccine, designed to increase the immune response and minimize the impact of influenza infections in the population. The vaccines are designed to induce both humoral and cellular immunity, providing long-term protection, given the limitations of previous vaccination strategies that targeted the humoral response. Evoking T cells from memory in conjunction with the development of antibodies is essential for long-term immunity and emphasizes the advancing knowledge regarding the respiratory system's activity in neutralizing infectious diseases like influenza (Glezen et al., 2016). Such synchronization between anatomical features and immune reactions explains the broader picture of the respiratory system as not only a conduit for air but as an active agent in defense health mechanisms.

Importance of defense mechanisms

The respiratory system employs a variety of defense mechanisms to protect from the constant barrage of pathogens, environmental pollutants, and particulate matter. The first defense is physical, the anatomical structures such as the nasal passages, trachea, and bronchial tree, lined with mucus and cilia. They trap dust and microorganisms, making them available for removal by the action of ciliary movement and sneezing. The mucociliary escalator is essential in that the air entering the lungs is relatively clean and unobstructed. The function of these physical barriers cannot be overstated, as they prevent many potential dangers from entering the respiratory tract, thereby reducing the likelihood of infection and inflammation. Beyond these physical barriers, the respiratory system also relies on innate immune mechanisms that provide additional protection. Immunocompetent cells, like macrophages and neutrophils, are strategically located in respiratory tissues and are capable of responding rapidly to any pathogenic challenge. When they encounter pathogens, these cells have the capacity to initiate inflammatory reactions that are specifically geared towards neutralizing and clearing the threat. While inflammation is essential for the clearance of pathogens, it also underscores the complexity of respiratory defense mechanisms and how they can, at times, be tissue-damaging if left unchecked. Recent evidence suggests that a balanced inflammatory response is necessary; for example, the NF-κB pathway plays a crucial role in regulating inflammation. Yet, hyperactivation results in chronic inflammatory disease for most respiratory conditions, and therefore, sensitive modulation of these defenses is necessary (Arulselvan et al., 2016).

Furthermore, the antioxidative activity of the respiratory system serves as an intrinsic defense mechanism against oxidative stress due to environmental toxins and pathogen-related challenges. Zinc, a trace element of critical significance, has the capability of enhancing immune function and functioning as an antioxidant key in preventing cell damage during respiratory insufficiency. It assists in maintaining protein stability and overcoming oxidative stress by eliminating free radicals, as well as modulating key signaling pathways, thereby safeguarding cellular integrity (Jarosz et al., 2017). Such antioxidative protection is crucial to the health of respiratory tissue, thereby preventing inflammatory diseases associated with chronic exposures. The richness and complexity of such defense mechanisms underscore the respiratory system's adaptability and its ability to survive, underscoring the need for continued research to optimize therapeutic interventions in respiratory health.

4.1. Anatomy of the Respiratory System

Learning Outcome

1. Major components of the respiratory system
2. Role of the upper and lower respiratory tracts
3. Interaction with other body systems

The respiratory system's anatomy is intricate, enabling not only gas exchange but also defense against microorganisms. The key structures of the system are the trachea, bronchi, and alveoli, which function in distinct ways. The trachea, supported by C-shaped rings of cartilage, is the principal airway to transport air from the larynx to the lungs. When air is inhaled into the lungs, the trachea splits into two major bronchi, which in turn split into secondary and tertiary bronchi, providing a vast surface area for gas exchange. This anatomical configuration is paramount to adequate airflow. Also, it plays a role in particulate matter and pathogen trapping, highlighting the respiratory system's inbuilt defense mechanisms that complement immune processes along lung-associated tissues, e.g., bronchus-associated lymphoid tissue (BALT) (Dalamani et al., 2006). The alveoli, or little air sacs of the lung, are the location of gas exchange and are centrally located in the bodys defense mechanisms. Alveolar structure consists of a fragile air-blood membrane that facilitates the exchange of oxygen and carbon dioxide in a very efficient manner by diffusion. There are numerous small blood vessels surrounding the alveoli so oxygen can be transferred into the blood and carbon dioxide can be removed. The alveolus is lined with a liquid film of surfactant that reduces surface tension, thereby enabling the stability and function of the alveoli. In addition to this, the surfactant also plays immunomodulatory roles through sequestration of pathogens and destruction, and thus constitutes a first line of defense against inhaled peril (Hegermann et al., 2020). Underpinning thus alveoli structure and function is central to understanding their function in respiratory disease and health. The co-operation between the structural components of the respiratory apparatus and its defense mechanisms is vital for maximum respiratory function. The presence of lymphocytes and macrophages in lung tissue enhances the immunity against infecting pathogens within the respiratory system. Compartmentalization of bronchus-associated lymphoid tissue (BALT) into B and T cell regions facilitates a specific immune response, which makes it possible to have an effective response to infection. Aside from immune cell activity, the intrinsic function of the alveolar epithelial glycocalyx also involves preserving the alveolar surface from pathogens and maintaining mucosal integrity. This multifaceted anatomy refers not only to respiratory function in the form of how the respiratory system can respire, but also refers to its complex nature in protection against disease, where structural and cellular elements are involved in respiratory health (Dalamani et al., 2006; Hegermann et al., 2020).

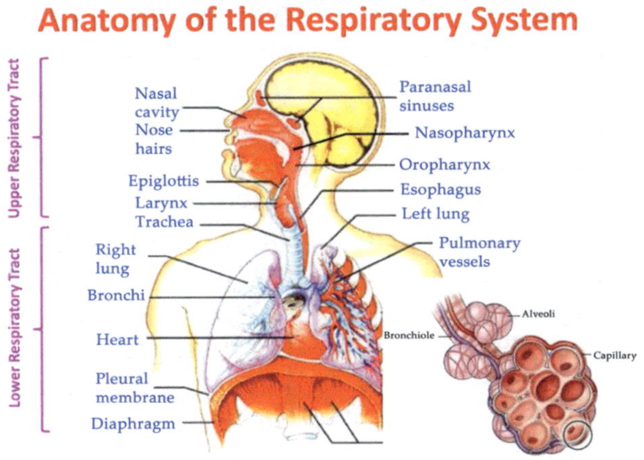

Figure 4.2. Anatomy of the respiratory system.

Source: https://external-content.duckduckgo.com/iu/?u=https%3A%2F%2Fimage1.slideserve.com%2F2044613%2Fanatomy-of-the-respiratory-system-l.jpg&f=1&nofb=1&ipt=6d00bfc159527a2101d03aee6a18f1862869e4f0e0767bc5cd336f63392bc0f9

4.1.1. Major Components of the Respiratory System

The human respiratory system is primarily composed of a chain of significant anatomical structures that are vital for both pathogen defense and gas exchange. The nasal cavity, the pharynx, and the larynx are the components of the upper respiratory tract, which function not only as air passages but also act as a barrier to foreign matter and microbes. The nasal cavity, lined by mucous membranes and cilia, filters, humidifies, and warms air going into the lungs, capturing and destroying pathogens before they reach the lower respiratory system. The larynx, below the pharynx, not only helps produce voice but also prevents food and other foreign substances from being inhaled into the trachea, contributing to the protective mechanisms of the respiratory system. In the lower respiratory system, the trachea, bronchi, and alveoli are the primary structures with gas exchange. The trachea divides into the bronchi, which branch further into smaller bronchioles in a sequential manner, ultimately ending in the alveolar sacs where oxygen and carbon dioxide gas exchange occurs. Alveoli are vital because they possess a large surface area as well as thin walls that facilitate effective gas diffusion. However, these structures are prone to a variety of pathogens, and therefore, effective defense mechanisms are critical. The respiratory epithelium produces mucus, an integral component that traps dust particles and microorganisms on inhalation, and is pivotal in the mucociliary clearance system, reliant on ciliary action for removal of stranded pathogens, contributing to the defense system's effectiveness. Mucus is a significant factor in maintaining respiratory efficiency and health. It consists primarily of glycoproteins of mucus named mucins, MUC5AC, and MUC5B, that are vital to lung protection. The balance of mucus secretion and ciliary movement is a single protective mechanism that prevents lung infection and inflammation. In disorders such as muco-obstructive airway disease, abnormalities in mucus composition can disrupt the protective mechanism, rendering the host susceptible to infection and chronic inflammation. As stated in recent studies, understanding the molecular and cellular processes of mucus dynamics is an essential step for building therapies against respiratory infections, particularly about newly appearing pathogens like SARS-CoV-2 (V'kovski et al., 2020) and the role of mucus in the respiratory defense mechanism (Ridley et al., 2018).

4.1.2. Role of the Upper and Lower Respiratory Tracts

The upper respiratory tract comprises vital structures such as the nasal cavity, pharynx, and larynx, each serving a critical function in defending the body against airborne pathogens. The primary function of these structures is to filter, warm, and humidify the air before it enters the lower respiratory tract. The lining of the upper respiratory tract is covered with ciliated epithelial cells that trap foreign particles and pathogens on mucus. The mucociliary escalator system is a crucial component of respiratory health, constantly clearing away debris to prevent infection. In addition, immune cells contained in this tract serve as an immediate local defense against invading pathogens. This type of immediate immune response is significant because the upper respiratory tract experiences a high frequency of exposure to various invading pathogens, including viruses that cause upper respiratory infections. As such, its role in overall defense mechanisms cannot be underestimated. Transiting to the lower respiratory tract, the trachea, bronchi, and lungs, the defense mechanisms are more complex. In this instance, the contribution of the bronchial epithelium is crucial, primarily through the secretion of antimicrobial agents and the induction of immune cells. Alveoli, the minute air sacs in the lungs, facilitate gas exchange and also serve as sites for immune responses. Within the alveolar lumina, macrophages are present that move to sense and engulf pathogens, also ensuring respiratory health. The lower respiratory tract is thus not only an airway conduit but a significant location for both gas exchange and immune vigilance. Further, coordination of the upper and lower respiratory tracts adds to the efficacy of the overall system as a defense mechanism against pathogens, as evidenced by research indicating that immune reactions within the upper tract can influence lower tract immunity, with evidence of a coordinated defense tactic against respiratory pathogens. Coordination of immune reaction between the upper and lower respiratory tracts illustrates the complexity of the body's defense against such infections within the respiratory tract. As is the nature of foods like Nutrimune®, claimed to enhance immune defense against gastrointestinal and upper respiratory infections, research verifies the relationship between them. The European Food Safety Authority group reviewed evidence for Nutrimune®, which suggested that, although some research indicated a positive effect on immune defense, disparities and a lack of replicable outcomes rendered its overall effectiveness questionable (Allergies et al., 2017). These findings justify further examination of the interaction between various factors in the respiratory tracts, revealing that even though the upper and lower tracts possess distinctive functions, their functions are combined in providing broad defense against respiratory pathogens (Nutri EPDP et al., 2017).

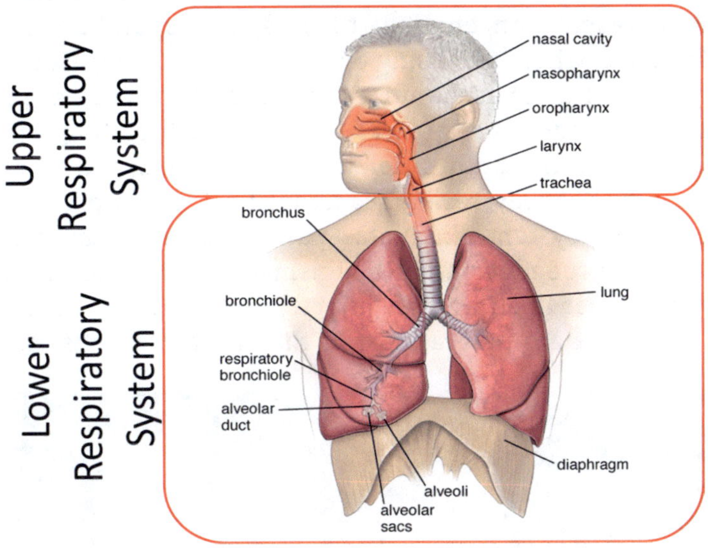

Figure 4.3. Role of the upper and lower respiratory tracts.

Source: https://external-content.duckduckgo.com/iu/?u=https%3A%2F%2Fblogs.gwu.edu%2Fsmhs-histology%2Ffiles%2F2022%2F10%2FPicture12.png&f=1&nofb=1&ipt=6e7881372a3b4c2daafb898f37ef506ee4fb2282f4afdbd9a821492a5f00b910

4.1.3. Interaction With Other Body Systems

The circulatory and respiratory systems cooperate closely with each other to highlight the intricate relationship in human anatomy. The air breathed into the lungs results in oxygen being exchanged for carbon dioxide in the alveoli, a process that relies on the normal functioning of both systems. The oxygenated blood is distributed through the pulmonary veins to the heart, which distributes the oxygenated blood throughout the body. This discussion not only indicates the respiratory system's important role in oxygenating blood but also homeostasis through the control of blood pH levels. The collapse of any part of this cooperative process can lead to profound derangements of physiological processes, i.e., hypoxia or respiratory acidosis, illustrating just how interconnected body systems are in their role of guarding against environmental insult and therefore emphasizing the respiratory system's role as a vital defense process against pathogen and toxin contaminants in inspired air. The immune system serves as another vital protective layer that acts in cooperation with the respiratory system. The airway is lined with a vast array of immune cells that trap pathogens and facilitate their elimination. An example is mucociliary clearance, a protective mechanism that removes pathogens and debris from the respiratory tract, which illustrates the interaction between goblet cells that secrete mucus and ciliated epithelial cells. During infections such as COVID-19, the interaction is increased even further, as the immune response must respond rapidly to pathogens like SARS-CoV-2. Research indicates that an effective immune response is crucial in limiting viral replication and transmission, highlighting the importance of both innate and adaptive immunity in preventing severe respiratory complications (Philip V'kovski et al., 2020). Thus, not only does the immune system protect the respiratory tract, but it also acts in collaboration with it to neutralize the adversary, demonstrating synergistic biological defense mechanisms. The neuroendocrine system also affects respiratory function and defense mechanisms. Neurotransmitters and hormones can adjust the depth and rate of respiration, enabling the body to respond to changes in carbon dioxide and oxygen levels. For instance, when exercising or during altitude adjustment, the brain sends the message of a rise in respiratory rate to account for increased oxygen requirements. Additionally, the hypothalamus participates in autonomic responses that regulate breathing rates in states of infection or stress and therefore enhance the body's defense mechanisms (Hu et al., 2020). Additionally, hormonal responses may affect airway resistance as well as mucus production, thereby dictating how effectively the respiratory system eliminates pathogens. This complex interaction between the respiratory system and neuroendocrine mechanisms further underscores the intricate nature of the body's response to protect itself against injury, demonstrating that the respiratory system is not an independent entity but an integral part of the broader defense mechanism.

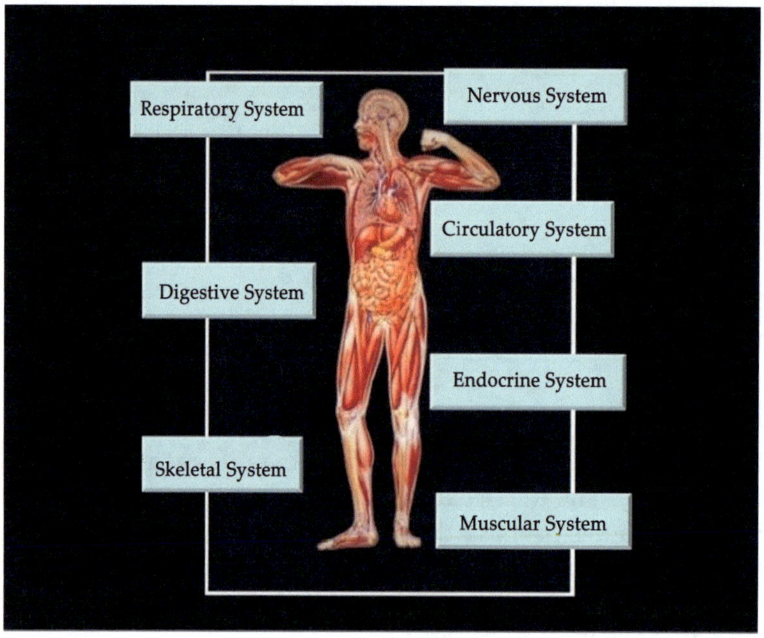

Figure 4.4. Respiratory tract interaction with other body systems.

Source: https://external-content.duckduckgo.com/iu/?u=https%3A%2F%2Fimage.slidesharecdn.com%2Fsysteminteractions-121120150308-phpapp01%2F95%2Fsystem-interactions-10-638.jpg%3Fcb%3D1353424245&f=1&nofb=1&ipt=85a5bcc6e8bac82347ec31faf51fd9bb5a45afb7e8e4b3d9986942e0c249157b

Test Your Knowledge

1. What are the major components of the respiratory system?
2. What is the role of the upper and lower respiratory tracts?

4.2. Physical Barriers

Learning Outcome

1. Nasal hairs and mucous membranes
2. Cilia and their function in trapping particles
3. The role of the cough reflex

The respiratory system relies on a series of physical barriers that function to protect the body from pathogens and particulate matter from the external world. These barriers include structural components like the nasal mucosa, epithelium, and mucociliary escalator. The nasal passages, lined with a ciliated epithelium, function to trap particulate substances and invading pathogens entering the airway in mucus. All of this mucus is being secreted by the goblet cells and acts as an adhesive trap to prevent harmful substances from being carried further down to the lower respiratory tract. Additionally, the cilia on the epithelial cells are beating in sync, actually moving the mucus up to the pharynx to be expelled or swallowed. These mechanisms constitute a critical first line of defense against inhaled pathogens, significantly reducing the load of infectious agents that penetrate further into the respiratory apparatus. In the context of the respiratory physical barriers, the role of the alveolar epithelium cannot be overstated. Alveoli, which are the sites of gas exchange, are lined by a thin layer of epithelial cells that not only facilitate the diffusion of oxygen and carbon dioxide but also provide a physical defense against invading pathogens. The alveolar epithelium is supported by the incorporation of surfactant proteins with bacteriostatic activity that help to stabilize alveoli. The alveolar epithelium works synergistically with the immune system by forming an unfavorable environment for the proliferation of pathogens. In instances where the physical barriers are breached by pathogens, they are typically confronted by alveolar macrophages that can engulf and kill invaders. Thus, the structure of the alveolar membrane serves a dual purpose: to facilitate gas exchange that is essential, and as an essential vital defense mechanism against potential invasions. Further, the physical barrier dynamics of the respiratory system are necessary to its defense mechanism. Pathogens like Salmonella enterica developed mechanisms to circumvent these barriers during passage through the respiratory tract. Since Salmonella is subjected to all the challenges posed by the biochemical and mechanical defense mechanisms, it employs sophisticated means of evading these barriers, just as it does with the gastrointestinal system's defense mechanisms (Bayard et al., 2018). Admiration for these encounters not only highlights the effectiveness of physical defenses but also makes one aware of how pathogens have adapted to exploit weaknesses within these defense systems. This host defense of the respiratory system, versus bacterial adaptability focuses on maintaining robust physical barriers in the respiratory system to reduce vulnerability to infection and ensure overall respiratory wellness.

4.2.1. Nasal Hairs and Mucous Membranes

The respiratory system possesses a sophisticated defense mechanism that is crucial for maintaining homeostasis and protecting against pathogens. Two of the most important defense mechanisms of this defense system are the mucous membranes and the nasal hairs, also known as vibrissae. Nasal hairs serve as the first line of defense against airborne particles, including dust, pollen, and microbes. These coarse hairs screen out large particles to keep them from moving further into the respiratory system. Furthermore, the omnipresent presence of mucous membranes within the nasal passage is crucial in this defense mechanism. The layer of mucus, combined with the action of cilia, serves to trap and remove entrapped particles from the respiratory tract. This first-line filtration system is essential in reducing the load of potential pathogens that can infect or cause respiratory illness, supporting the importance of such anatomical features in healthy respiration. The synergy between nasal hairs and mucous membranes enhances natural immune defense in the respiratory tract. Mucous membranes produce mucus, a thick liquid that not only traps smaller particles but also contains antimicrobial components that efficiently inactivate pathogens. If pathogens or irritants make contact with the mucous layer, immune cells within the membrane can identify and respond to the foreign substance. The immune response is essential in preventing respiratory infections and maintaining overall respiratory health. During periods of health emergencies, such as the COVID-19 pandemic, the function of these defenses becomes more prevalent, with increased vigilance regarding airborne transmission. The effectiveness with which nasal defenses capture pathogens highlights the significance of means to strengthen these defenses. Some topical preparations that induce local immunity and pathogen trapping have been examined as potential prophylactic measures, highlighting the protective function of mucous membranes at the site of crisis in the respiratory system (Ivanova et al., 2022). The protective function of nasal hairs and mucous membranes is further augmented by understanding their anatomical and biological concordance with the respiratory system. This continuous interaction between such defenses and external environmental agents is a vital component of disease prevention. For instance, poisonous pollutants and viral infections can compromise the integrity of these defenses, leading to compromised respiratory health. In addition, conditions such as allergy or chronic rhinitis can compromise the natural working of the nasal hairs and mucous membranes, making people more susceptible to infections. To counter these vulnerabilities, ongoing research attempts to develop pharmaceutical interventions that can enhance the function of such mucosal barriers. For example, the development of self-defense systems against respiratory infections is becoming increasingly important, particularly in light of recent global health emergencies. Hence, learning and developing nasal hairs and mucous membranes is crucial, as it provides valuable information regarding novel therapeutic strategies, affirming their vital role in the respiratory defense system (Yadav et al., 2023).

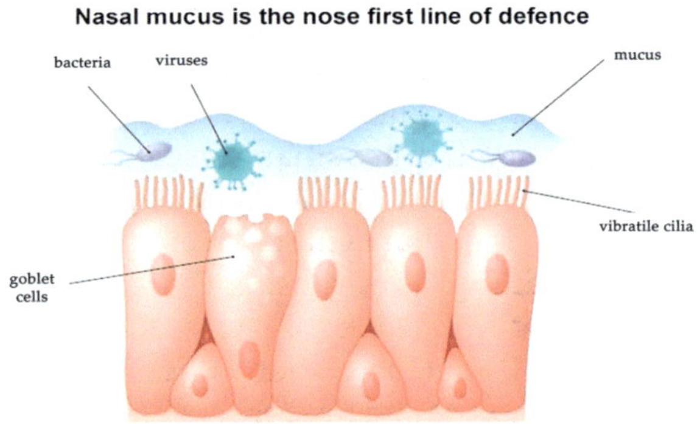

Figure 4.5. Nasal mucous is the nose first line of defence.

Source: https://ik.imagekit.io/rinosol2act/come_funziona_il_naso/nasal-mucus.jpg?updatedAt=1630005969699&tr=w-1200,h-675,fo-auto

4.2.2. Cilia and Their Function in Trapping Particles

In the intricate system of the respiratory tract, cilia play a crucial role in defending against foreign bodies and invading bacteria. Cilia are the tiny, hair-like projections that line the respiratory tract and perform a coordinated sweeping motion, enabling them to clear away dust inhaled. Cilia are essential in trapping inhaled impurities, bacteria, and mucus by rhythmic motion, carrying these trapped substances efficiently upward toward the pharynx, where they can be swallowed or coughed up. This function is essential because uneventful breathing relies on having unobstructed airways free of harmful particulates that could desecrate lung function. By performing this crucial function, cilia serve as the primary defense mechanism, reaffirming their significance in the respiratory defense system. The presence of pathogens, such as Pseudomonas aeruginosa, can potentially impair the functioning of the cilia in the respiratory system critically. In the case of patients suffering from illnesses such as cystic fibrosis, the thick mucus blocks the normal flow of cilia, providing an opportunity for pathogens to persist and causing recurrent infections. P. aeruginosa's genomic flexibility enhances its virulence so that it can withstand the unfavorable respiratory environments that are common in compromised lungs. Ciliary function and microbial colonization are coupled when examining conditions that inhibit mucociliary clearance. In a case where cilia are unable to trap and remove microbes effectively, the lungs become susceptible to infection, exacerbating illness problems such as COPD. Thus, the cilia-microbe interaction suggests the importance of maintaining practical ciliary function to ensure respiratory well-being. Adding to the complexity of the airways' defense mechanism is small airways disease (SAD), which is typically associated with chronic obstructive pulmonary disease (COPD). Inflammation and plugging of mucus within the small airways can inhibit the action of cilia, aggravating the progression of respiratory disease. Furthermore, the interaction with emphysema diseases helps to illustrate the multiplicity of mechanisms by which airway remodeling can be achieved. The functional presence of cilia is necessary to effectively counter pathological processes, lest loss of function leads to debris and bacterial accumulation in the airways. Cilia, through the clearance of particles, contribute to maintaining the health of the airways as well as suppressing exacerbations in the case of SAD. Therefore, ciliary function must be preserved to eliminate the impact of respiratory illnesses and provide robust defenses within the respiratory system.

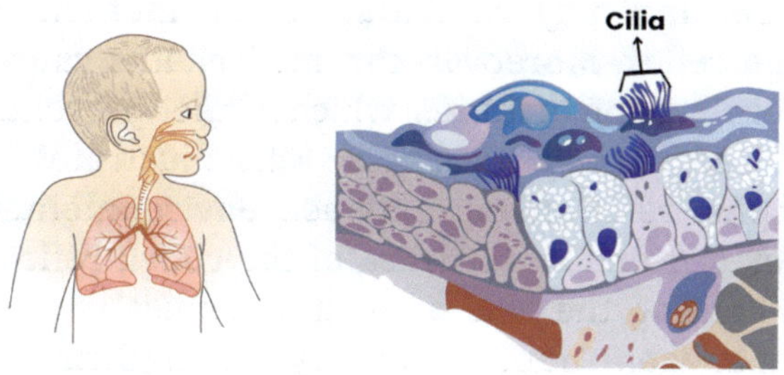

Figure 4.6. Cilia in lungs.

Source: https://images.examples.com/wp-content/uploads/2024/05/Cilia-in-Lungs.png

4.2.3. The Role of the Cough Reflex

The reflex of coughing is a critical protective mechanism of the respiratory tract, whose primary function is to protect the airways from harmful irritants and eliminate secretions. The reflex of coughing is brought about by stimulation of sensory receptors within the airways that are sensitive to multiple stimuli, such as smoke, dust, and even causative agents of infectious diseases. When activated, a coordinated chain of muscular and nervous events is triggered, culminating in the forceful expulsion of air from the lungs. In addition to removing foreign particles, this rapid expulsion also serves to flush out pathogens, thereby minimizing the risk of infection. Through the promotion of airway clearance, the cough reflex is an essential process in preserving respiratory well-being and maintaining the freedom of delicate lung structures from occlusive material. The efficacy of the cough reflex can be significantly impaired in chronic respiratory illness to render individuals more susceptible to infection and other diseases. For example, exposure to environmental irritants such as tobacco smoke has been found to predispose immune responses, leading to the development of chronic obstructive pulmonary disease (COPD) and other lung diseases. The alterations in immune response lead to exaggerated mucosal inflammation, which weakens the natural defense mechanism of the respiratory system and may contribute to an inefficient cough reflex. Moreover, chronic irritants cause hypersecretion of mucus, which further prevents adequate airway clearance. This illustrates a complex relationship between environmental exposures and the efficacy of the cough reflex, highlighting the role of such dynamics within the management of respiratory health (Strzelak et al., 2018).

The cough reflex also plays a role in the public health context, specifically in relation to alcohol consumption-related behaviors and tobacco exposure. Alcohol consumption, as with tobacco, has risks that can compromise respiratory function and, in turn, the effectiveness of cough reflexes. Excessive alcohol consumers may have impaired respiratory muscle function and thus, impaired ability to cough effectively. The additive nature of these lifestyle habits emphasizes the interdependence of health habits and the respiratory defense mechanisms. Intervening in such public health issues can enhance global respiratory health as well as cough reflex functioning. By increasing the awareness of the ill effects substances like alcohol and tobacco pose on the respiratory defense, health education can construct healthier environments and offer support to the critical role of mechanisms like coughing in protecting respiratory integrity (Jürgen Rehm et al., 2017).

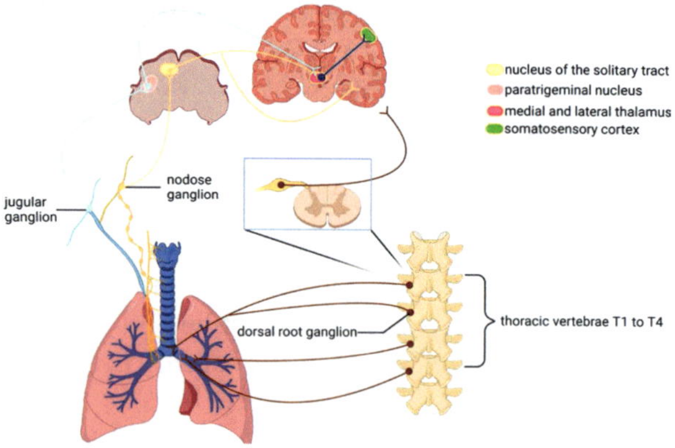

Figure 4.7. The role of the cough reflex.

Source: https://media.springernature.com/lw1200/springer-static/image/art%3A10.1007%2Fs12264-023-01104-y/MediaObjects/12264_2023_1104_Fig4_HTML.png

Test Your Knowledge

1. Explain about nasal hairs and mucous membranes.
2. What are cilia and their function in trapping particles?

4.3. Immune Response in the Respiratory System

Learning Outcome

1. Overview of the immune cells involved
2. Mechanisms of inflammation in response to pathogens
3. Role of antibodies in respiratory defense

The immune defense of the respiratory system is a complex organization of cellular and humoral defenses that combat pathogens invading the airways. At the heart of this defense strategy are several hundred immune cells, including macrophages, neutrophils, and lymphocytes, that work together to detect and eliminate foreign invaders. These immune cells are strategically positioned within the respiratory system, with a notable predominance in organs such as the bronchus-associated lymphoid tissue (BALT). BALT plays a crucial role in the early immune response by facilitating the activation of T and B cells to increase the body's ability to recognize and respond to pathogens in the respiratory tract. Additionally, research highlights how mathematical models can mimic the dynamics of immune interaction during viral infections and how such responses are driven by significant parameters, particularly during the onset of disease (Giegold et al., 2018).

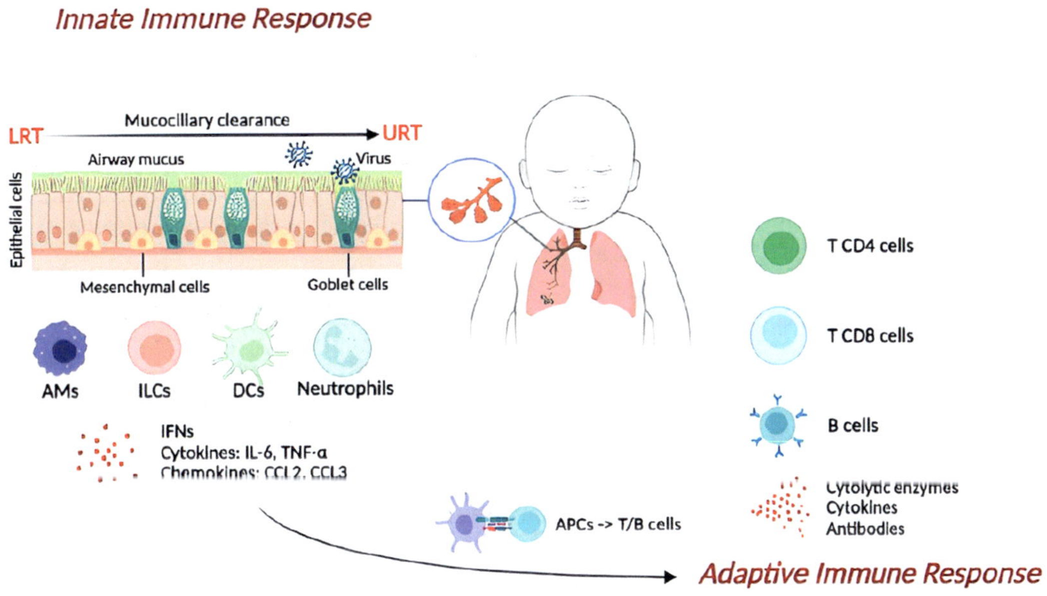

Figure 4.8. Immune response in the respiratory system.

Source: https://www.mdpi.com/ijms/ijms-25-06178/article_deploy/html/images/ijms-25-06178-g001.png

In addition to cellular immunity, the respiratory system also relies on humoral processes to provide resistance against pathogens. The mucosal surface of the respiratory tract contains immunoglobulins, particularly secretory IgA, which plays a vital role in neutralizing pathogens prior to their ability to cause infections. The antibody plays a crucial role in preventing the attachment of bacteria and viruses to mucosal surfaces and clearing them from the system. Furthermore, the topological organization of immune structures in the respiratory system, specifically BALT, provides a dynamic battlefield upon which immune cells can interact. The distinct regions within these structures contain specialized cells that respond to various stimuli, thereby enhancing immunity.

As noted with the case of bird research, the interaction between such regions and their respective functions should be taken into account while establishing immune responses across different situations (Dalamani et al., 2006). Of particular significance is the flexibility of the immune response in the respiratory tract to various pathogens and environmental stress. The development of a memory immune response enables quicker and more effective responses to reinfection with identical or very similar pathogens. Flexibility is significant in the regulation of recurrent respiratory infections, which, if not kept under control, can lead to chronic respiratory diseases. Mathematical modeling of the dynamics of viral infections and immune responses helps one understand these processes in detail. The models can further clarify differences in immune responses between the respiratory tract regions, posing significant questions regarding why specific pathogens preferentially infect the upper or lower respiratory systems. The insights derived from these models will not only enhance our current understanding of respiratory immunology but may also inform future drug development aimed at improving immune resilience in the respiratory system (Giegold et al., 2018).

4.3.1. Overview of the Immune Cells Involved

The respiratory tract is equipped with an intricate network of immune cells to ensure homeostasis and adequate protection against infectious agents. Alveolar macrophages are among these, and they play a crucial role in pulmonary immunity as they phagocytose inhaled particles, pathogens, and cellular debris. Alveolar macrophages can migrate across the alveolar space and have the unique function of initiating inflammatory responses when invading organisms exist. When stimulated, they release a variety of cytokines that control the activity of other immune cells, forming a complex series of defenses tuned to the threat posed by respiratory pathogens. The organization of such immune responses ultimately contributes to the integrity of the epithelial barrier and overall lung health, establishing the importance of alveolar macrophages in the respiratory immune landscape, as suggested by the complex interactions with the microbiota that influence immune system programming (Brown et al., 2016). In addition to macrophages, dendritic cells play a crucial role in the immune response of the respiratory system. These antigen-presenting cells are located in the airway epithelium, where they engulf and process antigens of airborne pathogens. When activated, these cells migrate to adjacent lymph nodes to interact with naïve T cells, directing them into effector populations capable of mounting a tailored immune response. This is crucial for the establishment of adaptive immunity, as it provides protection against repeated infections. Memory T cells created through such an interaction offer long-lasting protection. Furthermore, dendritic cells regulate cooperation between innate and adaptive immunity by secreting an array of cytokines that stimulate or inhibit inflammation, thereby regulating the balance necessary for proper lung protection and promoting recovery from respiratory distress (Aderem et al., 2012). However, another exceedingly crucial player in respiratory immunity is the role of neutrophils, which are often the first to be summoned to the sites of lung infection or inflammation. These cells possess an exceptionally swift recruitment to pulmonary tissues upon receiving activation cues from injured tissues and macrophages. Neutrophils have several mechanisms for protecting the lungs, including phagocytosis, secretion of reactive oxygen species, and formation of neutrophil extracellular traps that ensnare pathogens. However, the incessant recruitment and activation of neutrophils can lead to tissue injury if poorly regulated, which implies a double-edged sword in their role in the pulmonary defense mechanism. Their recruitment and function can be radically altered in chronic inflammatory disorders, such as COPD, revealing a complex interaction between immune cell activities and lung health that requires further investigation (Aderem et al., 2012).

4.3.2. Mechanisms of Inflammation in Response To Pathogens

The immune response elicited during the process of encountering pathogens, particularly in the respiratory system, plays a critical role in maintaining host integrity. Pioneering this response is inflammation, a complex process that enables the marking of immune cells at sites of infection. Upon entry, pathogens activate an array of pattern recognition receptors (PRRs) on immune cells, resulting in the release of pro-inflammatory cytokines. These cytokines, including interleukins and tumor necrosis factor-alpha, play a crucial role in amplifying the inflammatory response, promoting vascular permeability, and facilitating the entry of fluid and immune cells into infected tissues. Local inflammation not only neutralizes and clears the pathogens but also instigates the mechanisms of tissue repair once the threat has been removed.

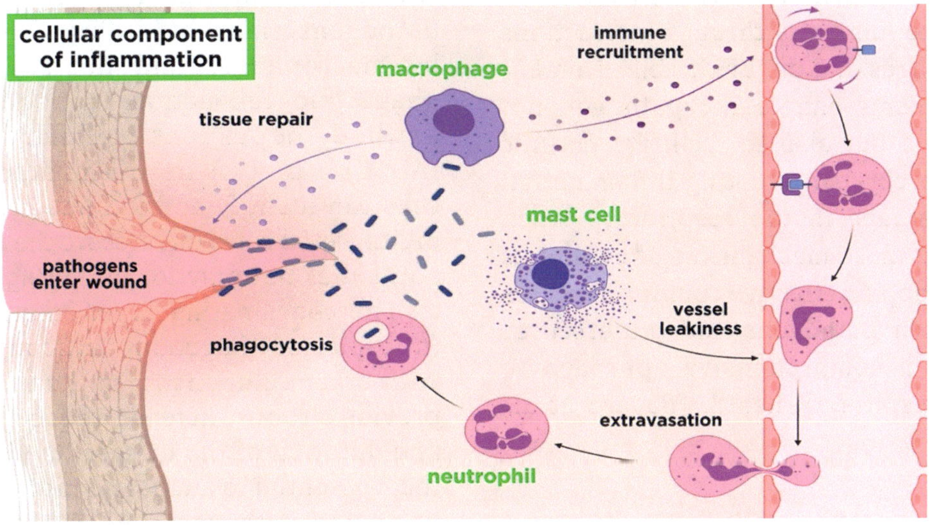

Figure 4.9. Mechanisms of inflammation in response to pathogens.

Source: https://i.ytimg.com/vi/yIMz9pkT9xQ/maxresdefault.jpg

The , delicate equilibrium of inflammation is a testament to the importance of such mechanisms in protecting the respiratory system from a myriad of infectious agents. Resident microbiota within the respiratory system further complicates the tale of inflammation and pathogen reaction. These microorganisms contribute to host defense mechanisms by forming a barrier that prevents pathogen colonization while simultaneously modulating the inflammatory response through disease tolerance pathways. Sympty is an intricate interplay wherein the microbiota not only enhances physical barriers but also reduces the inflammatory response when it encounters pathogens. Specifically, some resident microbiota can interfere with the pathogen-host interaction by modulating immune responses in a manner that maintains a minimal inflammatory state, thereby preventing overestimation of tissue injury. This concept of co-immunity describes how host defense is a bidirectional process, with both the immune system and microbiota collaborating effectively to manage the response to respiratory pathogens (Abt et al., 2017). Moreover, pathogens have developed sophisticated evasion strategies that complicate the inflammatory response. For instance, the Gram-negative bacterium Salmonella enterica demonstrates this through multiple mechanisms that undermine host defenses. Upon invasion, Salmonella can manipulate inflammatory pathways, thereby altering the host immune response to its advantage. This manipulation involves evading initial physical barriers, such as mucus and epithelial barriers, as well as escaping innate immunity through interactions with macrophages and dendritic cells. Notably, these mechanisms enable the pathogen not only to survive but also to facilitate chronic infections, thereby perpetuating inflammation and tissue damage in the respiratory tract. Understanding these mechanisms of evasion is crucial in developing effective countermeasures to combat such pathogens and underscores the need for a comprehensive approach to maintaining respiratory health (Bayard et al., 2018).

4.3.3. Role of Antibodies in Respiratory Defense

The respiratory tract is one of the primary portals of entry for pathogens, making effective immune responses crucial for maintaining health. Antibodies, especially immunoglobulin A (IgA), play a crucial role in respiratory defense by neutralizing airborne pathogens and preventing their binding to mucosal surfaces. Present in high levels in respiratory secretions, such as saliva and mucus, IgA acts as a first line of defense by binding to viruses and bacteria, thereby stopping them from infecting epithelial cells. This is particularly important in protecting against respiratory viruses such as influenza and coronaviruses that can cause severe respiratory illness. One of the primary challenges that IgA addresses is through agglutination, in which multiple pathogens are brought together, making it easier for them to be removed by immune cells in the respiratory tract, thereby enhancing overall respiratory integrity and well-being. Moreover, the effectiveness of antibodies in respiratory defense is not solely based on their capacity to neutralize; they also play a significant role in initiating other immune system responses. When attached to pathogens, antibodies can activate the complement cascade, a series of protein activations that enhance the immune response. Complement proteins can opsonize pathogens, marking them for destruction by macrophages and neutrophils through phagocytic cell action. Antibodies facilitate antibody-dependent cellular cytotoxicity (ADCC), a process in which natural killer (NK) cells can identify and kill infected cells. These multifaceted roles underscore the importance of antibodies not only for inhibiting infection but also for coordinating larger immune responses. In respiratory infections, antibody interactions with other components of the immune system provide a robust defense, reducing the severity and duration of the disease. In viral infections, their potential to adapt and modify against new upcoming pathogens underscores the role of antibodies further. Notably, the evolution of variants of concern, as has occurred with SARS-CoV-2, presents challenges to antibody-mediated immunity. Because such variants are capable of altering their antigenic properties, pre-existing antibodies may become ineffective. However, evidence has shown that the immune system is capable of modifying by mechanisms such as affinity maturation, whereby B cells producing antibodies can modify so that they can recognize such variants better (Alessandro M Carabelli et al., 2023). Moreover, specific immune reactions enabled by MDA5, a viral RNA-sensing receptor that triggers the production of type I interferons, may help sustain a heightened immune status (Antônio Dias et al., 2018). The collaborative action among antibodies and other immunity components in this process is a testament to their indispensable function in the respiratory organs' defense mechanisms against infection.

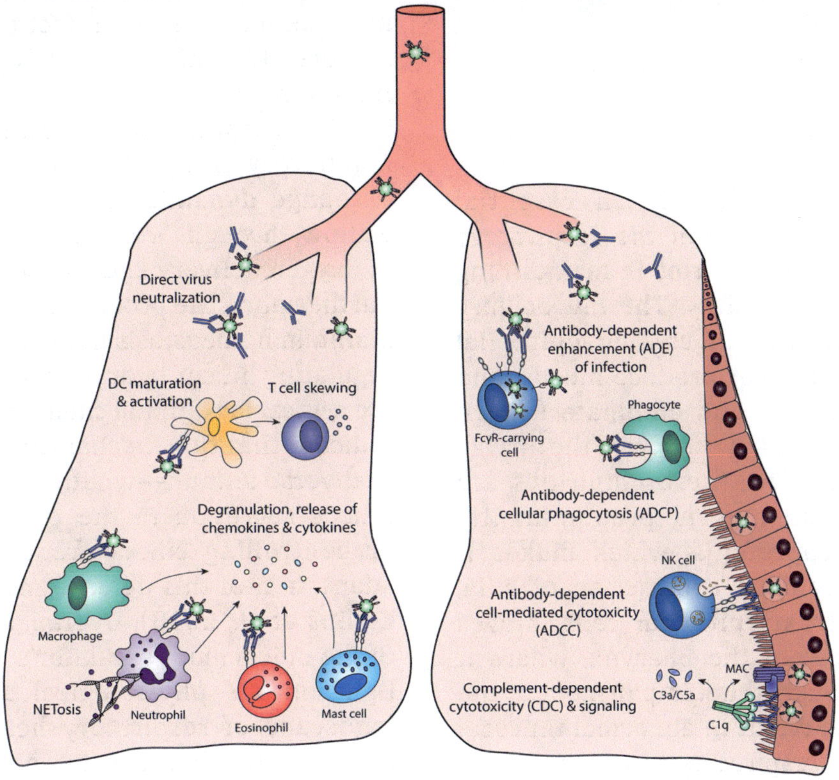

Figure 4.9. Role of antibodies in respiratory defense.

Source: https://www.frontiersin.org/files/Articles/432851/fimmu-10-00548-HTML/image_m/fimmu-10-00548-g001.jpg

Test Your Knowledge

1. What are the mechanisms of inflammation in response to pathogens?
2. What is the role of antibodies in respiratory defense?

4.4. Mucociliary Escalator

Learning Outcome

1. Function of mucus in trapping pathogens
2. Mechanism of ciliary movement
3. Importance of the mucociliary escalator in health

The mucociliary escalator is an essential protective mechanism within the respiratory system that plays a pivotal role in maintaining the pulmonary tract healthy. The mucociliary escalator is comprised of ciliated epithelial cells and goblet cells that produce mucus, and they cooperate to trap and eliminate foreign particles, bacteria, and irritants from the airway pathway. When inhaled, these impurities are coated with mucus that is predominantly composed of glycoproteins, which makes it thick. The synchronized contraction of cilia, which protrude from epithelial cells, moves mucus upward toward the pharynx, where it is swallowed or coughed up. Impairment of the process is likely to result in abnormal mucosal immunity, causing respiratory diseases such as COPD and asthma. These diseases underscore the importance of the proper functioning of the mucociliary apparatus in ensuring airway clearance and protection against respiratory pathogens. The effectiveness of the mucociliary escalator can be influenced by numerous factors, including lifestyle, biological, and environmental factors. For instance, exposure to infections, smoke, and pollutants can decrease ciliary function or alter mucus properties, which leads to reduced clearance efficiency. In patients with compromised mucociliary function, the severity of pulmonary infections is significantly heightened. Additionally, cystic fibrosis is among the conditions that pose a special challenge because it leads to the production of abnormally thick mucus that cilia cannot move effectively. Consequently, such patients frequently suffer from recurrent infections and airway obstruction, highlighting the need to maintain mucociliary function. Therapeutic interventions, such as the use of N-acetylcysteine, have been studied to enhance the mucolytic effectiveness of mucus and thereby restore escalator function and reduce rates of infection in susceptible subjects (Aldini et al., 2018). In addition to infection control, the mucociliary escalator is also responsible for maintaining overall respiratory system function. It assists the gas exchange dynamics by ensuring unrestricted airflow through, which is of great significance in oxygen delivery and carbon dioxide removal. Furthermore, the process of escalation serves to maintain homeostasis in the respiratory tract by regulating mucus hydration and viscosity, which are critical for optimal ciliary movement. Studies indicate that this mechanism's ability to adapt to diverse stimuli—whether through increased mucus secretion in the presence of irritants or controlling ciliary frequency beat—is an adaptation of this defense mechanism (Amélie Collins et al., 2018). Overall, an understanding of the mucociliary escalator's complexity sheds light on the physiological and pathological landscape of respiratory health, highlighting its crucial role in the body's defense mechanism.

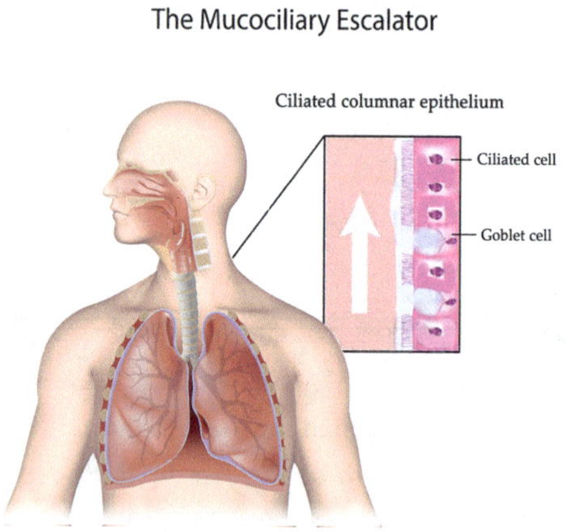

Figure 4.10. The mucociliary escalator.

Source: https://d38zjy0x98992m.cloudfront.net/aee97d2d-b1d8-4c43-a2dc-66e9f164bd90/mucociliary_escalator_xlarge.jpg

4.4.1. Function of Mucus in Trapping Pathogens

The respiratory system plays a role in defense against pathogens, and this is mainly accomplished by the activity of mucus, a viscoelastic secretion by airway epithelial goblet cells and submucosal glands. Mucus is a viscoelastic substance that contains a combination of various antimicrobial proteins and immune mediators, present in high titers, which act synergistically to trap inhaled pathogens, such as bacteria, viruses, and fungi. By ensnaring these invaders, mucus prevents them from binding to epithelial cells and initiating infections. The physical properties of mucus enable it to establish an impediment that physically stops pathogens while simultaneously providing a vehicle for immobilizing such harmful agents. The success of this trapping mechanism is a testament to the importance of mucus in respiratory function and to the fact that mucus serves as a first line of defense in the body's immune system. Effective mucociliary clearance, and thus effective pathogen trapping, relies upon coordinated motion of the cilia that line the airways.

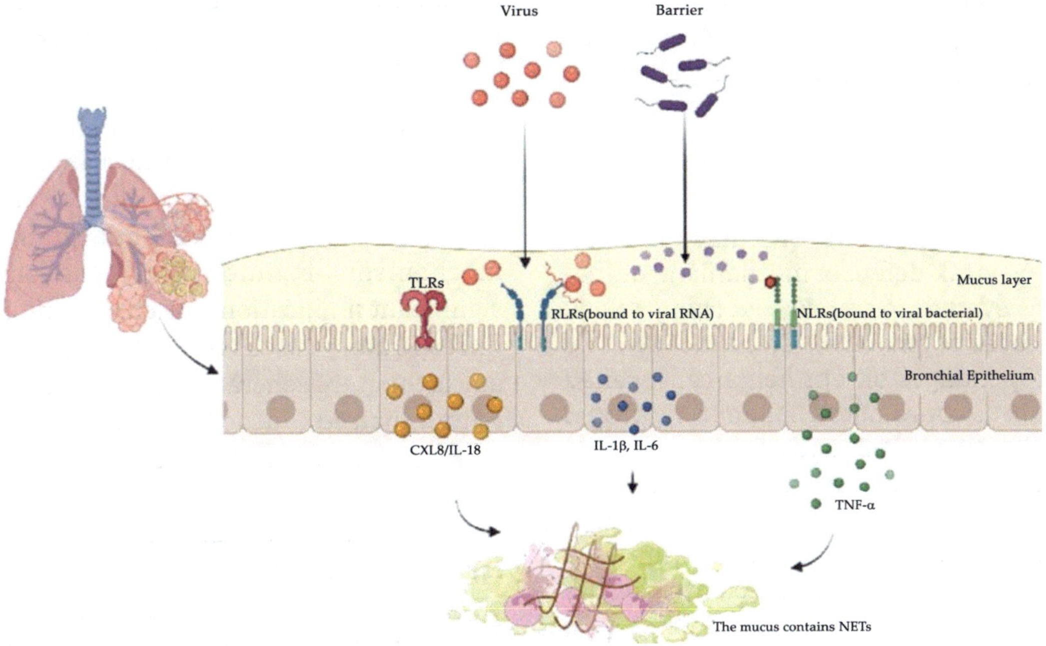

Figure 4.12. Function of mucus in trapping pathogens.

Source: https://ars.els-cdn.com/content/image/1-s2.0-S1567576923007592-gr3.jpg

These hairlike structures facilitate the upward transport of mucus, clearing trapped pathogens and debris from the lungs and along to the pharynx, from which they are removed or swallowed. This active mechanism not only clears filth but also maintains mucus in working order for the long term. The presence of neutrophils constitutes a second line of defense: as they are entrapped, neutrophils are capable of forming neutrophil extracellular traps (NETs), which further immobilize and kill microbes using their DNA and antimicrobial proteins (Rąpała-Kozik et al., 2013). The interaction between mucus production and ciliary motion is thus essential for a successful respiratory defense. In diseases like cystic fibrosis, however, the mucus and respiratory systems are markedly impaired. Thickened mucus due to cystic fibrosis transmembrane conductance regulator (CFTR) gene mutations in patients with cystic fibrosis is hard to move. The defective mucus hinders mucociliary clearance, allowing for an environment that promotes bacterial proliferation and chronic infection (Luan et al., 2018). With their accumulation of pathogens, the bacteria come into contact with neutrophils, which can trigger inflammation and secondary lung injury. The combined action of abnormal mucus and immune response is what goes on to illustrate the complexity of respiratory defense and points to the true significance of successful treatment that seeks to restore mucociliary function. Lastly, understanding the multidimensional role of mucus lies at the core of conceptualizing ways to bolster the respiratory system's immune defenses against the threat of pathogens.

4.4.2. Mechanism of Ciliary Movement

The intricate equipment of ciliary motion serves as a vital defense mechanism of the respiratory system, primarily working to rid airway surfaces of pathogens and toxicants. The hair-like appendages on epithelial cells, called cilia, beat in a coordinated manner to propel mucus droplets packed with debris towards the throat, where they are either swallowed or coughed out. This ciliary movement occurs in a metachronal rhythm, allowing waves of motion to transport mucus efficiently across the airway linings. Perhaps most interestingly, the airway surface liquid (ASL) is a bicameral system, comprising a thicker, more viscous mucous layer on the surface and a thinner, less viscous periciliary layer beneath, which creates an optimal microenvironment for ciliary performance. It is the new research that has demonstrated the dynamic interplay between these layers, so complementing our knowledge of ciliary movement and its absolute significance in mucociliary clearance (Albers et al., 2008).

Central to the success of ciliary movement are the unique structure and beat cycle of the cilia themselves. Each cilium is composed of a core of microtubules arranged in a specific manner that enables successful oscillation. Coordination of the beat of cilia is not haphazard, but is instead developed by multiple mechanical properties, including the viscoelasticity of the mucus that covers them and the forces on cilia exerted as it travels. Current evidence shows that both the elastomeric nature of mucus and the frequency of beat of cilia increase the efficiency of mucociliary clearance. It is evident that optimal ciliary function can be affected in various pathological states and plays a role in diminished mucociliary clearance, leading to secondary respiratory complications (Cortegiani et al., 2019).

As knowledge of ciliary movement becomes more profound, it is of utmost importance for therapeutic intervention in chronic respiratory disease. Furthermore, understanding the mechanisms behind ciliary movement has significant implications for clinical interventions in respiratory diseases. Diseases such as COPD and asthma are generally believed to be associated with impaired mucociliary clearance, and thus increased infection risk and exacerbations. New treatments, such as HFNT, aim to enhance airway hydration and optimize the microenvironment for ciliary function. HFNT delivers humidified oxygen, which sets the rheological properties of the mucus at their best and enhances the function of the cilia. In the dynamic respiratory environment, the integration of ciliary dynamics-related results into the therapeutic pipeline can significantly improve patient outcomes. From prioritizing ciliary movement mechanisms, future research can enable the realization of targeted interventions to alleviate the burden of respiratory diseases and optimize more beneficial airway functioning (Cortegiani et al., 2019).

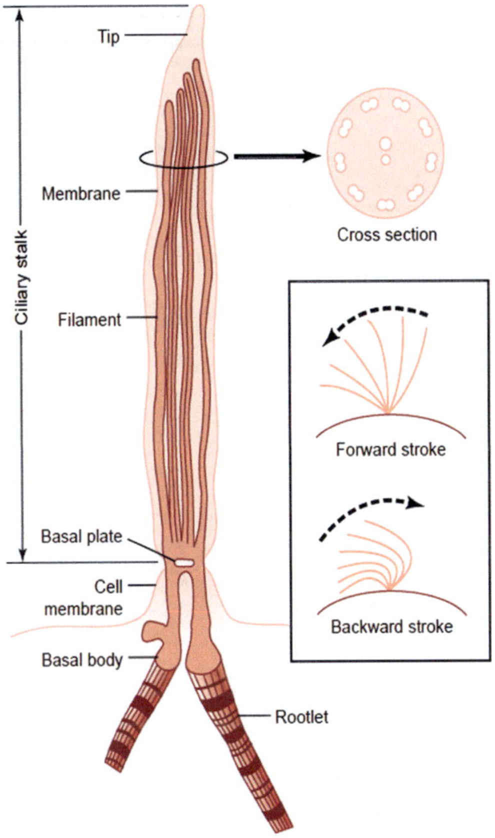

Figure 4.12. Mechanism of ciliary movement.

Source: https://img.brainkart.com/imagebk20/QUIOVnM.png

4.4.3. Importance of the Mucociliary Escalator in Health

The mucociliary escalator is a defense mechanism of the respiratory system, comprising primarily ciliated epithelial cells and goblet cells that produce mucus. This unique apparatus is responsible for trapping and expelling infective agents, particles, and irritants inhaled in the respiratory airways. Through coordinated rhythmic beating of the cilia, these cells propel mucus toward the pharynx, where it can be swallowed or expelled by coughing. This continuous process not only maintains a patent airway but also prevents the accumulation of potentially pathogenic material, which can initiate infection and respiratory disease. A functioning mucociliary escalator is of utmost importance in maintaining pulmonary health, particularly in individuals exposed to environmental toxins, allergens, or infectious substances that can compromise respiratory function and overall well-being. This process is crucial in daily life and disease prevention. Mucociliary escalator impairment could bring about severe health issues in the shape of chronic bronchitis and pneumonia. Tobacco smoking, respiratory infections, and air pollutants possess the ability to harm cilia activity and mucus secretion, resulting in a decrease in clearance efficiency. For instance, exposure to cigarette smoke decreases ciliary beat frequency, leading to mucus accumulation in the airways. This pooling can potentially facilitate bacterial growth and lead to secondary infections, thereby exacerbating underlying conditions. Such vulnerability is particularly highlighted in vulnerable individuals, such as in the situation of individuals with pre-existing lung disease, for instance, asthma or chronic obstructive pulmonary disease (COPD), as documented by historical records on respiratory disease relating to socioeconomic determinants in populations under such disease, as outlined in Chadwick et al., (2006). Additionally, understanding the mechanisms of the mucociliary escalator function is crucial for developing targeted therapies to improve respiratory health. The latest discoveries of cell research have revealed some types of cells that function to provide integrity and functionality to the airway epithelium, as evidenced by research that has illustrated the bronchial epithelium's complexity (Januskevicius et al., 2024). By establishing the specific functions of these cell types, researchers can develop new techniques for restoring mucociliary function in patients with diseases. This could be the basis for new therapeutic strategies to enhance mucosal immunity and mucus clearance. Thus, the functioning and integrity of the mucociliary escalator are not only significant at the individual level but also paramount in reducing the total burden of respiratory diseases in populations at risk from infectious and environmental hazards.

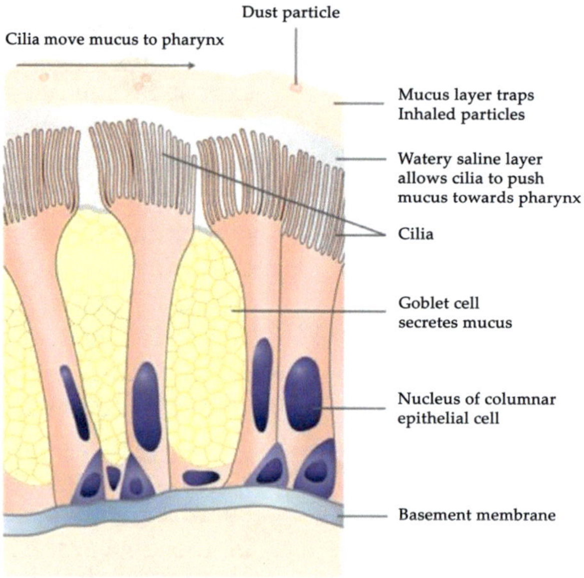

Figure 4.13. Importance of the mucociliary escalator in health.

Source: https://www.researchgate.net/profile/Alexandra-Laniece/publication/331485670/figure/fig17/AS:732574066438147@1551670676970/The-mucociliary-escalator-is-a-defense-mechanism-of-the-bronchi-the-ciliated-cells-beat.jpg

Test Your Knowledge

1. What is the function of mucus in trapping pathogens?
2. What is the mechanism of ciliary movement?

4.5. Role of Alveolar Macrophages

Learning Outcome

1. Function and location of alveolar macrophages
2. Mechanism of pathogen clearance
3. Interaction with other immune cells

Alveolar macrophages are a vital component of the respiratory system's defense mechanism as the frontline defense against airborne pathogens and particulate impurities. Resident in the alveolar spaces of the lungs, these immunocompetent cells can detect and respond to a wide range of pathogen types, including viruses, bacteria, and allergens. Their primary function is in phagocytosis, where they ingest and digest pathogens, and release inflammatory mediators upon ingestion that help target other immune cells towards the infected area. Such an acute inflammatory response initiated by alveolar macrophages plays a crucial role in regulating the immune profile throughout the lungs and hence aiding adequate clearance of pathogens without exacerbating tissue damage. The role of alveolar macrophages extends beyond the mere clearance of pathogens; they are also involved in maintaining pulmonary homeostasis. By releasing cytokines and growth factors, these macrophages promote tissue regeneration and healing following injury or infection. For instance, they coordinate the inflammatory process by releasing interleukins and tumor necrosis factors, which recruit other immune cells while also facilitating the resolution of inflammation. Aside from that, their interaction with different cell types, like lymphocytes and epithelial cells, indicates their contribution to mass immune reactions and the regulation of innate as well as adaptive immunity. Recent research has emphasized alveolar macrophages' role in the context of newly emerging respiratory diseases, including viral infections like COVID-19. Alveolar macrophages have also been shown to play a vital role in the host immune response against severe acute respiratory syndrome coronavirus 2 (SARS-CoV-2) infection, directing inflammatory responses that have a significant impact on disease outcomes. Release of pro-inflammatory cytokines by these macrophages results in the cytokine storm phenomenon due to the hyperstimulated immune response, leading to acute respiratory distress syndrome (ARDS) and other complications. An appreciation for the dual function of alveolar macrophages—protective as well as potentially pathogenic—can inform therapeutic strategies aimed at enhancing host resistance to respiratory infections (Hu et al., 2020; Cuadrado et al., 2020).

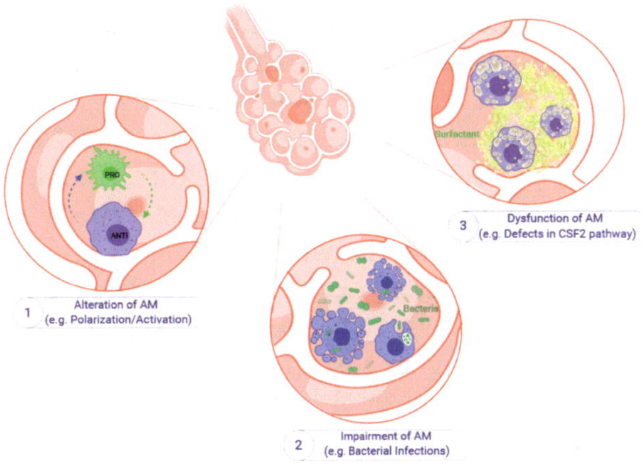

Figure 4.14. Role of alveolar macrophages.

Source: https://pub.mdpi-res.com/ijms/ijms-22-03308/article_deploy/html/images/ijms-22-03308-g001.png?1627940242

4.5.1. Function and Location of Alveolar Macrophages

The position and role of alveolar macrophages suggest the critical function that these cells have in respiratory defense mechanisms. Positioned within the alveolar spaces of the lungs, the specialized immune cells serve as the initial defense against airborne pathogens and particulate contaminants. Strategically located, they are positioned to effectively monitor and respond to a range of threats, including bacteria, viruses, and damaged cells. Alveolar macrophages also possess distinct features that enable them to recognize, engulf, and kill such noxious entities. Through phagocytosis, not only do they eliminate the pathogens, but they also play a role in organizing a more widespread immune response. This attribute is crucial, as the lungs are constantly exposed to environmental insults that compromise respiratory health. Apart from serving as defenders, alveolar macrophages are also tasked with maintaining pulmonary homeostasis. In addition to their direct destruction of pathogens, the cells control inflammation by releasing cytokines that modulate immune responses. For instance, they release signaling molecules that promote or suppress inflammation based on the context of the microbial invasion. However, some environmental toxins, such as persistent organic pollutants like PBDEs, impair the ability of alveolar macrophages to release cytokines. Experiments have shown that these chemicals cause a significant decline in the release of pro-inflammatory cytokines by macrophages, resulting in a higher susceptibility to respiratory disease (Hennigar et al., 2010). This highlights the delicate balance that alveolar macrophages must achieve to maintain lung function and respond to pathogenic agents. The intricate interaction between alveolar macrophages and respiratory epithelial tissues also highlights their significant contribution to lung defense. Respiratory tract lining epithelial cells present a physical barrier as well as secretory products, which activate alveolar macrophages upon inflammation. The interaction between these two cell populations enables localized inflammation and tissue repair after infection or injury. To facilitate this process, alveolar macrophages play a central role in both the adaptive and innate immune responses, enabling the lung tissue to heal and function effectively. The wound-healing mechanisms of lung tissue highlight how macrophage participation can play a positive role in epithelial repair processes through cytokine production and cell-to-cell contact (Chanson et al., 2018). In this way, the multi-functionality of alveolar macrophages not only protects lungs from acute harm but also facilitates longer-term tissue health and recuperation.

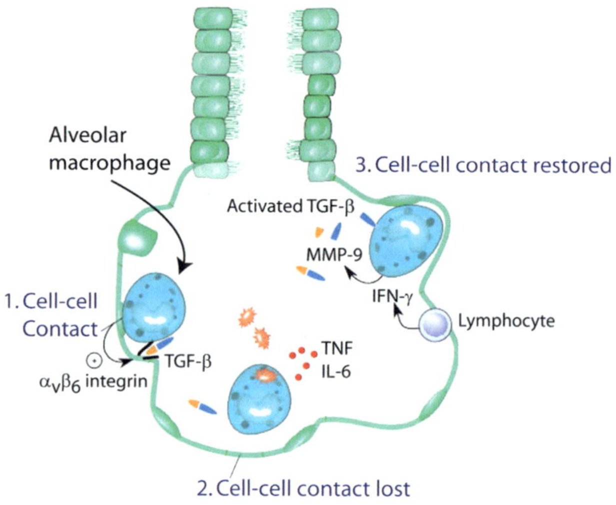

Figure 4.15. Function and location of alveolar macrophages.

Source: https://www.cell.com/cms/10.1016/j.immuni.2006.03.008/asset/3c887ade-b7cc-4976-bbee-258e068ec972/main.assets/gr1_lrg.jpg

4.5.2. Mechanism of Pathogen Clearance

The respiratory system employs a multi-dimensional set of mechanisms to enable the efficient elimination of pathogens, which, if not eliminated, will present an egregious challenge to overall health. At the forefront of this protection are the physical defenses offered by the respiratory epithelium, characterized by cilia and mucus. Mucus traps pathogens drawn into the airways, while cilia, by rhythmic motion, propel the trapped invaders down to the pharynx, where they may be swallowed or expectorated. This mucociliary escalator is an essential part of clearing pathogens before they can cause infection. The effectiveness of this first line of defense is supplemented by the presence of antimicrobial peptides and enzymes in the mucus that assist in degrading bacterial and viral particles, thereby minimizing the potential for pathogenesis. Besides the chemical and mechanical defenses, the immune system has an intrinsic role in clearing out respiratory pathogens. Cells such as macrophages and neutrophils form the first line of adaptive defense, responding rapidly to microbial invasion. Upon recognizing the pathogen, the activated macrophage can induce an inflammatory response that recruits additional immune cells and releases cytokines to further amplify the inflammatory environment. This activation plays a crucial role in modulating the efficacy of pathogen clearance through phagocytosis as well as the release of reactive oxygen species. In addition, organized compartments, such as bronchus-associated lymphoid tissue (BALT), play a critical role in the organized immune response, as both B and T lymphocytes are in their correct positions to respond against pathogens when they are repeatedly exposed or chronically infected (Dalamani et al., 2006). Furthermore, the enhancement of immune reactions within the respiratory tract is not solely dependent on cell-mediated mechanisms; humoral reactions also significantly contribute to the elimination of pathogens. Secretory IgA, one of the predominant antibodies found in mucosal surfaces, is a critical antibody that inactivates pathogens and prevents their adherence to epithelial cells. The level of IgA in respiratory secretions plays a crucial role in infection control by its capacity to neutralize infections caused by many pathogens, including viruses and bacteria. Additionally, the compartmentalization of immune components in the respiratory tissue ensures that local immune responses are tightly regulated. An understanding of dynamic interactions among heterogeneous immune cells and humoral components ensures an intimate knowledge of pathogen elimination mechanisms (Brown et al., 2014). The multidisciplinary nature of this approach highlights the importance of both innate and adaptive immunity in defending the respiratory system.

4.5.3. Interaction With Other Immune Cells

Such interaction between other immune cells is essential in the respiratory system's defense strategies so that there is a synergistic response to the pathogen. In the lung, specific structures such as bronchus-associated lymphoid tissue (BALT) serve as the key link that coordinates these immune interactions. BALT has typical populations of B and T lymphocytes, which play a crucial role in initiating the adaptive immune response. In microbial invasion, BALT facilitates the activation and proliferation of these lymphocytes, leading to enhanced antibody and cytokine production. This compartmentalized specialty is engineered to provide a tailored immune response, offering efficient protection against respiratory infection without incurring collateral damage to host tissues. Additionally, the presence of macrophages in the interstitial spaces of the lung interacts with lymphocytes via phagocytosis of bacteria and antigen presentation, thereby bridging innate and adaptive immunity in the respiratory tract, as noted in the modulation of immune responses in structures such as BALT (Dalamani et al., 2006). Moreover, the interactions of the respiratory immune system include not only lymphocytes and macrophages but also epithelial cells, the frontline of defense against airborne pathogens. Current evidence indicates that respiratory epithelial cells have the capacity to modulate immune responses by controlling the behavior of invading immune cells. For instance, under exposure to pathogens such as Neisseria meningitidis, epithelial cells undergo alterations in gene expression that affect host defense mechanisms. These events promote the recruitment of immune cells to the point of infection and the production of pro-inflammatory cytokines, thus augmenting the innate immune response. Of particular interest are the differential responses between pathogens, as reflected by the activity of Neisseria lactamica compared to that of N. meningitidis, which demonstrate how varying levels of immune modulation can manifest as different clinical presentations. This suggests the crucial role of communication between immune cells and epithelial cells in coordinating a coordinated defense mechanism against respiratory pathogens (Hibberd et al., 2011).

In addition to local interactions, systemic signaling through cytokines and chemokines plays a central role in the recruitment and activation of immune cells in the respiratory defense mechanism. For example, when an infection occurs, macrophages and dendritic cells produce a variety of signaling molecules that facilitate the recruitment of neutrophils and lymphocytes to the site of inflammation. Recruitment is crucial for the rapid immobilization of pathogens, as neutrophils are fast in reaching and destroying intruders. The communication between these immune cells is not entirely one-way; the activated lymphocytes can also produce cytokines to activate macrophages and cause further inflammatory responses, having a feedback mechanism which rectifies the local immune environment. The differential balance of pro-inflammatory and anti-inflammatory signals also governs the resolution of these interactions, ultimately determining whether the response subsides or leads to chronic inflammation. These complex interactions underscore the dynamic nature of the respiratory immune system, highlighting the crucial role of coordinated cellular dialogues in maintaining respiratory health and mitigating pathogenic insults (Dalamani et al., 2006).

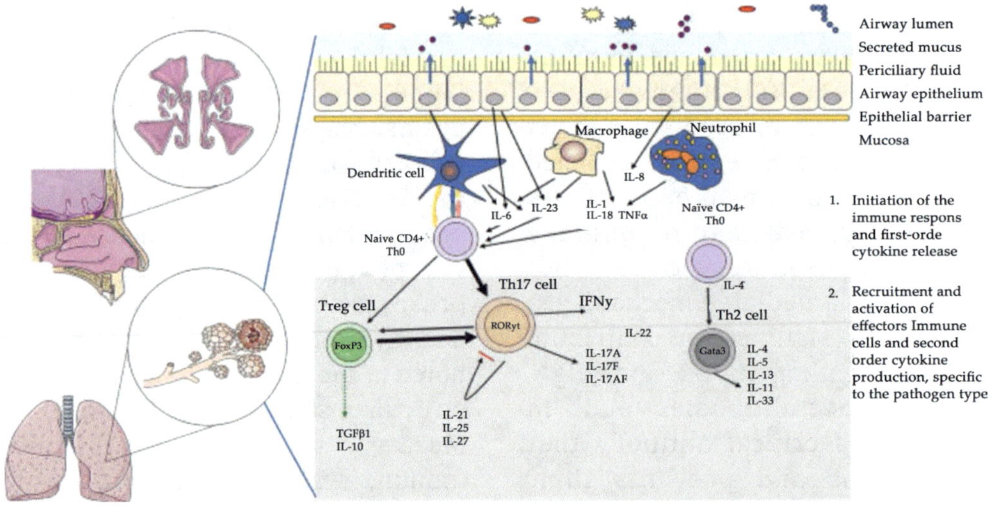

Figure 4.15. Interaction with other immune cells role in the respiratory systems defense mechanisms.

Source: https://media.springernature.com/lw685/springer-static/image/chp%3A10.1007%2F978-3-031-74853-0_5/MediaObjects/607708_1_En_5_Fig1_HTML.png

Test Your Knowledge

1. What are the function and location of alveolar macrophages?
2. What is the mechanism of pathogen clearance?

4.6. Impact of Environmental Factors

Learning Outcome

1. Effects of pollution on respiratory defense
2. Influence of smoking on defense mechanisms
3. Role of allergens in respiratory health

Environmental factors strongly impact the respiratory system's defense mechanisms across various species. The atmospheric structure, including oxygen levels and the presence of pollutants, directly impacts respiratory function and efficiency. For instance, individuals residing at high altitudes have reduced oxygen levels, which trigger their respiratory physiology to undergo adaptive changes. This mechanism demonstrates how environmental stress can lead to the evolution of respiratory mechanisms that enable maximum oxygen intake, regardless of unfavorable conditions. Through this, the resilience and adaptability of the respiratory system reflect its intrinsic relation with ambient environmental parameters, exhibiting survival tactics against various ecological niches. Moreover, temperature differences significantly influence the respiratory defense mechanisms employed by organisms. Extreme temperatures have been found to facilitate elevated metabolic rates, which in turn lead to increased oxygen demand. This is best exemplified in birds, whose habitats involve climatic and altitudinal variation. Structural adaptation in the lungs, such as the alveolar surface area, allows birds to extract oxygen even at hypoxic altitudes successfully. These adaptations not only enhance their overall respiratory effectiveness but also function as primary evolutionary defenses against environmental stressors that they face within their ecosystems. The interplay between temperature and the respiratory system highlights the significance of environmental factors in shaping physiological traits that enhance survival.

Finally, the presence of pollutants in environmental media presents an additional challenge to the respiratory system, which demands robust defensive adaptations. Pollutants inflict significant damage on lung tissues and impair respiratory efficiency, leading to the development of mechanisms that confer resistance. Organisms employ various means to resist airborne toxins, including increased mucous production and the induction of immune mechanisms. For example, migratory birds flying over urbanized regions have elevated levels of respiratory protective mechanisms to resist pollutants during their migration. These adaptations not only play a role in preserving respiratory health but also show the immediate influence of environmental pressures on the biological process. Combined, the impact of environmental factors such as altitude, temperature, and pollutants reveals the intricate relationship between an organism's environment and its respiratory protective responses, providing a broader ecological context in which these adaptations are found (Brown et al., 2014; Altshuler et al., 2006).

4.6.1. Effects of Pollution On Respiratory Defense

The respiratory system possesses inherent defense mechanisms designed to protect against hostile environmental conditions, including pollutants. However, exposure to air pollution severely compromises these protective mechanisms. It has been confirmed through scientific studies that particulate matter, wonderful particles, is capable of inducing inflammatory responses in lung epithelial cells. For instance, Urban Air Particles of Buenos Aires (UAP-BA) have exhibited proinflammatory activity, which was particularly demonstrated through their conditioned media, which reduced cell viability and elevated the generation of reactive oxygen species (O2-) and inflammatory cytokines, such as IL-8. These findings illustrate the paradoxical defense of the lung; while it initially attempts to repel inhaled irritants, repeated exposure can lead to long-term inflammation and damage, thereby compromising the very defenses designed to safeguard respiratory well-being (Astort et al., 2014).

The health inequalities linked to air pollution underscore a pressing need for targeted interventions to curb them. Populations residing in urban communities, with low socioeconomic status being the most vulnerable, have disproportionately higher levels of exposure to toxic pollutants. The American Lung Association has recognized these disparities, highlighting the importance of scientific research in guiding community interventions to reduce these exposures. Legislation has been passed since the initial stages of air pollution to mitigate air pollution, yet the exposed communities continue to have high health impacts. Evidence has elucidated the correlations between socioeconomic factors and the prevalence of respiratory disease exacerbated by pollution. Resolution of these inequalities demands not only educated awareness but also the formulation of policies for cleaner air as well as protection against the prohibitive effects on the populations affected by respiratory barriers (Association, 2001).

Additionally, the complexity of air pollution, which impacts respiratory health, demands an extensive understanding of the mechanisms. The poisons in various pollutants may generate a cascade of biological responses, like the discharge of proinflammatory mediators, resulting in cellular damage and compromised pulmonary defense. Current research indicates that the soluble fractions of pollutants are capable of amplifying the impact of airborne particles and making the process of the lungs constructing a proper response even more complicated. When inflammation progresses to become a chronic condition, the respiratory epithelium, a critical component of innate immunity, is disrupted, making the body vulnerable to infection and chronic respiratory disease. Therefore, an interdisciplinary strategy through public health interventions and community engagement is necessary to counteract the harmful effects of pollution on respiratory protection (Astort et al., 2014).

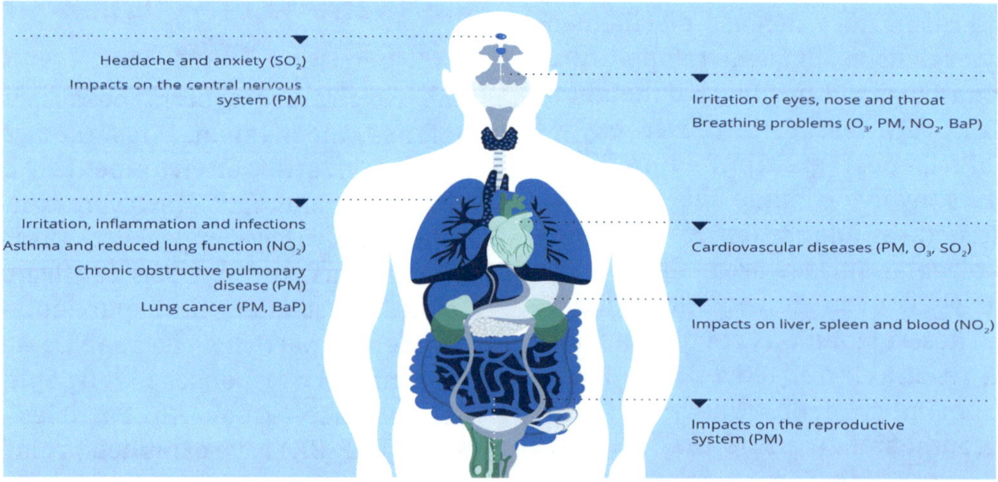

Figure 4.16. Effects of pollution on respiratory defense.

Source: https://i0.wp.com/O_2foreveryone.com/wp-content/uploads/2025/01/How-Does-Air-Pollution-Impact-Respiratory-Health.png?fit=800%2C387&ssl=1

4.6.2. Influence of Smoking On Defense Mechanisms

Smoking affects the respiratory system by causing widespread alterations in its defense mechanisms, ultimately leading to adverse health effects. The human respiratory system has various defense mechanisms, like mucociliary clearance and immune mechanisms, that are responsible for clearing inhaled pathogens and particulates. Cigarette smoke, however, subjects the system to a deluge of harmful chemicals, which leads to alterations in the operational mechanism of these protective mechanisms. Especially, cigarette smoking causes damage to cilia, the hair-like projections that transport mucus and trapped impurities out of the airways.

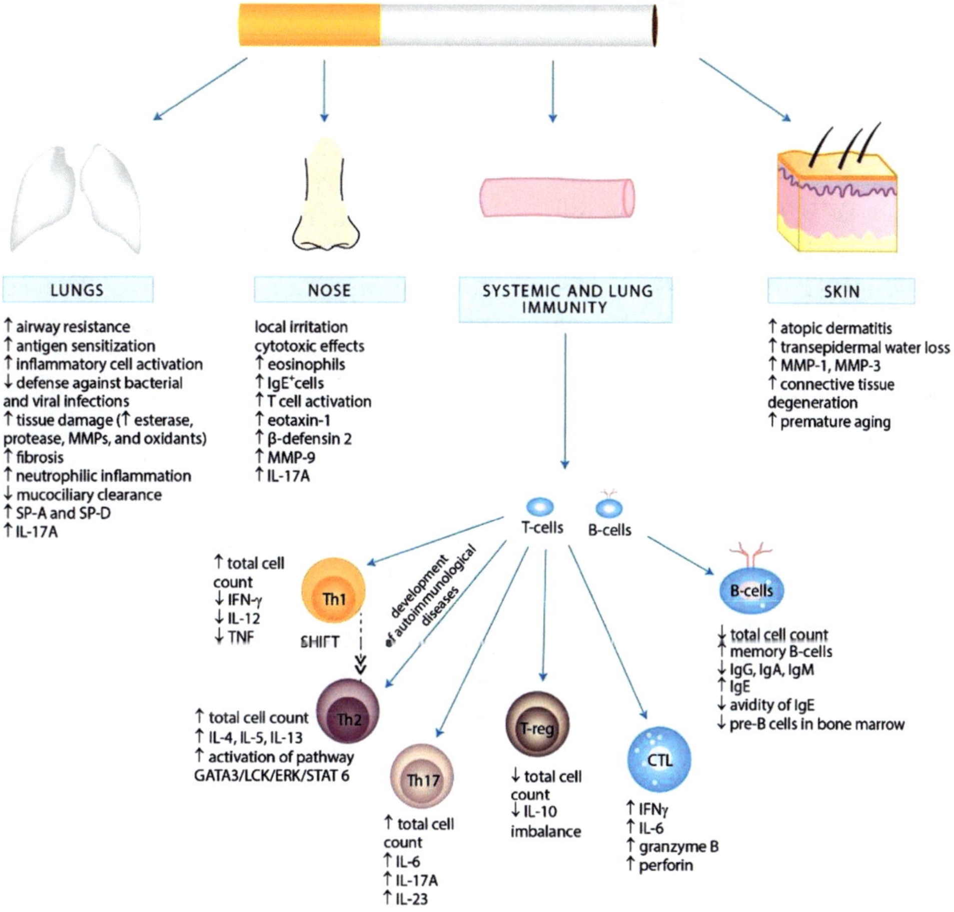

Figure 4.17. Tobacco smoke induces and alters immune responses in the lung.

Source: https://www.mdpi.com/ijerph/ijerph-15-01033/article_deploy/html/images/ijerph-15-01033-g001.png

This dysfunction reduces mucociliary clearance efficiency, making people more susceptible to respiratory infections and chronic diseases like COPD and lung cancer. Consequently, the efficiency of such natural defenses against environmental toxins is significantly compromised, giving prominence to a harmful cycle initiated by smoking that compromises lung health as a whole. Moreover, the toxic effects of smoking also affect the immune responses of the respiratory apparatus. Consumption of tobacco smoke releases numerous reactive oxygen species (ROS) that can cause oxidative stress, a condition that suppresses the body's ability to battle infection effectively. Higher levels of ROS can induce inflammation and tissue damage in the lungs, as well as impair immune function. The immune function of the immune system to detect and kill pathogens is compromised, which in turn results in long-term inflammatory responses in the respiratory tract. The chronic nature of ROS, as noted by researchers, can lead to DNA damage and cell apoptosis, increasing the likelihood of respiratory disease. As also highlighted in the literature, the rise in oxidative stress markers directly correlates with compromised sperm function, with more systemic implications (Dutta et al., 2019). The systemic impact of these changes due to smoking are widespread and point toward the importance of especially tailored interventions that will facilitate the enhancement of respiratory protection. Additionally, smoking significantly alters the secretion and production of immunologic factors throughout the respiratory tract. For instance, it alters cytokine levels and other molecules that regulate immune responses. Smokers have abnormal alveolar macrophage function, which is significant in recognizing and responding to pathogens in the lungs. Such abnormality leads to impaired clearance of bacteria and other pathogens, placing smokers at risk for respiratory tract infections, such as pneumonia. Research emphasizes the role of such changes as essential factors in the emergence of long-term respiratory complications. In addition, the chronic inflammation of inflammatory mediators and toxic agents that are characteristic of cigarette smoke can exacerbate existing respiratory disease. The cumulative effect demonstrates the necessity of public health interventions aimed at reducing the prevalence of smoking, thereby ensuring the efficacy of the respiratory system's defense mechanisms (Visseren et al., 2021).

4.6.3. Role of Allergens in Respiratory Health

Allergens have a crucial function in respiratory wellness, particularly with regard to the increasing prevalence of allergic disease across the world. Allergens, such as pollen, mould spores, and dust mites, provoke immune responses that compromise the integrity of the respiratory system. A case in point is the pollen grains of most vegetation, which contain proteolytic enzymes proven to compromise the respiratory epithelial barrier. Research has shown that pollen proteases in species like Kentucky bluegrass and white birch specifically target the anchorage of columnar respiratory cells, leading to increased susceptibility to infections such as those caused by alphaherpesvirus. This connection between exposure to allergens and the consequent harm to the respiratory epithelium illustrates how allergens can compromise the protective functions of the respiratory system, thereby exacerbating asthma and rhinitis (Gevaert et al., 2019).

The immune response to allergens also contributes to the sophistication of respiratory disease. Exposure to allergenic substances triggers the immune system to activate pathways that can lead to inflammation and tissue remodeling. Specifically, cytokines generated in the context of allergies can trigger profound transformations of the airway epithelium, contributing to hyperresponsiveness and chronic inflammation. Not only does this enhance the symptoms of those suffering from allergies, but it can also result in long-term complications, such as airway obstruction and diminished lung function. The necessity of preserving optimal immune system function becomes a pivotal focus in treating allergic disease. Nutrition, as an immune-modulating component, may also play a significant potential role in exacerbating or abating these allergic responses (Albers et al., 2017).

Thus, the interaction between allergens and the immune system identifies their respective critical functions in pulmonary wellness. In addition, the realization of the interaction between environmental determinants and pulmonary wellness also emphasizes the imperative for effective public health intervention. Interventions to minimize exposure to identified allergens can significantly maximize respiratory health benefits. For example, interventions that reduce airborne pollen or manage indoor allergens, such as dust mites, can help reduce allergic responses. Educational public campaigns aimed at sensitizing communities on the avoidance of allergens, as well as the requirement for immune nurturing through healthy eating, are imperative. Such programs would enable individuals to improve their respiratory health in the face of unavoidable allergen exposure. Finally, the intricate relationship between allergens and the mechanisms of respiratory protection necessitates an integrated strategy involving research, prevention, and therapeutic approaches to ensure respiratory health (Gevaert et al., 2019; Albers et al., 2017).

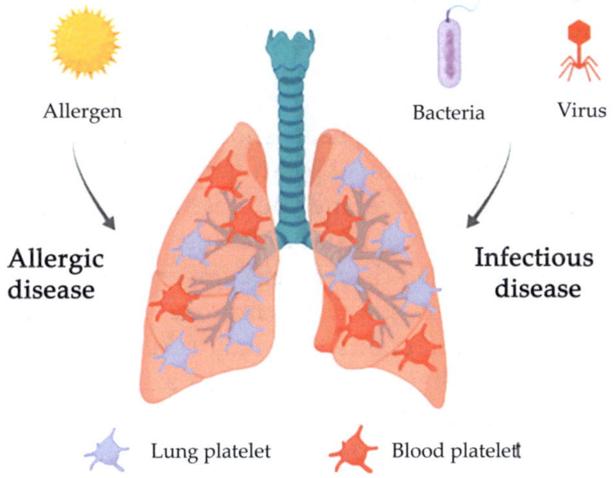

Figure 4.18. Role of allergens in respiratory health.

Source: https://www.mdpi.com/ijms/ijms-20-01730/article_deploy/html/images/ijms-20-01730 g001.png

Test Your Knowledge

1. What are the effects of pollution on respiratory defense?
2. What is the role of allergens in respiratory health?

SUMMARY

An examination of the defense mechanisms of the respiratory system reveals that these intricate processes are essential for maintaining homeostasis and protecting against many pathogens. The respiratory epithelium, with its intricate ciliary and mucous-secreting cell arrangement, serves as the initial defense, trapping airborne pathogens and particulates. Furthermore, the stimulation of Toll-like receptors (TLRs) in epithelial cells demonstrates that innate immunity is extremely rapid in responding to potential threats. For instance, TLR4 plays a critical role in recognizing microbial products. As such, they induce the production of antimicrobial peptides, such as beta-defensins, which play a critical role in modulating inflammation and tightening the epithelial layer against both endogenous and exogenous insults, as supported by the findings of Pace et al. (Aderem et al., 2012). Aside from these expressions, synergistic interactions between various immune cells and epithelial tissues also underscore the adaptive roles of the respiratory system. Exposure to bacteria can induce extensive modifications in gene expression and hence enhance the host's defense. A comparison of the impact of *Neisseria meningitidis* with *Neisseria lactamica* on respiratory epithelial cells highlights differential host responses to bacterial invasion and colonization. While N. meningitidis has been shown to suppress host defense genes, *N. lactamica* appears to have a positive modulation of pro-inflammatory responses, thus establishing a complex interaction between microbial presence and the host immune response. This information also further demystifies the intricacies of respiratory defense mechanisms and the potential vulnerabilities through which pathogens enter, thereby circumventing these mechanisms (Hibberd et al., 2011). Finally, however, the robustness of the respiratory system's defense mechanisms is most critical, particularly in preventing infections that may result in significant morbidity and mortality. Chronic obstructive pulmonary disease (COPD), for example, is characterized by diminished pulmonary defenses, which enhance bacterial colonization and modify disease course. The reduced expression of key antimicrobial peptides, such as HBD2, in COPD patients is only one indication of the adverse impact chronic inflammation and environmental exposures, such as cigarette smoking, have on lung health. Explain these alterations in addition to clarifying the respiratory disease pathophysiology and opening up possibilities for therapeutic interventions that restore and enhance the native immune potential of the respiratory system, as in the latest findings (Aderem et al., 2012).

The respiratory system employs a series of defense mechanisms that are designed to exclude noxious pathogens and irritants from reaching the airways. The mucociliary escalator is a primary defense system, consisting primarily of cilia and epithelial secreted mucus. Cilia beat rhythmically and continuously to move mucus, which traps dust particles and pathogens, toward the pharynx. This procedure not only aids in the clearance of debris but also as an immunological barrier. Additionally, the epithelial cells possess special receptors, specifically the transient receptor potential ankyrin 1 (TRPA1) channel, which serves as a sensory signal for irritants inhaled. Stimulation of this pathway can elicit a protective cough reflex and bronchoconstriction, thus illustrating the intricate interplay between structural and cellular defense mechanisms in the respiratory system (Tekulapally et al., 2024).

The other significant component of the defense against respiratory infections is the immune response, which involves both innate and adaptive mechanisms. The complement system is a pivotal element in this respect, serving as a component of innate immunity that can provide an immediate response to inhaled pathogens. The recognition of microbes activates complement proteins, facilitating opsonization, chemotaxis, and the formation of the membrane attack complex, all of which contribute to the induction of inflammation and pathogen destruction. Importantly, while the complement system is defensive against infection, it also possesses the ability to exacerbate disease states, such as those caused by viral infections like COVID-19. This dualism reminds us of the need for a sufficiently balanced response to prevent overinflammation that is causative of respiratory distress (Xiao et al., 2024).

Lastly, the role of immune cells contributes significantly to the richness of the respiratory system's defense capacity. Cells such as macrophages, neutrophils, and dendritic cells act in concert to monitor and respond to potential harm. Alveolar space macrophages are essential for the phagocytosis of pathogens and debris, serving as the initial first responders in the respiratory tract environment. Complementary to these cells, dendritic cells present antigens to T cells, thereby promoting the interaction between innate and adaptive immunity. Finally, the cooperative action of these immune components and the intricate signaling pathways employed confer a robust protection against environmental toxins without compromising the integrity of respiratory function. This multifaceted approach serves to illustrate the sophistication and versatility of the respiratory system in its ability to protect itself against a wide variety of insults.

KEY TERMS FROM THIS CHAPTER

- Mucociliary clearance
- Goblet cells
- Cough reflex
- Alveolar macrophages
- IgA antibodies
- Bronchus-associated lymphoid tissue (BALT)
- Antimicrobial peptides
- Reflex bronchoconstriction
- Inflammatory response
- Complement system
- Cilia
- Mucus
- Sneezing
- Respiratory epithelium
- Lymphoid tissue
- Surfactant proteins
- Nasal hairs
- Phagocytosis
- Histamine release
- Oxidative burst

CRITICAL THINKING QUESTIONS

1. **Which of the following cells plays a key role in phagocytosis within the alveoli?**
   a. Type I pneumocytes
   b. Goblet cells
   c. Alveolar macrophages
   d. Ciliated epithelial cells
2. **What is the primary function of the mucociliary escalator in the respiratory tract?**
   a. Produce surfactant
   b. Trap and remove inhaled particles and pathogens
   c. Facilitate gas exchange
   d. Detect airborne allergens
3. **Which type of cell secretes mucus in the respiratory tract?**
   a. Clara cells
   b. Goblet cells
   c. Type II pneumocytes
   d. Basal cells
4. **The cough reflex is primarily mediated by stimulation of which type of receptor?**
   a. Chemoreceptors in the medulla
   b. Stretch receptors in alveoli
   c. Irritant receptors in the airway epithelium
   d. Baroreceptors in the carotid sinus
5. **Which of the following provides the first line of defense in the upper respiratory tract?**
   a. Ciliated epithelium and mucus
   b. Alveolar macrophages
   c. Surfactant production
   d. Antibodies in blood

Short Answer Questions

1. What is the primary physical barrier that prevents pathogens from entering the respiratory tract?
2. Describe the role of mucus in respiratory defense.
3. What type of cells are responsible for the mucociliary escalator function?
4. Name the immune cells that act as the first line of cellular defense in the alveoli.
5. What is the role of surfactant proteins in respiratory immunity?

Answer to Critical Thinking Questions

1. (c) 2. (b) 3. (b) 4. (c) 5. (a)

REFERENCES

1. Chiu, L., Bazin, T., Truchetet, M., Schaeverbeke, T., Delhaes, L., & Pradeu, T. (2017). Protective microbiota: From localized to Long-Reaching Co-Immunity. *Frontiers in Immunology, 8.* https://doi.org/10.3389/fimmu.2017.01678Aderem, A., Biragyn, A., Bruno, A., Busacker, A., Kato, A., Cozens, A. L., Montalbano, A. M., et al. (2012). Beta defensin-2 is reduced in central but not in distal airways of smoker COPD patients. https://core.ac.uk/download/12212627.pdf (accessed on 16th June 2025).
2. Albers, R., App, H., Barton, J., Blake, D., et al. (2008). Modelling mucociliary clearance. https://core.ac.uk/download/pdf/97255.pdf (accessed on 16th June 2025).
3. Albers, R., Bourdet-Sicard, R., Braun, D., Calder, P. C., et al. (2017). Monitoring immune modulation by nutrition in the general population: Identifying and substantiating effects on human health. https://core.ac.uk/download/85214747.pdf (accessed on 16th June 2025).
4. Aldini, G., Altomare, A., Baron, G., Vistoli, G., Carini, M., Borsani, L., & Sergio, F. (2018). N-acetylcysteine as an antioxidant and disulphide breaking agent: The reasons why. *Free Radical Research, 52*, 751–762. https://doi.org/10.1080/10715762.2018.1468564 (accessed on 16th June 2025).
5. Altshuler, D. L., & Dudley, R. (2006). The physiology and biomechanics of avian flight at high altitude. https://core.ac.uk/download/4887664.pdf (accessed on 16th June 2025).
6. American Lung Association. (2001). Urban air pollution and health inequities: A workshop report. https://core.ac.uk/download/323074325.pdf (accessed on 16th June 2025).
7. Arkenberg, A., Bleakley, B., Bodenmiller, B., Brunelli, R., Chakravortty, D., Cherayil, B. J., Constantinidou, C., et al. (2011). The production and detoxification of a potent cytotoxin, nitric oxide, by pathogenic enteric bacteria. https://core.ac.uk/download/2781215.pdf (accessed on 16th June 2025).
8. Arulselvan, P., Tangestani Fard, M., Tan, W. S., Gothai, S., Fakurazi, S., Norhaizan, M. E., & Kumar, S. (2016). Role of antioxidants and natural products in inflammation. *Oxidative Medicine and Cellular Longevity, 2016.* https://doi.org/10.1155/2016/5276130 (accessed on 16th June 2025).
9. Astort, F., Maglione, G. A., Orona, N. S., Saldiva, P. H., et al. (2014). Direct and indirect air particle cytotoxicity in human alveolar epithelial cells. https://core.ac.uk/download/159293549.pdf (accessed on 16th June 2025).
10. Bayard, J. B., & Ramos Morales, F. (2018). Molecular mechanisms used by *Salmonella* to evade the immune system. https://core.ac.uk/download/222572248.pdf (accessed on 16th June 2025).
11. Bresson, J. L., Burlingame, B., Dean, M., et al. (2017). 'Nutrimune®' and immune defense against pathogens in the gastrointestinal and upper respiratory tracts: Evaluation of a health claim pursuant to Article 14 of Regulation (EC) No 1924/2006. https://core.ac.uk/download/84493852.pdf (accessed on 16th June 2025).
12. Brown, A. J. P., Brown, G. D., Gow, N. A. R., Netea, M. G., et al. (2014). Metabolism impacts upon *Candida* immunogenicity and pathogenicity at multiple levels. https://core.ac.uk/download/25497610.pdf (accessed on 16th June 2025).

13. Brown, G. D., Hardison, S. E., & Plato, A. (2014). Pattern recognition receptors in antifungal immunity. https://core.ac.uk/download/29151173.pdf (accessed on 16th June 2025).

14. Brown, R. L., & Clarke, T. B. (2016). The regulation of host defenses to infection by the microbiota. https://core.ac.uk/download/77016328.pdf (accessed on 16th June 2025).

15. Carabelli, A. M., Peacock, T. P., Thorne, L., Harvey, W. T., Hughes, J., de Silva, T. I., Peacock, S. J., et al. (2023). SARS-CoV-2 variant biology: Immune escape, transmission and fitness. *Nature Reviews Microbiology.* https://doi.org/10.1038/s41579-022-00841-7 (accessed on 16th June 2025).

16. Chadwick, D., & Goode, J. (2006). Innate immunity to pulmonary infection. https://www.semanticscholar.org/paper/2c26421da70058363c6fc1cbab6f73ba023dfff8 (accessed on 16th June 2025).

17. Chanson, M., Martin, P. E., O'Shaughnessy, E. M., Watanabe, H., et al. (2018). Connexin communication compartments and wound repair in epithelial tissue. https://core.ac.uk/download/293885271.pdf (accessed on 16th June 2025).

18. Collins, A., Weitkamp, J. H., & Wynn, J. L. (2018). Why are preterm newborns at increased risk of infection? *Archives of Disease in Childhood: Fetal & Neonatal, 103*, F391–F394. https://doi.org/10.1136/archdischild-2017-313595 (accessed on 16th June 2025).

19. Cortegiani, A., Gregoretti, C., & Spoletini, G. (2019). Physio pathological rationale of using high-flow nasal therapy in the acute and chronic setting: A narrative review. https://core.ac.uk/download/224993362.pdf (accessed on 16th June 2025).

20. Cuadrado, A., Pajares, M., Benito, C., Jiménez-Villegas, J., Escoll, M., Fernández-Ginés, R., García-Yagüe, Á. J., et al. (2020). Can activation of NRF2 be a strategy against COVID-19? *Trends in Pharmacological Sciences, 41*, 598–610. https://doi.org/10.1016/j.tips.2020.07.003 (accessed on 16th June 2025).

21. Dalamani, G., Kaspers, B., & Reese, S. (2006). The avian lung-associated immune system. https://core.ac.uk/download/12174987.pdf (accessed on 16th June 2025).

22. Dias, A. G., Sampaio, N. G., & Rehwinkel, J. (2018). A balancing act: MDA5 in antiviral immunity and autoinflammation. *Trends in Microbiology, 27*, 75–85. https://doi.org/10.1016/j.tim.2018.08.007 (accessed on 16th June 2025).

23. Dutta, S., Majzoub, A., & Agarwal, A. (2019). Oxidative stress and sperm function: A systematic review on evaluation and management. *Arab Journal of Urology, 17*, 87–97. https://doi.org/10.1080/2090598x.2019.1599624 (accessed on 16th June 2025).

24. EFSA Panel on Dietetic Products, Nutrition, and Allergies; Heinonen, M. (2017). 'Nutrimune®' and immune defense against pathogens in the gastrointestinal and upper respiratory tracts: Evaluation of a health claim pursuant to Article 14 of Regulation (EC) No 1924/2006. https://core.ac.uk/download/224638622.pdf (accessed on 16th June 2025).

25. Gevaert, K., Impens, F., Laval, K., Nauwynck, H., et al. (2019). Pollens destroy respiratory epithelial cell anchors and drive alpha herpesvirus infection. https://core.ac.uk/download/222452376.pdf (accessed on 16th June 2025).

26. Giegold, M. (2018). Modeling of the immune response during virus infection of the human respiratory tract. https://core.ac.uk/download/pdf/289960831.pdf (accessed on 16th June 2025).

27. Glezen, R., Hartshorn, K., Hufford, M., Jin, H., Jordan, J., Luo, D., Mosmann, T., et al. (2016). Influenza and memory T cells: How to awake the force. https://core.ac.uk/download/84594764.pdf (accessed on 16th June 2025).

28. Hegermann, J., Kuebler, W. M., Lopez-Rodriguez, E., Matuszak, J., et al. (2020). On top of the alveolar epithelium: Surfactant and the glycocalyx. https://core.ac.uk/download/323256852.pdf (accessed on 16th June 2025).

29. Hennigar, S. R. (2010). Exposure to polybrominated diphenyl ethers (PBDEs) suppresses the release of pro-inflammatory products by alveolar macrophages *in vitro*. https://core.ac.uk/download/215515896.pdf (accessed on 16th June 2025).

30. Hibberd, M. L., Kroll, J. S., Langford, P. R., Li, D., et al. (2011). Genome-wide expression profiling reveals suppression of host defense responses during colonization by *Neisseria meningitidis* but not *N. lactamica*. https://core.ac.uk/download/13115586.pdf (accessed on 16th June 2025).

31. Higham, A., Quinn, A. M., Delfini Cançado, J. E., & Singh, D. (2019). The pathology of small airways disease in COPD: Historical aspects and future directions. *Respiratory Research, 20*. https://doi.org/10.1186/s12931-019-1017-y (accessed on 16th June 2025).

32. Hu, B., Guo, H., Zhou, P., & Shi, Z. L. (2020). Characteristics of SARS-CoV-2 and COVID-19. *Nature Reviews Microbiology, 19*, 141–154. https://doi.org/10.1038/s41579-020-00459-7 (accessed on 16th June 2025).

33. Ivanova, N., Sotirova, Y., Gavrailov, G., Nikolova, K., & Andonova, V. (2022). Advances in the prophylaxis of respiratory infections by the nasal and the oromucosal route: Relevance to the fight with the SARS-CoV-2 pandemic. *Pharmaceutics, 14*, 530–530. https://doi.org/10.3390/pharmaceutics14030530 (accessed on 16th June 2025).

34. Januskevicius, A., Vasyle, E., & Malakauskas, K. (2024). Asthma: A new approach to the bronchial epithelium. *Pulmonology and Allergology*. https://www.semanticscholar.org/paper/0c0fee4e3b5abb1efc1e882f4937be416821bc16 (accessed on 16th June 2025).

35. Jarosz, M., Olbert, M., Wyszogrodzka, G., Młyniec, K., & Librowski, T. (2017). Antioxidant and anti-inflammatory effects of zinc. Zinc-dependent NF-κB signaling. *Inflammopharmacology, 25*, 11–24. https://doi.org/10.1007/s10787-017-0309-4 (accessed on 16th June 2025).

36. Jurado-Martín, I., Sainz-Mejías, M., & McClean, S. (2021). *Pseudomonas aeruginosa*: An audacious pathogen with an adaptable arsenal of virulence factors. *International Journal of Molecular Sciences, 22*, 3128–3128. https://doi.org/10.3390/ijms22063128 (accessed on 16th June 2025).

37. Luan, X. J. (2018). Effect of bacteria on airway submucosal glands liquid secretion in swine. https://core.ac.uk/download/226146030.pdf (accessed on 16th June 2025).

38. Rąpała-Kozik, M., & Zawrotniak, M. (2013). Neutrophil extracellular traps (NETs): Formation and implications. https://core.ac.uk/download/53115269.pdf (accessed on 16th June 2025).

39. Rehm, J., Gmel, G., Gmel, G., Hasan, O. S. M., Imtiaz, S., Popova, S., Probst, C., et al. (2017). The relationship between different dimensions of alcohol use and the burden of disease—An update. *Addiction, 112*, 968–1001. https://doi.org/10.1111/add.13757 (accessed on 16th June 2025).

40. Ridley, C., & Thornton, D. J. (2018). Mucins: The frontline defense of the lung. *Biochemical Society Transactions, 46*, 1099–1106. https://doi.org/10.1042/bst20170402 (accessed on 16th June 2025).

41. Strzelak, A., Ratajczak, A., Adamiec, A., & Feleszko, W. (2018). Tobacco smoke induces and alters immune responses in the lung triggering inflammation, allergy, asthma and other lung diseases: A mechanistic review. *International Journal of Environmental Research and Public Health, 15*, 1033–1033. https://doi.org/10.3390/ijerph15051033 (accessed on 16th June 2025).

42. Tekulapally, K. R., Lee, J. Y., Kim, D. S., Rahman, M. M., Park, C. K., & Kim, Y. H. (2024). Dual role of transient receptor potential ankyrin 1 in respiratory and gastrointestinal physiology: From molecular mechanisms to therapeutic targets. *Frontiers in Physiology, 15.* https://www.semanticscholar.org/paper/5f10a35c1575f05d633bf8ea38c69d25802d5c15 (accessed on 16th June 2025).

43. V'kovski, P., Kratzel, A., Steiner, S., Stalder, H., & Thiel, V. (2020). Coronavirus biology and replication: Implications for SARS-CoV-2. *Nature Reviews Microbiology, 19*, 155–170. https://doi.org/10.1038/s41579-020-00468-6 (accessed on 16th June 2025).

44. Visseren, F. L. J., Mach, F., Smulders, Y. M., Carballo, D., Koskinas, K. C., Bäck, M., Bénétos, A., et al. (2021). 2021 ESC guidelines on cardiovascular disease prevention in clinical practice. *European Heart Journal, 42*, 3227–3337. https://doi.org/10.1093/eurheartj/ehab484 (accessed on 16th June 2025).

45. Xiao, M. T., Ellsworth, C. R., & Qin, X. (2024). Emerging role of complement in COVID-19 and other respiratory virus diseases. *Cellular and Molecular Life Sciences: CMLS, 81.* https://www.semanticscholar.org/paper/0a656c1a3ef1b7ad03f0037a8d3bc42da6be88dc (accessed on 16th June 2025).

46. Yadav, P., Azam, M., Ramesh, V., & Singh, R. (2023). Unusual observations in leishmaniasis—An overview. *Pathogens, 12*, 297–297. https://doi.org/10.3390/pathogens12020297 (accessed on 16th June 2025).

DIAGNOSTIC METHODS IN LUNG DISEASES

5

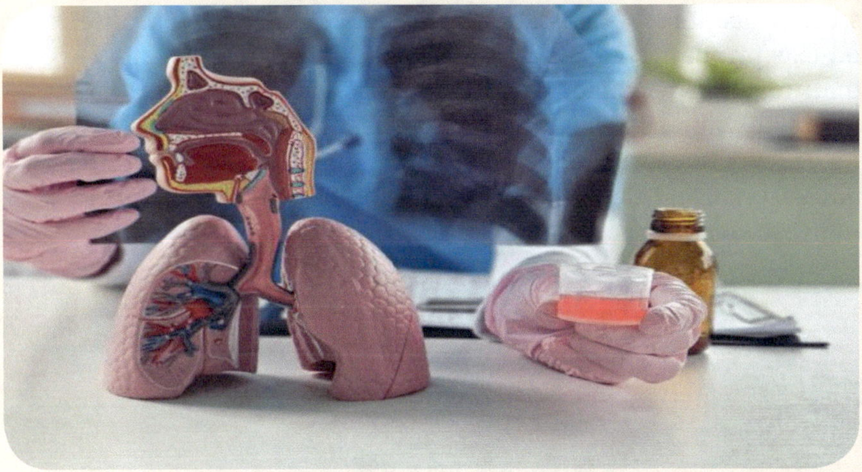

LEARNING OBJECTIVES

After studying this chapter, you will able to:

1. Discuss clinical evaluation of lung diseases
2. Explore imaging techniques
3. Explain pulmonary function tests (PFTs)
4. Identify the laboratory tests
5. Define endoscopic procedures
6. List the advanced diagnostic techniques

Introduction

A thorough understanding of the diagnostic methods employed in lung disease is essential for effective patient management and treatment planning. The severity of lung disease, ranging from broad categories of diseases such as asthma to more precise disease processes like interstitial lung disease, requires a systematic approach to diagnosis. A meticulous examination of the patient's history, clinical presentation, and imaging studies is typically the first step in the diagnosis process. But as the diseases of the lung become increasingly complex, the diagnostic techniques must also become more sophisticated. This has resulted in the addition of newer imaging modalities and interventions that enhance diagnostic accuracy, thereby impacting treatment strategies. Therefore, a multidimensional approach in diagnosis becomes essential in understanding the unique clinical nuances of lung disease management. The application of high-resolution computed tomography (HRCT) has revolutionized the practice of diagnostic respiratory medicine. Its ability to clearly define lung structures allows for improved diagnosis of various lung pathologies. Specifically, HRCT can elucidate radiological patterns that are of most tremendous significance in distinguishing the diverse types of diffuse parenchymal lung disease (DPLD) and establishing an elementary understanding of a patient's condition. As suggested by (Cancellieri et al., 2001), the timing and selection of diagnostic procedures are primarily influenced by the outcome of HRCT, alongside patient-specific factors such as immunological status and clinical course. The integration of radiological assessment within the overall diagnostic process thus accentuates its pivotal role in establishing appropriate therapy plans for patients with lung disease. Despite advancements in non-invasive diagnostic methods, there are cases when invasive approaches are necessary for accurate diagnosis. Transbronchial cryobiopsy is one such option, and it serves as a valuable alternative to routine surgical biopsies for patients with fibrosing interstitial lung disease. The recent research highlights the procedures' diagnostic performance and safety profile, and recorded sensitivities have achieved exceptional levels, as expressed in Caminati et al. (2019). Further, when conducted under ideal conditions in specialized units, cryobiopsy has exhibited a low rate of complications, thereby solidifying its position as a valuable tool in the respiratory clinician's arsenal. The ongoing examination of its efficacy underscores the need for ongoing research into existing and emerging diagnostic modalities, ensuring that healthcare providers can offer accurate and timely diagnoses for a range of lung diseases.

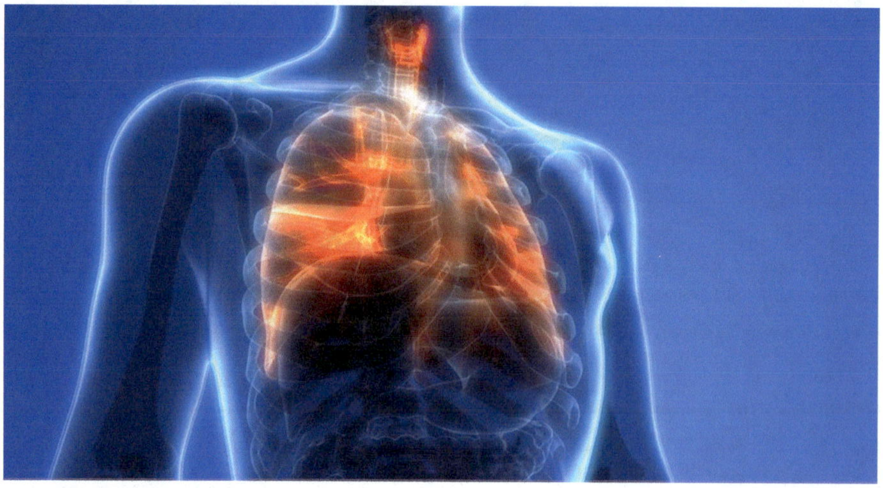

Figure 5.1. Diagnostic methods in lung diseases.

Source: https://www.hopkinsmedicine.org/-/media/images/health/_-images-to-be-filed/humanbodyrespiratorysystemhero.jpg?h=500&iar=0&mh=500&mw=1300&w=1297&hash=6A8EAB22FC40E2CEAEBB5354FE1A77CF

Importance of diagnosing lung diseases

The importance of adequate diagnosis of lung diseases cannot be overstressed, as early detection has a significant impact on shaping patient outcomes and the efficacy of treatment. From asthma and COPD to lung cancer and infections, each of these conditions requires particular diagnostic approaches to enable timely and appropriate management. For instance, conditions like lung cancer are highly reliant on the correct diagnosis of stage and type of cancer, which directly affects the treatment available and outcome. Misdiagnosis in such cases leads to severe complications, including disease progression and mortality at a high rate. The results of such research point out the dire need for effective diagnostic modalities in primary and tertiary care centers, where delayed diagnosis leads to adverse outcomes for the critically ill patients, as indicated by the shocking mortality rates against underdiagnosed diseases like melioidosis (Subbalaxmi et al., 2023). Furthermore, understanding the epidemiology and clinical presentation of lung diseases will aid in enhancing diagnosis. For instance, illnesses such as melioidosis typically present with nonspecific symptoms, which are easily confused with other conditions, thus complicating diagnosis. In a case study of melioidosis employing a retrospective observational approach, the majority of patients were reported to have presented with respiratory symptoms. Still, some were not diagnosed with suffering from this potentially lethal illness until it was too late (Subbalaxmi et al., 2023). The ongoing presence of these problems suggests the role of advanced diagnostic techniques as well as the clinician's perception of disease-specific characteristics. Implementing comprehensive training sessions for healthcare providers incorporating the recognition of diverse presentations can render early diagnosis and intervention possible, ultimately reducing morbidity and mortality from lung disease. Furthermore, incorporating evidence-based clinical quality measures into the diagnosis and treatment of lung disease can substantially streamline care processes and enhance patient outcomes. As highlighted in studies of lung cancer treatment pathways, identifying and monitoring clinical variation can streamline care delivery. By monitoring performance through feedback dashboards and quality measures, clinicians actively engage in tracking their performance and identifying opportunities for improvement. Such a systematic process not only ensures adherence to best practices but also allows for timely interventions among patients, tailoring treatment methods according to their individual needs. Thus, an ongoing emphasis on the advancement of diagnostic methods and the establishment of robust quality improvement initiatives is crucial to managing the complex problems presented by lung diseases, ultimately enhancing health outcomes for those affected.

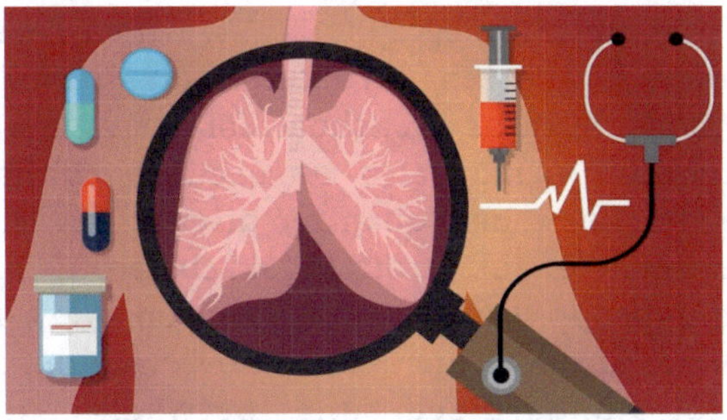

Figure 5.2. Diagnosing lung diseases.

Source: https://cdn2.hubspot.net/hubfs/3306744/dreamstime_s_60695157-min.jpg

Overview of common lung diseases

Lung diseases are a diverse group of disorders of pulmonary function and overall health. The most prevalent of them are chronic obstructive pulmonary disease (COPD), asthma, and interstitial lung diseases (ILD). COPD is characterized by airflow limitation and is predominantly caused by smoking and air pollution, and presents with chronic cough and exertional dyspnea. Asthma, on the other hand, is a reversible obstructive disease often triggered by allergens, physical activity, or environmental exposures, characterized by wheezing and shortness of breath. The nature of these diseases requires an understanding of etiology and pathophysiology, as accurate diagnosis is a prerequisite for effective treatment, which may include drug therapy and non-drug therapy, to enhance the quality of life for patients. Interstitial lung diseases (ILDs) are a broad range of lung conditions that cause inflammation and scarring of the lung tissue. According to studies conducted in Malta, the prevalence of ILD has been estimated at 24.9 per 100,000 population, indicating a significant public health importance. All these establish the absence of ILD. Various diagnostic instruments are used to determine the presence of ILD, ranging from pulmonary function tests to advanced imaging modalities, such as computed tomography scans, which reveal fibrosis in the lung structure. More invasive methods, such as bronchoalveolar lavage and lung biopsy, may also be used to confirm the diagnosis and quantify disease severity. Treatment of ILD is often corticosteroid- and immunosuppression-based; however, follow-up regimes for these therapies are overwhelmingly under-standardized, and between-center practice proves highly inconsistent, impacting outcomes for patients. This points to a need for improvement in diagnostic methods in the clinic (Fenech et al., 2012). The pathogenesis of lung disease in relation to exosomes has been described in recent research, which has improved our understanding of disease processes. These nanoscale vesicles are loaded with biomolecules such as proteins, lipids, and RNAs and serve as central tools of cell-to-cell communication. Notably, exosomal microRNAs (miRNAs) have shown promise as biomarkers of various pulmonary diseases, and with the interest they hold in non-invasive diagnosis. This new idea implies that exosomes have the ability to effectively reflect disease states and can help in the diagnosis of disease at an early stage and tracking. By incorporating exosome analysis into their routine diagnostic protocols, clinicians can improve the early diagnosis and management of lung diseases, thereby providing timely interventions and achieving better clinical outcomes (Adcock et al., 2016). Emphasis on both traditional and new diagnostic techniques is crucial to support advancing patient care in lung disease.

5.1. Clinical Evaluation

Learning Outcome

1. Patient history and symptom assessment
2. Physical examination techniques
3. Role of clinical judgment in diagnosis

Clinical evaluation of lung disease plays a crucial role in the development of a proper diagnosis, as it encompasses a thorough patient history, physical examination, and diagnostic testing. It serves as the foundation upon which other diagnostic procedures are undertaken. Patient history can reveal likely risk factors such as smoking, environmental exposure, and past respiratory infections. In addition, a physical examination also enables clinicians to detect wheezing, crackling, or diminished breath sounds, which will impact the selection of advanced tests subsequently. The incorporation of these early findings not only guides the choice of advanced modalities but also raises clinical suspicion for specific diseases, allowing for targeted diagnosis. Furthermore, the ability to pair patients' symptoms and their clinical background accentuates the importance of a systematic evaluation, thereby becoming a vital part of the entire lung condition diagnostic process. In addition to the pivotal role by the clinical assessment, current diagnosis methods have evolved significantly, and with the integration of advanced technologies that enhance diagnostic accuracy for a broad spectrum of lung diseases. Techniques such as imaging examinations, i.e., chest X-rays and computed tomography scans, provide critical visual information regarding lung architecture. Additionally, advances in cryobiopsy procedures have focused on highlighting the efficiency of obtaining lung tissue samples for histopathological examination. Importantly, cryobiopsies are notable for the larger tissue samples that tend to retain adequate alveolar structure, thereby minimizing artifacts associated with traditional biopsy procedures (Griff et al., 2019). The integration of newer imaging technologies with clinical evaluation enables a deeper understanding of pulmonary pathologies, leading to more accurate and prompt diagnoses, and ultimately improving patient outcomes. Apart from this, special emphasis should be placed on the need for continually evolving better diagnostic tools, especially in the context of infectious diseases such as tuberculosis. The traditional laboratory diagnostic tests, despite being the gold standard, are prone to prolonging the time to diagnosis and treatment, thereby aggravating the disease burden among affected populations. The importance of fast point-of-care tuberculosis diagnosis tests is exemplified by the current methods, which hinder timely detection and subsequent care (Harari et al., 2012). Innovative strategies, such as novel biomarker development and rapid testing modalities, are required to enhance early case detection and adherence to treatment, particularly in resource-limited settings. A thoughtful examination of these developments not only highlights the imperative need for effective diagnostics but also underscores the synergy between clinical evaluation and evolving technologies in the quest to improve the management of lung disease.

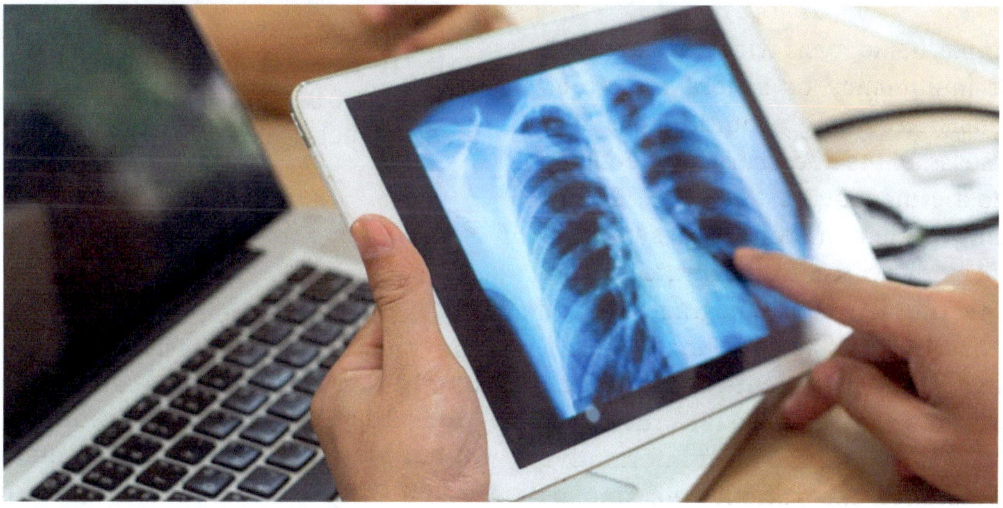

Figure 5.3. Clinical evaluation of lung diseases.

Source: https://www.niehs.nih.gov/sites/default/files/health/assets/images/lung_disease_og.jpg

5.1.1. Patient History and Symptom Assessment

In diagnosing lung disease, careful patient history and symptom assessment are essential in making an accurate diagnosis. A comprehensive patient history examines several factors, including past respiratory illnesses, exposure to environmental toxins, and family medical history, with a particular focus on hereditary lung diseases. For instance, asthma or chronic obstructive pulmonary disease (COPD) in the patient or among his family members might be a good marker for genetic susceptibility to airflow obstruction or an allergic response. In addition, occupational risks, such as those encountered by workers engaged in construction or industrial settings, can increase the risk of acquiring diseases like pneumoconiosis or silicosis, thereby contributing to the clinical progression of treatment undertaken by medical practitioners during symptom examination and the formulation of follow-up diagnostic measures. Therefore, a detailed patient history forms the foundation of individualized diagnosis plans (Chopra et al., 2020). Symptom assessment is crucial in diagnosing lung disease and should involve both quantitative and qualitative evaluations of patient-reported symptoms. The traditional metrics, such as cough, dyspnea, and sputum production, must be characterized based on their onset, duration, and severity. Moreover, it is essential to differentiate between acute and chronic respiratory symptoms because chronic presentations of symptoms may presage diagnoses such as interstitial lung disease or lung cancer. Also, symptoms that are closely related—such as chest pain, tiredness, and even systemic presentation in the form of fever or loss of weight—are very helpful in providing key clues in shortlisting the differential diagnoses.

For example, hemoptysis with chronic cough can suggest malignancy or severe infections like tuberculosis. Accordingly, multidimensional symptom assessment is necessary to effectively guide diagnostic maneuvers (Su et al., 2020). By integrating patient history and symptom scores, the provider can create a strategic plan for further testing, such as imaging tests or pulmonary function tests, to confirm diagnoses. By identifying trends in patient-reported data, healthcare workers can maximize the ordering of diagnostic tests that yield the most informative results. For instance, the patient who smokes with severe exertional dyspnea can qualify for direct spirometry to ascertain the lung function and screen for the potential of COPD. Moreover, identifying red flags, such as unexpected weight loss or new symptoms, in an older adult can lead to early interventions. Thus, the integration of patient history and symptom evaluation not only contributes to higher diagnostic accuracy but also results in better clinical outcomes through tailored healthcare interventions formulated based on the individualized needs of each patient (Chopra et al., 2020).

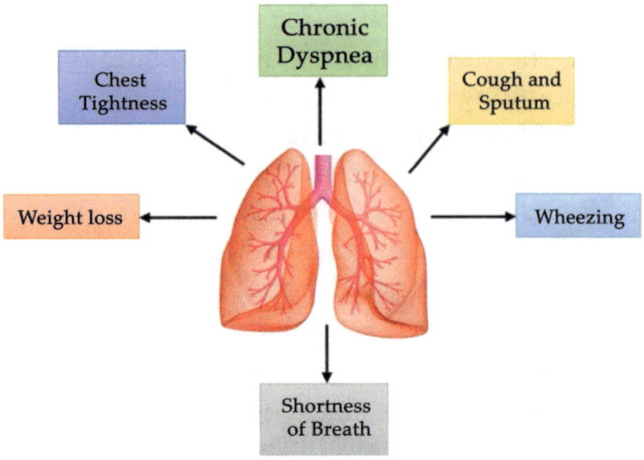

Figure 5.4. Patient history and symptom assessment of lung diseases.

Source: https://media.springernature.com/lw685/springer-static/image/chp%3A10.1007%2F978-981-33-6827-9_1/MediaObjects/503167_1_En_1_Fig2_HTML.png

5.1.2. Physical Examination Techniques

Physical examination skills are a key part of the diagnostic evaluation for lung disease, complementing advanced imaging and laboratory testing. Inspection is a crucial initial step in a thorough examination, during which clinicians observe the patient for signs of respiratory distress, chest movement symmetry, and abnormal movement that may indicate underlying disease. Patient monitoring of accessory muscle use and respiratory pattern may detect diseases such as pneumonia or chronic obstructive pulmonary disease. Additionally, color anomalies such as cyanosis may indicate severe hypoxia. Skilled physical examination skills enable doctors to construct a working diagnosis, which is essential before proceeding to more invasive investigations or interventions. Palpation is also a key method used in the clinical assessment of patients suspected of having lung disease. By lightly pressing the thoracic wall, doctors can evaluate tactile fremitus, which is decreased in pleural effusion but increased in lung consolidation.

Palpation of the lung apex can also identify any abnormal masses or lymphadenopathy that may compromise lung function. Auscultation is the second procedure, following palpation, which gathers vital information by auscultating breath sounds. Wheezes, crackles, or diminished breath sounds alert the clinician to possible bronchial obstruction, pulmonary edema, or other pathologic mechanisms responsible for lung pathology. Together, these physical examination techniques provide a systematic process for identifying and learning about lung disease. Physical examination findings must be integrated into diagnostic reasoning for efficient management of lung diseases.

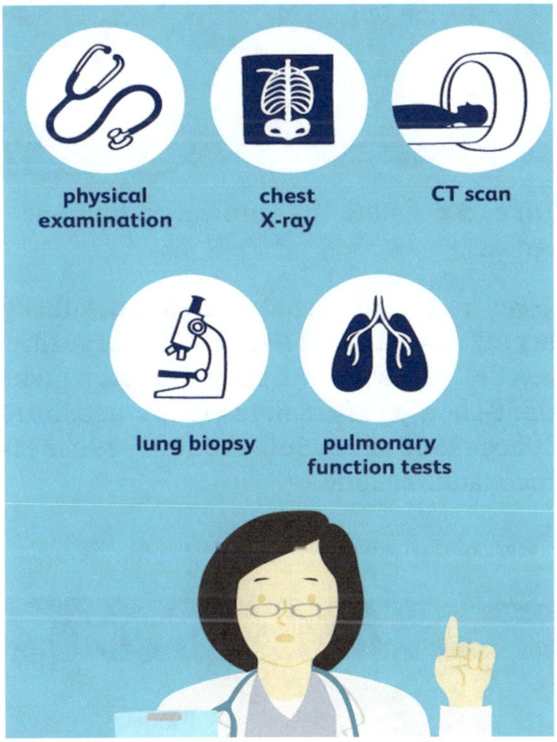

Figure 5.5. Physical examination techniques of lung diseases.

Source: https://www.verywellhealth.com/thmb/jY2gGnmo7WFu6qs1P4uWCNsr4b0=/1500x0/filters:no_upscale():max_bytes(150000):strip_icc()/diagnosis_05-ef6311502b9e413fa59c4872492c4a7b.jpg

For instance, a patient with clinical suspicion of tuberculosis may exhibit typical signs identified through these examination techniques, which can guide further diagnostic work-up. The 2007 WHO algorithm for the diagnosis of smear-negative pulmonary tuberculosis illustrates the significant interaction among clinical history, physical exam findings, and confirmatory testing (Cattamanchi et al., 2012). By integrating physical exam results and related laboratory or imaging tests, a clearer understanding of the patient's disease can be established, ultimately leading to more effective treatment modalities. Hence, physical examination techniques remain ineliminable when it comes to diagnosing and treating patients with lung pathology and become the foundation for an effective diagnostic process (Kitsiou et al., 2013).

5.1.3. Role of Clinical Judgment in Diagnosis

Clinical judgment plays the most crucial role in diagnosing lung diseases, as it has a direct impact on patient outcome and the appropriateness of diagnostic strategies. The physician is required to integrate data from patient histories, physical examinations, and diagnostic testing to arrive at a well-supported conclusion. The clinical process of judgment entails not only symptom assessment but also the context in which the presentation occurs. Recognition of the intricacies of a patient's health status, i.e., any underlying medical conditions or recent respiratory disease, enables clinicians to differentiate among conditions like bronchitis and pneumonia. Such differentiation is essential; e.g., pneumonia may require further imaging and potential antibiotics, but uncomplicated acute bronchitis is less likely to, highlighting the necessity of clinicians applying judgment to avoid unnecessary treatments that may lead to complications or antibiotic resistance (Cui et al., 2020).

Another key aspect of applying clinical judgment is integrating modern diagnostic technologies with traditional examination techniques. Emergent conditions, such as SARS-CoV-2, impose the need for flexible and adaptive clinical thinking in the face of shifting circumstances. Imaging modalities such as chest X-rays and CT scans have become more widespread and informative during outbreaks of respiratory illness; it remains for clinicians to decide when such technology is indicated. For example, ultrasound demonstrated great utility in COVID-19 diagnosis because it is safe and portable, signaling the importance of timely and prudent clinical judgment in optimizing diagnostic pathways (Cui et al., 2020). The ability to combine clinical acumen with technology ultimately optimizes diagnostic accuracy in lung disease. Moreover, effective communication is a crucial aspect of clinical judgment in the process of diagnosing lung disease. Effective communication with patients not only helps in acquiring appropriate clinical information but also serves as one means of creating a patient satisfaction-enhancing therapeutic relationship. Overprescription and the consequent misuse of antibiotics can occur if the pervading misimpression that antibiotics are a magic bullet for respiratory infections continues to exist. Therefore, a clear definition of the distinction between viral and bacterial infections is necessary. In addition, if a cough persists, such as in the case of acute bronchitis, doctors must use their best judgment to determine whether to pursue further treatment. This emphasis on communication makes patients aware of their diseases, the reasoning behind diagnostic choices, and the management of their care, which empowers them in the healthcare process (Bartlett et al., 2001).

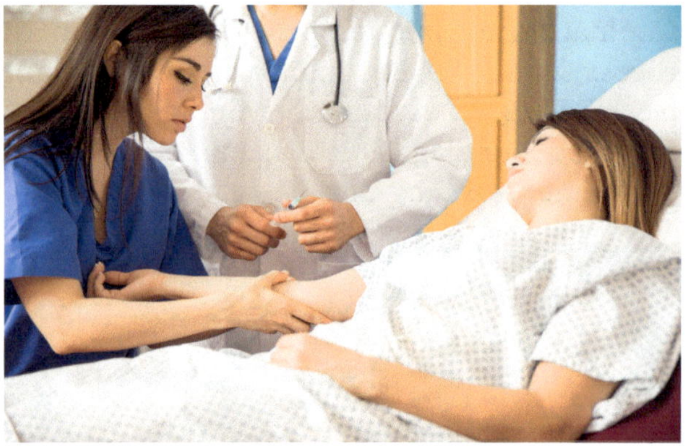

Figure 5.6. Role of clinical judgment in diagnosis.

Source: https://external-content.duckduckgo.com/iu/?u=https%3A%2F%2Fnursethink.com%2Fimages%2Fnurse-and-doctor-giving-patient-shot.jpg&f=1&nofb=1&ipt=aee5be179dc30acb4a86532220560fa75d06ee49bc8e1c767f6cb5add52e26dd

Test Your Knowledge

1. What are the physical examination techniques
2. What is the role of clinical judgment in diagnosis

5.2. Imaging Techniques

Learning Outcome

1. Chest X-rays and their diagnostic value
2. Computed Tomography (CT) scans
3. Magnetic Resonance Imaging (MRI) applications

Imaging modalities play a prominent role in the diagnostic assessment of lung diseases, providing essential information about the pulmonary tissue's anatomical and pathological status. Of all the imaging modalities employed, CT stands out due to its excellent resolution and ability to depict lung anatomy and fine details. With this modality, it is pretty simple to differentiate among various lung pathologies, like malignancies, interstitial lung diseases, and infections. Additionally, advancements in CT imaging technology, such as HRCT scans, enhance the detection of subtle changes in lung architecture, thereby facilitating early diagnosis and management of conditions like pulmonary fibrosis and emphysema. The integration of newer imaging modalities into routine practice has significantly enhanced lung pathology quantification and treatment process guidance, underscoring the role of a multidisciplinary team in diagnosis and management. Though conventional imaging techniques still form a component of lung disease assessment, newer technology, such as autofluorescence imaging (AFI), is increasingly becoming more prevalent. AFI leverages the intrinsic autofluorescence properties of biological tissues, providing a non-destructive technique for imaging cell and subcellular structures in the absence of exogenous contrast agents. This technique has been widely applied in a multitude of medical uses, including the diagnosis of lung disease, where it aids in identifying atypical tissue characteristics associated with pathological conditions. For instance, studies have established that methods of AFI can provide surrogate markers for disease states, enabling clinicians to visualize the demarcation of lung lesions during procedures such as bronchoscopies. With growing maturity of the technology, its potential for enhancing diagnostic accuracy in lung disease is excellent, though there is a need for standardization over a variety of applications to realize its best clinical benefit (Aigner et al., 2020). Cryobiopsy is another new imaging technique that complements traditional diagnostic modalities in pulmonary and pleural diseases. This technique, which involves sampling tissue through cryogenic freezing, has proven more diagnostic than routine transbronchial biopsies, particularly in cases involving interstitial lung diseases and tumors. Studies show that specimens obtained through cryobiopsy were larger and had better representative alveolar architecture, providing more morphological information about different lung conditions (Griff et al., 2019). Additionally, the discovery of new evidence demonstrating its equivalence to standard flexible thoracoscopy for pleural lesions highlights its utility and versatility in clinical practice. As the field of pulmonary medicine continues to grow and mature, practices like cryobiopsy will become second nature, enabling us to diagnose and treat end-stage lung disease properly.

5.2.1. Chest X-Rays and Their Diagnostic Value

The method of chest X-rays remains a cornerstone in the diagnostic evaluation of lung disease, providing valuable information that informs clinical decision-making. Being a non-invasive imaging method, chest X-rays are commonly the first investigation done on patients with respiratory signs. Their worth is not only in the diagnosis of obvious disorders such as pneumonia, tuberculosis, and lung cancerbut also because they can reveal hidden abnormalities through , but also in revealing hidden abnormalities through the indication of consolidation signs, effusions, or infiltrates.

Furthermore, advancements in radiographic technique have enhanced image quality and diagnostic sensitivity, thereby making the detection of subtle changes that can improve prognostic assessment in various pulmonary conditions. Hence, while not diagnostic, chest X-rays are part of an overall diagnostic process and contribute to the foundation of facts from which a more in-depth investigation would be warranted. While extremely useful, the interpretation of chest X-rays demands a keen awareness of both normal and abnormal pulmonary anatomy. Radiologists and clinicians must consider a number of variables, such as the patient's clinical history and presentation, before adequately assessing findings. For instance, the finding of a nodular opacity may indicate malignancy, which would require further extensive workup in the form of CT scans or biopsies. In settings with enormous burdens of disease such as tuberculosis, the utility of chest X-rays in prompt diagnosis cannot be overstated, as evidence from studies examining evaluation of smear-negative pulmonary tuberculosis illustrates; these highlight the significant role of radiographs in facilitating the timely and effective initiation of therapy in high-risk groups (Cattamanchi et al., 2012). Hence, accurate interpretation is essential, as misdiagnosis can lead to inappropriately treated patients and poorer outcomes. The limitations of chest X-rays should also be acknowledged, particularly when used in the context of more subtle lung disease. Although valuable for initial impressions, X-rays may be insensitive to specific processes, such as early interstitial lung disease or occult changes in the parenchyma of VAP. Recent studies indicate that pulmonary function tests and blood gas analysis are typically needed for comprehensive evaluation, especially in critical care settings. Moreover, sole reliance on radiographic characteristics without supporting clinical manifestations may compromise the validity of the diagnosis (Cilloniz et al., 2019). Therefore, while chest X-rays are an integral building block in the diagnosis of pulmonary illness, they are best served by being situated within a broader clinical framework that includes other types of diagnostic modalities. This stratified approach maximizes patient management to be evidence-based and directed towards particular clinical disease states.

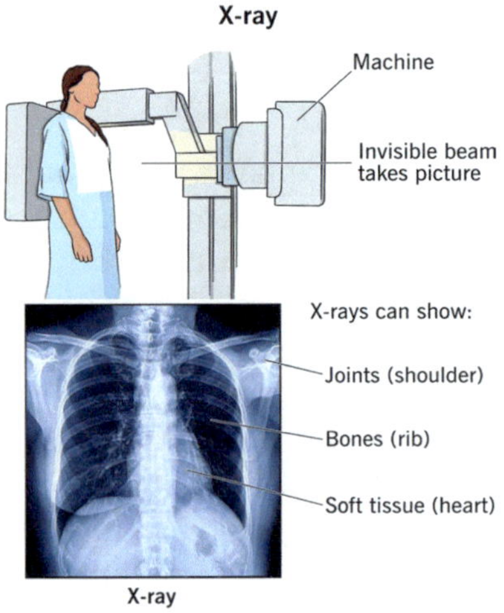

Figure 5.7. Chest X-rays and their diagnostic value.

Source: https://my.clevelandclinic.org/-/scassets/images/org/health/articles/21818-x-ray

5.2.2. Computed Tomography (CT) Scans

Computed Tomography (CT) scans are a diagnostic tool that has become a fundamental part of diagnosing various lung diseases, offering enhanced visualization of pulmonary structures compared to conventional imaging methods. The technology enables a detailed assessment of lung architecture, with the potential to identify potential abnormalities, such as tumors, infections, or COPD. One of the key advantages of CT scans is that they are capable of providing cross-sectional imaging, which allows for the assessment of complex structures and the diagnosis of abnormalities not visible on standard chest X-rays. Thus, CT scans are vital in achieving a proper and timely diagnosis, which in turn dictates the treatment and management plan for affected patients. The application of contrast-enhanced CT scans, particularly in the detection of pleural malignancies, highlights the subtle nature of this modality. In a study assessing CT performance in routine clinical practice, the sensitivity for detecting pleural malignancies was 58%, with even lower sensitivity when performed by non-thoracic specialist radiologists (53%) compared to specialist thoracic radiologists (68%) (Alexander et al., 2017).

While CT scans are beneficial in the detection of malignancies, the findings point to the fact that utilization of CT findings in isolation for a conclusive diagnosis may not be sufficient. Therefore, correlating CT findings with clinical assessments and other diagnostic procedures, such as biopsies or pleural sampling, would be necessary to yield optimal patient care and disease management. Despite their advantages, CT scan success is limited by technology capabilities and potential misinterpretation in non-specialist settings. The above study demonstrates that specialist reporting significantly contributes to diagnostic outcomes, highlighting the importance of expertise in CT image interpretation (Alexander et al., 2017). Additionally, while CT scans yield superb imaging, they are not riskless and carry the threat of exposure to ionizing radiation, which must be weighed against the benefit of accurate diagnosis. On a day-to-day basis, as in clinical practice, patient history, clinical presentation, and other diagnostic modalities must be considered in conjunction with CT findings, adopting a comprehensive approach to lung disease diagnosis and optimizing patient outcomes in the complex realm of respiratory medicine.

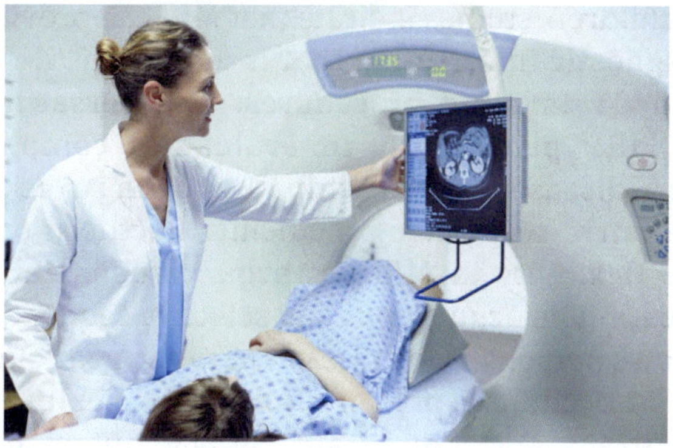

Figure 5.8. Computed tomography (CT) scans.

Source: https://www.health.com/thmb/YS4wUCB92en5gnvigWN98_ZgFMI=/5121x0/filters:no_upscale():max_bytes(150000):strip_icc()/ctscan-GettyImages-493216325-63c244b9138f460f8529ecf076166864.jpg

5.2.3. Magnetic Resonance Imaging (MRI) Applications

The incorporation of Magnetic Resonance Imaging (MRI) into diagnostic tools for lung disorders represents a significant advancement in imaging technology. Historically, X-ray and CT scans have dominated lung imaging, but now MRI's ability to offer both morphological and functional information without the risks from ionizing radiation is added to the medical field. This aspect is especially beneficial for susceptible groups like children, pregnant women, and young adults, where radiation exposure has significant implications. Additionally, the visualization of soft tissues and respiratory mechanics that MRI facilitates enhances the diagnostic accuracy of conditions such as cystic fibrosis and pulmonary embolism, making it a first-line imaging modality in these cases. With advancements in MRI technology, its role is increasing, with a focus on the necessity to adapt clinical routines to incorporate this novel diagnostic method (Hebestreit et al., 2011). MRI may serve both as an alternative and as an adjunct to conventional imaging methods for general diagnosis of lung diseases. In diagnosing tumors and pneumonia in children, studies indicate that MRI can provide diagnostic information that is as good as X-ray and CT imaging procedures. The versatility of MRI, particularly in evaluating complex lung diseases, aligns with its growing role in pediatric respiratory medicine. Furthermore, the flexibility in MRI protocols through rapid breath-hold acquisitions and selective sequences allows personalized assessment to each patient's unique clinical presentation. This flexibility positions MRI not as an adjunct, but rather as a significant component in the diagnosis of lung disease, evolving towards a deeper understanding of pulmonary disease (Hebestreit et al., 2011). However, despite these advances, ongoing investigations into the clinical utility of MRI in certain situations, such as interstitial lung disease, remain. Although MRI has potential to provide additional information that may complement studies and clinical practice, its use in routine assessments is not yet established. The challenge posed by motion artifacts and the requirement of complex imaging protocols further complicate its use in this setting. With continuing technical improvements, developments such as motion-compensated imaging and self-navigated sequences may improve the practicality of MRI in the clinical setting. Lastly, while MRI is highly promising for the diagnosis of lung disease, it is still important to regularly evaluate and confirm its effectiveness in order to realize optimum benefit (Hebestreit et al., 2011).

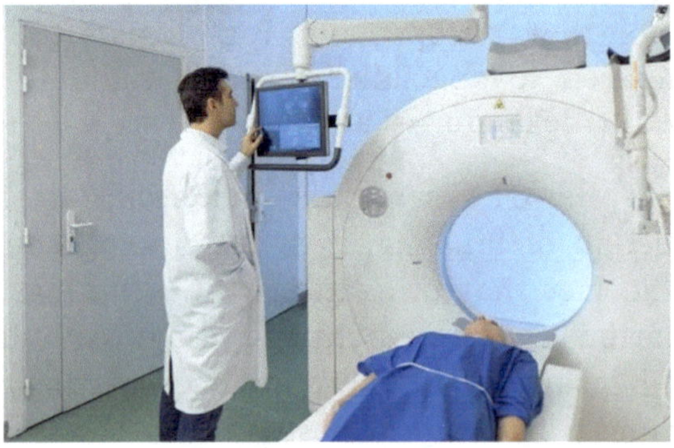

Figure 5.9. Magnetic resonance imaging (MRI).

Source: https://www.news-medical.net/image-handler/picture/2016/11/MRI_shutterstock_509318605.jpg

Test Your Knowledge

1. What are computed tomography (CT) scans?
2. What are the magnetic resonance imaging (MRI) applications?

5.3. Pulmonary Function Tests (PFTs)

Learning Outcome

1. Spirometry and its significance
2. Diffusion capacity testing
3. Bronchodilator response assessment

Pulmonary Function Tests (PFTs) play a significant role in the diagnostic evaluation of lung disease, as they provide valuable information about respiratory function. These tests assess various pulmonary mechanics, including airflow rates, lung volumes, and gas exchange efficiency, thereby facilitating the accurate diagnosis of conditions such as asthma, chronic obstructive pulmonary disease (COPD), and restrictive lung disease. The essence of this diagnostic technique is measurements such as Forced Vital Capacity (FVC) and Forced Expiratory Volume in one second (FEV1), the combination of which determines the level of airflow blockage. Increased levels of these indicators might be consistent with normal respiratory function, but below-normal levels generally necessitate additional investigation. Hence, interpretive findings generated by PFTs are not only crucial for determining the presence of pulmonary conditions but also for assessing disease progression and the outcome of therapy in patients.

Applications of PFTs extend beyond basic pulmonary assessment; they are pivotal in identifying underlying genetic conditions, such as Alpha-1 Antitrypsin Deficiency (AATD). In a separate study, an interdisciplinary protocol was employed to maximize AATD screening among PFT-outpatients, yielding significant gains in detection. Initially, only 5.9% of the PFT-outpatients eligible for AATD screening were actually tested, but following staff education and the implementation of a systematic protocol, this increased to 66.7%. The study highlighted the importance of identifying irreversible airflow obstruction on PFTs, a prerequisite for immediate AATD screening. This is an indication of the potential of PFTs as a gateway to identify genetic susceptibility to chronic respiratory disease, and further ensure prompt intervention and management in at-risk populations (Vazquez et al., 2023). Additionally, advances in pulmonary diagnostics reinforce the connection between systemic diseases and lung disorders, and further support the use of PFTs as part of a comprehensive evaluation in patients. For instance, the relationship between rheumatoid arthritis (RA) and interstitial lung disease (ILD) is better known, wherein PFTs have been instrumental in establishing pulmonary involvement in RA patients.

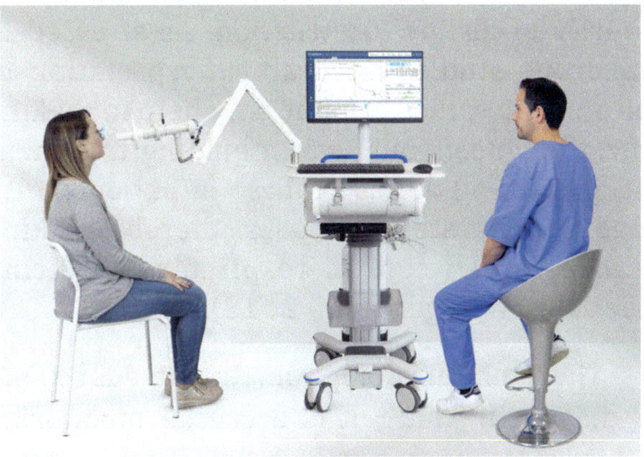

Figure 5.10. Pulmonary function tests (PFTs).

Source: https://www.cosmed.com/images/03_product_item/quark_pft/quark_pft_panel.jpg

The research has demonstrated that increased biomarkers associated with the onset of lung disease are typically identifiable through simultaneous testing, thereby enhancing the overall diagnostic system. By integrating PFT results with novel markers and clinical data, clinicians can develop individualized therapeutic programs for RA and related pulmonary diseases. The ongoing refinement of diagnostic methods validates the potential of PFTs to offer helpful information, which ultimately enhances our understanding of the multifaceted nature of lung diseases (England et al., 2019).

5.3.1. Spirometry and Its Significance

Spirometry is a quantitative element in the diagnosis and therapy of lung disease, particularly in the evaluation of asthma and chronic obstructive pulmonary disease (COPD). As a test of lung function, it measures the volume of air that can be inhaled and exhaled, thus providing essential information on lung capacity and function. The outcome from spirometry is most often expressed in terms of forced expiratory volume in one second (FEV1) and forced vital capacity (FVC), both of which play critical roles in determining the severity of airflow obstruction. As stressed in numerous studies, accurate interpretation of spirometric values can not only help in making a firm diagnosis but also in guiding treatment and predicting disease course in patients with various respiratory diseases, thereby making it an essential tool in respiratory medicine (Leopoldo N Segal et al., 2018).

The significance of spirometry extends beyond its diagnostic value; it is a crucial monitoring tool for disease management. Regular spirometry testing enables clinicians to track changes in lung function over time, allowing for the early identification of exacerbations or deterioration in individuals with chronic lung disease. Early treatment can follow as a result of this proactive approach, minimizing the severity of symptoms and improving quality of life. Spirometry can also be important in patient education, enabling individuals better to understand their illness and aid in medication compliance. Increased patient understanding can also enable patients to adopt lifestyle modifications that positively impact their respiratory health, thereby highlighting the role of the test in comprehensive patient management (Rosenkranz et al., 2015). Within the context of evolving clinical paradigms, there is a growing appreciation for the significance of individualized medicine in respiratory care, which spirometry can support. By coupling spirometric data with clinical observation and patient symptoms, clinicians can develop individualized treatment protocols that address specific pathophysiologic characteristics of lung disorders. New developments center on the more nuanced application of spirometry, such as its use in conjunction with imaging techniques to enhance our understanding of complex disease phenotypes. This combined approach emphasizes the significance of spirometry not only as a diagnostic measure but also as a foundation that forms a comprehensive image of respiratory well-being, ultimately leading to improved clinical results for patients suffering from lung disease (Leopoldo N Segal et al., 2018).

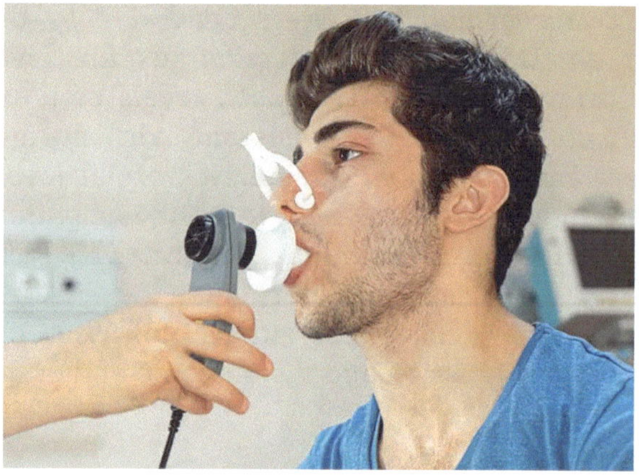

Figure 5.11. Spirometry.

Source: https://media.post.rvohealth.io/wp-content/uploads/2020/09/732x549_THUMBNAIL_Spirometry.jpg

5.3.2. Diffusion Capacity Testing

Among the various tests used to assess lung function, diffusion capacity testing is particularly important in detecting gas exchange defects associated with a broad spectrum of pulmonary diseases. Diffusion capacity testing is a specific test that measures the ability of the lungs to exchange gases from the alveoli into the bloodstream, for example, oxygen and carbon dioxide. By highlighting the efficiency of alveolar-capillary diffusion, diffusion capacity testing provides insight into conditions like interstitial lung disease (ILD) and chronic obstructive pulmonary disease (COPD). Results are generally expressed in terms of diffusing capacity for carbon monoxide (DLCO) and reflect both surface area available for gas exchange and alveolar membrane permeability. The clinical relevance of diffusion capacity testing goes beyond its direct quantification of gas transfer effectiveness; it also has a prognostic impact on the timely diagnosis and treatment of several lung disorders.

For example, research has demonstrated that early and precise detection of ILD by diffusion capacity testing significantly decreases diagnostic delay, which is essential in enhancing patient outcomes. Retrospective cohort analysis revealed that early notification of ILD features observed on diffusion capacity testing was associated with highly correlated pulmonary referrals, resulting in timelier intervention for affected patients (Adegunsoye et al., 2019). This highlights the importance of measuring diffusion capacity as part of a comprehensive pulmonary evaluation. Diffusion capacity measurements also can detect underlying pathophysiologic processes causing certain pulmonary disorders. Plasma B-type natriuretic peptide (BNP) alterations in AECOPD, although primarily linked with heart failure, have an indirect relationship with pulmonary function as observed in the dynamics of exacerbation (Hasegawa et al., 2014). Alterations in diffusion capacity are an expression of mechanical and gas-exchange-based impairments common to AECOPD, reflecting the multidimensional nature of pulmonary assessment. Overall, tests of diffusion capacity remain a cornerstone of the diagnostic toolkit for lung disease, underpinning both short-term and long-term patient management pathways.

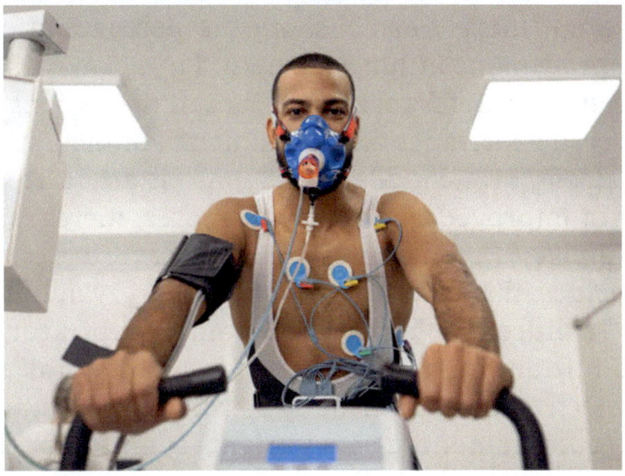

Figure 5.12. Lung diffusion testing.

Source: https://media.post.rvohealth.io/wp-content/uploads/2021/10/mid_adult_man_taking_cardiopulmonary_stress_test_in_clinic-732x549-thumbnail-732x549.jpg

5.3.3. Bronchodilator Response Assessment

Measurement of bronchodilator response is a critical component of diagnosing several lung diseases, with asthma and chronic obstructive pulmonary disease (COPD) being the most prominent among them. The procedure involves measuring lung function both before and after administering a bronchodilator medication, which enables clinicians to assess the reversibility of airway obstruction. In asthma patients, the reaction to bronchodilators is typically vigorous, reflecting the intrinsic airway inflammation and hyperreactivity. In contrast, patients with COPD may exhibit a limited reaction due to structural changes in the lungs. An effective response to a bronchodilator is conventionally interpreted as a rise in forced expiratory volume in one-second (FEV1) of at least 12% and 200 mL following the administration of a bronchodilator.

Understanding the extent of this response is essential, as it assists in differentiating asthma from other obstructive airway diseases and guides the appropriate management approach. The assessment criteria of bronchodilator response are not merely establishing the percentage of improvement in lung function. Physicians also evaluate relief from symptoms and the patient's overall experience after treatment. For instance, a strong bronchodilator response is associated with improved quality of life scores, increased exercise tolerance, and reduced exacerbations. Besides this, the assessment is very valuable in children, where overlapping respiratory conditions can complicate exact diagnosis. Objective measurement by spirometric findings is complemented by patient symptoms to offer total evaluation, which is critical in tailoring treatment regimens. The response to bronchodilators is a dynamic indicator that mirrors the pathophysiology of lung disease, particularly when bronchial spasm and inflammation are common, highlighting its clinical utility. Over the past few years, improvements in the techniques of assessment have significantly improved the evaluation of responsiveness to bronchodilators. New tools such as impulse oscillometry and exhaled nitric oxide testing provide additional ways to fully evaluate airway dynamics and inflammation in asthmatics and COPD patients. They are particularly beneficial for those who may not be able to perform standard spirometry. In addition, bronchodilator responsiveness is increasingly applied in combination with other parameters to conduct the multidimensional evaluation of lung function. Response modifiers are age, smoking history, and comorbidities, and thus, by being part of clinical assessment, allow for more nuanced analysis of patient data, ultimately resulting in enhanced diagnostic accuracy and enhanced management practice customized to individual lung pathologies, thereby making bronchodilator response a central element of respiratory diagnostics as part of the broader context of lung disease management.

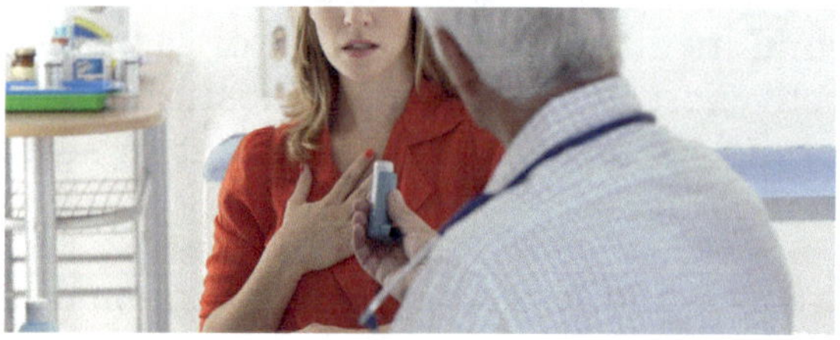

Figure 5.13. Response to bronchodilators in patients with bronchiectasis.

Source: https://external-content.duckduckgo.com/iu/?u=https%3A%2F%2Fbronchiectasisnewstoday.com%2Fwp-content%2Fuploads%2F2016%2F06%2Fshutterstock_174164669-1400x480.jpg&f=1&nofb=1&ipt=d53b5037c6fa7845788270a8caae48759c5efdb294ad9796009c1be3a6a6739d

Test Your Knowledge

1. What is spirometry, and explain its significance?
2. What is diffusion capacity testing?

5.4. Laboratory Tests

Learning Outcome

1. Blood tests for inflammatory markers
2. Sputum analysis and culture
3. Arterial blood gas (ABG) analysis

In diagnosing lung disease, laboratory testing plays a crucial role in making accurate diagnoses and determining the most effective therapy. They provide information that cannot be obtained with routine imaging alone. For instance, testing of sputum is vital to make a diagnosis of infections like TB, where point-of-care rapid diagnostic tests are largely unavailable. The reference laboratory tests for TB can include several investigations that last weeks, emphasizing the urgency and precision needed in diagnosis. Such delays can hinder effective treatment and prolong transmission in communities, thereby making TB control worldwide even more challenging (Harari et al., 2012). Thus, ongoing advancements in laboratory methods are crucial for maximizing early detection rates, which will facilitate effective intervention and prevent the spread of diseases. Moreover, biomarkers have also proven to be potential markers for differentiating various lung conditions, such as cancers like SCLC and NSCLC. The launch of new tests, such as the Elecsys neuron-specific enolase (NSE) enzyme immunoassay, marks outstanding progress on the diagnostic horizon for lung cancer. The specific test is highly sensitive and specific, offering precise measurements of NSE levels in serum samples related to the disease's extent (SF et al., 2003). The use of precise laboratory tests to assess biomarkers enables clinicians to make more informed patient management decisions. Not only does this enhance diagnostic outcomes, but it also aids in the monitoring of treatment efficacy and the detection of disease recurrence in lung cancer patients. Lastly, the integration of laboratory tests in the diagnosis of lung disease reinforces the necessity of combined healthcare disciplines. As technology continues to advance, the likelihood of more timely and pervasive diagnostic tools becomes increasingly promising. However, issues of resource distribution, technical capacity, and the fair distribution of these tests remain key determinants affecting their successful application. Investors will need to prioritize investments in laboratory infrastructure and undertake research to create a wider range of diagnostic tests, especially for complex and high-burden conditions such as TB and lung cancer. Ultimately, expanded laboratory testing capacity will become a critical factor in achieving enhanced health outcomes, and patients will receive timely and appropriate interventions necessary for effective management of lung disease.

5.4.1. Blood Tests For Inflammatory Markers

The diagnosis of lung disease has also improved immensely with the application of blood work for inflammatory markers, which are critical in the evaluation of most pulmonary diseases. Traditional diagnostic methods, such as spirometry, primarily evaluate lung function rather than disease activity and often require supporting indicators for a comprehensive examination. Blood tests for inflammatory markers, such as cytokines and acute phase reactants, provide a measurable picture of the underlying inflammatory processes that characterize diseases like COPD and asthma. This paradigm shift towards biomarker use is indicative of the growing appreciation for the fact that inflammation plays a pivotal role in lung disease pathophysiology, so that there can be earlier diagnosis, assessment of the severity of functional impairment, and prediction of therapeutic response, thus enhancing patient care in general (Conti et al., 2016).

Among all lung diseases, the use of biomarkers through blood tests represents a significant leap forward in the clinical arena. Compared to traditional invasive procedures, blood tests provide a less invasive means of quantifying inflammatory activity, which is crucial in disease development and response to therapy. Quantification of specific inflammatory markers provides valuable prognostic information that contributes to individualized therapeutic plans, leading to improved patient outcomes. For instance, an increase in specific cytokines can correlate with disease exacerbations in conditions such as COPD, prompting changes in therapeutic strategies. Additionally, the field is also making advances in proteomics, which enables the detection of varied protein profiles corresponding to different inflammatory reactions, further enhancing the predictive capability of such blood tests (Conti et al., 2016). The application of blood tests for inflammation markers not only increases the diagnostic accuracy but also does away with the access barrier commonly encountered in routine pulmonary assessments. Its use as a test fluid is particularly worthwhile because blood is non-invasive in nature and can be performed in various environments, including remote regions where standardized pulmonary testing may not be readily available. Advances in analyte stabilization methods and detection systems over the past few years have enhanced the reliability and utility of these tests in clinical practice. Although traditional techniques, such as bronchoalveolar lavage, remain central to specific investigations, blood tests hold promise for less expensive, more widespread, and more cost-effective diagnostic approaches in the management of lung disease. The studies undertaken in this area aim to position the test as an essential element in standard clinical evaluation, thereby supplementing traditional models of diagnosis with new, biomarker-based information.

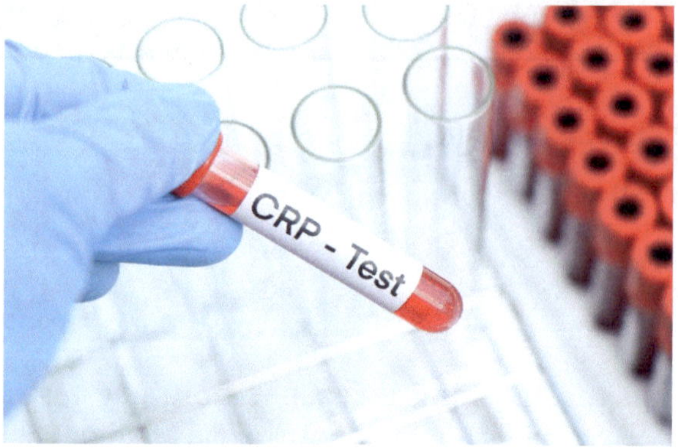

Figure 5.14. Inflammatory markers used in blood tests.

Source: https://external-content.duckduckgo.com/iu/?u=https%3A%2F%2Ffirebasestorage.googleapis.com%2Fv0%2Fb%2Fglycan-age.appspot.com%2Fo%2Fscience-magazine-articles-inflammation-markers-in-blood-tests-1-blobid8.jpg%3Falt%3Dmedia%26token%3D6bf735fa-5bc8-4f39-b5c9-2e67fcc99fcc&f=1&nofb=1&ipt=1b82b4546494f0b4a5d8d75b407b8a9a40ffa67848aa82950cb1c5cb0e03ea9b

5.4.2. Sputum Analysis and Culture

Sputum culture and analysis are crucial tools in the diagnostic arsenal for lung diseases, particularly pulmonary infections. Sputum collection, or mucus expectorated from the airways, can yield important information about the presence of inflammation or pathogens in the lungs. For tuberculosis (TB), the sputum examination is especially critical since control of the spread of the disease largely depends on early diagnosis. Current practice is inclined toward laboratory-based diagnostic procedures, such as microscopy and culture tests. Since TB is known to spread stealthily, a good sputum test can accelerate diagnosis and allow care professionals to implement treatment measures that contain transmission risks within communities, necessitating high precision and accessibility in the test methods (Harari et al., 2012). Sputum test methods have evolved with the integration of advanced diagnostic techniques. Historical sputum culture will take weeks to yield a diagnosis, but advances in mass spectrometry have enabled faster identification of mycobacterial species. With the application of electrospray ionization tandem mass spectrometry, scientists have been able to detect characteristic profiles that identify *Mycobacterium tuberculosis* from non-tuberculous mycobacterial strains. This evolution not only enhances sensitivity and specificity compared to conventional techniques but also streamlines the diagnostic process, enabling clinicians to accurately diagnose TB-positive patients more rapidly. As noted in some of the studies, including case-control assessment, this rapid diagnostic approach reiterates the importance of promoting sputum examination techniques in increasing patient outcomes and reducing lung disease burden, such as TB (Janiszewska-Drobinska et al., 2013).

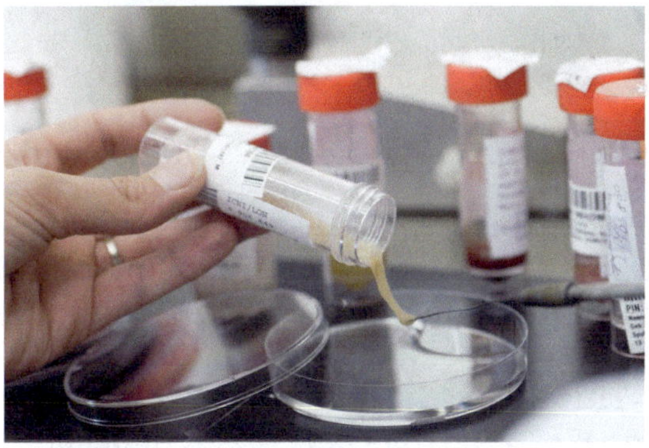

Figure 5.15. Sputum analysis and culture.

Source: https://external-content.duckduckgo.com/iu/?u=https%3A%2F%2Fwww.empr.com%2Fwp-content%2Fuploads%2Fsites%2F7%2F2019%2F10%2FSputum.Culture_SS_SS2302943.jpg&f=1&nofb=1&ipt=e921c367dc3ef2c5a4b6c77d2de2e0ec3693fac305b2c4015b810a8b0359e84f

The role of advanced sputum analysis and culture extends beyond patient-level treatment to global health programs. Effective detection and treatment of latent and active TB are integral components of public health programs aimed at eradicating the disease.

As healthcare systems strive to implement rapid and accurate diagnostic tests, the economic implications of sputum analysis must be addressed. Investment in their development and spread will likely come at considerable cost savings in terms of earlier treatment, decreased rates of transmission, and associated health costs of later disease stages. Lastly, sputum analysis and culture are foundations for the science of diagnostic equipment for lung disease, enhancing patient-centered care as well as overall public health gains through earlier and more precise detection and disease control.

5.4.3. Arterial Blood Gas (ABG) Analysis

The measurement of arterial blood gases (ABG) is a significant diagnostic tool in the diagnosis of lung illness. Through the measurement of oxygen, carbon dioxide, and blood pH, ABG measurement provides valuable information regarding the pulmonary and metabolic condition of an individual. It is particularly vital in disease conditions such as chronic obstructive pulmonary disease (COPD), acute respiratory distress syndrome (ARDS), and status asthmaticus.

The results thus derived can help determine whether the patient is experiencing respiratory acidosis or alkalosis, which will inform clinical maneuvers such as ventilatory support or oxygen therapy. Moreover, interpretation of ABG can reflect the adequacy of gas exchange through the lungs, which plays a critical role in monitoring the course of illness and the effectiveness of treatment, thereby revealing its value in offering effective management of respiratory diseases. With clinical assessment and ABG analysis, it helps in determining the appropriate staging and management plans for lung illnesses. For instance, in long-term respiratory diseases, assessment of blood gases can help medical professionals determine the severity of a patient's condition, allowing them to take appropriate action accordingly. As defined in existing literature, guaranteed access to the like diagnostic technology can close the gap in care for chronic diseases so that therapeutic interventions are closer to patient needs. The electronic integrated COPD proforma for emergency departments emphasizes adherence to guidelines and the implementation of timely interventions based on ABG findings to achieve better patient outcomes. Following a thorough review of implementation challenges, clinical consensus arises regarding the application of ABG analysis in routine practice in emergency settings, solidifying its value as a diagnostic tool for lung disease (Issac et al., 2022).

The integration of ABG analysis into routine care for lung disease patients can also enhance health care management in general (and particularly in complex symptom cases). By identifying certain abnormalities in gas exchange, clinicians can individualize treatment regimens to address both symptomatic and physiological aspects of respiratory illness. In extreme cases such as severe equine asthma syndrome, familiarity with the blood gas profile will have a significant impact on environmental manipulations as well as pharmacologic management. This multi-factorial therapeutic approach, combined with ongoing monitoring through ABG analysis, provides a comprehensive picture of patient care, aiming not only to improve lung function but also to enhance quality of life. As this discipline continues to evolve, ongoing research continues to consolidate the role of arterial blood gas analysis in enhancing diagnostic rates and patient outcomes in the case of lung diseases (Simões et al., 2020).

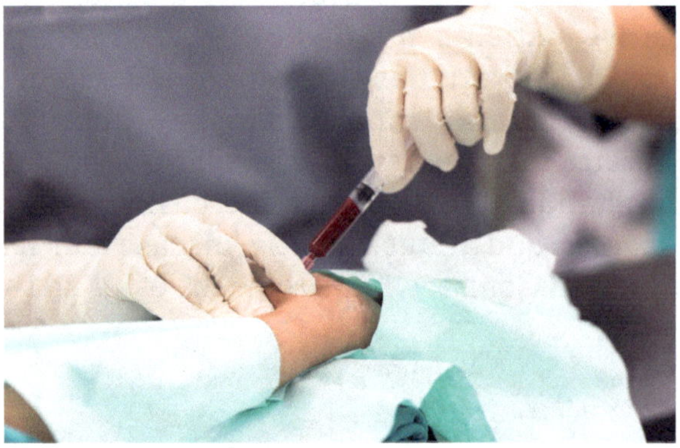

Figure 5.16. Arterial blood gas (ABGs) analysis.

Source: https://external-content.duckduckgo.com/iu/?u=https%3A%2F%2Fnurseslabs.com%2Fwp-content%2Fuploads%2F2020%2F09%2Farterial-blood-gas-collection.jpg&f=1&nofb=1&ipt=41945f5cf88af376a0a8ff6bbb64dddd7dbe7c9892b1b5e9abb7920ccd00ecb0

Test Your Knowledge

1. What are the blood tests for inflammatory markers?
2. Discuss sputum analysis and culture.

5.5. Endoscopic Procedures

Learning Outcome

1. Bronchoscopy and its diagnostic uses
2. Endobronchial ultrasound (EBUS)
3. Thoracoscopy for pleural disease evaluation

Endoscopic procedures are now at the forefront of diagnostic equipment for lung disease, particularly in assessing and managing conditions such as lung cancer, infections, and interstitial lung disease. These techniques employ techniques such as bronchoscopy, endobronchial ultrasound, and video-assisted thoracoscopic surgery to allow direct visualization of the respiratory tract and the collection of tissue samples. Bronchoscopy, for example, enables clinicians to examine the bronchial tree and biopsy abnormal-appearing lesions, facilitating the early diagnosis of cancer. In addition, advances in imaging technology have enhanced the success of these procedures, allowing for real-time assessment of abnormalities with minimal patient discomfort and reduced recovery time. Endoscopic procedures thus form the basis for the trend towards higher accuracy and less invasive diagnostic tests within pulmonary medicine.

The role of autofluorescence (AF) imaging in enhancing endoscopic procedures has been a concern in recent years, as it is a label-free method for assessing lung tissue. Properties of endogenous fluorophores in AF enable clinicians to differentiate between pathological and normal tissues, thereby supplementing conventional bronchoscopic techniques. AF imaging continues to evolve as a tool in lung disease; however, its utility is most readily appreciated in other areas where it has attained clinical value. A good example is its utility in differentiating parathyroid and thyroid tissue intraoperatively, illustrating its application in preventing errors secondary to anatomical misidentifications. By integrating AF imaging into routine endoscopic evaluation, immense potential is realized to increase diagnostic accuracy and improve patient management in lung disease compared to conventional methods (Aigner et al., 2020). As progress is made in the field, there remains an essential need for standardized protocols and rigorous training on endoscopic techniques. The increasing sophistication of lung disease diagnosis requires healthcare practitioners to be well-versed in these new technologies and be brought in line with safety standards. Facilities need to prioritize the development of training programs that combine technical proficiency with interpretive skills, enabling clinicians to utilize new methodologies to their best advantage. In addition, continuous research and development would be necessary to evolve the techniques further and determine long-term effectiveness in clinical application. A joint effort in this direction of education and advancement will not only enhance diagnostic capacity but also usher in better treatment interventions for lung diseases, resulting in better care for patients in pulmonary medicine (Ndongo et al., 2010).

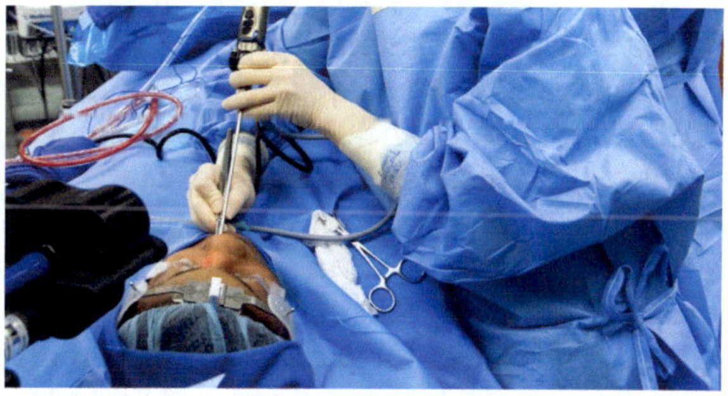

Figure 5.17. Endoscopy procedure.

Source: https://external-content.duckduckgo.com/iu/?u=http%3A%2F%2Fwww.healthylifecentar.com%2Fwp-content%2Fuploads%2F2019%2F06%2FGuest-Post.jpg&f=1&nofb=1&ipt=3b8ccc22e40c872c399e0e54a3c988fefe2edbc1c5f1a38c561401ffedf805c0

5.5.1. Bronchoscopy and Its Diagnostic Uses

Bronchoscopy is a crucial diagnostic technique in evaluating various lung diseases, allowing for direct visualization of the airways and the collection of tissue samples. The less invasive procedure enables clinicians to examine abnormalities, such as tumors, infections, and inflammation, within the bronchial tubes. The technique involves the use of a bronchoscope, a slender, pliable tube equipped with a camera and light delivery, for direct visualization of the bronchial tree in real-time. Furthermore, bronchoscopy can be combined with other interventions, such as bronchoalveolar lavage (BAL), which maximizes diagnostic yield by allowing the sampling of lung fluids. This role is of particular importance in the identification of infectious pathogens, such as Mycobacterium gordonae, as evidenced by studies proving the identification of this pathogen from BAL samples after bronchoscopy intervention. These findings underscore the value of bronchoscopy in the effective diagnosis of lung illnesses. Bronchoscopy has a role beyond viewing; it also includes therapeutic procedures, hence making it an essential instrument in the treatment of lung illnesses. Aside from diagnostic, procedures can be utilized to deliver interventions like stenting and laser ablation to palliate obstructive symptoms caused by tumors or other lesions. In addition, technological advances in imaging technologies, such as autofluorescence (AF) imaging, have enhanced the detection of precancerous changes in bronchial tissue, thereby facilitating earlier intervention and improved outcomes for patients. The potential application of AF techniques in bronchoscopy highlights a growing emphasis on integrating novel diagnostic modalities into existing procedures. However, as emphasized through research, standardization of protocols is crucial to maximize clinical return and ensure patient safety, given the variability of methods applied across specialties (Aigner et al., 2020). Whereas its advantages are significant, its issues and close attention to patient parameters and procedure risk cannot be overlooked. The procedure may not be feasible in all patients, especially those with acute respiratory distress or with other medical conditions putting the patient at increased procedural risk. Furthermore, strict adherence to reprocessing guidelines and monitoring regimens is crucial for the prevention of potential infection related to bronchoscopy. A retrospective analysis identified a pseudo-outbreak of *Mycobacterium gordonae* linked to environmental contamination and emphasized the importance of rigorous infection control measures following bronchoscopic procedures (Cottarelli et al., 2016). As the medical community continues to uncover innovative diagnostic applications for bronchoscopy, further research and development of safety protocols will be essential in optimizing outcomes while reducing risks for patients undergoing lung evaluations.

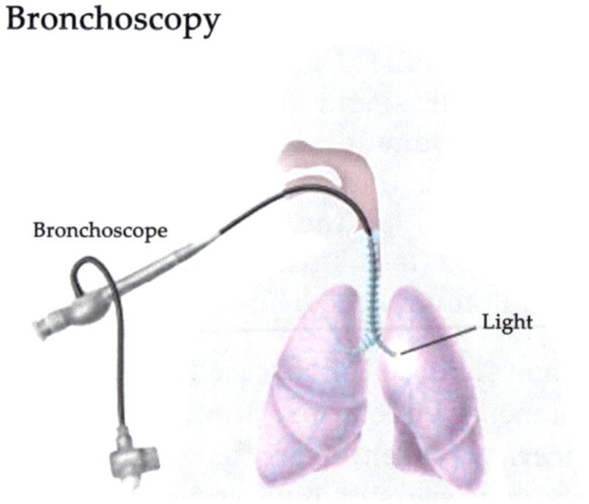

Figure 5.18. Bronchoscopy and its diagnostic uses.

Source: https://external-content.duckduckgo.com/iu/?u=https%3A%2F%2Fwww.lungevity.org%2Fsites%2Fdefault%2Ffiles%2Fillustrations%2Fbronchoscopy.png&f=1&nofb=1&ipt=b1833e85fae663fa3eae50a283a0ff515eecb5fee7c0ab2d5b54c88b877dd048

5.5.2. Endobronchial Ultrasound (EBUS)

Endobronchial ultrasound (EBUS) is now a central diagnostic technology for lung disease, enabling the precise evaluation of mediastinal and hilar lymph nodes. This less invasive procedure enhances the detection of lung cancer and other pulmonary diseases by utilizing bronchoscopy in conjunction with real-time ultrasound imaging. Since professionals can visualize bronchial anatomy and surrounding tissue, they can correctly localize lymph nodes potentially with pathologic changes. These are especially useful in staging lung carcinoma and the diagnosis of illnesses such as sarcoidosis and tuberculosis. For example, one study of 159 patients undergoing EBUS-TBNA presented that the test had an impressive diagnostic accuracy of 83% for benign granulomatous disease, highlighting its ability to diagnose a range of lung pathologies (Abu-Hijleh et al., 2015). The benefit of EBUS is particularly significant in its ability to improve patient outcomes through enhanced diagnostic precision. The procedure reduces reliance on more invasive procedures, such as mediastinoscopy, which carries an increased risk profile and attendant complications. Of particular note is the implication that EBUS-TBNA allows for the taking of multiple samplesthereby increasing the possibility of a definitive diagnosis. Retrospectively, 84% of patients were accurately diagnosed with EBUS-TBNA, being an effective option for both malignant and benign pathology (Abu-Hijleh et al., 2015). Additionally, the advent of other techniques such as ultrasound-guided transbronchial cryobiopsy promises improved diagnostic yield in mediastinal lesions over the conventional EBUS-TBNA, with a diagnostic yield of 91.2%. Despite the advances provided by EBUS, there continue to be hindrances to its application and the interpretation of findings, particularly in the context of certain malignancies and less common pulmonary diseases. Sampling method variability and operator experience may affect the diagnostic results. In addition, although EBUS offers better access to areas that were previously considered challenging to reach, the learning curve associated with this technique requires extensive operator training to optimize its advantages. Continued research and development of EBUS applications will be necessary to overcome these challenges, enabling clinicians to apply this method to its diagnostic best within the evolving scope of lung disease management.

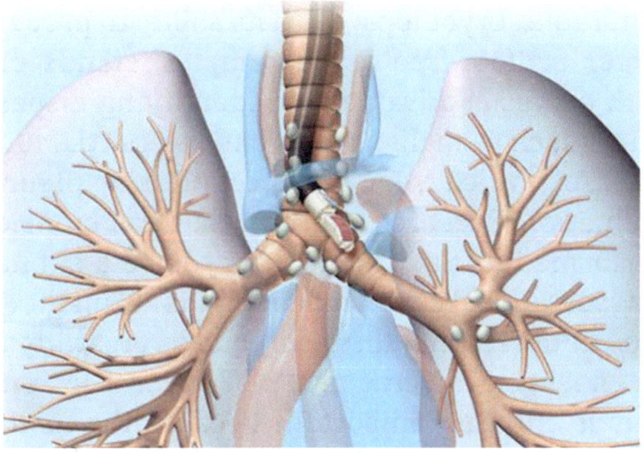

Figure 5.19. Endobronchial ultrasound (EBUS).

Source: https://external-content.duckduckgo.com/iu/?u=https%3A%2F%2Fpulmonarypracticeassociates.com%2Fwp-content%2Fuploads%2F2018%2F11%2FEndobronchialUltrasound-img.jpg&f=1&nofb=1&ipt=e2d48812b10dc0c80c2b16c456d4f7df4800b4c995d4d239286a0e6e3dbb2d56

5.5.3. Thoracoscopy For Pleural Disease Evaluation

Thoracoscopy or video-assisted thoracic surgery (VATS) is a pillar of minimally invasive diagnostic procedures for pleural disease evaluation. Its utility lies in providing direct visualization and biopsy of the pleural space, which is particularly useful when traditional imaging modalities are insufficient for making a specific diagnosis. By employing a thoracoscope, patients can not only assess pleural effusions and masses but also obtain histological samples for histopathological assessment. The method is crucial in distinguishing between benign and malignant pleural conditions, which can have far-reaching implications for management plans. By way of illustration, thoracoscopy has been discovered to improve diagnostic yield in patients with pleural effusions whose etiology cannot be determined, facilitating interventions immediately that can improve patient outcomes. The use of advanced techniques, such as cryobiopsy, enhances the efficiency of thoracoscopy in evaluating pleural conditions. Cryobiopsy, with its ability to procure larger artifact-free tissue samples, stands out with a special advantage in identifying disease states such as malignancies and interstitial lung diseases, which frequently occur during pleural evaluation. Research indicates that cryobiopsies performed during thoracoscopy have a similar diagnostic yield compared to traditional methods, thus underscoring the technique's versatility in diagnosing a diverse array of pleural lesions. This is clinically important because the ability to accurately characterise pleural abnormalities facilitates targeted therapy and comprehensive patient care strategies (Griff et al., 2019). As the technique and methodologies are changing every day, thoracoscopy still remains at the pinnacle of pleural disease evaluation. In addition, the application of imaging modalities, such as MRI, alongside thoracoscopy complements the diagnostic approach for pleural malignancies. Ongoing research discovers that semi-objective biomarkers from contrast-enhanced MRI, such as early contrast enhancement (ECE), are beneficial for tumor characterization and also assist in thoracoscopic procedures. This multimodal approach enhances the sensitivity of pleural malignancy detection, particularly in cases of minimal pleural thickening that may not be easily demonstrated on routine imaging (Alexander et al., 2018). By integrating these advanced imaging modalities with thoracoscopic intervention, physicians can make more accurate diagnoses and implement targeted therapeutic interventions to achieve improved patient outcomes in the management of pleural disease. The complementarity of surgical evaluation and imaging diagnostics highlights the need for ongoing research and innovation in lung disease diagnostics.

Test Your Knowledge

1. What is bronchoscopy, and explain its diagnostic uses?
2. What is endobronchial ultrasound (EBUS)?

5.6. Advanced Diagnostic Techniques

Learning Outcome

1. Genetic testing for hereditary lung diseases
2. Biomarkers in lung disease diagnosis
3. Artificial intelligence in diagnostic imaging

The evolving diagnostic environment for lung disease calls for the use of innovative methods to enhance early detection and treatment effectiveness. Traditional techniques such as chest X-rays and sputum testing are usually late or inadequate in reflecting pulmonary conditions, particularly in multi-factorial conditions such as tuberculosis. Advances currently highlight a shift to new methods aimed at instant and accurate diagnosis. As emphasized in current literature, the development of new screening tests for active tuberculosis and drug-resistant *M. tuberculosis* reflects the ongoing effort towards increased accuracy and accessibility, which remains a significant concern with global health initiatives aimed at controlling respiratory infections (Harari et al., 2012). Therefore, integrating these new processes into practice can significantly alter patient outcomes by better handling lung disease. Among the emerging technologies used in pulmonary diagnosis is autofluorescence imaging (AFI) that relies on the inherent fluorescent properties of biological tissues for non-invasive assessment. Although used predominantly in ophthalmology, increasing interest in AFI has led to experimental research in other clinical specialties, including pulmonology. Recent reviews have highlighted significant developments in AF technologies, emphasizing their ability to provide real-time visualization of respiratory tissues without the need for invasive sampling (Aigner et al., 2020). This shift toward non-invasive methods not only enhances the comfort of patients but also enables quicker diagnoses, particularly for lung cancer and other respiratory malignancies. With the medical profession further optimizing and simplifying AF methods, there is a genuine hope that these will become more relevant in respiratory diagnosis. Furthermore, overcoming the present barriers to the widespread application of high-tech diagnostic strategies calls for not just technological advancements but also a revolution in healthcare infrastructure. The installation of sophisticated diagnostic devices requires proper investment in training medical specialists and enhancing existing diagnostic centers. Technique variability and the lack of standard protocols are two issues that must be addressed to render output consistent. Mutual coordination between researchers, clinicians, and policymakers is necessary to ensure the common purpose of optimal maximization of lung disease diagnostics. As recognized in the debates around tuberculosis tests, striking a balance between test sensitivity and affordability, as well as accessibility, is essential to provide equitable healthcare delivery (Harari et al., 2012). By implementing an integrated approach to diagnostics, the clinical community can work towards improved lung condition management.

5.6.1. Genetic Testing For Hereditary Lung Diseases

Genetic testing for inherited lung disease is an essential addition to the family of diagnostic methods, providing more accurate information to patients and clinicians regarding respiratory conditions. Genetic testing that identifies genetic mutations associated with diseases such as cystic fibrosis, alpha-1 antitrypsin deficiency, and primary pulmonary hypertension can facilitate earlier diagnosis and more targeted treatment protocols. This forward-thinking approach enables clinicians to initiate preventive strategies and interventions much earlier in the disease process, often even before clinical symptoms have developed. Additional investigation into genetic markers not only improves diagnostic accuracy but also enhances the potential for personalized medicine, with treatments that are specifically adapted to the genetic defects present in unique patients, facilitating more integrated practices aligned with the greater emphasis on predictive healthcare practices in numerous fields, as the direction of past research (Bubnov et al., 2015). Secondly, genetic testing enables the assessment of risk for hereditary lung disease in at-risk groups, thereby maximizing familial screening programs. Relatives of individuals diagnosed with such a genetic disease can derive significant advantages from the same and undergo early intervention with ongoing monitoring. Identification of at-risk individuals allows for lifestyle modification, regular monitoring, and early therapeutic interventions to minimize or avoid the effects of genetic lung disease. However, the ethical implications and concerns of genetic testing cannot be overlooked. Consent, privacy, and potential genetic discrimination are concerns that must be addressed carefully. The healthcare system must develop a robust set of guidelines to ensure that genetic information is handled responsibly, maintaining the confidentiality of the patient while offering helpful diagnostic services (Bhatia et al., 2013). As genetic research continues to advance, so does the technology that facilitates genetic testing. Next-generation sequencing technologies, combined with sophisticated bioinformatics software, enable comprehensive genetic testing that was previously impossible. These technological advancements not only enhance the sensitivity and specificity of genetic tests but also their accessibility and cost-effectiveness for their incorporation into widespread clinical practice. The integration of these technologies into routine diagnostic practice can revolutionize the management of inherited lung disease, with a vast advantage to patient outcomes. Lastly, ongoing collaboration among geneticists, pulmonologists, and other clinicians is crucial for the successful implementation and use of genetic tests in the treatment of hereditary lung disease. This cross-disciplinary solution will ensure that both the scientific and practical methods of this diagnostic method are tackled appropriately, paving the way for the design of tailored patient care solutions (Bubnov et al., 2015).

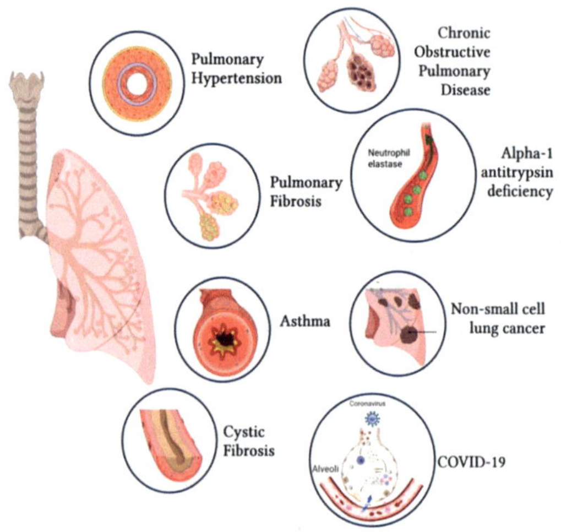

Figure 5.20. Genetic testing for hereditary lung diseases.

Source: https://www.mdpi.com/cells/cells-11-00984/article_deploy/html/images/cells-11-00984-g001.png

5.6.2. Biomarkers in Lung Disease Diagnosis

Biomarker discovery has transformed the practice of lung disease diagnosis, enabling the more precise and earlier measurement of respiratory diseases. Biomarkers, such as proteins, metabolites, or genetic markers, provide valuable insights into disease mechanisms and progression. Measurement of some cytokines in bronchoalveolar lavage fluid, for instance, has been helpful in the diagnosis of asthma and chronic obstructive pulmonary disease (COPD). The significance of these biomarkers, however, lies not only in diagnosis but also in their promise to guide personalized therapeutic interventions. As researchers seek to determine the molecular underpinnings of pulmonary conditions, the ongoing discovery and verification of novel biomarkers promise to enhance diagnostic accuracy and facilitate early intervention, hence optimizing patient outcomes. When infectious lung diseases, such as tuberculosis, are involved, the application of biomarkers in diagnostics becomes increasingly significant. Conventional diagnostic methods typically involve extensive laboratory procedures, resulting in delayed diagnosis and limited treatment windows. Emerging technologies in biomarker discovery aim to overcome these challenges; however, providing reliable point-of-care tests is a complex endeavor.

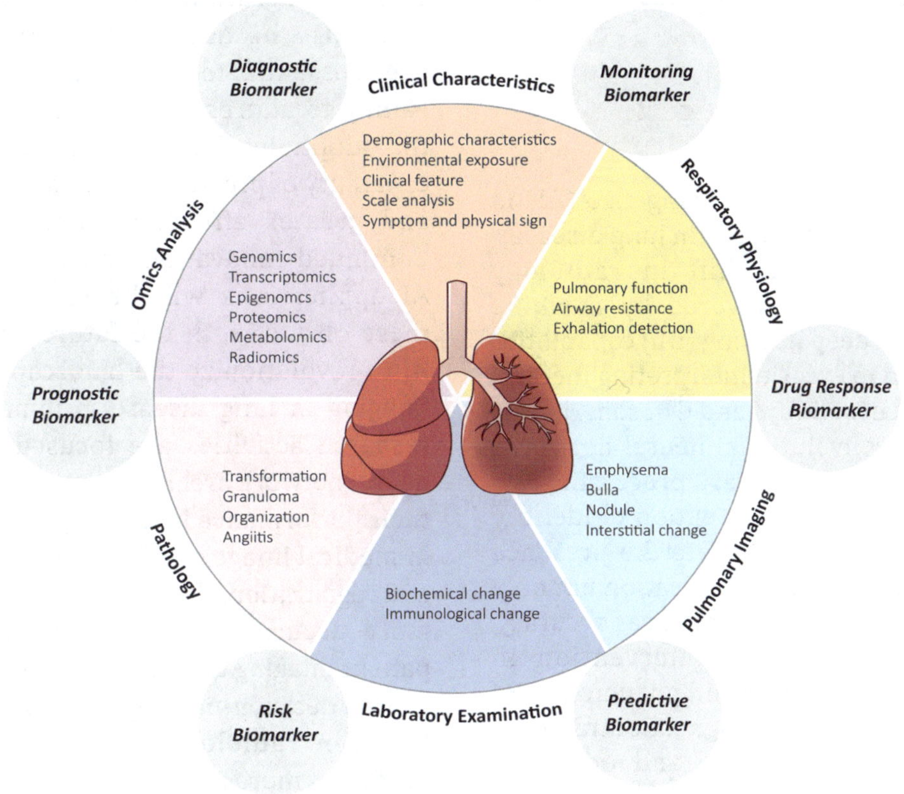

Figure 5.21. Biomarkers in lung disease diagnosis.

Source: https://onlinelibrary.wiley.com/cms/asset/77b61889-6b03-479e-a34b-ada534bef06f/ctd211-fig-0001-m.png

For instance, although numerous new tests have been designed for latent tuberculosis screening and the detection of drug resistance, they require further validation before being used in routine clinical settings. As quoted in the literature, the absence of , practical, rapid diagnostic tools directly impacts tuberculosis control, highlighting continued study of new biomarkers and new diagnostic technologies to try to combat this persistent global health burden (Harari et al., 2012). Salivary diagnostics is a new area of research for lung disease biomarkers, presenting a non-invasive option to existing diagnostic testing. Saliva collection is less susceptible to contamination and also has a high potential to increase accessibility in resource-poor populations. Advances in salivary analytical and stabilizing technology have enabled the detection of promising biomarkers employing genomic, transcriptomic, proteomic, and metabolomic techniques with success. Transcriptomic analysis, most importantly, has been reported in recent studies to have high sensitivity and specificity in disease detection in lung diseases. Utilizing advancements in biomarker science, salivary diagnostics has the potential to revolutionize patient screening and monitoring of respiratory diseases, providing practitioners with the necessary tools to enhance early detection and targeted treatment strategies (Bonne et al., 2012).

5.6.3. Artificial Intelligence in Diagnostic Imaging

The application of artificial intelligence (AI) in diagnostic imaging, particularly in lung diseases, represents a paradigm shift in radiology processes. AI systems powered by machine learning (ML) and deep learning (DL) capabilities have been shown to excel in interpreting medical images, such as chest X-rays and CT scans. In this field, primarily, convolutional neural networks (CNNs) have surpassed the rest, processing raw images without human intervention to identify prominent features that indicate the presence of pulmonary diseases. This innovation not only speeds up diagnosis but also enhances accuracy, which is critical for early intervention in diseases such as lung cancer and pneumonia. By complementing traditional diagnostic strategies, AI reduces diagnostic errors and enhances patient management, ultimately leading to improved clinical outcomes and effectiveness in healthcare settings (Bartoszek et al., 2025).

Although considering the significant advantages provided by AI in diagnostic imaging, certain challenges must be addressed to utilize its potential in clinical use fully. Reliance on robust, heterogeneous training data sets is most critical; such data sets enable the AI systems to generalize across various population groups and disease presentations. The interpretability of the model is also an important challenge; clinicians must understand how AI arrives at its recommendations before they will accept them. Integration with existing workflows must also be addressed, since simplicity of use is essential for overall clinician acceptance. Failing to address these obstacles could delay the adoption of AI technologies, despite their capability of providing more accurate diagnoses and greater efficiency (Jiang et al., 2010). Continued innovation and rigorous testing of AI applications will be vital to overcoming these obstacles. In the future, the potential of AI to revolutionize the landscape of diagnostic imaging in lung disease is immense. Ongoing research activities are focused on enhancing neural network architectures, thereby improving their performance in not only diagnosis but also in medical image segmentation, edge detection, and registration. These measures aim to provide more accurate and quantitative analysis of patient imaging data, thereby further supporting clinical decision-making. Moreover, collaboration between radiologists and AI systems will produce a more efficient synergy, with AI serving as a valuable resource that supplements, rather than replaces, human intelligence. Ultimately, as problems related to data quality, system integration, and interpretability are overcome, the enhanced role of AI in diagnostic imaging will be a factor leading to better patient outcomes for lung disease therapy (Bartoszek et al., 2025).

Test Your Knowledge

1. Explain Genetic testing for hereditary lung diseases.
2. What are the biomarkers in lung disease diagnosis?

SUMMARY

The evolution of diagnostic methods in lung disease has considerably expanded the ability to assess and manage respiratory diseases effectively. Traditional physiological testing has provided the foundation for understanding conditions such as asthma and chronic obstructive pulmonary disease (COPD). More recent developments, however, have established comprehensive diagnostic pathways that encompass more than physiological parameters. For instance, the COPD and Asthma Rotterdam Integrated Care Approach (CORONA) places particular emphasis on an integrated assessment that includes not only biomedical markers but also behavioral markers, reflecting the overall state of health of the patients. An overall outlook encourages a patient-centered approach, and consequently, better treatment results and improved quality of life in patients with lung diseases (Braunstahl et al., 2015). Furthermore, advances in imaging modalities such as probe-based confocal endomicroscopy are revolutionizing the diagnosis of diffuse parenchymal lung diseases. With this modality, doctors can image elastin structures directly in real-time within alveoli, allowing early and accurate assessment of lung pathology. By applying automated algorithms to estimate structural parameters, researchers have shown that these methods are capable of rapidly distinguishing various lung diseases from normal tissue. The quantitative assessment of elastin thickness and connectivity reveals statistically significant differences among patient groups compared to normal controls, which provides a promising direction for future research and clinical applications (Behr et al., 2020). In summary, the incorporation of novel diagnostic methods in lung disease assessment underscores the ongoing need for innovation within pulmonology. As clinicians and investigators investigate and develop these techniques, the possibility exists to significantly streamline the diagnostic process and improve patient outcomes. The insights gained from comprehensive diagnostic protocols and sophisticated imaging technology not only augment clinical knowledge but also provide opportunities for personalized treatment strategies. In the future, it is crucial for healthcare professionals to adopt these advancements, enabling patients to receive the most accurate diagnoses and effective treatment plans available. It's only through such forward-thinking strategies that lung diseases can be adequately treated, despite their complexity, ultimately resulting in better health for those affected.

Several methods are used in the diagnosis of lung disease to ascertain the extent and nature of pathology within the pulmonary system. Traditional imaging systems, such as chest X-rays and computed tomography (CT) scans, provide the initial steps toward determining abnormalities. These modalities enable clinicians to visualize central thoracic cavity structures, which allows for identification of tumors, infection, and other abnormalities. However, while imaging is an essential element, it most often requires supplemental evidence in the form of invasive tests. For instance, bronchoscopy, which involves direct visual inspection of the airways, can facilitate biopsies, thereby providing a definitive diagnosis. Such a synergy of imaging and invasive techniques exemplifies the multidimensional approach required for effective diagnosis of lung disease. The effectiveness of pulmonary examinations has been significantly enhanced through the development of new diagnostic techniques. Cryobiopsy, the new method, differs from conventional biopsies because it retains larger tissue samples of the lung that are less prone to artefacts. The most recent data indicate that cryobiopsies have higher diagnostic yield for malignancy and interstitial lung disease compared to conventional methods, thus showing its scope of more uses in clinical practice. The application of this technique in pleural lesion diagnosis has been as accurate as flexible thoracoscopy, highlighting its multi-use advantage. With advancing technology and diagnostic tools, the flexibility and specificity of measures like cryobiopsy will predict better patient outcomes and more tailored treatment protocols, with emphasis on a transition towards more sophisticated methods in pulmonology (Griff et al., 2019). Additionally, the incorporation of immunological tests significantly enhances the diagnostic accuracy of lung diseases. The tests have gained increased application in the detection of viral infections that would complicate respiratory pathology. Specifically, studies have illustrated the application of seroepidemiological methods for detecting herpesvirus infections in sea turtles, also linking viral presence with respiratory diseases (Jacobson et al., 2001). This approach, in addition to aiding understanding of infection dynamics, also guides therapeutic management in affected groups. The ability to identify specific pathogens through targeted diagnostics enhances knowledge of disease etiology, allowing for the treatment of patients on an individual basis. More and more, with advancements in the area, the synergism of several diagnostics will further streamline the evaluation process and give clinicians a solid decision-making base in lung disease treatment.

KEY TERMS FROM THIS CHAPTER

Chest X-ray
Pulmonary function tests (PFTs)
Bronchoscopy
Arterial blood gas (ABG) analysis
Thoracentesis
Mantoux test (Tuberculin test)
Diffusing capacity for carbon monoxide (DLCO)
Ventilation-perfusion (V/Q) scan
Capnography
Magnetic Resonance Imaging (MRI)
CT scan (Computed Tomography)
Spirometry
Sputum analysis
Pulse oximetry
Lung biopsy
Peak expiratory flow rate (PEFR)
Polysomnography
Pleural fluid analysis
Chest ultrasound
Exhaled nitric oxide test

CRITICAL THINKING QUESTIONS

1. **Which of the following is the gold standard imaging technique for detecting pulmonary embolism?**
   a. Chest X-ray
   b. High-resolution CT scan
   c. Ventilation-perfusion (V/Q) scan
   d. CT pulmonary angiography
2. **Which pulmonary function test parameter is most helpful in diagnosing obstructive lung disease?**
   a. Total lung capacity (TLC)
   b. Forced expiratory volume in 1 second (FEV_1) / Forced vital capacity (FVC) ratio
   c. Residual volume (RV)
   d. Diffusing capacity for carbon monoxide (DLCO)
3. **Which diagnostic procedure allows direct visualization and biopsy of the airways?**
   a. Thoracentesis
   b. Bronchoscopy
   c. Pleural biopsy
   d. Sputum cytology
4. **What does a chest X-ray typically show in a patient with lobar pneumonia?**
   a. Hyperinflation
   b. Homogeneous consolidation in a lobe
   c. Pleural effusion only
   d. Diffuse interstitial infiltrates
5. **In which lung disease is a DLCO (diffusing capacity of the lung for carbon monoxide) test most likely to be reduced?**
   a. Asthma
   b. Chronic bronchitis
   c. Pulmonary fibrosis
   d. Emphysema

Short Answer Questions

1. What is the primary imaging technique used to evaluate lung pathology?
2. Which pulmonary function test measures the amount of air a patient can forcibly exhale in one second?
3. Name the diagnostic procedure used to obtain lung tissue samples via a bronchoscope.
4. Which test is commonly used to detect pulmonary embolism?
5. How does a chest X-ray help differentiate between pneumonia and pleural effusion?

Answer to Critical Thinking Questions

1. (d)   2. (b)   3. (b)   4. (b)   5. (c)

REFERENCES

1. Albers, R., App, H., Barton, J., Blake, D., et al. (2008). Modelling mucociliary clearance. https://core.ac.uk/download/pdf/97255.pdf (accessed on 16th June 2025).
2. Albers, R., Bourdet-Sicard, R., Braun, D., Calder, P. C., et al. (2017). Monitoring immune modulation by nutrition in the general population: Identifying and substantiating effects on human health. https://core.ac.uk/download/85214747.pdf (accessed on 16th June 2025).
3. Aldini, G., Altomare, A., Baron, G., Vistoli, G., Carini, M., Borsani, L., & Sergio, F. (2018). N-acetylcysteine as an antioxidant and disulphide breaking agent: The reasons why. *Free Radical Research, 52*, 751–762. https://doi.org/10.1080/10715762.2018.1468564 (accessed on 16th June 2025).
4. Altshuler, D. L., & Dudley, R. (2006). The physiology and biomechanics of avian flight at high altitude. https://core.ac.uk/download/4887664.pdf (accessed on 16th June 2025).
5. American Lung Association. (2001). Urban air pollution and health inequities: A workshop report. https://core.ac.uk/download/323074325.pdf (accessed on 16th June 2025).
6. Arkenberg, A., Bleakley, B., Bodenmiller, B., Brunelli, R., Chakravortty, D., Cherayil, B. J., Constantinidou, C., et al. (2011). The production and detoxification of a potent cytotoxin, nitric oxide, by pathogenic enteric bacteria. https://core.ac.uk/download/2781215.pdf (accessed on 16th June 2025).
7. Arulselvan, P., Tangestani Fard, M., Tan, W. S., Gothai, S., Fakurazi, S., Norhaizan, M. E., & Kumar, S. (2016). Role of antioxidants and natural products in inflammation. *Oxidative Medicine and Cellular Longevity, 2016.* https://doi.org/10.1155/2016/5276130 (accessed on 16th June 2025).
8. Astort, F., Maglione, G. A., Orona, N. S., Saldiva, P. H., et al. (2014). Direct and indirect air particle cytotoxicity in human alveolar epithelial cells. https://core.ac.uk/download/159293549.pdf (accessed on 16th June 2025).
9. Bayard, J. B., & Ramos Morales, F. (2018). Molecular mechanisms used by *Salmonella* to evade the immune system. https://core.ac.uk/download/222572248.pdf (accessed on 16th June 2025).
10. Bresson, J. L., Burlingame, B., Dean, M., et al. (2017). 'Nutrimune®' and immune defense against pathogens in the gastrointestinal and upper respiratory tracts: Evaluation of a health claim pursuant to Article 14 of Regulation (EC) No 1924/2006. https://core.ac.uk/download/84493852.pdf (accessed on 16th June 2025).
11. Brown, A. J. P., Brown, G. D., Gow, N. A. R., Netea, M. G., et al. (2014). Metabolism impacts upon *Candida* immunogenicity and pathogenicity at multiple levels. https://core.ac.uk/download/25497610.pdf (accessed on 16th June 2025).
12. Brown, G. D., Hardison, S. E., & Plato, A. (2014). Pattern recognition receptors in antifungal immunity. https://core.ac.uk/download/29151173.pdf (accessed on 16th June 2025).
13. Brown, R. L., & Clarke, T. B. (2016). The regulation of host defenses to infection by the microbiota. https://core.ac.uk/download/77016328.pdf (accessed on 16th June 2025).
14. Carabelli, A. M., Peacock, T. P., Thorne, L., Harvey, W. T., Hughes, J., de Silva, T. I., Peacock, S. J., et al. (2023). SARS-CoV-2 variant biology: Immune escape, transmission and fitness.

Nature Reviews Microbiology. https://doi.org/10.1038/s41579-022-00841-7 (accessed on 16th June 2025).

15. Chadwick, D., & Goode, J. (2006). Innate immunity to pulmonary infection. https://www.semanticscholar.org/paper/2c26421da70058363c6fc1cbab6f73ba023dfff8 (accessed on 16th June 2025).
16. Chanson, M., Martin, P. E., O'Shaughnessy, E. M., Watanabe, H., et al. (2018). Connexin communication compartments and wound repair in epithelial tissue. https://core.ac.uk/download/293885271.pdf (accessed on 16th June 2025).
17. Collins, A., Weitkamp, J. H., & Wynn, J. L. (2018). Why are preterm newborns at increased risk of infection? *Archives of Disease in Childhood: Fetal & Neonatal, 103*, F391–F394. https://doi.org/10.1136/archdischild-2017-313595 (accessed on 16th June 2025).
18. Cortegiani, A., Gregoretti, C., & Spoletini, G. (2019). Physio pathological rationale of using high-flow nasal therapy in the acute and chronic setting: A narrative review. https://core.ac.uk/download/224993362.pdf (accessed on 16th June 2025).
19. Cuadrado, A., Pajares, M., Benito, C., Jiménez-Villegas, J., Escoll, M., Fernández-Ginés, R., García-Yagüe, Á. J., et al. (2020). Can activation of NRF2 be a strategy against COVID-19? *Trends in Pharmacological Sciences, 41*, 598–610. https://doi.org/10.1016/j.tips.2020.07.003 (accessed on 16th June 2025).
20. Dalamani, G., Kaspers, B., & Reese, S. (2006). The avian lung-associated immune system. https://core.ac.uk/download/12174987.pdf (accessed on 16th June 2025).
21. Dias, A. G., Sampaio, N. G., & Rehwinkel, J. (2018). A balancing act: MDA5 in antiviral immunity and autoinflammation. *Trends in Microbiology, 27*, 75–85. https://doi.org/10.1016/j.tim.2018.08.007 (accessed on 16th June 2025).
22. Dutta, S., Majzoub, A., & Agarwal, A. (2019). Oxidative stress and sperm function: A systematic review on evaluation and management. *Arab Journal of Urology, 17*, 87–97. https://doi.org/10.1080/2090598x.2019.1599624 (accessed on 16th June 2025).
23. EFSA Panel on Dietetic Products, Nutrition, and Allergies; Heinonen, M. (2017). 'Nutrimune®' and immune defense against pathogens in the gastrointestinal and upper respiratory tracts: Evaluation of a health claim pursuant to Article 14 of Regulation (EC) No 1924/2006. https://core.ac.uk/download/224638622.pdf (accessed on 16th June 2025).
24. Gevaert, K., Impens, F., Laval, K., Nauwynck, H., et al. (2019). Pollens destroy respiratory epithelial cell anchors and drive alpha herpesvirus infection. https://core.ac.uk/download/222452376.pdf (accessed on 16th June 2025).
25. Giegold, M. (2018). Modeling of the immune response during virus infection of the human respiratory tract. https://core.ac.uk/download/pdf/289960831.pdf (accessed on 16th June 2025).
26. Glezen, R., Hartshorn, K., Hufford, M., Jin, H., Jordan, J., Luo, D., Mosmann, T., et al. (2016). Influenza and memory T cells: How to awake the force. https://core.ac.uk/download/84594764.pdf (accessed on 16th June 2025).
27. Hegermann, J., Kuebler, W. M., Lopez-Rodriguez, E., Matuszak, J., et al. (2020). On top of the alveolar epithelium: Surfactant and the glycocalyx. https://core.ac.uk/download/323256852.pdf (accessed on 16th June 2025).

28. Hennigar, S. R. (2010). Exposure to polybrominated diphenyl ethers (PBDEs) suppresses the release of pro-inflammatory products by alveolar macrophages *in vitro*. https://core.ac.uk/download/215515896.pdf (accessed on 16th June 2025).

29. Hibberd, M. L., Kroll, J. S., Langford, P. R., Li, D., et al. (2011). Genome-wide expression profiling reveals suppression of host defense responses during colonization by *Neisseria meningitidis* but not *N. lactamica*. https://core.ac.uk/download/13115586.pdf (accessed on 16th June 2025).

30. Higham, A., Quinn, A. M., Delfini Cançado, J. E., & Singh, D. (2019). The pathology of small airways disease in COPD: Historical aspects and future directions. *Respiratory Research, 20*. https://doi.org/10.1186/s12931-019-1017-y (accessed on 16th June 2025).

31. Hu, B., Guo, H., Zhou, P., & Shi, Z. L. (2020). Characteristics of SARS-CoV-2 and COVID-19. *Nature Reviews Microbiology, 19*, 141–154. https://doi.org/10.1038/s41579-020-00459-7 (accessed on 16th June 2025).

32. Ivanova, N., Sotirova, Y., Gavrailov, G., Nikolova, K., & Andonova, V. (2022). Advances in the prophylaxis of respiratory infections by the nasal and the oromucosal route: Relevance to the fight with the SARS-CoV-2 pandemic. *Pharmaceutics, 14*, 530–530. https://doi.org/10.3390/pharmaceutics14030530 (accessed on 16th June 2025).

33. Januskevicius, A., Vasyle, E., & Malakauskas, K. (2024). Asthma: A new approach to the bronchial epithelium. *Pulmonology and Allergology*. https://www.semanticscholar.org/paper/0c0fee4e3b5abb1efc1e882f4937be416821bc16 (accessed on 16th June 2025).

34. Jarosz, M., Olbert, M., Wyszogrodzka, G., Młyniec, K., & Librowski, T. (2017). Antioxidant and anti-inflammatory effects of zinc. Zinc-dependent NF-κB signaling. *Inflammopharmacology, 25*, 11–24. https://doi.org/10.1007/s10787-017-0309-4 (accessed on 16th June 2025).

35. Jurado-Martín, I., Sainz-Mejías, M., & McClean, S. (2021). *Pseudomonas aeruginosa*: An audacious pathogen with an adaptable arsenal of virulence factors. *International Journal of Molecular Sciences, 22*, 3128–3128. https://doi.org/10.3390/ijms22063128 (accessed on 16th June 2025).

36. Luan, X. J. (2018). Effect of bacteria on airway submucosal glands liquid secretion in swine. https://core.ac.uk/download/226146030.pdf (accessed on 16th June 2025).

37. Rąpała-Kozik, M., & Zawrotniak, M. (2013). Neutrophil extracellular traps (NETs): Formation and implications. https://core.ac.uk/download/53115269.pdf (accessed on 16th June 2025).

38. Rehm, J., Gmel, G., Gmel, G., Hasan, O. S. M., Imtiaz, S., Popova, S., Probst, C., et al. (2017). The relationship between different dimensions of alcohol use and the burden of disease—An update. *Addiction, 112*, 968–1001. https://doi.org/10.1111/add.13757 (accessed on 16th June 2025).

39. Ridley, C., & Thornton, D. J. (2018). Mucins: The frontline defense of the lung. *Biochemical Society Transactions, 46*, 1099–1106. https://doi.org/10.1042/bst20170402 (accessed on 16th June 2025).

40. Strzelak, A., Ratajczak, A., Adamiec, A., & Feleszko, W. (2018). Tobacco smoke induces and alters immune responses in the lung triggering inflammation, allergy, asthma and other lung diseases: A mechanistic review. *International Journal of Environmental Research and Public Health, 15*, 1033–1033. https://doi.org/10.3390/ijerph15051033 (accessed on 16th June 2025).

41. Tekulapally, K. R., Lee, J. Y., Kim, D. S., Rahman, M. M., Park, C. K., & Kim, Y. H. (2024). Dual role of transient receptor potential ankyrin 1 in respiratory and gastrointestinal physiology: From molecular mechanisms to therapeutic targets. *Frontiers in Physiology, 15.* https://www.semanticscholar.org/paper/5f10a35c1575f05d633bf8ea38c69d25802d5c15 (accessed on 16th June 2025).

42. V'kovski, P., Kratzel, A., Steiner, S., Stalder, H., & Thiel, V. (2020). Coronavirus biology and replication: Implications for SARS-CoV-2. *Nature Reviews Microbiology, 19,* 155–170. https://doi.org/10.1038/s41579-020-00468-6 (accessed on 16th June 2025).

43. Visseren, F. L. J., Mach, F., Smulders, Y. M., Carballo, D., Koskinas, K. C., Bäck, M., Bénétos, A., et al. (2021). 2021 ESC guidelines on cardiovascular disease prevention in clinical practice. *European Heart Journal, 42,* 3227–3337. https://doi.org/10.1093/eurheartj/ehab484 (accessed on 16th June 2025).

44. Xiao, M. T., Ellsworth, C. R., & Qin, X. (2024). Emerging role of complement in COVID-19 and other respiratory virus diseases. *Cellular and Molecular Life Sciences: CMLS, 81.* https://www.semanticscholar.org/paper/0a656c1a3ef1b7ad03f0037a8d3bc42da6be88dc (accessed on 16th June 2025).

45. Yadav, P., Azam, M., Ramesh, V., & Singh, R. (2023). Unusual observations in leishmaniasis—An overview. *Pathogens, 12,* 297–297. https://doi.org/10.3390/pathogens12020297 (accessed on 16th June 2025).

PNEUMONIAS, LUNG ABSCESS, AND BRONCHIECTASIS

6

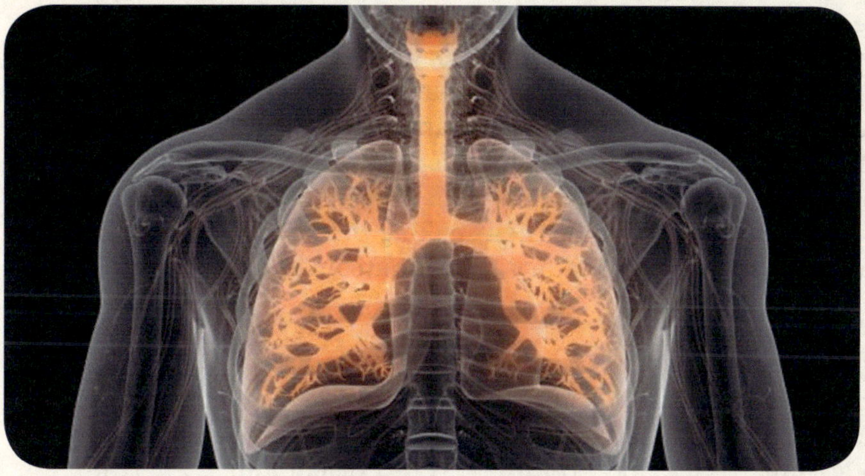

LEARNING OBJECTIVES

After studying this chapter, you will be able to:

1. Explain the types of pneumonia
2. List the causes and risk factors
3. Describe the symptoms and diagnosis
4. Discuss about lung abscess: definition and causes
5. List the symptoms and treatment of lung abscess
6. Explore bronchiectasis: overview and causes

Introduction

The respiratory system is a complex network tasked with vital functions, including gas exchange, host defense against pathogens, and the facilitation of debris removal. Among the various conditions affecting the system, pneumonias, lung abscesses, and bronchiectasis are notable due to their prevalence and potential severity. Pneumonias, which are most often due to infection, have the potential to provoke disseminated inflammatory responses, leading to significant morbidity. Lung abscesses are localized collections of pus within the lung tissue, typically secondary to aspiration or pneumonia, and present special diagnostic and therapeutic challenges. Finally, bronchiectasis is an abnormal permanent widening of the bronchi and is typically secondary to chronic infections or underlying diseases, which increase symptoms and cause a decline in pulmonary function. Grasping the subtleties of these conditions entails an awareness of their etiology, clinical presentation, and therapeutic options. Recent advances in diagnostic methods have revolutionized the treatment of pulmonary infections, particularly with the use of rapid sequencing technologies. The traditional culture-based model of diagnosis has been found to be time-consuming and often inadequate for the timely identification of pathogens in lower respiratory tract infections (LRI) (Mu et al., 2021). For instance, a clinical metagenomics assay has proven to be more sensitive and specific than conventional culture methods, dramatically reducing turnaround times. In addition to accelerating the detection of bacterial pathogens responsible for diseases such as pneumonia and lung abscesses, it enhances the potential for targeted therapy. Consequently, the utilization of rapid diagnostics has the potential to stimulate improved patient outcomes by allowing improved antimicrobial stewardship through the early de-escalation of the treatments as a function of effective identification of the pathogen. Beyond advances in diagnostics, imaging modalities play significant roles in the diagnosis of respiratory disorders. A variety of tools, including chest X-rays, computed tomography (CT), and lung ultrasound, provide specific data on pulmonary pathology, particularly in cases of acute respiratory failure (Chiumello et al., 2019). These modalities are beneficial in medical practice for arriving at proper diagnoses, follow-up, and treatment planning of diseases such as bronchiectasis and lung abscesses. However, the current lack of standardized guidelines for imaging utilization highlights a critical gap, necessitating further research to optimize clinical benefits. Comprehensive imaging strategies not only enhance understanding of disease severity but also facilitate better decision-making processes in managing these complex lung conditions, ultimately improving respiratory health outcomes.

Definition of Pneumonia

The term pneumonia encompasses a range of inflammatory conditions that affect the lung parenchyma, but most frequently result from infectious etiologies. Pneumonia can be caused by bacteria, viruses, fungi, or atypical pathogens, which infect lung tissue and produce severe presentations. Infection with these agents results in alveolar consolidation and impaired gas exchange, and typically presents as respiratory distress. The World Health Organization is concerned about pneumonia as a global health issue, particularly in vulnerable groups such as children and the elderly. The disease not only leads to acute respiratory presentation but also has potential grave complications, which makes it a cause for investigation of its clinical image and pathogenesis (Smiyan et al., 2023). Community-acquired pneumonia (CAP) is the most frequent and is a significant public health concern. It typically occurs outside the hospital and is most likely to occur in those with host factors of risk, such as smoking, immunosuppression, or chronic pulmonary disease. The presentation may range from mild to severe and includes fever, cough, chest pain, and dyspnea. Diagnostic approaches often rely on imaging techniques, such as chest X-rays or computed tomography, along with immunological testing, in an attempt to identify etiologic agents. Literature at hand offers proof that pneumonia remains a leading cause of morbidity and mortality, emphasizing the necessity of effective prevention techniques and treatment strategies (Smiyan et al., 2023). Moreover, identification of atypical pneumonia induced by unconventional pathogens enriches the context of pneumonia's complexity. In addition to classical types of pneumonia, recent studies have identified strong associations between systemic illnesses and pulmonary complications, such as lung involvement in rheumatoid arthritis and other connective tissue diseases. This highlights the way in which latent systemic inflammation can exacerbate pulmonary manifestations, demonstrating the multifactorial nature of pneumonia. The challenge in pneumonia diagnosis, especially among those with comorbid conditions, necessitates vigilant evaluation of clinical signs and symptoms in tandem with high-tech imaging. In addition, the cross-relation between pneumonia and other lung diseases, like bronchiectasis, highlights the complexity of lung disease that clinicians must address. Integrating clinical, radiological, and biochemical investigations in a holistic setting may enhance the accuracy of therapy, thereby improving patient outcomes.

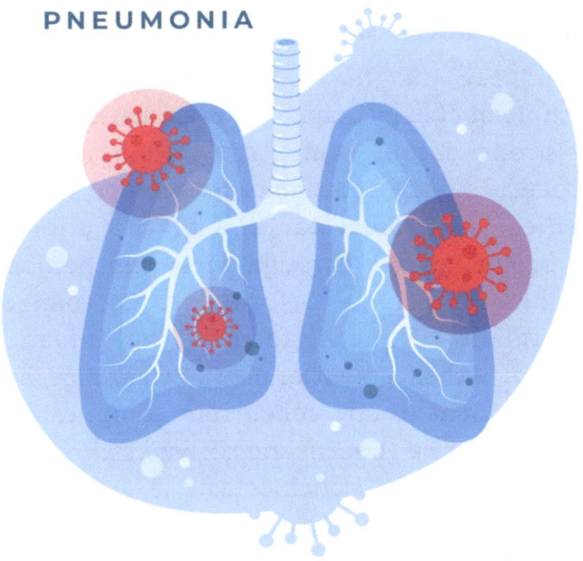

Figure 6.1. Understanding pneumonia.

Source: https://www.omegahospitals.com/blog/storage/2024/09/3724991-765x765.jpg

Overview of Lung Abscess

Lung abscesses are localized collections of pus within lung tissue, typically secondary to an infectious process. Such abscesses can occur secondary to infection with various pathogens, including bacteria, fungi, or parasites, and are frequently associated with predisposing conditions such as aspiration, immunosuppression, or lung disease. Primarily, anaerobic bacteria, typically found in the oral pharynx, are the primary culprits, particularly in patients with poor oral hygiene or a history of aspiration. The clinical presentation is likely to include cough, fever, chest pain, and pleuritic pain, which may mimic pneumonia. Early detection is critical, as delayed treatment can result in sequelae such as sepsis or bronchopleural fistulas, necessitating a proper evaluation of patients presenting with respiratory symptoms and potentially exhibiting unusual imaging findings. It is fundamental imaging applied in diagnosing lung abscesses, with chest X-rays and CT scans being the essential tools employed. These modalities can also show typical features such as a thick-walled abscess filled with necrotic material and pus. It should be noted that high-resolution CT scans also provide secondary information concerning the morphology of the abscess and associated bronchiectasis or consolidation, which are essential in planning the treatment. The treatment varies depending on the etiology and is based primarily on antibiotics. Where the abscess is extensive or treatment with medicine fails, surgery will be necessary. A new discovery documented in recent literature is the prevalence of methicillin-resistant Staphylococcus aureus (MRSA) as a causative agent, particularly in cases of severe necrotizing pneumonia, which necessitates close observation of current-day patterns of resistance in clinical practice (Leung et al., 2024). The course of lung abscesses is mainly governed by prompt diagnosis, appropriate antimicrobial therapy, and any underlying comorbidities that may complicate the recovery. While most patients can be successfully managed with antibiotics and supportive care, severe cases may require prolonged treatment or surgery, which has inherent risks. Of note, results may be dictated to a large extent by the patient's age, general state of health, and underlying diseases of the lungs, if any. Moreover, maintaining a healthy oral status, detecting aspiration symptoms early, and ensuring prompt medical attention are key aspects of prevention and management strategies. With the emergence of new bacterial threats and evolving patterns of resistance, more studies are being conducted, and clinicians must remain vigilant, adjusting treatment modalities accordingly to achieve the most optimal patient outcomes for lung abscess treatment (Jo et al., 2025).

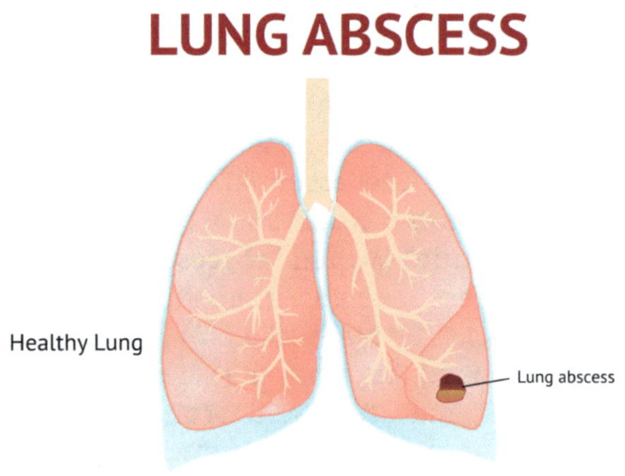

Figure 6.2. Lung abscess.

Source: https://dada2.org/wp-content/uploads/2023/06/Lung-Lung-Abscess-scaled.jpeg

Explanation of Bronchiectasis

Bronchiectasis is a chronic pulmonary disease characterized by the abnormally permanent dilation of the bronchial airways, which recurrent infections, inflammation, or obstruction within the lungs can cause. Bronchiectasis is often accompanied by various forms of lung disease, including recurrent bronchial infections, which can produce severe respiratory symptoms. In patients with STAT3 hyperimmunoglobulin E syndrome (STAT3-HIES), bronchiectasis frequently develops as a consequence of recurrent pneumonia and lung abscesses, leading to chronic cough, sputum production, and exacerbation of lung function impairment. The architectural changes in the bronchial tubes impair the effectiveness of mucus removal, predisposing patients to recurrent infections and an inflammatory response, thereby establishing a vicious cycle of illness that worsens overall respiratory health (Mahdaviani et al., 2023).

Moreover, the clinical presentation of bronchiectasis relies on a blend of imaging exams and patient history assessment, enabling clinicians to formulate a particular treatment regimen. High-resolution CT scans are necessary to visualize the aforementioned anatomical changes of bronchiectasis, including airway dilation, extent, and distribution.

These imaging tests are subsequently complemented by diagnostic examinations, such as bronchoscopy, which can be employed to procure biopsy specimens or remove foreign bodies. The understanding of the etiology of bronchiectasis through these mechanisms enables clinicians to formulate customized treatment regimens, focusing on infection control, enhancement of airway clearance, and management of any concurrent complications that may arise (Chernekhovskaya et al., 2023). Management of bronchiectasis is generally a multidisciplinary process that encompasses both pharmacological and non-pharmacological interventions.

Antibiotic treatment may be helpful in patients in order to conquer chronic infection, while inhaled treatments can assist in mucus removal. In severe cases with significant structural lung damage in patients, surgery may be indicated, particularly with localized bronchiectasis and lung abscesses. In instances such as STAT3-HIES, surgical treatment may be necessary to prevent life-threatening complications due to uncontrolled pulmonary infection. Yet, these interventions are not without risk, requiring the precise selection of patients and proper preoperative evaluations to optimize results while avoiding complications (Mahdaviani et al., 2023).

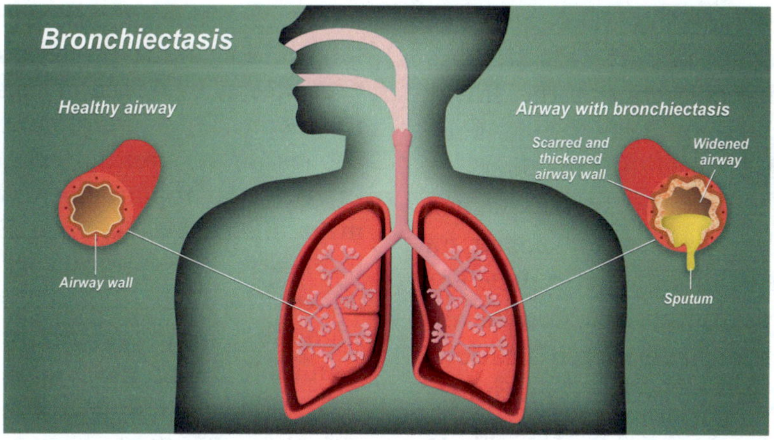

Figure 6.3. Bronchiectasis.

Source: https://www.svhlunghealth.com.au/Images/UserUploadedImages/3452/8_SVH_Lung_Health_Bronchiectasis_final_1080p.jpg

6.1. Types of Pneumonia

Learning Outcome

1. Community-Acquired Pneumonia (CAP)
2. Hospital-Acquired Pneumonia (HAP)
3. Aspiration Pneumonia

Pneumonia, categorized primarily by the etiologic pathogen and site of acquisition, occurs in various forms. Perhaps the most common are bacterial and viral pneumonias, each with typical pathogens and clinical presentation. Bacterial pneumonia, most commonly caused by Streptococcus pneumoniae or Haemophilus influenzae, is typified by the onset of acute fever, chills, and productive cough. On the other hand, viral pneumonia, typically caused by influenza viruses or coronaviruses, tends to present with an insidious onset of less severe respiratory symptoms that may progress into complications, such as hypoxia. The diagnostic workup for differentiating these forms of pneumonia often involves imaging studies, such as chest X-rays or CT scans, which show characteristic patterns of pulmonary opacities according to the nature and severity of the infection and enable appropriate, specific therapy promptly.

Another form is atypical pneumonia, which is typically caused by less common pathogens, such as Mycoplasma pneumoniae and Chlamydia pneumoniae. This form of pneumonia is also referred to as walking pneumonia because it typically presents with milder symptoms that do not require hospitalization. They may present with a nonproductive cough, low-grade fever, and nonspecific malaise; therefore, clinicians should include this in their differential diagnoses, especially in younger age groups. The impaired respiration present in atypical pneumonia may progress to bronchiectasis—a condition of pathological bronchial dilation—if left untreated, making early intervention necessary. Measures for early detection and management of atypical forms can significantly reduce the likelihood of chronic respiratory issues. Additionally, pneumonia may also arise due to primary immunodeficiencies (PIDs), which weaken the immune system's capacity to fight off infection. PID patients, who have a vast array of genetic disorders, are prone to having repeated respiratory infections, e.g., pneumonias. The impact of such infections is severe, as they specifically target the lower respiratory system, leading to conditions such as bronchitis, pneumonia, and bronchiectasis. Presentations in the respiratory system in such patients can also vary extensively based on the degree and type of immunodeficiency. For instance, while upper respiratory infections are more common, lower respiratory complications have a profound impact on patients' morbidity and mortality. Therefore, it is crucial to understand the intricate interaction between pneumonias and inherent immunologic flaws in order to improve therapy outcomes, especially in hospitals where respiratory examinations are routinely carried out on immunocompromised individuals (Jeseňák et al., 2014).

6.1.1. Community-Acquired Pneumonia (CAP)

Community-acquired pneumonia (CAP) is a public health concern and one of the leading causes of morbidity and mortality worldwide. CAP is an inflammation of the lung parenchyma due to pathogens acquired outside a healthcare facility and can range from mild to severe. The major pathogens recognized to cause CAP typically are Streptococcus pneumoniae, Haemophilus influenzae, and the atypical pathogens Mycoplasma pneumoniae and Chlamydophila pneumoniae. Several factors predispose to CAP, including age, comorbid disease, and lifestyle, e.g., smoking. With its widespread incidence, especially among high-risk patient groups such as the elderly and those with chronic diseases, understanding the pathophysiology and treatment of CAP is critical to improving patient outcomes and optimizing treatment strategies. The relationship between periodontal disease and pulmonary status has generated significant interest, particularly regarding the occurrence of CAP. Clinical studies reveal that periodontitis patients are likely to present increased susceptibility to lung diseases like pneumonia. Specifically, the presence of evidence of periodontal pathogens in respiratory samples was demonstrated, suggesting a potential role of these pathogens in the pathogenesis of pneumonia. The mechanisms by which such pathogens can be implicated in respiratory infections are through adhesion and invasion of respiratory pathogens, immune modulation, and inflammation in lung tissues. It is such a connection that necessitates possessing periodontal health as a preventive action against lung disease. Lastly, the findings suggest a multidisciplinary approach in the treatment of CAP involving dental hygiene and routine periodontal therapy, which may reduce pneumonia incidence among infected individuals (Zhang et al., 2024).

Most critical in treating CAP is combating the spreading issue of antibiotic resistance with the rising rate of resistant strains of bacteria. The World Health Organization has reported a growing concern regarding antibiotic resistance, which makes infections, including CAP, harder to treat. The issue necessitates exploring new treatment methods to enhance the effectiveness of existing antibiotics. Recent advancements in nanotechnology provide promising avenues for more effective targeting of antibacterial drugs. By employing new drug delivery systems, such as liposomes and polymeric nanoparticles, researchers aim to enhance drug solubility and targeting activity while minimizing side effects. This novel method can not only improve the therapeutic effects of CAP but also combat antibiotic resistance by maximizing the pharmacological properties of existing drugs (Eleraky et al., 2020). With this, ongoing research in this field is an essential part of the advancement of the management of Community-Acquired Pneumonia and to the protection of public health from new bacterial threats.

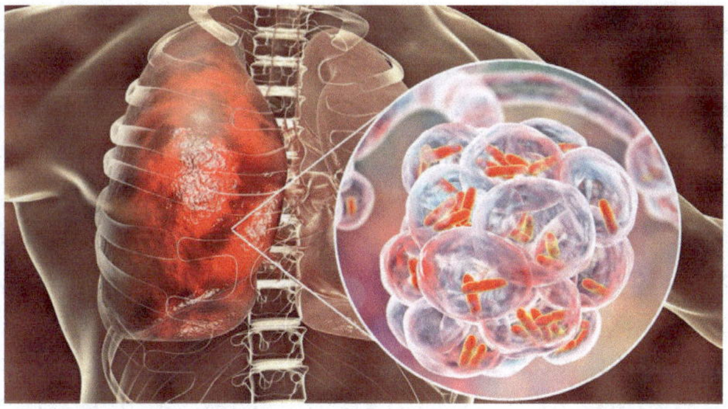

Figure 6.4. Community-acquired pneumonia (CAP).

Source: https://ai-care.id/photos/Healthpedia%20Sistem%20Pernapasan/621dae8b395d7.jpg

6.1.2. Hospital-Acquired Pneumonia (Hap)

The Hospital-Acquired Pneumonia (HAP) syndrome is a grave condition in health-care settings, particularly among high-risk patient populations such as the elderly and the comorbid. Unlike community-acquired pneumonia, HAP develops in an individual who is most often already seriously ill and hospitalized with other illnesses, which renders it particularly sinister. Diagnosis of HAP is reliant on a thorough assessment of clinical symptoms, radiological appearance, and examination of potential risk factors related to the hospital environment. A high index of suspicion is therefore necessary to differentiate HAP from other respiratory infections that have similar presentations, in order to implement timely and appropriate interventions.

Apart from this, the complexity of HAP underscores the need for strict adherence to infection control measures in hospitals, which are critical in reducing incidence rates and optimizing patient outcomes, especially in high-risk groups (Avari et al., 2020).

A multifaceted approach to empirical antibiotic therapy for the range of pathogens most frequently linked with such infections is necessary for the management of HAP. Treatment regimens in everyday use typically comprise a combination of beta-lactam antibiotics and macrolides, reflecting the need to cover both common bacterial pathogens and atypical ones. It is essential, nonetheless, to individualize therapy based on patients' clinical course and evolving microbiological data. In particular, the implementation of clinical practice guidelines, such as the care bundle for community-acquired pneumonia, can significantly enhance HAP management and is a priority in acute care hospitals (Avari et al., 2020).

Repeated biomarker measurements, such as C-reactive protein, can be helpful in monitoring the response to treatment and in identifying patients who are at a higher risk of complications or death. Education plays a central role in hospital-acquired pneumonia control, according to the relationship between education and outcome. Courses aimed at enhancing knowledge of respiratory infections among healthcare professionals, such as the curriculum developed by ERS for postgraduate training, can equip clinicians with the understanding they need to combat HAP more effectively. An educated health care workforce is better positioned to implement evidence-based practice standards and establish care standards that minimize the risk of HAP.

Moreover, patient and family awareness campaigns, addressing both medical staff and patients and their families, can aid in prevention. Ultimately, a combined strategy of education, targeted therapy, infection control practices, and quality control will be required to moderate the impact of HAP within healthcare systems, thereby improving overall patient safety and quality of care.

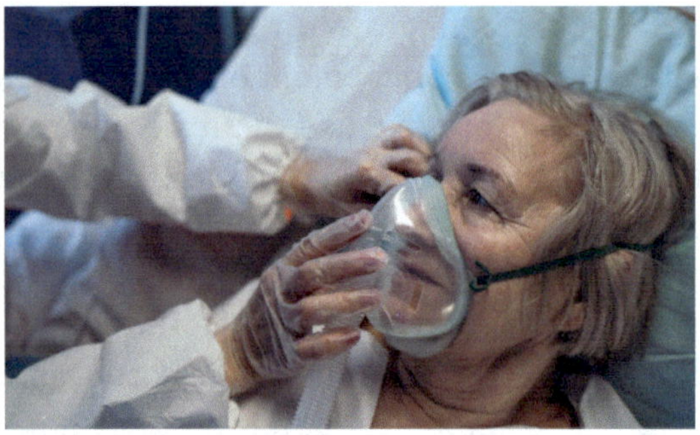

Figure 6.5. Hospital-acquired pneumonia (HAP).

Source: https://drgalen.org/uploads/blog-uploads/1705062256.png

6.1.3. Aspiration Pneumonia

Aspiration pneumonia results when foreign material, most commonly oral or gastric contents, is aspirated into the respiratory tree and leads to infection and inflammation. The condition occurs most frequently in individuals with impaired swallowing mechanisms, such as those affected by neurologic disorders, altered consciousness, or advanced age. The developing infection is most frequently found in dependent regions of the lungs and may provide an ideal environment for both aerobic and anaerobic bacteria to proliferate. Clinically, aspiration pneumonia can present with various signs and symptoms such as cough, fever, and the production of foul sputum, typically suggesting the presence of anaerobic infections. Given the seriousness of this condition, accurate diagnosis and early intervention are necessary to minimize morbidity and mortality from this form of pneumonia. To effectively treat aspiration pneumonia, clinicians would consider a myriad of parameters that encompass the overall health of patients, comorbidities, and the nature of the aspirate. Broad-spectrum antibiotics typically make up the first line of treatment, commonly chosen to address polymicrobial flora usually involved in this syndrome, including both anaerobic and aerobic bacteria. In more severe cases, hospitalization may be necessary to provide intravenous antibiotics and supportive care, such as oxygen therapy or mechanical ventilation, if respiratory failure occurs. Additionally, prevention of recurrence through position change during feeding, swallowing therapy, and dietary modification is also necessary, especially in populations who are at higher risk, such as the elderly or those with neurological impairment. The epidemiology of aspiration pneumonia highlights its significance in certain patient populations, such as those with chronic diseases or impaired immunocompetence. As studies show, diabetics, patients with chronic lung disease, or critically ill patients are at higher risk for aspiration pneumonia and complicate their management as well. In addition, the cycle of such pneumonias may become a vicious cycle of deteriorating pulmonary function and infection. Chronic obstructive pulmonary disease and drug abuse disorders are typically comorbid with risks of aspiration pneumonia and are challenging to treat. Therefore, proper assessment and targeted interventions are a pillar to effective treatment, making the need for awareness level elevation among medical personnel paramount (Currie et al., 2010; Kousha et al., 2011).

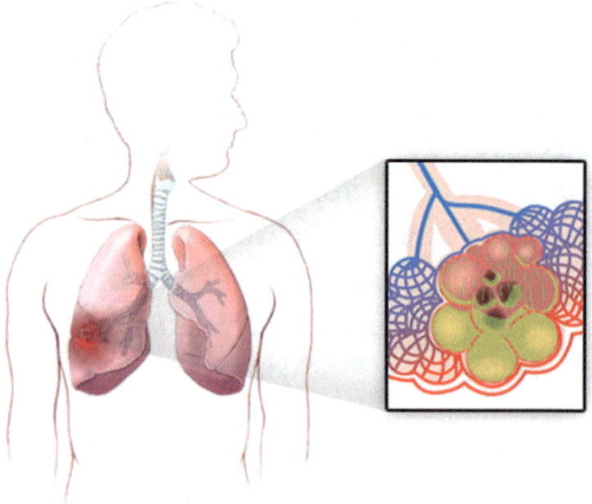

Figure 6.6. Aspiration pneumonia.

Source: https://www.manhattanprimarycaredoctorsnyc.com/wp-content/uploads/2021/12/Aspiration-pneumonia.jpg

Test Your Knowledge

1. What is community-acquired pneumonia (CAP)?
2. What is hospital-acquired pneumonia (HAP)?

6.2. Causes and Risk Factors

Learning Outcome

1. Infectious Agents (Bacteria, Viruses, Fungi)
2. Environmental Factors (Pollution, Smoking)
3. Underlying Health Conditions (COPD, Immunosuppression)

A proper understanding of the etiology and risk factors for pneumonia, lung abscesses, and bronchiectasis is crucial for optimal prevention and control. Infections with a range of infectious pathogens, including bacteria, viruses, and fungi, cause pneumonias, of which pneumococcal pneumonia is one of the leading bacterial causes. Further, some risk factors such as old age, smoking, and chronic respiratory conditions significantly increase the likelihood of acquiring these infections. For instance, individuals with impaired lung function or congenital lung disorders are typically exposed to heightened vulnerabilities.

Moreover, poor oral hygiene has also been linked to cases of lung abscesses, particularly when oral pathogens enter the respiratory tract and lead to abscesses and complicating factors (Sperling et al., 2024). The intricate relationship between numerous causes and host factors points to the multidimensional aspect of such diseases and the application of multifaceted measures in managing respiratory health. For abscesses of the lung, specific factors predisposing them need to be valued. Previous abnormalities in lung architecture are some of those factors, and they are significantly crucial in providing favorable ground for the formation of abscesses. Ventilator-associated pneumonia is another crucial risk factor, especially in critically ill patients, as mechanical ventilation dependence may lead to aspiration and subsequent development of lung abscesses. More recent research also suggests that electronic cigarette use may be an emerging risk factor, though further studies are needed to establish a direct relationship (Sperling et al., 2024). These donations underscore the importance of closely monitoring patients with such risk factors and implementing preventive measures to minimize their likelihood of developing severe pulmonary complications. Additionally, the complications of viral infections, particularly those caused by SARS-CoV-2, have emerged as a concerning risk factor in the development of secondary infections such as lung abscesses. COVID-19 recovered patients can have a compromised immune system, making they susceptible to bacterial or fungal infections even if their histories were otherwise healthy. The establishment of the bacterial flora following viral infections can significantly influence pulmonary health, which can compromise the otherwise healthy individual's ability to develop lung disease. These developing patterns must be identified by healthcare professionals to apply appropriate therapeutic interventions and treatments, including pulmonary rehabilitation, to control the potential complications of such respiratory infections. This shifting risk factor landscape necessitates an adaptive treatment and prevention protocol tailored to the target needs and condition of the patients.

6.2.1. Infectious Agents (Bacteria, Viruses, Fungi)

Identification of the causative infecting organisms of respiratory diseases is crucial in the treatment of pneumonias, lung abscesses, and bronchiectasis. Bacteria, viruses, and fungi play various roles in these conditions, influencing the clinical approach in diagnosis and treatment. Bacterial pneumonia, such as that caused by organisms like Streptococcus pneumoniae, can lead to widespread inflammation and formation of pus within the lung, severely compromising respiratory function. Viral infections like influenza and COVID-19 can complicate or even precipitate pneumonia, further complicating the clinical picture. The union of viral and bacterial infections has been particularly known to precipitate a secondary bacterial infection, hard to manage. By identifying the specific infectious agent, healthcare providers can tailor treatment methods to minimize morbidity and mortality associated with these conditions, ultimately improving patient outcomes in a clinical setting. In addition to viruses and bacteria, fungi are also significant pathogens in the etiology of pneumonia, particularly among individuals with compromised immune systems.

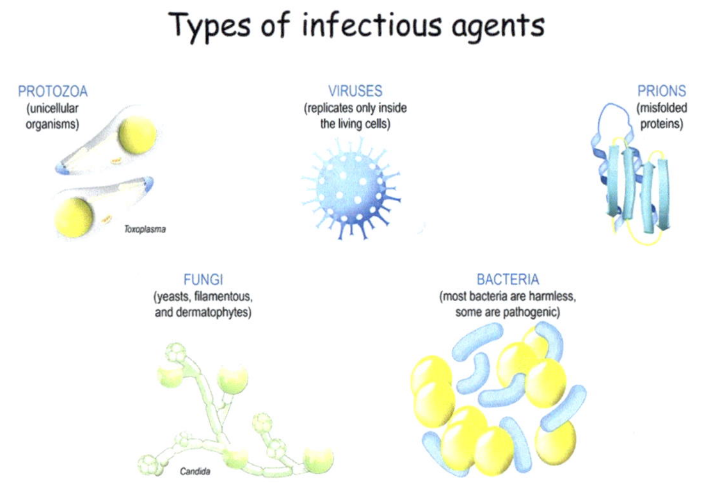

Figure 6.7. Infectious agents.

Source: https://thumbs.dreamstime.com/b/pathogen-infection-prions-viruses-to-bacteria-fungi-unicellular-organism-pathogens-types-infectious-agents-organisms-203146313.jpg

Fungal pneumonia caused by pathogens such as *Pneumocystis jirovecii* and *Aspergillus* is characterized by its diagnostic and therapeutic complexities. Fungal pneumonias, unlike bacterial infections, would have an insidious onset and are tricky to diagnose if not specifically diagnosed. The frequency of fungal infection in patients with related underlying illnesses, such as HIV/AIDS or patients undergoing chemotherapy, underlines the need for a clear awareness of diverse infectious agents. Moreover, the therapeutic regimens for fungal pneumonias are typically quite different from those for pneumonias caused by bacteria or viruses. They can include the use of antifungal drugs. Heightened awareness of such pathogens underscores the importance of clinicians being sensitive to the diagnosis and management of pneumonia among heterogeneous populations. With the increasing sophistication of infection-causing agents, research advances are crucial for optimizing diagnostic and therapeutic approaches for pneumonia, lung abscess, and bronchiectasis. The advent of innovations like deep learning has shown promise in enhancing diagnostic accuracy, as evidenced by the latest studies employing Convolutional Neural Networks (CNNs) to diagnose pneumonia from chest X-rays. By using sophisticated algorithms, doctors can rapidly and accurately differentiate among subtypes of pneumonia, improving care based on individual patient profiles. This technological innovation has particularly been crucial in controlling pneumonia's high morbidity and mortality rates, as seen in the shocking statistics reporting around 4 million deaths annually from the illness (Kautsar et al., 2024). As the scientific world continues to learn about the complexities of infectious agents, whatever they discover will undoubtedly enhance patient care and clinical practice for pneumonia and its complications (Aadarsh, 2024).

6.2.2. Environmental Factors (Pollution, Smoking)

Environmental causes, notably pollution and smoking, are significant in the etiology and severity of several respiratory illnesses, including pneumonias, bronchiectasis, and lung abscesses. Smoking and air pollution have the potential to produce chronic inflammation of the lungs, which considerably impacts immune status and resistance to infection. For example, smoking is an established risk factor for the development of chronic obstructive pulmonary disease (COPD), and this may also place individuals at risk for lung infections such as pneumonia and abscesses. Adverse air, caused by pollution, particularly in urban areas, is also to blame for exacerbating respiratory illnesses and increasing the risk of infection. This complex interaction between smoking, air pollution, and respiratory disease highlights the necessity for a comprehensive strategy to reduce exposure to such harmful environmental forces to improve patients' outcomes for chronic lung disease. The impact of environmental forces is not confined to purely direct damage to the lungs, as smoking and air pollution can also induce alterations in lung architecture and function, resulting in disease states such as bronchiectasis. Chronic inflammation resulting from prolonged exposure to noxious environmental agents has been demonstrated by studies to lead to persistent alterations in the elasticity and architecture of the bronchi. bronchiectasis, involving irreversible bronchial dilation and cough, is closely associated with recurrent infection of the lungs that can be triggered by such environmental factors. Cumulatively, these conditions create a double hit scenario in the majority of patients; smokers with a history of respiratory infections experience heightened risks of developing severe complications. Accordingly, examining the intersection of smoking, environmental air pollution, and pre-existing lung disease is relevant to understanding the pathophysiology of bronchiectasis and other pulmonary diseases. Innovative approaches to mitigating the effects of environmental exposures consider their broader biological impacts, particularly on inflammation and oxidative stress pathways. More recent evidence suggests that dietary patterns rich in antioxidants and nutrients can help buffer some of the adverse effects of smoking and air pollution on lung function. For instance, the Mediterranean diet has been shown to have protective effects against the progression of COPD by reducing systemic inflammation, demonstrating the role of nutritional interventions. Also, exploration of the field of nutriepigenomics suggests potential mechanisms by which certain foods may modulate the genetic expression of susceptibility to lung disease. This emphasizes the need for an overall strategy that combines lifestyle modifications, such as diet and smoking, in order to address the adverse effects of environmental factors on pneumonias, lung abscesses, and bronchiectasis, thereby improving patient outcomes overall (Mar Cín-Hinojosa et al., 2021; Kim, 2022).

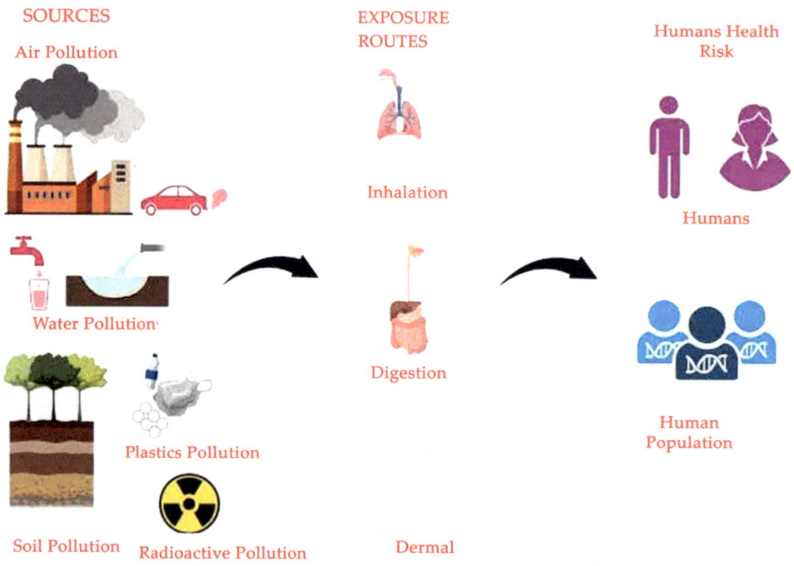

Figure 6.8. Environmental factors.

Source: https://ars.els-cdn.com/content/image/1-s2.0-S0375674223001723-gr3.jpg

6.2.3. Underlying Health Conditions (COPD, Immunosuppression)

Chronic Obstructive Pulmonary Disease (COPD) is a common underlying health condition that significantly increases the risk and severity of respiratory infections such as pneumonia and lung abscesses. COPD has an intrinsic, chronic airway inflammation with resultant structural changes and impaired lung function. This ongoing airway inflammation creates an environment that favors colonization and infection with a variety of pathogens. In patients with COPD, chronic inflammation-mediated airway damage is a continuous process that diminishes the body's resistance to infection. Research shows that such a history of COPD poses a higher risk for lung cancer, complicating clinical management of these patients and highlighting the relationship between chronic lung ailments and increased susceptibility to lung infections (Kim, 2022). Immunosuppression is yet another very critical underlying health condition that seriously affects lung health, particularly when it relates to pneumonias and bronchiectasis. Individuals with compromised immune systems are less able to effectively respond to infection, thus being prone to both usual and atypical causes of pneumonia. This vulnerability also leads to the formation of lung abscesses, as some bacteria can proliferate out of control in immunocompromised conditions. In addition, the presence of bronchiectasis complicates the clinical presentation because the condition itself is characterized by compromised and enlarged airways that promote bacterial colonization. Evidence also shows that patients with bronchiectasis and other chronic respiratory diseases have increased morbidity due to persistent infections, further highlighting the importance of frequent observation and severe management of individuals with immune compromise (N/A, 2022). The synergy between chronic conditions such as COPD and immunosuppression underscores the necessity of personalized treatment protocols in managing pneumonias, lung abscesses, and bronchiectasis. In particular, individuals with these chronic conditions require close observation and forward-thinking risk management of potential infections. Healthcare practitioners must identify the specific problems these patients present, employing a combination of antimicrobial therapy targeting specific pathogens and supportive treatment to optimize pulmonary function and overall health. As research evolves, there will be a greater appreciation for the two-way interaction between underlying states and respiratory infections, necessary to optimize patient care and maximize therapeutic protocols in routine practice (Kim, 2022; N/A, 2022).

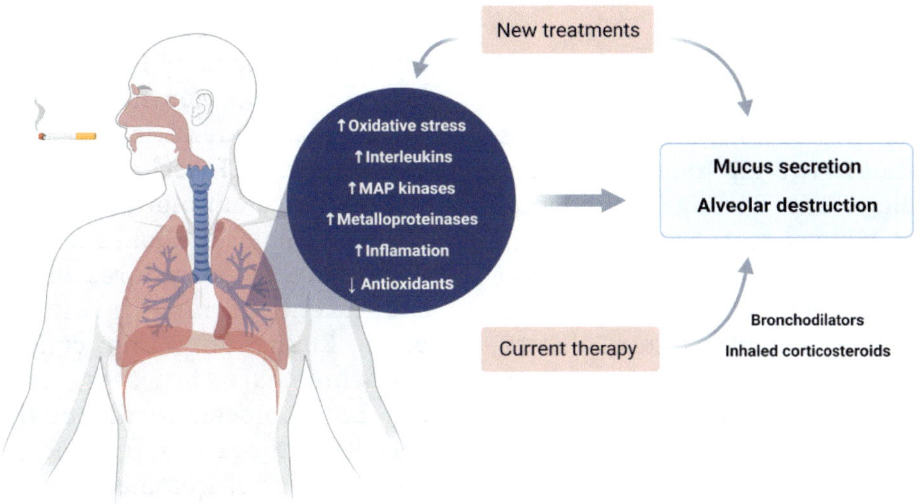

Figure 6.9. Underlying health conditions (COPD, Immunosuppression).

Source: https://pub.mdpi-res.com/pharmaceuticals/pharmaceuticals-14-00979/article_deploy/html/images/pharmaceuticals-14-00979-ag.png?1632648627

Test Your Knowledge

1. What are the infectious agents?
2. What are the environmental factors?

6.3. Symptoms and Diagnosis

Learning Outcome

1. Common Symptoms of Pneumonia
2. Diagnostic Tests (Chest X-ray, Sputum Culture)
3. Differentiating Between Pneumonia and Other Conditions

Symptoms of bronchiectasis, lung abscesses, and pneumonias can overlap to a great extent, presenting a diagnostic dilemma for doctors. Some standard clinical features are chronic cough, at times productive of purulent sputum, fever, chills, and dyspnea. In pneumonia, particularly with viral infections like COVID-19, the rapid onset of symptoms, including myalgias and fatigue, apart from respiratory symptoms, is frequent. The severity of such symptoms may vary depending on the etiologic agent and the patient's overall health condition. Lung abscesses may also be accompanied by local manifestations, such as pleuritic chest pain and significant weight loss, which can aid in their distinction from pneumonia. As the clinical presentation of such respiratory illnesses can be highly heterogeneous, careful history and physical examination are precious resources for clinicians in reaching a diagnosis. Diagnostic imaging is also crucial in diagnosing pneumonia, lung abscesses, and bronchiectasis, which helps in delineating underlying pathological alterations. For example, chest X-rays are usually used as a first screening because they are easily accessible and inexpensive, but they can detect abnormalities in only 75% of RT-PCR positive COVID-19 infections, thus alone being insufficient. On the other hand, HRCT provides greater sensitivity and specificity, revealing characteristic patterns such as ground-glass opacities and traction bronchiectasis, which are associated with diseases like idiopathic nonspecific interstitial pneumonia (iNSIP) (Rahman et al., 2025). While lung abscesses may be viewed as round, cavitary lesions on imaging, bronchiectasis is typically characterized by bronchial dilatation and structural changes that can be easily delineated by an HRCT. Thus, it is essential to incorporate sophisticated imaging modalities into the diagnostic workup for a proper identification and diagnosis, followed by management. Laboratory investigations remain an essential component of diagnosing respiratory diseases, particularly in distinguishing between infectious and non-infectious etiologies. In pneumonias, identification of pathogens by culture and PCR techniques allows treatment with targeted antibiotic therapy. For COVID-19, RT-PCR remains the gold standard for diagnosis, with imaging procedures used to determine the extent of lung involvement (Rahman et al., 2025). For other conditions, such as bronchiectasis, however, sputum analysis can be employed to detect the presence of specific pathogens and guide the appropriate management of treatment. As identified in the literature, the timing of chronicity and symptom progression may be helpful; for instance, patients with idiopathic nonspecific interstitial pneumonia typically exhibit subacute symptoms, characterized by bilateral reticular opacities and ground-glass opacities (Jo et al., 2025). Thus, a multidisciplinary approach integrating clinical evaluation, imaging, and laboratory investigations is essential for a correct diagnosis and successful intervention in the management of such respiratory diseases.

6.3.1. Common Symptoms of Pneumonia

Pneumonia is a serious respiratory illness characterized by lung parenchymal inflammation, most commonly caused by infection. Typical features are a productive cough that may yield sputum, fever, chills, and dyspnea. These symptoms occur as the body tries to combat the causative infectious agents of the disease. The cough can be dry or productive, and when productive, often yields yellow, green, or even rust-brown sputum, depending on the attendant inflammatory processes. Systemic symptoms, such as fever and chills, are also superimposed on localized respiratory distress as a secondary effect of the body's inflammatory response to pneumonia. Symptoms can, in elderly patients and those with comorbid illness, be atypical so that they require astute clinical judgment to diagnose. These signs are important for the effective management and early intervention to prevent complications due to the disease. There are other signs in pneumonia patients that imply severe infection or complications. Discomfort upon deep breathing or cough can imply pleuritic involvement, where the pleura, or lung lining, is inflamed. Additionally, shortness of breath is a concerning symptom that requires medical attention at the earliest opportunity, as it may indicate deteriorating respiratory failure. There usually are accompanying fatigue and malaise that accompany the more obvious symptoms, which will cause patients to have a hard time doing simple activities. Such systemic presentation emphasizes the potential of pneumonia to impact the quality of life of a patient significantly. In specific immunocompromised populations, such as STAT3 hyperimmunoglobulin E syndrome patients, pneumonia has been observed to recur and have other consequences such as lung abscesses, as noted in Mahdaviani et al., (2023). This highlights the importance of early detection of such signs to prevent the disease from evolving into advanced forms. In conjunction with the characteristic signs of pneumonia, diagnostic imaging plays a significant role in elucidating the extent of lung involvement. High-resolution computed tomography may reveal abnormalities, such as bronchiectasis or lung abscess, which can complicate the clinical situation and render management difficult. Those with protracted or severe courses should be carefully assessed for structural abnormality or secondary infection, which could exacerbate their condition. In addition, the presentation of pneumonia in patients with underlying conditions, such as COPD, can be markedly unusual. Balkissoon (2019) points out the concurrent epidemic existence of bronchiectasis in patients with COPD, with heightened intensity of symptoms and respiratory infections. This emphasizes the clinician's requirement to adopt a holistic evaluation approach, such that etiologies of respiratory distress are optimally managed in therapeutic paradigms.

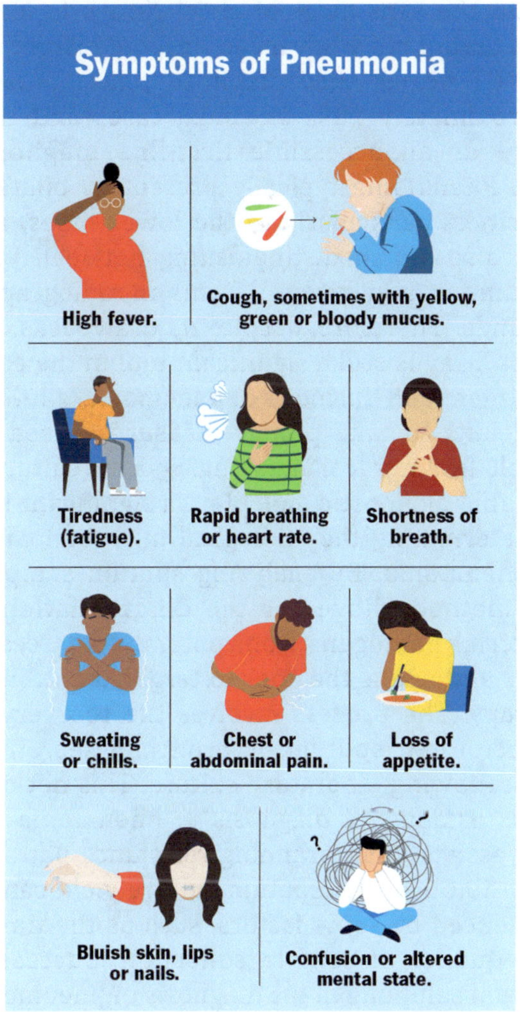

Figure 6.10. Common symptoms of pneumonia.

Source: https://my.clevelandclinic.org/-/scassets/images/org/health/articles/4471-pneumonia-02

6.3.2. Diagnostic Tests (Chest X-Ray, Sputum Culture)

In the diagnostic evaluation of pneumonia, chest X-ray imaging is a cornerstone but necessary test. Offering a speedy assessment of lung anatomy, it may identify necessary abnormalities associated with pneumonia, including infiltrates, consolidations, and, in some cases, effusions. While the sensitivity of chest X-rays is lower than that of more advanced imaging techniques like CT scans, they diagnose pneumonia in approximately 75% of actual cases and thus serve as an accessible first-line diagnostic tool. Pneumonia typically present as bilateral opacities, particularly in the lower lobes, and may also aid in distinguishing between viral pneumonia and bacterial forms on radiographic grounds. Therefore, despite its drawbacks, the chest X-ray is still a significant tool in the early treatment and diagnosis of pneumonia, allowing clinicians to take proper measures based on visible findings from imaging. Sputum culture, a valuable diagnostic tool, plays a significant role in determining the etiological microbial cause of pneumonia. By analyzing sputum samples, the method allows for the differentiation of bacterial pathogens from potential sources of virus and opens the door to targeted antibiotic therapy. The process involves the recovery of expectorated sputum or bronchial secretions and following laboratory culture. This not only helps establish a diagnosis of pneumonia but also assists in determining resistance patterns to antibiotics. The sputum culture yield can be influenced by some factors, such as the timing and quality of sample collection. Successful sputum sampling in the diagnosis of pneumonia can significantly enhance clinical outcomes by ensuring that proper antibiotic regimens are administered at the right time, thereby reducing the risk of complications (Rahman et al., 2025). The use of chest X-rays and sputum cultures together is an exhaustive diagnostic approach to managing pneumonia and other pulmonary disorders. While the chest X-ray provides an outline of the lungs' pathological status, sputum culture indicates the precise infectious organism involved. Together, these tests not only expedite the diagnosis but also inform subsequent treatment planning, a particularly significant point in advanced illness, where delays can lead to considerable morbidity. Furthermore, refinements in imaging technology and microbiological techniques continue to improve these diagnostics, rendering them more accurate and cost-effective. As our knowledge on respiratory infections advances, the synergistic application of these imaging modalities will continue to progress, eventually enhancing patient outcomes in the context of pneumonia, lung abscess, and bronchiectasis (Rahman et al., 2025).

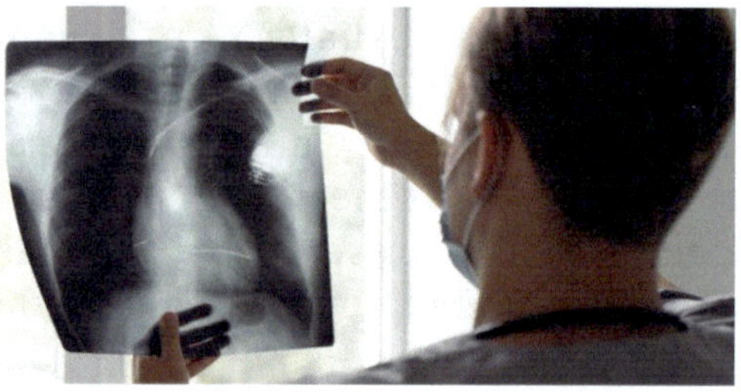

Figure 6.11. Diagnostic tests (Chest X-ray, Sputum culture) of pneumonia.

Source: https://max-website20-images.s3.ap-south-1.amazonaws.com/Pneumonia_d7585eafca.jpg

6.3.3. Differentiating Between Pneumonia and Other Conditions

A precise distinction between pneumonia and other respiratory illnesses is imperative for accurate diagnosis and management. Pneumonia can often manifest with symptoms resembling those of lung abscesses and bronchiectasis, such as chronic cough, fever, and dyspnea. However, the pathophysiological process behind such conditions is distinctly different. For instance, bronchiectasis involves the chronic dilatation of the bronchi, often accompanied by chronic infection and inflammation, which complicate the clinical presentation with more enduring symptoms than pneumonia. Lung abscess, by contrast, involves localized pus in the lung parenchyma after pneumonia, for which separate diagnostic imaging is needed to confirm its presence. The overlap in clinical presentation requires clinicians to conduct extensive testing, including imaging and microbiological studies, for an unequivocal diagnosis and to shift treatment strategies accordingly. Infectious etiologies that contribute to the differential diagnosis of pneumonia, such as acute bronchitis, further complicate the diagnosis. For Pseudomonas aeruginosa pneumonia, for instance, previous lung infections are pertinent, especially for individuals with bronchiectasis. Pseudomonas is said to be a common pathogen among patients with bronchiectasis, particularly during episodes of exacerbation, thereby increasing morbidity and complicating modalities of treatment (N/A, 2022). Recognition of the pathologic history of lung infections in the patient is vital, as a chronic bacterial infection, such as Pseudomonas, can lead to recurrent pneumonia, which may initially be misdiagnosed as a benign infection. Thus, scrutiny of the patient's prior state of health and respiratory history can highlight nuances of differences between pneumonia, bronchiectasis, and other lung infections. Diagnostic imaging techniques are imperative in their ability to detect the fine differences between pneumonia and other lung diseases. Chest X-rays are typically the first diagnostic tool used to detect pneumonia, revealing infiltrates that correspond to the infection. Yet, HRCT scans are vital in the diagnosis of bronchiectasis as they are capable of showing bronchial dilatation and thickening, which are pathognomonic of the disease. Additionally, lung abscesses appear as focal areas of abnormal density or empyema on imaging. As conditions such as lung cancer also manifest with non-specific respiratory symptoms (Kim, 2022), it becomes increasingly important to deal with diagnosis using a polyvalent approach incorporating clinical history, microbiologic data, and advanced imaging modalities. This detailed analysis effectively discriminates between pneumonia and other respiratory diseases, ensuring that suitable patients receive early treatment.

Test Your Knowledge

1. What are the common symptoms of pneumonia?
2. What are the diagnostic tests?

6.4. Lung Abscess: Definition and Causes

Learning Outcome

1. Pathophysiology of Lung Abscess
2. Common Causes (Aspiration, Infections)
3. Risk Factors for Developing Lung Abscess

Lung abscesses are collections of pus in the pulmonary parenchyma that are localized, typically due to infection. They are characteristically demarcated by necrosis of lung tissue, most often due to bacterial pathogens such as anaerobic bacteria, Staphylococcus aureus, and other gram-negative bacilli. Although the prevalence of lung abscesses is not high, their presence can be a sign of underlying health issues in the patient, especially in those with weakened immune systems or chronic lung conditions. Moreover, individuals with risk factors such as previous lung disease, poor teeth, or aspiration pneumonitis are at an increased risk of acquiring lung abscesses because these conditions offer a pathway for the pathogens to enter the lung, infecting the region and triggering the formation of an abscess (Lee et al., 2011). The formation of lung abscesses is typically a multifactorial process. Anaerobic oral cavity bacteria most commonly aspirate into the lungs and infect them, especially during a period of altered consciousness or a swallowing defect. Other causes include neoplasm or foreign body obstruction of the bronchus with subsequent stagnant environment for infection. Certain pneumonias, such as aspiration pneumonia, can result in abscess formation due to bacterial proliferation in necrotic tissue. This is further exacerbated by the fact that comorbid conditions, such as diabetes or malignancy, develop and may weaken the body's immune defenses, making them prone to dangerous infections (Lee et al., 2011). Understanding the etiology of lung abscesses is very important for appropriate management and treatment. The approach typically involves the prescription of broad-spectrum antibiotics, which have to be tailored based on the presumed pathogen. In some cases, most notably when the abscesses are large or significantly have a marked mass effect, intervention through surgery may be indicated. It is noteworthy that imaging post-therapy, such as chest CT scans, is very important in assessing the resolution of the abscesses and residual lung tissue damage. It has also been established in research that changes can persist even after treatment within the lung parenchyma, highlighting the importance of careful follow-up and monitoring (Lee et al., 2011). This is to avoid complications such as the development of bronchiectasis, which can be a consequence of chronic lung infection and further complicate the patient's respiratory status.

6.4.1. Pathophysiology of Lung Abscess

Understanding the pathophysiology of lung abscess is crucial for comprehending its clinical significance and therapeutic approach, particularly in relation to pneumonia and bronchiectasis. A lung abscess is when localized collections of pus occur within the pulmonary parenchyma, typically as a complication of a bacterial infection, such as aspiration pneumonia or anaerobic infections. It arises due to the complex interaction of host defense mechanisms and microbial virulence factors. Primary lung injury allows infecting pathogens to proliferate, leading to tissue necrosis and the formation of a purulent-filled, necrotic cavity. While lung abscesses may form on previously healthy lungs, underlying diseases like bronchiectasis predispose the development of lung abscesses due to impaired airway function and an inability to expel secretions, thereby creating a fertile environment for bacterial proliferation and successful invasion of lung tissue. The clinical presentation of lung abscess tends to be indistinguishable from that of typical pneumonia, making early detection challenging. Patients may experience nonspecific symptoms, such as malaise, fever, and cough, which can mislead clinicians into underestimating the condition's severity. Actually, the initial presentation of lung abscess might not be differentiated from typical pneumonia, as seen in cases where a fever of uncertain origin was noted weeks before diagnosis. Imaging studies, particularly chest X-rays and computed tomography scans, are critical in the detection of lung abscesses, which create distinctive cavitary lesions that distinguish them from pneumonia. In certain instances, as outlined in specific case reports, delayed treatment and diagnosis can lead to serious morbidity. Therefore, cautious diagnostic examinations are necessary to provide immediate and appropriate treatment policies for lung abscesses (Buntara et al., 2023). Treatment of lung abscess is multidisciplinary, with the use of antibiotic therapy combined with, in some instances, surgery.

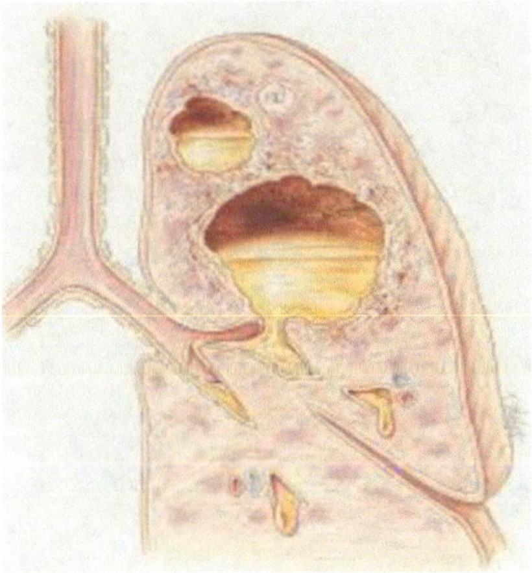

Figure 6.12. Pathophysiology of lung abscess.

Source: https://encrypted-tbn0.gstatic.com/images?q=tbn:ANd9GcT7H1m0I0lKrsceBOyZdO6P5pzP8QBj7DuskA&s

The antibiotic therapy is tailored to the microbiological profile of the infection, including any resistant bacteria, as seen in cases such as Staphylococcus spp. Surgical management has a role where medical treatment fails or when massive abscesses occur with complications such as empyema or severe respiratory compromise. Furthermore, the identification of the primary or secondary etiology of the abscess guides clinicians on how to monitor and prevent recurrence. This multifaceted treatment bears testimony to the complexity of the lung abscess and the importance of merging thorough clinical evaluations with cutting-edge diagnostic techniques to provide the best possible patient outcomes (Ayoub et al., 2024).

6.4.2. Common Causes (Aspiration, Infections)

An understanding of the most common causes of pneumonia, particularly aspiration and infection, is fundamental in the management of severe pulmonary complications like lung abscess and bronchiectasis. Aspiration pneumonia is the phenomenon where oropharyngeal material is aspirated into the lung accidentally, causing an infection that is primarily caused by anaerobic bacteria or pathogens from the oral cavity. It often occurs in patients with impaired consciousness or swallowing function, e.g., neurological diseases, or in the elderly. Related inflammation may compromise lung function, leading to complications such as lung abscesses, which are focal collections of pus within the pulmonary parenchyma. Clinicians are therefore required to be sensitive to identifying patients at risk of aspiration and initiating preventive maneuvers or prompt interventions. Infection of the lung can be caused by several etiologies, each with some specific challenges in management and treatment. Ventilator-associated pneumonia (VAP), for instance, is a common complication of the management of critically ill patients receiving mechanical ventilation. XDR organisms, such as Acinetobacter baumannii, are one manifestation of this imposing profile of infection due to their formidable antibiotic resistance patterns (Kumar et al., 2025). Thus, VAP patients can have unfavorable prognoses through increased hospital stays and increased morbidity. The multifaceted nature of the treatment required for such infections necessitates a multifaceted approach, with an emphasis on good critical care and effective antibiotics. Successful identification and treatment of the etiologic pathogens are crucial in preventing further progression, i.e., the development of lung abscesses, thereby highlighting the importance of strict adherence to infection control practices and vigilant monitoring in at-risk populations. Moreover, the emergence of atypical bacteria as etiologic agents in aspiration pneumonia cannot be assumed. There is proof that some organisms like Enterococcus faecium can be responsible for some severe health issues, especially in patients with a vast array of comorbid conditions like diabetes and drug abuse history (Asokan et al., 2024). In these cases, it happens that the bacteria will advance rapidly to develop a lung abscess, whose management and prognosis becomes difficult. Radiological evaluation is crucial in such situations, enabling the early diagnosis of abscess formations that require intensive treatment procedures. A tailored treatment protocol, including broad-spectrum antibiotics and drainage procedures, may be indicated to prevent complications arising from such severe infections. The complexity of the process underscores the importance of thorough patient assessment and individualized therapy regimens in managing pneumonia complications.

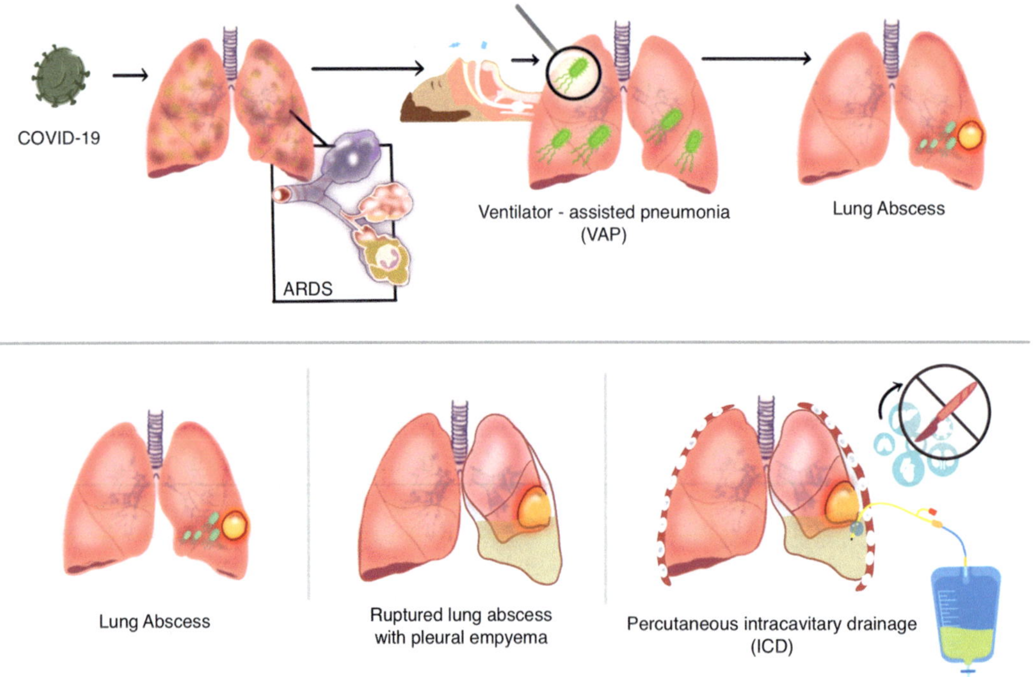

Figure 6.13. Infection associated lung abscess.

Source: https://pub.mdpi-res.com/jcm/jcm-13-06962/article_deploy/html/images/jcm-13-06962-ag.png?1734944524

6.4.3. Risk Factors For Developing Lung Abscess

The development of a lung abscess, a focal accumulation of pus within the lung parenchyma, can be significantly influenced by several risk factors. Foremost among them is the comorbid underlying condition that compromises the immune system, such as diabetes and chronic respiratory disease. Patients with underlying comorbidities are at increased risk for infections that lead to lung abscesses. The linkage between metabolic disturbances, such as diabetes, and lung infections highlights the importance of overall health in preventing or avoiding complications. To this, lifestyle influences, such as alcoholism and smoking, have also been known to contribute negatively to lung health, again elevating risk for lung abscess formation, particularly in populations with prior lung disease that diminishes lung defense and healing capacity. In the context of infectious pathogens, recognition of the etiologic pathogens in lung abscesses identifies their risk factors. Bacterial infection is most frequently identified as the etiology behind the formation of lung abscesses, and anaerobic oral cavity flora are some of the major culprits. Individuals with poor dental health or those who carry periodontal disease are often at risk of aspiration events, which can result in the introduction of these microbes into the lungs and lead to the development of abscesses. Importantly, studies have shown that the consumption of illicit substances will most likely predispose the patient to such infections, taking place, adding another layer to the clinical picture. As an instance, altered consciousness aspiration while under substances puts the patient at risk of introducing pathogens into the respiratory system. Awareness of these infection modes and associated behaviors is crucial in developing targeted prevention strategies for lung abscesses in populations at risk. Social determinants of health also play a deciding part in risk for lung abscess formation. Access to healthcare, socioeconomic status, and education level can potentially have a significant impact on an individual's health-seeking behavior, leading to delays in treatment and diagnosis of any potential infection. Individuals from lower socioeconomic groups may lack access to preventive healthcare services or be uninformed about how to maintain healthy airways, which contributes to their increased risk. Also, the present recommendations have made it clear that conditions such as bronchiectasis and chronic obstructive pulmonary disease (COPD) predispose individuals to the formation of lung abscess, particularly in populations already disadvantaged by health inequities in the system. This intertwining of social determinants with health outcomes in this case brings to the fore the significance of holistic strategies which address not just the medical factors but also the overall social setting behind lung abscess risk, as operationalized in more recent studies (Stuart G Tangye et al., 2022; Lewis P, 2020).

Test Your Knowledge

1. What is the pathophysiology of a lung abscess?
2. What are the risk factors for developing lung abscess?

6.5. Symptoms and Treatment of Lung Abscess

Learning Outcome

1. Clinical Presentation of Lung Abscess
2. Diagnostic Approaches (CT Scan, Bronchoscopy)
3. Treatment Options (Antibiotics, Surgery)

The presentation of a lung abscess is typically indicative of an underlying infection and may vary in its severity. Typical presentations are chronic cough, pyrexia, and purulent sputum production that may be odorous in anaerobic infections. Pleuritic chest pain and hemoptysis can also occur as the abscess grows larger. Weight loss and malaise can happen in some cases, reflecting systemic disease. When imaging is performed, most commonly chest X-rays or computed tomography scans, the finding of a cavitary lesion increases the suspicion for a lung abscess. Correct identification of these symptoms is crucial because early recognition and treatment of a lung abscess can have a profound impact on patient outcome, preventing potential complications, such as sepsis or chronic lung disease, that can arise from an untreated infection. When treating lung abscesses, the initial step is usually antibiotic therapy, which is initiated based on the suspected etiology of the infection. Broad-spectrum antibiotics would usually be recommended to cover a range of possible pathogens, including anaerobic bacteria, which are frequently causative agents in such abscesses, particularly in patients at risk for aspiration. Intervention is indicated in situations where the abscess is extremely large or is not yielding to medical treatment. This can be done through percutaneous drainage or surgical drainage to resect necrotic tissue. In severe cases, especially those with recurrent abscess formation or complications such as bronchopleural fistula, operative resection of the affected lung tissue may be required. Follow-up is crucial for assessing treatment outcomes and identifying potential recurrence or related complications. The coexistence of underlying conditions could significantly influence both symptoms and management of lung abscesses. For instance, patients with chronic lung diseases, immunocompromised states, or structural lung abnormalities might have unusual presentations or delayed disease. Natural history studies of respiratory disease identify not only the necessity of treating the abscess but also any predisposing factors, which may include poor lung hygiene or concurrent infection (Garmhausen et al., 2013). Additionally, understanding the interplay between co-morbid diseases, including sarcoidosis, highlights the importance of accurate imaging and early diagnosis to guide treatment and improve patient outcomes (Criado et al., 2010). Comprehensive management, therefore, requires a multidisciplinary approach that integrates medical treatment, surgical intervention, and management of comorbid conditions to minimize the risk of recurrence and achieve optimal healing.

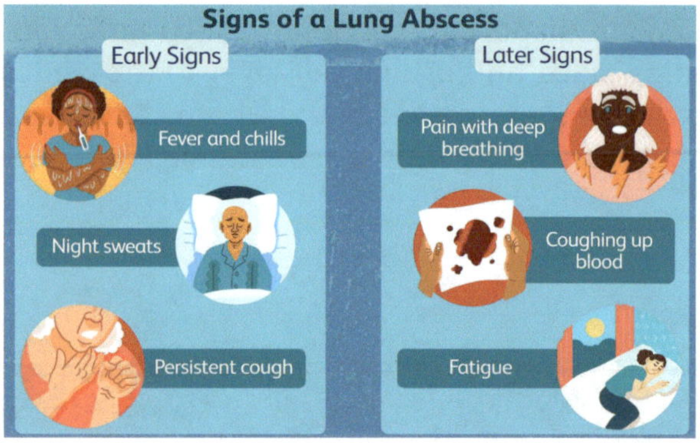

Figure 6.14. The symptoms of a lung abscess.

Source: https://www.verywellhealth.com/thmb/RbGhENLy4rbB-F2o6OhHtVMSns4=/1500x0/filters:no_upscale():max_bytes(150000):strip_icc()/lung-abscess-overview-4768089_final-8c6a0ccd797345289aa2dc0a5856d8e1.jpg

6.5.1. Clinical Presentation of Lung Abscess

The clinical presentation of lung abscesses is varied, and they often present in the context of a range of symptoms that may initially mimic other pulmonary conditions. Patients report cough, and it may be copious and foul-smelling, suggesting anaerobic bacterial infection. Fever, night sweats, and weight loss are also common, which together paint a picture consistent with a more ominous infectious process. As the abscesses develop, dyspnea becomes more likely, as well as chest pain, particularly if the abscess is peripheral in the lung. Complications of pleural effusion or development of empyema may also be present, resulting in worsening respiratory distress. Identification of these signs and their progression are critical since early diagnosis and treatment can make a tremendous difference in patient outcomes. Radiographic findings are crucial in the diagnosis of lung abscess, typically revealing a round, well-circumscribed opacity on a chest X-ray. The abscess can be surrounded by an associated consolidation that can be representative of accompanying pneumonia. Computed tomography (CT) can better delineate the size, location, and potential complications of the abscess, such as bronchiectasis or necrotizing pneumonia. In the majority of cases, the radiological evidence of visible air-fluid levels within the abscess cavity can be detected, lending impetus to the suspicion of an anaerobic infection. CT scanning is also capable of differentiating lung abscesses from other differential diagnoses, such as malignancy or granulomatous disease. As implied by some studies, the diagnosis of bronchiectasis has been associated with conditions such as activated phosphoinositide 3-kinase δ syndrome, which influences clinical management and highlights interconnected pathophysiologies that form the basis of respiratory disease (Coulter et al., 2016). Management of lung abscesses is grounded on both the identified causative organism and the underlying clinical context. Empirical antibiotic therapy most often encompasses anaerobic bacteria, which are typically caused by aspiration events in most cases. Surgical intervention may be indicated if the patient develops severe disease or remains unresponsive to conservative treatment. Underlying immunocompromised conditions, for example, may complicate the clinical presentation and necessitate a more aggressive therapeutic approach. As with other respiratory infections, identifying and treating any potential contributing factors, such as intravenous drug use or chronic aspiration, is necessary for optimal recovery. Furthermore, recognizing that pulmonary complications, including the development of lung abscesses, can present as extraintestinal manifestations of more extensive systemic disease can enhance clinical acumen (Harbord et al., 2015). Multidisciplinary evaluation, including pulmonology and infectious diseases consultants, is generally beneficial to the delivery of comprehensive care.

6.5.2. Diagnostic Approaches (Ct Scan, Bronchoscopy)

In the imaging of lung diseases, such as pneumonias and lung abscesses, radiologic imaging plays a central role, most notably through the use of computed tomography (CT) scans. CT scans can provide detailed cross-sectional images of the lungs, which allow for the accurate evaluation of different lung conditions. They are invaluable to determine the presence of consolidation, cavitary lesions, and interstitial changes, which are most often indicative of pneumonia or lung abscess. Furthermore, CT scans can enable the assessment of complications such as bronchiectasis through the definition of the structural defect of the airways. The sensitivity of CT imaging is such that it allows doctors to detect abnormalities that may not be visible using plain chest X-rays, ultimately guiding treatment and improving patient outcomes. Hence, the incorporation of CT scans into the diagnostic criteria significantly enhances the clinician's ability to identify and differentiate between various pulmonary disorders effectively. Bronchoscopy is a critical diagnostic method when faced with complex presentations of pneumonia, lung abscess, and bronchiectasis. This minimally invasive procedure provides direct visualization of the lung parenchyma and airways, enabling doctors to obtain biopsy samples and sputum cultures directly from sites of potential infection. Refractory pneumonia can also be distinguished by bronchoscopy, allowing for the differentiation between infectious and non-infectious processes. For instance, in cases where a lung abscess is suspected, bronchoscopy can give essential information regarding the presence of necrotizing tissue or unusual pathogens like mycobacteria or fungi. It is also highly valuable in patients presenting with bronchiectasis, as it can reveal focal inflammation changes or obstructions that cause recurrent infections. Consequently, bronchoscopy is a highly valuable resource in the methodical diagnosis of respiratory disorders. The combination of bronchoscopy and CT imaging is a true example of the multidisciplinary approach, enhancing the diagnosis of complex lung disease. For example, in pulmonary enteric adenocarcinoma (PEAC) patients, imaging may initially suggest pneumonia and guide the diagnostic suspicion towards a neoplastic process when standard therapeutic maneuvers remain ineffective (Luo et al., 2024). Further, CT scans are also helpful in identifying fluid collections suggestive of lung abscess or empyema, as observed in patients with significant risk factors such as obesity and asthma (Chiji-Aguma et al., 2024). Such instances can be confirmed by bronchoscopy to determine the nature of these fluid collections, thus enabling appropriate interventions. Lastly, the integration of these diagnostic imaging modalities not only allows precise identification of underlying conditions but also aids in individualizing patient-specific treatment regimens, thereby improving overall management outcomes in pneumonia, lung abscess, and bronchiectasis.

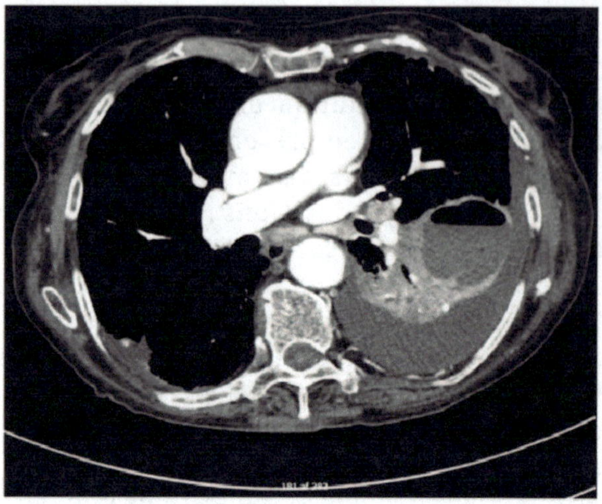

Figure 6.15. CT Scan of lung abscess.

Source: https://www.researchgate.net/profile/Andreas-Floe/publication/378524660/figure/fig2/AS:11431281227036564@1709394993361/Computed-tomography-image-in-horizontal-plane-illustrating-a-lung-abscess.png

6.5.3. Treatment Options (Antibiotics, Surgery)

Management through treatment of pneumonias, lung abscesses, and bronchiectasis is primarily comprised of the administration of antibiotics and surgery based on the condition and severity of the diseases. Antibiotics constitute the first line of treatment, particularly for bacterial infections causing respiratory disorders. For instance, in the case of lung abscesses, one should administer empirical antibiotics with a broad spectrum against the pathogens, gram-positive and gram-negative bacteria as well as anaerobic bacteria. A good example is in studies that demonstrated the importance of effective antibiotic therapy in diabetic patients, wherein Klebsiella pneumoniae was isolated with higher frequency, emphasizing the importance of targeted therapy (Md. Alam et al., 2025). Application of the appropriate antibiotics at the right time not only provides relief but also prevents further progression of the disease. In some instances where antibiotics alone may fail, surgery is an option. Surgical operations, such as lobectomy or drainage procedures, are particularly indicated for abscesses that do not respond to antibiotics within a reasonable time period, such as in individuals with severe infections. A case study of one such patient involves a pregnant woman who underwent emergent right lower lobectomy to treat a refractory pulmonary abscess, showing how crucial surgery is in the treatment of complicated infections (Hino et al., 2024). Coupling the use of surgical techniques with antibiotic therapy guarantees a multipronged approach to treatment that allows for the effective treatment of extensive lung infection with minimized risks of complications. The use of these therapies—surgery and antibiotics—alongside each other is made with close consideration of the patient's general health status, comorbidities, and specific clinical conditions. In cases where immunocompromised individuals or those with pre-existing pulmonary conditions are concerned, therapeutic management should be individually tailored to account for the complex interactions among the involved pathogens. With the assistance of multidisciplinary collaboration among pulmonologists, surgeons, and other physicians, treatment plans in patients can be individually fashioned to provide optimal patient outcomes. Lastly, a balanced process that combines both pharmacological and surgical aspects must be followed for the effective treatment of pneumonia, lung abscesses, and bronchiectasis to enhance patient recovery and quality of life.

Test Your Knowledge

1. Illustrate the clinical presentation of lung abscess.
2. What are the diagnostic approaches?

6.6. Bronchiectasis: Overview and Etiology

Learning Outcome

1. Definition and Pathophysiology of Bronchiectasis
2. Causes (Cystic Fibrosis, Infections)
3. Risk Factors (Genetic, Environmental)

Bronchiectasis, characterized by the permanent and abnormal dilation and inflammation of the bronchi, has a significant impact on respiratory well-being. As the compromised airways are unable to effectively remove mucus, infection and ongoing damage in a vicious circle ensue. Bronchiectasis is etiologically multifactorial, with infectious causes, immune deficiencies, and other associated conditions being of first rank. Typically associated with chronic lung infection, such as pneumonia, those with underlying diseases such as cystic fibrosis or primary immunodeficiency disorders (PIDs) are also predisposed. Such underlying causes underscore the need for early treatment and diagnosis in an effort to limit disease progression and improve quality of life in individuals affected. Unraveling the complex relationship between bronchiectasis and the causative factors is critical to creating effective treatment plans. In recent clinical studies, a strong association has been established between primary immunodeficiency diseases such as Common Variable Immunodeficiency (CVID) and bronchiectasis. These conditions are more likely to be precipitated by chronic lung disease, of which bronchiectasis is a part, following frequent infections and autoimmune responses in the airways. Importantly, in CVID patients, there is a high prevalence of chronic lung disease, and among these, bronchiectasis is one of the predominant manifestations. The compromised immune response not only facilitates the development of bronchiectasis but also complicates the treatment of underlying infections, with patients being prone to not responding favorably to standard antibiotic therapy. The relationship between bronchiectasis and immunodeficiency highlights the need for careful evaluation and treatment regimens tailored to these patients' unique challenges, underscoring the importance of collaboration between immunologists and pulmonologists in the coordination of care. Additionally, bronchiectasis can also arise from other non-infectious factors, such as genetic predisposition, exposure to environmental toxins, and post-infectious pathology.

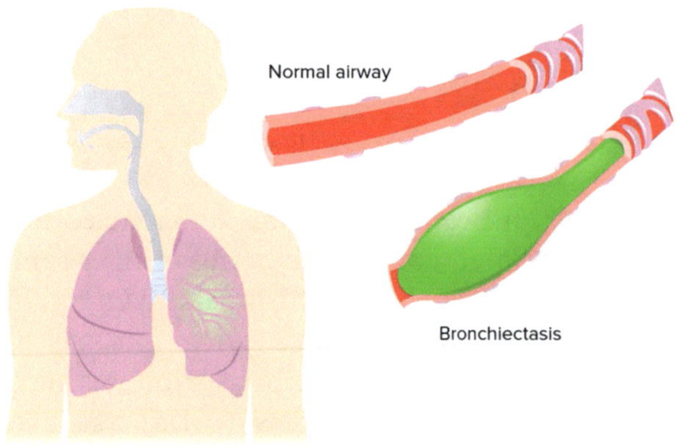

Figure 6.16. Overview of bronchiectasis.

Source: https://cdn.lecturio.com/assets/Bronchiectasis-pathophysiology-1200x861.png

Occupational and urban exposures to environmental toxins have a propensity to exacerbate respiratory diseases and airway inflammation. Genetic predispositions, such as gene mutations in cystic fibrosis or familial bronchiectasis, are also commonly found in patients with a history of chronic, recurrent respiratory infections. Management strategy calls for a multi-disciplinary approach, not only the treatment of infections and symptomatic relief, but also intervention on the environmental and genetic origins of the disease. An understanding of these diverse causes fosters a more comprehensive concept of bronchiectasis, thereby enhancing patient management and directing future research into its multifactorial pathophysiology and better therapeutic options.

6.6.1. Definition and Pathophysiology of Bronchiectasis

Bronchiectasis is a chronic respiratory illness characterized by abnormal and irreversible dilation of the bronchial airways, resulting in impaired clearance of secretions, chronic infection, and inflammation. This pathological condition typically arises following a sequence of airway damage and inflammation, most often precipitated by infections or other insults such as cystic fibrosis, allergic bronchopulmonary aspergillosis, or recurrent episodes of pneumonia. This generates a vicious cycle in which airway obstruction, mucus plugging, and bacterial colonization increase local inflammation and aggravate symptoms, while further injuring the bronchi walls. Patients of bronchiectasis are usually characterized by chronic coughing, sputum production, recurrent lung infection, and hemoptysis in some cases. The long-term consequences of bronchiectasis include the development of respiratory failure and impaired quality of life, making knowledge of its pathophysiology crucial to effective treatment in the context of concurrent pulmonary diseases. The underlying pathophysiological mechanisms of bronchiectasis are multifaceted and complex. Initially, a precipitating factor, such as an infection or an autoimmune disorder, impairs the integrity of the airway epithelium, which subsequently triggers a cascade of inflammatory processes. With advancing inflammation, deteriorative alterations in the airway walls, i.e., disruption of the bronchial smooth muscle and elastin fibers, cause dilation and deformity of the airway. Consequently, this altered morphology contributes to further compromise of mucociliary clearance, thereby putting patients at risk for chronic bacterial infections. Of particular significance is the fact that the presence of certain pathogens, most notably Pseudomonas aeruginosa, can sustain ongoing inflammation and exacerbate airway injury. This sustaining vicious cycle of injury and infection highlights the critical need to understand the pathophysiologic events of bronchiectasis to inform therapeutic approaches aimed at both infection control and airway inflammation. The diagnosis of bronchiectasis is primarily established through high-resolution computed tomography (CT) scans, which reveal the classic morphological features of the airways.

The radiologic patterns on CT scans are essential in establishing the diagnosis, particularly abnormalities of airway dilatation, non-tapering of airways, and irregularity of bronchial walls. Nevertheless, recent evidence emphasizes the need for standardized lung volume control during CT scan acquisition, as airway diameters can vary with lung inflation status and potentially compromise diagnostic sensitivity. Finally, new developments in automated image analysis software are unlocking more objective measurements of bronchial size, allowing for more accurate bronchiectasis diagnoses. For the best use of such advancements, the generation of accurate radiological definitions and sex- and age-adjusted reference values becomes essential. Such a sensitive method of diagnosing bronchiectasis will enhance clinical practice, particularly in the early diagnosis and intervention of this chronic disease in cases of pneumonia and other lung diseases (Johkoh et al., 2021; Tiddens HA et al., 2020).

6.6.2. Causes (Cystic Fibrosis, Infections)

Cystic fibrosis (CF) is a classic example of how inherited diseases can increase susceptibility to severe lung conditions, including pneumonia and bronchiectasis. CF occurs due to mutations in the cystic fibrosis transmembrane conductance regulator (CFTR) gene, leading to the secretion of thick, adhesive mucus that clogs the airways and provides a route for chronic infection. Over time, the chronic infection and inflammation cycle induced by pathogens such as Pseudomonas aeruginosa not only exacerbates lung injury but also causes bronchiectasis, characterized by the dilation and inflammation of airway conduits. Such a pathological environment excellently illustrates the close interaction of genetic predisposition and resultant infectious complications, which must be constantly controlled by medical interventions to herald improved outcomes in patients suffering from the condition. Infection is a predisposing cause for the development and worsening of lung disease, especially in patients with an underlying condition like CF or bronchiectasis. Respiratory tract infection is typically the clinical presentation in such patients, and there is a cyclical mechanism whereby infection causes lung tissue damage, with subsequent infection. The recurrent character of bacterial colonization in cystic fibrosis lungs necessitates extreme antibiotic treatment; as a regrettable consequence, indiscriminate use induces antibiotic resistance, an emerging issue of concern in the medical community. Also worth mentioning is that most respiratory infections of childhood are viral and usually harmless but have significant potential to evolve into more severe complications among vulnerable populations, demonstrating the need for vigilant clinical evaluation and management options (Montalto et al., 2005). The interaction between environmental conditions and lung infections reinforces the multifaceted nature of illnesses affecting pneumonia and lung abscesses. The increased vulnerability of patients suffering from chronic pulmonary conditions, such as CF, to develop secondary infection must be addressed by prevention and intervention at the very onset of symptoms. Early diagnosis of infection can increase the success of treatment and prevent the exacerbation of lung injury. Technological innovations in diagnostic devices may facilitate earlier diagnosis of pneumonia and other pulmonary diseases, promoting timely interventions that can halt the adverse effects on pulmonary function (Devan et al., 2006). This understanding promotes an interdisciplinary approach to the treatment of pneumonic disease, lung abscess, and bronchiectasis, ultimately reducing morbidity and mortality rates among high-risk populations.

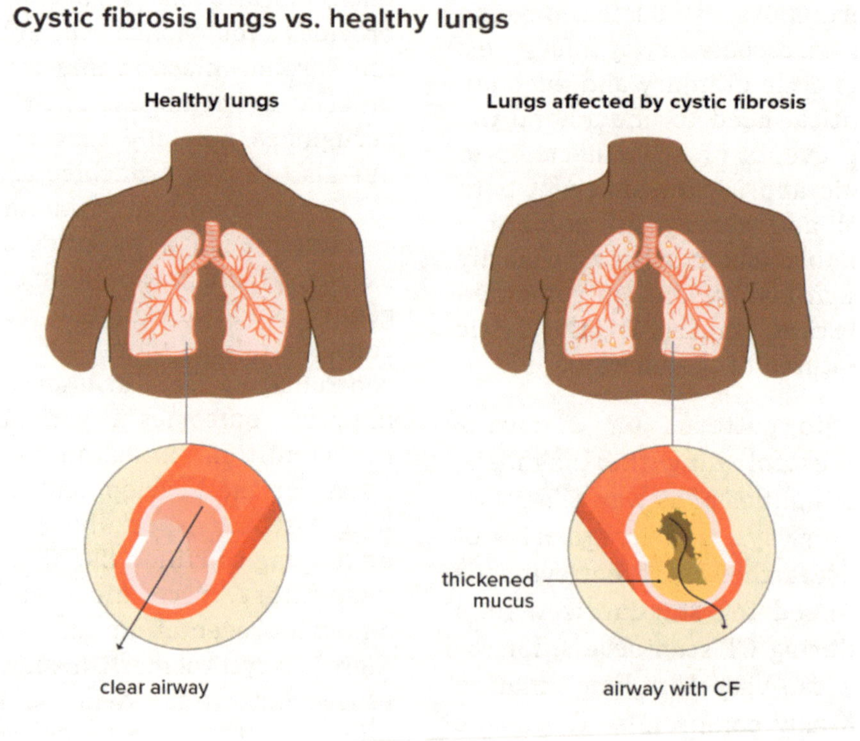

Figure 6.17. Cystic fibrosis in Lungs.

Source: https://media.post.rvohealth.io/wp-content/uploads/2023/07/3081005-cystic-fibrosis-lungs-1296x728-body.png

6.6.3. Risk Factors (Genetic, Environmental)

Understanding risk factors for pneumonias, lung abscesses, and bronchiectasis involves a detailed analysis of both genetic and environmental factors. Genetic predispositions can significantly increase an individual's susceptibility to respiratory ailments, particularly in those with inherited immunocompromised diseases. For instance, individuals with variable immunodeficiency disorders are disproportionately at risk of developing lung complications, including bronchiectasis and chronic lung disease, due to their affected immune functions that reduce their ability to combat infections. As such, these genetic disorders can create a convergence of risks that increase the likelihood of severe pulmonary disease development. Therefore, it is crucial to unravel the genetic etiology of such diseases in order to develop targeted prevention and treatment paradigms. Environmental factors also play a significant role in contributing to the risk profile for pneumonias, lung abscesses, and bronchiectasis. Exposures to allergens, irritants, and air pollutants can potentially exacerbate an existing lung disease or trigger an inflammatory one. They living in highly polluted city environments, for example, may have high rates of respiratory illness from chronic inflammation and injury caused by toxin-laden air breathed into the lungs. Occupational exposure, for example, from working in construction or manufacturing, contributes to particulates and chemical irritants that can dramatically impair lung function with repeated exposure. These environmental precipitants are significant to know because they have the potential to interact with genetic susceptibilities, thereby enhancing the risk of respiratory infections and declines in overall lung function. Furthermore, lifestyle decisions play a significant role in the development of risk factors for these respiratory diseases, particularly in conjunction with genetic and environmental factors. Smoking, for example, has been a proven first-order risk factor for several pulmonary diseases, including bronchiectasis. The toxic effects of tobacco smoke on lung tissue can impair respiratory defenses, increasing susceptibility to infection and inflammation. Similarly, inadequate nutrition, with deficiencies in key nutrients, can impair immune function, increasing vulnerability to pneumonia and other infections. As illustrated by the interaction between environmental factors and genetics, an integrated understanding of these closely related factors will be crucial to the development of effective public health interventions and personal health approaches for reducing the prevalence of pneumonias, lung abscesses, and bronchiectasis.

Test Your Knowledge

1. What is the pathophysiology of bronchiectasis?
2. What are the causes of bronchiectasis?

SUMMARY

The literature on pneumonias, lung abscesses, and bronchiectasis reveals that these respiratory diseases, despite their differing etiologies and pathophysiologies, share commonalities in pathophysiology and challenges in treatment. Pneumonias, for instance, can often be prevented by vaccination and prompt medical intervention, but may be complicated by concomitant conditions such as lung abscesses. The latter, usually a result of infection that may initially manifest as pneumonia, highlights the importance of early diagnosis and effective treatment. Advancements in advanced diagnostic modalities, such as metagenomic next-generation sequencing (mNGS), underscore the need to revise traditional treatment strategies to effectively respond to and address evolving trends in microbial infections (Zhang et al., 2025). Such multifaceted understanding is valuable in optimizing patient outcomes and can set the future research agenda for respiratory care. The multidimensional nature of bronchiectasis also contributes to clinical heterogeneity, as reflected in its heterogeneous pathophysiologies and presentations. Bronchiectasis patients generally have a unique constellation of chronic and acute exacerbation manifestations that demand special care approaches. Radiographic analysis by techniques such as the BEST-CT system reveals a high degree of heterogeneity of structural lung disease. It therefore highlights the relevance of individualized treatment regimens based on clinical phenotyping. The association of airway infections, such as those caused by Pseudomonas aeruginosa, with an increased severity of structural lung injury suggests a cycle that renders the disease challenging to treat (Pieters et al., 2024). Thus, detailed assessment and surveillance strategies are a part of effective long-term management of bronchiectasis. Ultimately, pneumonias, lung abscesses, and bronchiectasis require integrated medical therapy that encompasses prevention, early diagnosis, and novel therapeutic approaches. Awareness among practitioners about the interrelatedness of these disorders can optimize diagnosis and acute therapy, reducing morbidity and mortality rates of respiratory illness. As studies continue and novel diagnostic tests become part of the clinician's armamentarium, patient outcomes become increasingly likely to improve. Through ongoing development in our comprehension of these respiratory illnesses in the entirety of their complicated clinical settings, clinicians to provide more successful responses to the challenges created by pneumonia, lung abscess, and bronchiectasis and thereby further the specialty of pulmonary medicine in significant ways.

The differential presentations of pneumonia and their corresponding conditions require comprehensive knowledge for accurate diagnosis and management. Pneumonias can be either community-acquired or hospital-acquired, with different pathogens and treatment options. Detection of acute COVID-19 pneumonia is one of the significant advancements in the evaluation of pneumonia, which is associated with specific special imaging characteristics, such as organizing pneumonia that CT scans can identify. This particular strain can progress to acute respiratory distress syndrome in severe cases, and recognition of their presence emphasizes the need for rapid identification and treatment (Tcheroyan et al., 2025). Recognition of these characteristics not only allows timely treatment but also allows for the prediction of chronic complications that can arise following an acute attack. Lung abscesses are another essential feature of the clinical presentation of respiratory disease, typically a complication of aspiration of foreign material or pneumonia. Lung abscesses clinically present with a necrotic cavity in the lung parenchyma due to various infectious causes, mainly anaerobic bacteria. Early identification is essential because delayed treatment tends to make the condition worse and leads to severe morbidity. Wide-ranging imaging tests, including chest

X-rays and CT scans, play a significant role in providing information for differential diagnosis and management strategies. Notably, significant results from imaging will help discriminate between etiologies for lung abscesses, directly influencing treatment options, which underscores the relevance of advanced imaging modalities in improving clinical outcomes. Bronchiectasis, a chronic disease of abnormal dilation and damage of airways, can result from repeated infections, including pneumonia. These patients typically present with sputum production and chronic cough, which can significantly impact their quality of life. Pathophysiologic alterations seen in bronchiectasis include inflammation and structural alterations in the airways. Ideal diagnosis is often brought forth through recent case reports, as conditions like anti-melanoma differentiation-associated gene 5 (MDA5)- related interstitial lung disease may present together and complicate management (Yein et al., 2024). Therefore, a well-integrated strategy with a focus on early diagnosis and tailored treatment protocols is of utmost necessity to improve clinical results and minimize the risk of severe complications of such complex pulmonary disorders.

KEY TERMS FROM THIS CHAPTER

- Community-acquired pneumonia (CAP)
- Aspiration pneumonia
- Bronchopneumonia
- Empyema
- Anaerobic bacteria
- Bronchiectasis
- Varicose bronchiectasis
- Chronic productive cough
- Pus formation
- Air-fluid level
- Hospital-acquired pneumonia (HAP)
- Lobar pneumonia
- Interstitial pneumonia
- Lung abscess
- Necrotizing pneumonia
- Cylindrical bronchiectasis
- Saccular (cystic) bronchiectasis
- Hemoptysis
- Bronchial wall thickening
- Chest physiotherapy

CRITICAL THINKING QUESTIONS

1. **Which of the following organisms is the most common cause of community-acquired pneumonia?**
   a. Pseudomonas aeruginosa
   b. Streptococcus pneumoniae
   c. Staphylococcus aureus
   d. Klebsiella pneumoniae
2. **Which of the following is the hallmark feature of bronchiectasis?**
   a. Reversible airway obstruction
   b. Permanent dilation of bronchi
   c. Alveolar consolidation
   d. Pleural thickening
3. **What is the most common cause of lung abscess formation?**
   a. Viral infection
   b. Aspiration of oral anaerobic bacteria
   c. Fungal infection
   d. Autoimmune inflammation
4. **Which of the following symptoms is most characteristic of bronchiectasis?**
   a. Dry cough
   b. Productive cough with foul-smelling sputum
   c. Hemoptysis without cough
   d. Acute chest pain
5. **Which radiological finding is most typical for lung abscess?**
   a. Diffuse interstitial infiltrates
   b. Cavitary lesion with an air-fluid level
   c. Pleural effusion without cavitation
   d. Homogeneous lobar consolidation

Short Answer Questions

1. What is the most common bacterial cause of community-acquired pneumonia?
2. Which clinical feature is characteristic of lung abscess?
3. What is the typical radiologic finding in bronchiectasis?
4. Name two common risk factors for developing lung abscess.
5. Which pneumonia type is characterized by patchy involvement of one or more lobes?

Answer to Critical Thinking Questions

1. (b) 2. (b) 3. (b) 4. (b) 5. (b)

REFERENCES

1. Aadarsh, S. (2024). Automated pneumonia identification through CNN-based analysis. *International Journal of Scientific Research in Engineering and Management.* https://www.semanticscholar.org/paper/c2fc06577e28dd2f2892c1c4147eab5cb8fb5d37 (accessed on 16th June 2025).

2. Alam, N. M. S., Saqeb, N. K. M. N., Hossain, N. M. M., & Shikha, N. M. I. (2025). Clinical types and infective pattern of pyogenic neck abscess in diabetic patients. *Bangladesh Critical Care Journal, 13*(1), 23–29. https://doi.org/10.3329/bccj.v13i1.81301Asokan, D., Bawankar, N. S., Khadse, R. R., & Bhise, S. M. (2024). Unravelling the unusual: *Enterococcus faecium* in aspiration pneumonia complicated with lung abscess in a severely comorbid patient. *International Journal of Research in Medical Sciences.* https://www.semanticscholar.org/paper/be860b969c668f0eb5101edc06cfd6203b9e2a55 (accessed on 16th June 2025).

3. Attard Montalto, S. (2005). Respiratory infections in childhood: To use antibiotics or not? https://core.ac.uk/download/83019665.pdf (accessed on 16th June 2025).

4. Avari, M., & Brown, J. S. (2020). Management of community-acquired pneumonia: Essential tips for the physician on call. https://core.ac.uk/download/326711248.pdf (accessed on 16th June 2025).

5. Ayoub, A., Salhi, H., Najlae, Z., Ammor, A., & Benhaddou, H. (2024). Primary staphylococcal lung abscess: A rare situation in infants. *Cureus, 16.* https://www.semanticscholar.org/paper/ea233d5bf8089ab7a7f11a30a329430c9467acee (accessed on 16th June 2025).

6. Balkissoon, R. (2019). Journal club–Bronchiectasis/COPD overlap: Syndrome versus treatable trait? *Chronic Obstructive Pulmonary Diseases: Journal of the COPD Foundation.* https://www.semanticscholar.org/paper/1d18cc376a0db6bfaebf6de489468fa5ff8d8357 (accessed on 16th June 2025).

7. Borys, R., Szeliga, E., Wojtuń, K., Kużdżał, A., & Sawka, K. (2024). Lung abscess with pneumonia after SARS-CoV-2 infection–A case report. *European Journal of Clinical and Experimental Medicine.* https://www.semanticscholar.org/paper/b99270ebc6bc4eb59e9f50bd113226443968aefa (accessed on 16th June 2025).

8. Buntara, I., Hidayat, S. P., Buulolo, C. S., & Hendsun. (2023). Lung abscess preceded by fever of unknown origin: A case report. *International Journal of Advances in Medicine.* https://www.semanticscholar.org/paper/f36512b1387f2a73e07d4a0ee22a48b1377a9aec (accessed on 16th June 2025).

9. Chernekhovskaya, N. E., Korzheva, I., Vychuzhanina, N. V., & Volova, A. V. (2023). Middle lobe syndrome. *Filin's Clinical Endoscopy.* https://www.semanticscholar.org/paper/4ba1722c28ba4e519a051783ad085b498fb38193 (accessed on 16th June 2025).

10. Chiji-Aguma, J. C., Adeyemi, O. M., Osanoto, A. S., & Akanmode, A. M. (2024). Progression of community-acquired pneumonia in a morbidly obese patient with a history of vaping and asthma: A multidisciplinary approach to management. *Cureus, 16.* https://www.semanticscholar.org/paper/4589ab62178e3aa00a2602b35cb993838e6ae998 (accessed on 16th June 2025).

11. Chiumello, D., Sferrazza Papa, G. F., Artigas, A., Bouhemad, B., Grgic, A., Heunks, L., Markstaller, K., et al. (2019). ERS statement on chest imaging in acute respiratory failure. *European*

Respiratory Journal, 54, 1900435–1900435. https://doi.org/10.1183/13993003.00435-2019 (accessed on 16th June 2025).

12. Coulter, T., Chandra, A., Bacon, C. M., Babar, J., Curtis, J., Screaton, N., Goodlad, J. R., et al. (2016). Clinical spectrum and features of activated phosphoinositide 3-kinase δ syndrome: A large patient cohort study. *Journal of Allergy and Clinical Immunology, 139*, 597–606.e4. https://doi.org/10.1016/j.jaci.2016.06.021 (accessed on 16th June 2025).
13. Criado, E., Sánchez, M., Ramírez, J., Arguis, P., de Caralt, T. M., Perea, R. J., & Xaubet, A. (2010). Pulmonary sarcoidosis: Typical and atypical manifestations at high-resolution CT with pathologic correlation. *Radiographic, 30*, 1567–1586. https://doi.org/10.1148/rg.306105512 (accessed on 16th June 2025).
14. Currie, B. J., Ward, L., & Cheng, A. C. (2010). The epidemiology and clinical spectrum of melioidosis: 540 cases from the 20-year Darwin prospective study. *PLoS Neglected Tropical Diseases, 4,* e900–e900. https://doi.org/10.1371/journal.pntd.0000900 (accessed on 16th June 2025).
15. Devan, K. S. (2006). Expert system with an embedded imaging module for diagnosing lung diseases. https://core.ac.uk/download/301113939.pdf (accessed on 16th June 2025).
16. Eleraky, N. E., Allam, A., Hassan, S. B., & Omar, M. (2020). Nanomedicine fight against antibacterial resistance: An overview of the recent pharmaceutical innovations. *Pharmaceutics, 12*, 142–142. https://doi.org/10.3390/pharmaceutics12020142 (accessed on 16th June 2025).
17. Farr, A., Torres, A., Ringshausen, F. C., Blasi, F., Dimopoulos, G., Rohde, G., Migliori, G. B., et al. (2018). ERS syllabus for postgraduate training in respiratory infections: A guide for comprehensive training. https://core.ac.uk/download/195292060.pdf (accessed on 16th June 2025).
18. Garmhausen, D., Hagemann, T., Bieber, T., Dimitriou, I. M., Fimmers, R., Diepgen, T. L., & Novak, N. (2013). Characterization of different courses of atopic dermatitis in adolescent and adult patients. *Allergy, 68,* 498–506. https://doi.org/10.1111/all.12112 (accessed on 16th June 2025).
19. Harbord, M., Annese, V., Vavricka, S. R., Allez, M., Barreiro-de Acosta, M., Boberg, K. M., Burisch, J., et al. (2015). The first European evidence-based consensus on extra-intestinal manifestations in inflammatory bowel disease. *Journal of Crohn's and Colitis, 10*, 239–254. https://doi.org/10.1093/ecco-jcc/jjv213 (accessed on 16th June 2025).
20. Herzinger, J., Hytych, V., Mališ, J., Pavlíčková, K., Čermák, J., Demeš, R., Svoboda, P., et al. (2024). The role of thoracic surgery in the management of complicated acute and post-acute COVID-19 pneumonia (PASC). *Rozhledy v chirurgii: Mesicnik Ceskoslovenske Chirurgicke Spolecnosti, 103*(2), 57–64. https://www.semanticscholar.org/paper/64ec4dee3bbc490be514553887efffe674967163 (accessed on 16th June 2025).
21. Hino, H., Yasuhara, Y., Nakahata, K., Utsumi, T., Maru, N., Matsui, H., Taniguchi, Y., et al. (2024). Emergency right lower lobectomy for severe pulmonary abscess in a pregnant woman at the 25th week of gestation: A case report. *Surgical Case Reports, 10.* https://www.semanticscholar.org/paper/f53208d84500d89ed132a20ef65c70b39bee0573 (accessed on 16th June 2025).
22. Ho, H., & Cunningham-Rundles, C. (2020). Non-infectious complications of common variable immunodeficiency: Updated clinical spectrum, sequelae, and insights to pathogenesis. *Frontiers in Immunology, 11.* https://doi.org/10.3389/fimmu.2020.00149 (accessed on 16th June 2025).

23. Jeseňák, M., Bánovčin, P., Jesenakova, B., & Babušíková, E. (2014). Pulmonary manifestations of primary immunodeficiency disorders in children. *Frontiers in Pediatrics, 2.* https://www.semanticscholar.org/paper/33afec84dcba0468c554020b4c12883260ed02f9 (accessed on 16th June 2025).

24. Jo, Y. S., Lee, H. K., Park, S. H., Joh, J., Jang, H. J., & Park, J. S. (2025). Korean guidelines for diagnosis and management of idiopathic nonspecific interstitial pneumonia. *Tuberculosis and Respiratory Diseases, 88*, 237–246. https://www.semanticscholar.org/paper/b7a9b423104ac4fca9ff8a3fe5997572451ec54d (accessed on 16th June 2025).

25. Johkoh, T., Lee, K. S., Nishino, M., Travis, W. D., Ryu, J. H., Lee, H. Y., Ryerson, C. J., et al. (2021). Chest CT diagnosis and clinical management of drug-related pneumonitis in patients receiving molecular targeting agents and immune checkpoint inhibitors: A position paper from the Fleischner Society. *Radiology, 298*, 550–566. https://doi.org/10.1148/radiol.2021203427 (accessed on 16th June 2025).

26. Kautsar, M., & Khairunnisa, C. (2024). Characteristics and treatment of pneumonia patients at Cut Meutia General Hospital North Aceh in 2022. *Proceedings of Malikussaleh International Conference on Health and Disaster Medicine (MICOHEDMED).* https://www.semanticscholar.org/paper/19a3a353f68679572e8b6ca750e4e429439a7055 (accessed on 16th June 2025).

27. Kim, Y. (2022). Complex relationship between bronchiectasis and lung cancer. *Annals of the American Thoracic Society, 19*, 1455–1456. https://www.semanticscholar.org/paper/c2b26f06cd59f1f510c4870b8957de09ba1b1e7f (accessed on 16th June 2025).

28. Kousha, M., Tadi, R., & Soubani, A. O. (2011). Pulmonary aspergillosis: A clinical review. *European Respiratory Review, 20*, 156–174. https://doi.org/10.1183/09059180.00001011 (accessed on 16th June 2025).

29. Kumar, A., Chetiwal, R., Rana, N., Dubey, A., & Tanwar, S. (2025). Lung abscess complicating ventilator-associated pneumonia caused by extensively drug-resistant *Acinetobacter baumannii. Exploration of Medicine.* https://www.semanticscholar.org/paper/074abcddcfb660b4cba96e48d59ac4f4b8b7337a (accessed on 16th June 2025).

30. Lee, J., Koo, S., Park, K., Seo, Y. R., Kim, S. H., Kim, Y. K., Kim, K. U., et al. (2011). Analysis of lung parenchymal sequelae following treatment for lung abscess. *Tuberculosis and Respiratory Diseases, 71*, 438–444. https://www.semanticscholar.org/paper/885fa1daea964653226e2545dab4c658f751eb91 (accessed on 16th June 2025).

31. Leung, C. C. D., Chan, Y., Ho, M., Chan, M., Chen, C. H., Ngai, C. M., Chan, H. C. C., et al. (2024). A single lung abscess caused by Panton-Valentine leucocidin-producing methicillin-resistant *Staphylococcus aureus. Cureus, 16.* https://www.semanticscholar.org/paper/324d8d7f8e7bc15c483f0ca9d5bd35c05f31625c (accessed on 16th June 2025).

32. Lewis, P. (2020). Risk factor evaluation for methicillin-resistant *Staphylococcus aureus* and *Pseudomonas aeruginosa* in community-acquired pneumonia. *Annals of Pharmacotherapy, 55*, 36–43. https://doi.org/10.1177/1060028020935106 (accessed on 16th June 2025).

33. Luo, Z. H., Luo, X. Y., Luo, X. Q., Jin, A. F., & Zeng, Q. (2024). Case report: 18F-FDG PET/CT in pulmonary enteric adenocarcinoma. *Frontiers in Oncology, 14.* https://www.semanticscholar.org/paper/15a33258401b473f1780ff6319841b14012c6509 (accessed on 16th June 2025).

34. Mahdaviani, S., Ghadimi, S., Fallahi, M., Hashemi-Moghaddam, S. A., Chavoshzadeh, Z., Puel, A., Rezaei, N., et al. (2023). Interventional pulmonary procedures and their outcomes in

patients with STAT3 hyper IgE syndrome. *BMC Surgery, 23.* https://www.semanticscholar.org/paper/24c1ec17d88c5f4ef9fa9abe72b6885188d9ea8f (accessed on 16th June 2025).

35. Marín-Hinojosa, C., Eraso, C. C., Sánchez-López, V., Hernández, L. C., Otero-Candelera, R., & López-Campos, J. (2021). Nutri epigenomics and chronic obstructive pulmonary disease: Potential role of dietary and epigenetics factors in disease development and management. *The American Journal of Clinical Nutrition.* https://www.semanticscholar.org/paper/fceb8cd736deceb246aa61b96256a8c38a196a20 (accessed on 16th June 2025).

36. McCusker, C., Upton, J., & Warrington, R. (2018). Primary immunodeficiency. *Allergy Asthma and Clinical Immunology, 14.* https://doi.org/10.1186/s13223-018-0290-5 (accessed on 16th June 2025).

37. Mu, S., Hu, L., Zhang, Y., Liu, Y., Cui, X., Zou, X., Wang, Y., et al. (2021). Prospective evaluation of a rapid clinical metagenomics test for bacterial pneumonia. *Frontiers in Cellular and Infection Microbiology, 11.* https://doi.org/10.3389/fcimb.2021.684965 (accessed on 16th June 2025).

38. Panossian, A., Efferth, T., Shikov, A. N., Pozharitskaya, O. N., Kuchta, K., Mukherjee, P. K., Banerjee, S., et al. (2020). Evolution of the adaptogenic concept from traditional use to medical systems: Pharmacology of stress- and aging-related diseases. *Medicinal Research Reviews, 41,* 630–703. https://doi.org/10.1002/med.21743 (accessed on 16th June 2025).

39. Pieters, A. L. P., van der Veer, T., Meerburg, J. J., Andrinopoulou, E., Vd Eerden, M. M., Ciet, P., Aliberti, S., et al. (2024). Structural lung disease and clinical phenotype in bronchiectasis patients: The EMBARC CT study. *American Journal of Respiratory and Critical Care Medicine.* https://www.semanticscholar.org/paper/41570dd14024ac7370d7374da0d076f94a877b02 (accessed on 16th June 2025).

40. Pulmonary Infection Assembly of Chinese Thoracic Society. (2022). [Chinese expert consensus on the management of lower respiratory tract infections of *Pseudomonas aeruginosa* in adults (2022)]. *Zhonghua jie he he hu xi za zhi = Zhonghua jiehe he huxi zazhi = Chinese Journal of Tuberculosis and Respiratory Diseases, 45*(8), 739–752. https://www.semanticscholar.org/paper/97a247a51d1353ae90b48c5cbddc5ef5581fac4e (accessed on 16th June 2025).

41. Rahman, N. A., Amin, M., & Rosyid, A. (2025). Imaging techniques in COVID-19 diagnosis: Evaluating the role of chest X-ray, chest CT scan, and lung ultrasound in identifying key radiological features. *Coronaviruses.* https://www.semanticscholar.org/paper/d690b65da459a52d523ef2964b621795f283b4eb (accessed on 16th June 2025).

42. Smiyan, O., Taramak, L., Smiian, K., Vasilyeva, O., Loboda, A., Petrashenko, V., Moshchych, O., et al. (2023). Modern view from Ukraine on etiology, pathogenesis and clinical-diagnostic aspects of community-acquired pneumonia in children. *Eastern Ukrainian Medical Journal.* https://www.semanticscholar.org/paper/e0553743e87b650e272876936edcd67d1e98dbcc (accessed on 16th June 2025).

43. Sperling, S., Dahl, V. N., & Fløe, A. (2024). Lung abscess: An update on the current knowledge and call for future investigations. *Current Opinion in Pulmonary Medicine, 30,* 229–234. https://www.semanticscholar.org/paper/3e3b44daa9a3fab50b06c962545c5a1e2c1a3a89 (accessed on 16th June 2025).

44. Sun, Z., Liu, X., Wang, J., Wang, X., Liu, W., & Chen, Y. (2020). Computed tomography evaluation of airway changes in adult patients with COVID-19 pneumonia. *Journal of the College of Physicians and Surgeons--Pakistan: JCPSP, 30*(8), 785–789. https://www.semanticscholar.

org/paper/1fcaa8812c4149324b007edfbae605ddf3dd8518 (accessed on 16th June 2025).

45. Tangye, S. G., Al-Herz, W., Bousfiha, A., Cunningham-Rundles, C., Franco, J. L., Holland, S. M., Klein, C., et al. (2022). Human inborn errors of immunity: 2022 update on the classification from the International Union of Immunological Societies Expert Committee. *Journal of Clinical Immunology, 42*, 1473–1507. https://doi.org/10.1007/s10875-022-01289-3 (accessed on 16th June 2025).

46. Tcheroyan, R., Makhoul, P., & Simpson, S. (2025). An updated review of pulmonary radiological features of acute and chronic COVID-19. *Current Opinion in Pulmonary Medicine, 31*, 183–195. https://www.semanticscholar.org/paper/32d298213d1158294dcbc1a6af74e3c695a9b128 (accessed on 16th June 2025).

47. Tiddens, H. A. W. M., Meerburg, J. J., van der Eerden, M. M., & Ciet, P. (2020). The radiological diagnosis of bronchiectasis: What's in a name? *European Respiratory Review, 29*, 190120–190120. https://doi.org/10.1183/16000617.0120-2019 (accessed on 16th June 2025).

48. Vega, L., Calvo, I., Ibarguengoitia, O., Montero, D., García, C., Galíndez, E., Blanco, J., et al. (2021). AB0170: Rheumatoid arthritis associated lung disease: Experience in a biological therapy unit. *Annals of the Rheumatic Diseases, 80.* https://www.semanticscholar.org/paper/ec8e1240c6939b61c365b7d170e598a0b70415e6 (accessed on 16th June 2025).

49. Yaraghi, S., & Khosravi, F. (2024). Diagnosis of pneumonia from chest X-ray images using transfer learning and generative adversarial network. *International Journal of Innovative Science and Research Technology (IJISRT).* https://www.semanticscholar.org/paper/36809088790b62eb1d3c8379ec4d3299c395dbf4 (accessed on 16th June 2025).

50. Yein, K., Sadiq, S., Zeb, S., Ahmed, A., & Price, E. (2024). P029: Successful treatment of rapidly progressive MDA-5 with dual combination therapy as a bridge to lung transplantation. *Rheumatology.* https://www.semanticscholar.org/paper/1df59d5ee38ca5c2d0e6ae184c4f50a6d42f426c (accessed on 16th June 2025).

51. Zhang, R., Yu, J., Shang, X., Wang, Z., Li, H., & Cao, B. (2025). Heterogeneity in clinical patterns of adult lung abscess patients: An 8-year retrospective study in a tertiary hospital. *BMC Pulmonary Medicine, 25.* https://www.semanticscholar.org/paper/0599fde7b053d49c22ff122a175c410e85814d5b (accessed on 16th June 2025).

52. Zhang, Z., Wen, S., Liu, J., Ouyang, Y., Su, Z., Chen, D., Liang, Z., et al. (2024). Advances in the relationship between periodontopathogens and respiratory diseases (Review). *Molecular Medicine Reports, 29.* https://doi.org/10.3892/mmr.2024.13166 (accessed on 16th June 2025).

TUBERCULOSIS

7

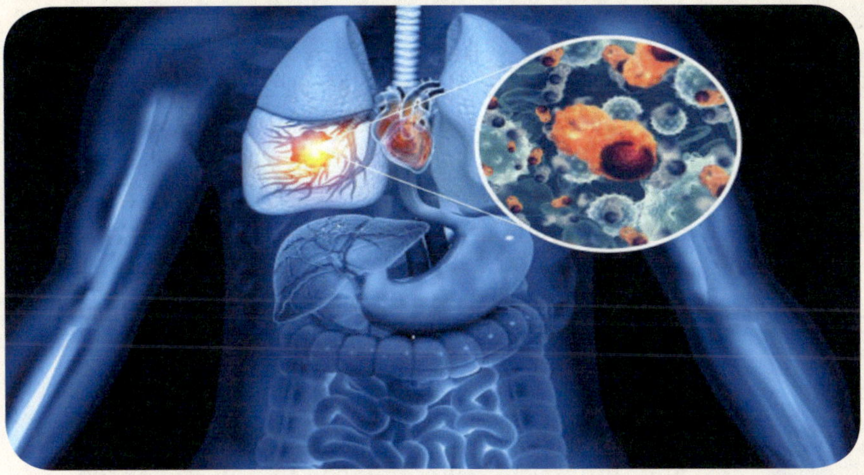

LEARNING OBJECTIVES

After studying this chapter, you will be able to:

1. List the causes and transmission
2. Describe symptoms and diagnosis
3. Focus on the treatment options
4. Explore the global impact
5. Explain the prevention strategies
6. Discuss the current research and developments

Introduction

Tuberculosis (TB) is the most significant public health problem in the world, affecting millions and representing an interrelated complex of medical, social, and cultural determinants. Characterized by its resilience and versatility, TB is primarily found in the lungs but has the potential to involve other body systems, thereby presenting a diverse range of clinical presentations. The disease is caused by the bacterium *Mycobacterium tuberculosis*, which is spread by droplet nuclei in the air when the infected person coughs or sneezes. The epidemiology of TB plays a highly crucial role in both prevention and treatment of the disease. It goes beyond merely clinical practice to encompass the socio-cultural settings that influence knowledge and attitudes towards the disease, and it establishes that firmly rooted convictions can affect disease control at community levels. Aside from the health determinants, sociocultural beliefs also play an role in determining how tuberculosis is perceived and managed in various populations.

Particularly within marginalized communities, like the Somali community, deeply rooted TB beliefs could hinder effective public health interventions. For instance, stigma for TB can prevent people from accessing proper medical treatment on time, as shown by a study uncovering the general knowledge of symptoms of TB among the population, but referring to myths surrounding its transmission and cure, which are bound to be written in cultural scripts (Gerrish et al.). These sociocultural dynamics hinder healthcare professionals, and therefore, public health campaigns should create community involvement and education to dissipate myths surrounding the disease and encourage active health-seeking behavior. Also, tuberculosis needs to be addressed by blending clinical practice with culturally modified models of providing healthcare.

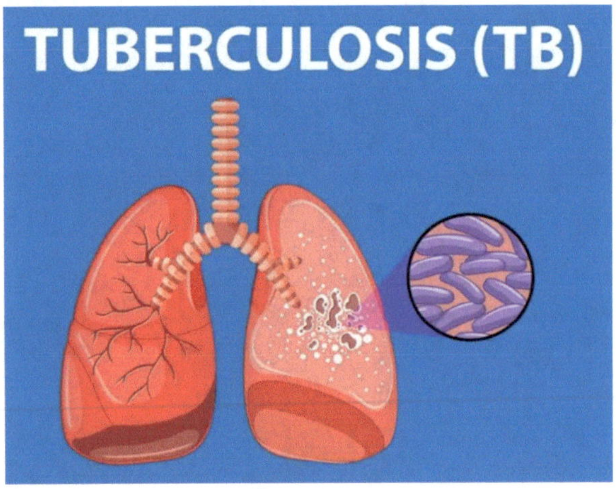

Figure 7.1. Tuberculosis.

Source: https://www.metropolisindia.com/upgrade/blog/upload/24/01/Tuberculosis1705674281.webp

Procedures such as sputum induction have been highlighted for their value in collecting diagnostic specimens without causing excessive discomfort to patients (Farrugia et al., 2013). This highlights the need for healthcare systems to balance their response to the diverse needs of TB populations. Through recognizing the interface between clinical practice and sociocultural sensitivity, public health interventions can be more effective in enabling access to care. Lastly, a refined strategy that respects and incorporates community beliefs while prioritizing scientific education can enhance awareness and effectiveness of treatment, as well as reduce the tuberculosis burden on a global level.

Definition of Tuberculosis

Tuberculosis (TB), one of the most contagious diseases and usually caused by *Mycobacterium tuberculosis*, has been a global public health issue for decades. TB has been known to affect the lungs but can also affect other parts of the body, leading to different clinical presentations. TB spreads through droplet infection when the infected person coughs or sneezes; hence, close contact with the patient is necessary to understand how it is transmitted. Beyond its infectious nature, tuberculosis has gained notoriety for unleashing widespread morbidity and mortality, particularly in low-resource settings, to justify the impetus for proper public health intervention. TB incidence is also aggravated by poor socioeconomic status, malnutrition, and co-infections such as HIV. With its ongoing persistence, there is extensive awareness of TB's definition and its implications in society that is vital to the development of plans to combat this public health threat.

The World Health Organization (WHO) recognizes tuberculosis as a significant communicable disease that contributes to causing incident cases and deaths worldwide. The disease exists in two primary forms: latent TB infection, where the bacteria are latent but no clinical symptoms are present, and active TB disease, with its clinical presentation of chronic cough, fever, and weight loss. This is important since people who have latent TB are not infectious but are at a higher risk of getting the active form if their immune systems are somehow weakened. The global burden of tuberculosis is staggering with tens of millions of new cases each year and a significant burden on healthcare systems, especially among the resource-poor countries. Providing a solution to the numerous factors of TB, from transmission patterns to health and social determinants, is crucial in developing focused treatments and interventions. Tuberculosis also has very tight links with antimicrobial resistance (AMR), further complicating the treatment and public health interventions. As antibiotic resistance grows, the resistant strains, such as multidrug-resistant TB (MDR-TB) and extensively drug-resistant TB (XDR-TB), are also posing significant challenges. Not only do resistant strains carry a higher risk of treatment failure, but they also require longer, more complex treatment durations, thereby inducing additional high patient burden and stress on healthcare resources. Understanding the definition of tuberculosis must factor in these dynamics of resistance since studies inform us that AMR is a leading cause of morbidity and mortality from the disease (Murray et al., 2022). Moreover, while scientists proceed to investigate the social determinants of health and TB outcomes' interaction, TB's definition has changed to encapsulate not only the bacterium but the broader concept of health equity and systemic factors that affect treatment access and disease management (Gravlee, 2020).

Historical context of the disease

The etiology of tuberculosis (TB) testifies to its widespread impact on societies through the centuries. Since its earliest known incidences in ancient cultures, such as Egypt and Greece, TB has had an effect on public health measures as well as social sentiment. The disease, when it was termed consumption due to its debilitating nature, used to be romanticized in literature and the arts as an indicator of its prevalence among artists and thinkers. But this charm drew attention from the bitter reality of high death rates attributed to TB. As urbanization and industrialization boomed in the 19th century, TB was a public health concern. The creation of high-density residential conditions facilitated the escalation of the diseases transmitted, prompting the healthcare authorities to pinpoint TB as a problem requiring immediate attention and intervention. The development of scientific understanding of tuberculosis accelerated during the late 19th and early 20th centuries. This period saw the identification of *Mycobacterium tuberculosis* by Robert Koch in 1882, marking a pivotal moment in medical history. Koch's discovery not only confirmed the bacteriological roots of the disease but also signified the advent of modern microbiology. The subsequent public health campaigns were directed to educate people about transmission and prevention, emphasizing sanitation, fresh air, and nutrition. These campaigns laid the basis for more structured disease management measures. Later breakthroughs in therapy, from sanatoriums to antibiotic therapies like streptomycin in the middle of the 20th century, transformed TB into an incurable disease that became a treatable condition and not one that eliminated inequalities of access to healthcare at the regional level. Besides, the social and economic impacts of tuberculosis cannot be overlooked. TB was stigmatized socially, which generally led to exclusion from society, particularly among people who had TB, as a result of community fear of contracting the disease. This discrimination was compounded by the socio-economic determinants that governed a person's access to healthcare, reflecting broader societal inequalities. The response to tuberculosis also catalyzed the development of healthcare policy and local governance institutions, based on the need for concerted public health action in the face of an epidemic. Understanding the intricate association between TB and socio-economic environments provides a clearer picture of issues of the times in controlling the disease, particularly in countries where access to treatment and resources remains in tatters. It serves to underscore the imperative of learning from history in the interest of informing current strategies for combating tuberculosis today, as the disease continues to pose one of the most significant challenges to public health globally.

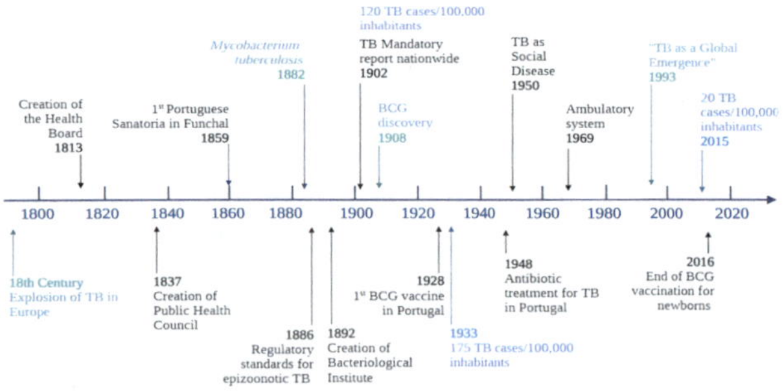

Figure 7.2. The historical context of tuberculosis (TB).

Source: https://pub.mdpi-res.com/world/world-06-00061/article_deploy/html/images/world-06-00061-ag-550.jpg?1746542429

Importance of studying Tuberculosis today

Understanding the significance of education on Tuberculosis (TB) in contemporary times requires a reflection on its profound impact on global public health. Despite medical science advances, TB remains a significant infectious disease, claiming nearly 1.5 million lives annually. The resurgence of TB across most parts of the globe, driven by factors like increased antibiotic resistance and socio-economic turbulence, necessitates ongoing research as well as intervention strategies. For example, the World Health Organization (WHO) stresses the fight against TB, particularly in areas of conflict where health systems are typically incapacitated, as in Ukraine. WHO took enormous funding and emergency interventions to ensure TB treatment during emergencies, urging resilience in public health infrastructure and the provision of vital medical services to vulnerable populations. With the changing global health landscape, the study of TB cannot be overstated and still necessitates a consistent focus and budget allocation. In addition to the overall public health issues, the study of Tuberculosis has significant socio-economic effects that require comprehension. TB disproportionately affects poor populations, further cementing the traps of poverty and limiting access to education and employment opportunities. The economic burden of TB includes healthcare costs, loss of productivity, and disability in the long term, which can stretch the healthcare systems and the national economy as well. The psychological effect on the individual, family, and community can lead to further mental health issues. According to studies, poor responses to TB can exacerbate mental illness, and the treatment needs to be integrated with both physical and psychological care. The WHO's funding initiatives, for example, in Ukraine, demonstrate the overlap between TB and mental health treatment, underscoring the need for comprehensive approaches that consider various factors of well-being throughout treatment and recovery. Lastly, the importance of studying Tuberculosis today also lies in the making of public health policies and holistic health systems. As countries strive to meet global health goals, the experience in the battle against TB can be leveraged in the prevention of other infectious diseases and public health emergencies. The shared human global history of battling against TB proves that nations and global institutions must collaborate to promote the struggle, resulting in advancements in diagnostics, treatment, and social mobilization. For instance, WHO's work in conflict-affected areas not only assists with emergency responses to TB but also assists with building the capacity of health systems to respond to a variety of public health needs. Facilitating continued research on TB can help stakeholders build resilience in their health infrastructure, expand access to treatment, and improve overall community health. Learning about TB thus not only addresses a vital health concern but also provides the foundation for sustainable gains that are healthy and resilient in the face of emerging global challenges.

7.1. Causes and Transmission

Learning Outcome

1. Bacterial agent: Mycobacterium tuberculosis
2. Modes of transmission
3. Risk factors for infection

The primary cause of tuberculosis (TB) is the *Mycobacterium tuberculosis* bacterium that primarily infects the lungs but can also infect other parts of the body. TB is transmitted from human to human through airborne droplets if an individual who has active pulmonary TB coughs, sneezes, or talks and releases infective droplets into the air. This type of transmission emphasizes the significance of close contact, as prolonged exposure to an infected individual significantly increases a person's risk of infection. Furthermore, are predisposed to being exposed based on social and environmental factors. For instance, children residing in densely populated settings such as orphanages are more prone to latent tuberculosis infection (LTBI), as evidenced by a study where 21.7% of the children in the orphanage tested positive for LTBI without having an active case, necessitating the use of particular screening practices (Mayangsari ASM et al., 2024). The dynamics of TB transmission are further complicated by other factors, such as nutritional status and a history of previous vaccination. Research indicates that children with no BCG vaccine scar, which is meant to provide some protection against TB, are likely to get infected with LTBI. More specifically, the absence of a BCG scar was identified as a risk factor, and an odds ratio of 2.29 also indicated an excellent correlation between non-vaccination and the prevalence of LTBI in vulnerable populations (Mayangsari ASM et al., 2024). The identification highlights the importance of vaccination campaigns as a prophylactic measure in controlling TB transmission, particularly in high-risk populations. In addition, malnutrition and stunting causes are also involved, as those children with an inadequate diet can have compromised immune systems, which predispose them to TB infection. Beyond individual factors, healthcare accessibility and societal structure are also among the determinants affecting TB transmission dynamics. Issues such as poor support from families and low socioeconomic status can create non-adherence to treatment, hence perpetuating TB transmission among communities. From studies that investigated barriers to successful TB treatment, determinants including older age, male sex, and lower education level correlate with a higher risk of treatment non-adherence, which subsequently informs ongoing transmission levels. These issues can be addressed in society through education campaigns and community support interventions, thereby ensuring higher adherence to treatment regimens for TB and consequently reducing transmission. With TB being one of the top global health concerns, the strategy of attempting to investigate both biological and societal determinants is essential for effective prevention and control of this infectious disease.

7.1.1. Bacterial Agent: Mycobacterium Tuberculosis

The etiological agent of tuberculosis (TB) and a global public health challenge is the disease bacterium *Mycobacterium tuberculosis*. It is a member of the family Mycobacteriaceae and possesses a unique cell wall that is highly lipophilic, rendering the bacterium virulent and antibiotic-resistant. *M. tuberculosis* is an intracellular pathogen that is highly efficient at infecting host macrophages, where it evades the host immune system. This ability to survive within phagocytic cells is key to its pathogenicity. Recent research has elucidated the intricate relationships between

M. tuberculosis and immunocompetent cells, particularly macrophages, as being pivotal to an understanding of these interactions and the development of improved therapeutic interventions for TB. The pathogenic mechanisms employed by M. tuberculosis underscore the complexity of host-pathogen interactions that contribute to disease formation and regulation. Gene regulation is at the heart of *M. tuberculosis* pathogenicity. Chromosome conformation capture technologies, such as Hi-C, have uncovered the three-dimensional structure of the bacterial genome, which plays a central role in understanding its gene regulation mechanisms. Comparative analyses between the virulent H37Rv and the avirulent H37Ra strains revealed dramatic differences in genome architecture, most probably contributing to virulence attenuation in H37Ra. For instance, H37Rv exhibits a larger size of chromosome interaction domains (CID) and gene expression profiles with distinct features that correlate with its virulent phenotype, whereas H37Ra displays a systemic reorganization of CIDs with an impact on virulence gene expression. These observations suggest that the genomic topological patterns may be key determinants of the pathogenic potential of *M. tuberculosis*, indicating possible directions for therapeutic intervention against TB (Mishra et al., 2025). Furthermore, the host-immune response interaction by *M. tuberculosis* is a central problem in TB pathogenesis. The *M. tuberculosis* secreted proteins, particularly early secretory antigen target 6 (ESTA6) and culture filtrate protein 10 (CFP-10), are crucial antigens for immunodiagnosis and understanding the mechanisms of immune evasion by the bacterium. Research has established that CFP-10 is highly efficacious in enhancing the phagocytic activity of murine macrophages, inducing the pro-inflammatory cytokines TNF-α and IL-6. The activation of the macrophages was regulated through mTORC2 pathway-dependent signaling mechanisms, which witness the sophistication of mechanisms adopted by *M. tuberculosis* in utilizing host immune responses for its survival. The information gained by studying these interactions and the molecular processes that are involved is critical in developing new immunotherapies and diagnostic reagents for the effective treatment of tuberculosis (Huang et al., 2025).

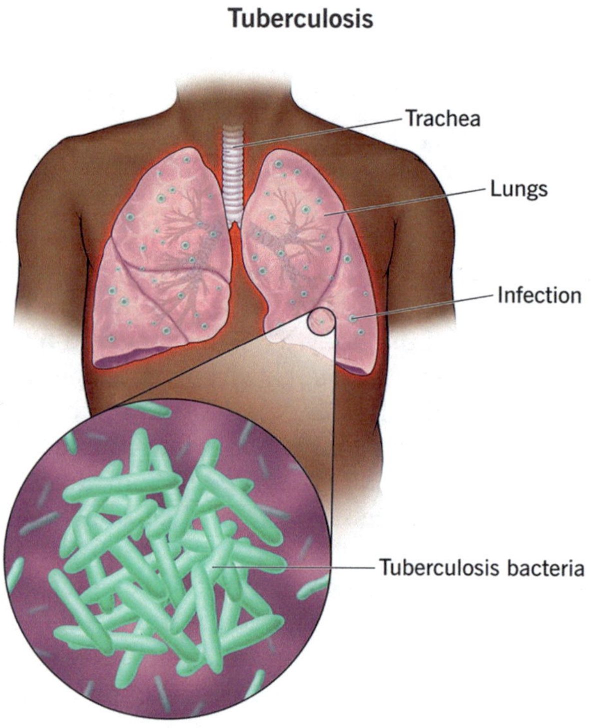

Figure 7.3. Bacterial agent: *Mycobacterium tuberculosis.*

Source: https://my.clevelandclinic.org/-/scassets/images/org/health/articles/11301-tuberculosis

7.1.2. Modes of Transmission

The modes of transmission of tuberculosis (TB) are fundamental to understanding its spread and disease control. TB is primarily transmitted through droplets in the air when a person with TB coughs or sneezes, expelling microscopic droplets that carry *Mycobacterium tuberculosis.* The droplets remain suspended in the air for a considerable time and are inhaled by people in contact. Thus, intimate contact in close quarters significantly increases the risk of transmission, particularly in crowded urban settings. Furthermore, host behavioral differences, social interaction, and public health infrastructure can influence the patterns of transmission, necessitating higher specificity in epidemiology modeling. With an emphasis on physical influence of these factors, scientists can develop more effective measures of controlling TB transmission within a population (Semianiv et al., 2024). The understanding of transmission of TB has been enhanced by the utilization of more advanced techniques, such as whole genome sequencing (WGS), which allows improved source tracking of infection and transmission pathways. A report spanning a decade in the eastern part of China illustrates this enhancement, where 2,114 *M. tuberculosis* strains were sampled and analyzed. Genetic clustering among the strains was identified in the study as indicative of recent transmission, with certain populations, such as students, showing higher rates of recent infection. This highlights the importance of targeting high-risk populations for intervention and developing strategies tailored to their specific circumstances (Yin et al., 2024). By using these techniques, public health workers are better equipped to accurately identify patterns of transmission and risk factors, enabling them to provide information that informs effective prevention strategies to curb TB outbreaks. Spatial patterns of TB transmission are also of significant concern for public health planning. Research has identified certain geographic areas as being at higher risk of *M. tuberculosis* transmission using techniques such as kernel density estimation and K-function analysis. In the same study in eastern China, locations such as Haizhou, Donghai, and Guanyun exhibited intense clustering of recent transmission cases. Public health authorities can apply targeted interventions, mobilizing the community and using communication appropriate to the locality, if mapped. These strategic measures enhance the efficiency of resource utilization, ensuring that efforts to curb TB transmission are focused and productive, thereby contributing to the overall goal of reducing TB incidence globally (Yin et al., 2024).

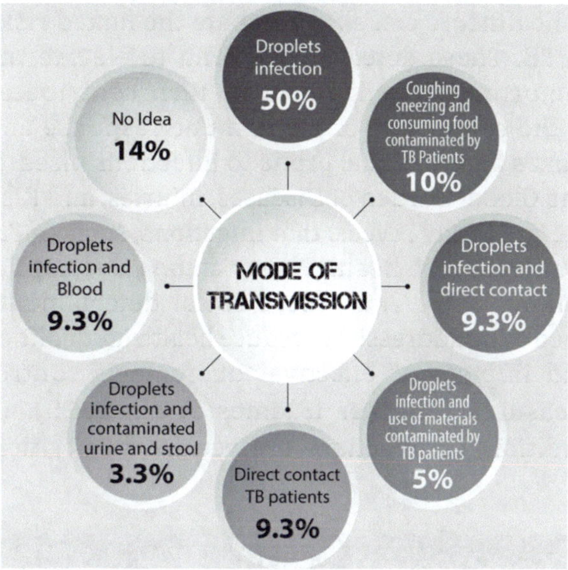

Figure 7.4. The modes of transmission of tuberculosis (TB).

Source: https://patientawareness.in/wp-content/uploads/2019/10/tuberculosis_img6.webp

7.1.3. Risk Factors For Infection

Understanding the risk factors for acquiring tuberculosis (TB) infection is crucial to its prevention and control. Among the most significant risk determinants is the health of an individual's immune system. The infant, for example, has been seen to be particularly vulnerable, with studies indicating that activation of the immune system could significantly increase the risk of acquiring TB disease. A case-control study demonstrated that the immune response elicited by cytomegalovirus (CMV) is associated with enhanced CD8+ T cell activation, equating to a double risk of TB diagnosis in infants. The above discovery highlights the importance of infant immune status, suggesting that immune response interventions could be a valuable strategy for curbing TB infections among children, particularly in TB-endemic areas (Julius Müller et al., 2019). Social determinants also play an essential role in susceptibility to TB infection. Poverty, housing, and poor access to healthcare can all exacerbate the linked risks of TB. These determinants tend to elevate the comorbidity level, which in turn contributes to the complexity of the immune response and makes an individual prone to infectious disease. The Global Burden of Diseases, Injuries, and Risk Factors Study reveals that infections, such as TB, remain severe health issues among developing communities. Thus, these social determinants need to be addressed to reduce health inequalities and implement effective tuberculosis control measures (Spencer L James et al., 2018). In addition, co-infections are yet another critical risk factor for tuberculosis. Diseases such as HIV and certain viral infections can potentially destroy immune defenses and thus contribute to increased risks of TB progressing from latent infection into active disease. Research has indicated that HIV co-infected individuals are at significantly increased risk of TB, which complicates their clinical management and disease outcomes. The combination of viral infections, immunocompromised states, and TB infection highlights the complexity of disease susceptibility. General strategies that encompass the prevention of TB, as well as the management of co-infection, are critical in the global fight against tuberculosis, enhancing patient outcomes and reducing transmission rates effectively (Julius Müller et al., 2019).

Test Your Knowledge

1. What is Mycobacterium tuberculosis?
2. What are the risk factors for infection?

7.2. Symptoms and Diagnosis

Learning Outcome

1. Common symptoms of Tuberculosis
2. Diagnostic tests and procedures
3. Challenges in diagnosing Tuberculosis

The clinical presentation of TB is often bewildering due to its nonspecific symptoms and polymorphism that overlap with other conditions. The patients typically present with chronic cough, often accompanied by hemoptysis, weight loss, and fever. The nonspecific presentation may lead to early misdiagnosis, particularly when fever of unknown origin (FUO) is being considered. Studies have found that in classical FUO patients, infectious diseases constitute a high proportion of the cases, with about 19.50% being due to tuberculosis. Thus, making the diagnosis of TB from the rest of the potential FUO causes requires accurate study of clinical features because TB presents a symptomatology that could be indistinguishable from cancer and other systemic illnesses (Zhou et al., 2020). Proper evaluation is of utmost importance, as early diagnosis directly influences the effectiveness of therapy and the outcome of patients. Diagnoses for tuberculosis are multifaceted and dependent upon a combination of clinical evaluation, radiographic examination, and microbiologic testing. Diagnosis of TB, in a significant number of instances, depends upon chest X-rays, which can detect typical features like cavitary lesions or infiltrates. Moreover, microbiological proof, as demonstrated by sputum smear microscopy, culture, and nucleic acid amplification tests, plays a vital role in establishing the diagnosis. As TB may masquerade as lymphoma and other infections, reliance on tests specific to tuberculosis must be employed to establish an accurate diagnosis (Zhou et al., 2020). Additionally, newer techniques such as polymerase chain reaction (PCR) can enhance detection, especially in smear-negative individuals. The application of these approaches enables clinicians to navigate the complexities in diagnosing TB when it coexists with other similarly occurring infectious diseases. With a rising number of cases being reported globally, the need for early and accurate tuberculosis diagnosis remains a priority. As presentations can progress to more complicated pulmonary complications if not addressed promptly, the implications of delayed diagnosis cannot be overstated. Moreover, the understanding that the majority of patients can initially experience nonspecific symptoms can lead to a more aggressive protocol in clinics. The interaction between systemic inflammation and the immune response, elucidated in other conditions such as COVID-19, emphasizes the need for careful monitoring of inflammatory markers, which could potentially be incorporated into TB diagnosis as well. Finally, increasing awareness of TB symptoms and maximizing diagnostic procedures will be crucial in the fight against the disease and preventing it from spreading within communities.

7.2.1. Common Symptoms of Tuberculosis

Tuberculosis (TB), a chronic infection caused primarily by Mycobacterium tuberculosis, presents with a range of symptoms, often of insidious onset. The most common presentation is a persistent cough lasting more than three weeks, occasionally accompanied by haemoptysis or dyspnoea. This respiratory involvement may also lead to chest pain and general malaise, and therefore, it is necessary for health workers to have a suspicion of TB, particularly in high-risk groups. Additionally, systemic manifestations such as fever, chills, night sweats, and unexplained weight loss may complicate the clinical picture. Identification of these symptoms at an early stage is crucial as they are indicators to doctors to initiate further investigation into the patients' health and exclude the possibility of TB infection, especially in endemic regions (Maharani PIP et al., 2021). Other than pulmonary manifestation, tuberculosis may infect other organ systems and extrapulmonary signs may complicate diagnosis. Abdominal tuberculosis is widespread, and it may present with nonspecific symptoms like abdominal pain, swelling, and gastrointestinal alteration. The patient may experience changes in appetite and weight loss secondary to chronic inflammatory processes or malabsorption. Although extrapulmonary TB is possibly more difficult to diagnose due to the nonspecificity of presentation, it is regularly necessary to consider TB in the setting of these presentations when epidemiology is considered. Failure to recognize these symptoms results in delays in treatment, generating more profound complications and a greater public health hazard (Debi et al., 2020). A well-rounded knowledge of the heterogeneous presentations of tuberculosis is thus vital in managing and treating the disease. Tuberculosis also produces musculoskeletal symptoms in some instances, particularly in disseminated or extra-pulmonary TB, with high morbidity. Symptoms may include spinal pain, joint swelling, and restricted motion, typically caused by inflammation such as osteomyelitis and septic arthritis. Such a complication is most frequent when the spine is involved, resulting in neurological compromise because of compression of adjacent structures. The nature of such musculoskeletal symptoms leads to the requirement that clinicians maintain a broad differential diagnosis when encountering patients with chronic pain and systemic symptoms. Given the high incidence of musculoskeletal TB as well as the high risk of serious consequences in case it is not treated, there is a need for healthcare providers to monitor closely these presentations among exposed populations, once more highlighting the need for early diagnosis and treatment (Maharani PIP et al., 2021).

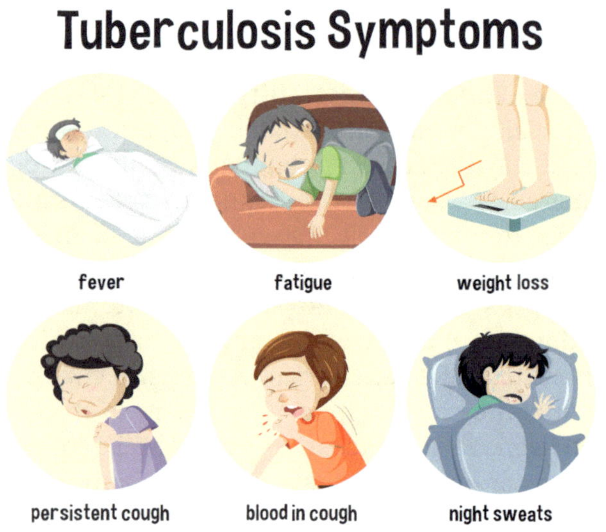

Figure 7.5. Common symptoms of tuberculosis.

Source: https://www.yashodahealthcare.com/blogs/wp-content/uploads/2023/04/Tuberculosis-scaled.jpg

7.2.2. Diagnostic Tests and Procedures

Effective diagnostic tests and examination methods are crucial in controlling tuberculosis (TB), as they determine treatment outcomes and the transmission of the infectious disease. Traditional diagnostic methods, such as sputum smear microscopy, culture, and chest X-rays, have long dominated TB diagnosis. However, such methods prove ineffective in terms of sensitivity, particularly in controlling extrapulmonary tuberculosis (EPTB) and in pediatric patients. A study from a tertiary care center revealed that while the vast majority of pediatric TB was EPTB, only 11.25% were confirmed microbiologically using advanced methods like CBNAAT, reflecting the limitations of the current practices. This emphasizes the urgency of novel diagnostic approaches that can enhance precision and accessibility in TB detection, particularly in economically deprived regions where TB incidence is significantly high (Ramanthan et al., 2025). The introduction of molecular diagnostic technology has been a significant landmark in TB detection, with the use of nucleic acid amplification tests (NAATs) as the primary driver. These tests give rapid results and greater sensitivity and specificity, which are very important in diagnosing pulmonary and EPTB forms of TB. Additionally, recent research indicates that breath analysis has enormous potential as a non-invasive diagnostic tool, which can bypass some of the shortcomings of the traditional sampling methods. Breath analysis, in its current state, is a nascent field that relies on the detection of specific biomarkers present in exhaled breath, a field of TB diagnosis that is also relatively new. However, the technology would need to undergo rigorous validation and standardization if it were to be acceptable and useful across a broad spectrum of clinical settings (Lotte W Nijman et al., 2025). These advancements are crucial for improved diagnosis, treatment initiation, and risk reduction for drug-resistant TB strains. Furthermore, diagnostic approaches must be complemented by a strong understanding of epidemiological and clinical contexts in which cases of TB are encountered. Socioeconomic determinants such as malnutrition and accessibility to healthcare cannot be overstated, especially in rural communities where the incidence of TB is exceptionally high. The recent evidence of frequent EPTB among affected children thus further supports this nexus, and targeted public health interventions are now amply justified. The integration of advanced diagnostics with nutritional management and health education at the community level would greatly enhance TB management outcomes. Streamlining diagnostic procedures, along with the fortification of intervention components, is necessary to counter the multifaceted challenges posed by TB, as well as to ensure timely and effective containment and treatment modalities (Ramanthan et al., 2025).

7.2.3. Challenges in Diagnosing Tuberculosis

Diagnosis of tuberculosis (TB) is challenging due to the existence of various factors that render it difficult to obtain a timely and correct diagnosis. Traditional procedures for TB diagnosis, such as smear microscopy and culture techniques, are insensitive for identifying active infections, particularly in individuals with low bacterial loads. Such a restriction is particularly problematic given that it's estimated that nearly one-third of the global population harbors the TB bacillus, *Mycobacterium tuberculosis*, and that its early detection is crucial to limiting its transmission. The fact that patients tend to come in with non-specific symptoms, such as cough and fever, contributes to the difficulties faced by healthcare professionals in making timely and effective diagnoses. Therefore, the delay in detecting active cases can lead to ongoing transmission between communities, particularly in high-burden populations. Another aspect to TB diagnosis is the emergence of antibiotic-resistant strains, which also calls for a shift towards more sophisticated testing techniques. Diagnostic tools available for use for tuberculosis are not as rapid and sensitive as needed to combat the current tuberculosis epidemic successfully.

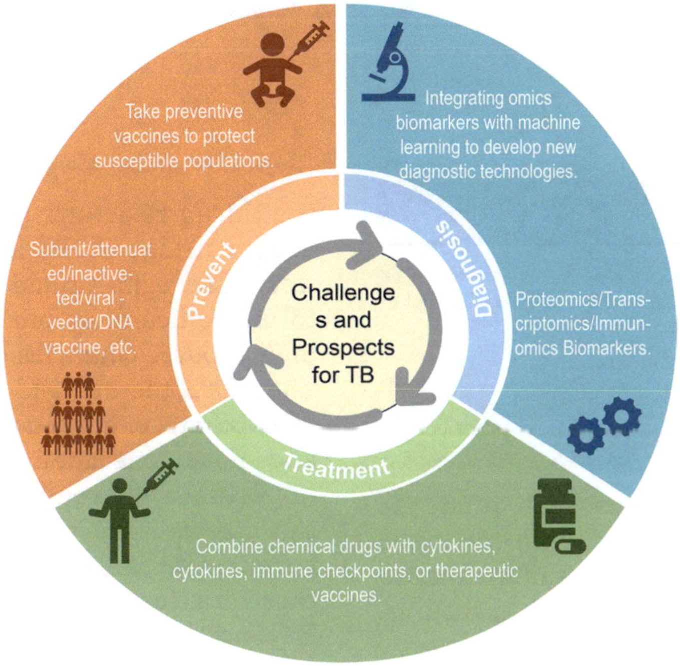

Figure 7.6. Challenges in diagnosing tuberculosis.

Source: https://onlinelibrary.wiley.com/cms/asset/dd99722f-074e-401b-847b-190a55231d0f/mCO$_2$419-fig-0003-m.jpg

Real-time Polymerase Chain Reaction (RT-PCR) promises quick and targeted diagnosis; however, it is often impeded by the waxy and resistant nature of the mycobacterial membrane, which prevents the amplification of sufficient genomic DNA. More recent approaches, like the employment of recombinant TDM-specific hydrolase (rTDMH) to facilitate rapid lysis of bacterial cells, have shown promise to enhance the efficiency of RT-PCR. By addressing these factors, it may be possible to create a more sensitive diagnostic tool to be able to play a vital role in the combat against TB and its entailments, such as morbidity and mortality rates. Apart from that, the combination of high-end diagnostic techniques, such as clinical metagenomic next-generation sequencing (mNGS), can revolutionize the field of TB diagnostics. This method enables a comprehensive examination of both microbial and host genomic material, providing information that cannot be obtained through traditional methods. While promising, the use of mNGS in clinical settings is burdened by several challenges, including the need for an expert knowledge base, expense, and integration with routine laboratory protocols. Success in this area is contingent upon overcoming these hurdles and providing assurance that healthcare systems will be positioned to facilitate long-term improvements in TB diagnostics. Thus, enhancing diagnosis capacity is not merely central to maximizing patient outcomes but also crucial in public health initiatives on controlling and eventually eliminating tuberculosis as a health crisis across the world (Chiu et al., 2019) (Bhatti et al., 2012).

Test Your Knowledge

1. What are the common symptoms of tuberculosis?
2. Write the challenges in diagnosing tuberculosis.

7.3. Treatment Options

Learning Outcome

1. Standard treatment regimens
2. Drug-resistant tuberculosis
3. Importance of adherence to treatment

Effective TB treatment has seen immense progress in the past decades, with increased impetus largely drawn from advancements in medical science and public health measures. The core of TB treatment remains the directly observed treatment short course (DOTS) scheme, with emphasis on patient adherence and correct drug usage. This strategy has achieved very high cure rates in most nations and, since the beginning of the 2000s, has been linked to a worldwide decline in the incidence of tuberculosis. However, the emergence of multidrug-resistant (MDR) and extensively drug-resistant (XDR) tuberculosis complicates treatment regimens and poses severe challenges to public health systems, particularly those of low-resource countries (Abubakar et al., 2012). Therefore, the demand for new strategies that incorporate enhanced diagnostic mechanisms and novel therapeutic drugs is of utmost importance in treating these new strains of the disease. The treatment of drug-resistant tuberculosis calls for an integrated approach that transcends normal treatment processes. Beyond the standard first-line antibiotics, MDR and XDR tuberculosis therapy typically involves the administration of second-line drugs, which could be more costly and less tolerable. To control effectively, health systems must provide sufficient laboratory facilities and drug resistance testing apparatus, particularly in high-endemicity settings where resistant strains are prevalent. The complexities of MDR and XDR treatment mirror the urgent need for improved health services (Abubakar et al., 2012). Improved healthcare infrastructure not only enhances patient outcomes but also mitigates the economic burden of lengthy treatment protocols and rising healthcare costs, underscoring the indispensable intersection of health policy and disease management. In addition, the prevention of developing and spreading drug-resistant tuberculosis necessitates robust public health measures in the form of education and awareness. The development of policies and interventions through the implementation of preventive strategies, such as vaccination, early diagnosis, and public awareness campaigns, can significantly reduce the rates of transmission. Collaboration among various stakeholders—governments, non-profit organizations, and international health agencies—is also necessary for implementing an effective package of interventions that addresses the complexity of tuberculosis and treatment. Knowledge-sharing initiatives, as are pursued in projects that assess the impact of TB on public health, can be leveraged to inform policy and maximize resource allocation. Therefore, a treatment strategy that is multi-faceted, with prevention, early detection, and improved care for drug-resistant cases, is pivotal in combating the epidemic of tuberculosis and ultimately achieving better health outcomes globally.

7.3.1. Standard Treatment Regimens

Control of tuberculosis (TB) has undergone significant transformation since its inception, with regular regimens now forming the foundation of successful control. The most universally used regimen of treatment is the combination of antibiotics administered over a period of six months, which includes isoniazid, rifampicin, ethambutol, and pyrazinamide, referred to as the RHZE regimen. The rationale for combination therapy is to prevent the emergence of drug-resistant organisms and to achieve a wider therapeutic effect by targeting multiple metabolic pathways of the *Mycobacterium tuberculosis* organism. The regimen must be strictly adhered to, as irregularity can lead to treatment failure and the emergence of multidrug-resistant tuberculosis (MDR-TB), necessitating more complex and more extended treatment regimens in the affected individuals. In multidrug-resistant TB, the regimens become complex and more individualized. In multidrug-resistant tuberculosis (MDR-TB) patients, shorter, modified regimens are useful. Studies have demonstrated high success rates with regimens such as the modified short-course regimen (mSCR) and BPaLM treatment, with mSCR achieving a success rate of approximately 90.7% in patients (Yatskevich et al., 2023). These regimens routinely employ active agents such as bedaquiline, linezolid, and levofloxacin, which have high activity against resistant strains. The reduced duration of the treatment regimens not only seeks to improve compliance but also reduces the potential for adverse effects, providing a promising alternative to conventional and prolonged treatments where extensive resistance is present. Greater research into treatment regimens for pre-XDR and MDR-TB patients has cast further illumination on the role of surgery in treatment regimens. A prospective investigation into adolescent MDR/pre-XDR TB highlighted the use of short-course chemotherapy—with accompanying surgical intervention—leading to successful outcomes in a significant majority of instances (Ovsyankina et al., 2024). Specifically, the evidence indicated that short-course chemotherapy was often sufficient, with relapse rates no different from continued chemotherapy. Therefore, the addition of surgery may be a valuable adjunct to drug treatment, catering to patients' differing needs and possibly lowering the overall drug-resistant tuberculosis burden. This combined approach underscores the need for individualizing treatment regimens based on patient-specific characteristics to optimize therapeutic outcomes.

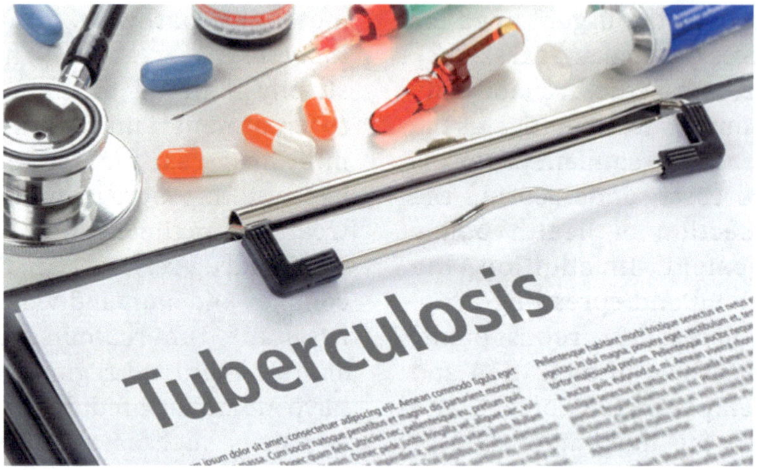

Figure 7.7. Standard treatment regimens for tuberculosis.

Source: https://hospitalhealthcare.com/wp-content/uploads/2023/03/Shorter-tuberculosis-treatment-strategy-non-inferior-to-standard-regimen.jpg

7.3.2. Drug-Resistant Tuberculosis

Drug-resistant tuberculosis (TB) poses an impressive threat to health systems around the world, being difficult to control and eliminate the infectious disease. Drug-resistant types, particularly multidrug-resistant tuberculosis (MDR-TB), occur primarily as a result of poor treatment regimens, antibiotic misuse, and prolonged exposure to anti-TB drugs. The World Health Organization (WHO) has reported an acute increase in MDR-TB infections, i.e., resistance to both isoniazid and rifampicin, the two most effective first-line medicines. This is not merely a product of medical misuse; it is also mixed up with socioeconomic factors that make it difficult to access proper medical care. With the advancement of drug resistance, the success probability of treatment declines, and there is a need for new strategies to combat this dynamic challenge (Jin D, 2025). Public health interventions and community engagement are interrelated in fixing the root causes of drug resistance. Molecular mechanisms of drug resistance in *Mycobacterium tuberculosis* are complex, with genetic mutation being the primary driver. These mutations can alter sites of antibiotic targets, reduce drug permeability, and enhance drug efflux through specialized pumps. Understanding these mechanisms is crucial for identifying new therapeutic strategies. New studies have unraveled how biofilm development is involved in the persistence of drug-resistant strains, making them less susceptible to immune responses and antibiotics too. Apart from this, the resistance mechanisms enable a subset of bacteria to survive after treatment, with implications for persistent transmission in communities. Due to these challenges, researchers are seeking adjunctive therapies that modulate the host immune response in conjunction with standard antibiotic regimens, emphasizing a more synergistic approach to treating drug-resistant tuberculosis (Omoteso et al., 2025). The multi-faceted approach has the potential to maximize therapeutic effect and enhance patient outcomes. Treating drug-resistant tuberculosis entails significant breakthroughs in drug discovery and delivery systems. Standardized regimens of MDR-TB are typically long treatment courses with less effective and more toxic second-line drugs. Recent breakthroughs in drug formulation and delivery, particularly the application of nanotechnology, offer promising means of maximizing the bioavailability of these treatments. Nanoparticle-based platforms can potentially facilitate target delivery, allowing therapeutic levels at infection sites more efficiently with fewer systemic side effects. In addition, personalized medicine approaches, founded on host and pathogen genomic information, enable individualized treatment regimens tailored to meet the unique needs of each patient. As we continue to face the dual challenge of drug-resistant TB and patient non-compliance, multidisciplinary collaboration and innovative research will be crucial in developing efficient, cost-effective, and sustainable solutions in the fight against this public health threat (Jin D, 2025; Omoteso et al., 2025).

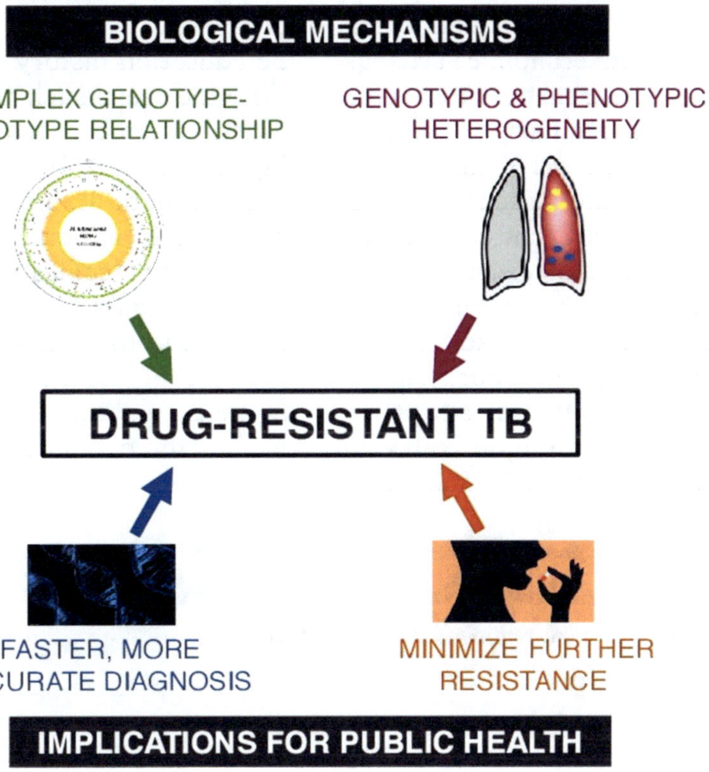

Figure 7.8. Drug-resistant tuberculosis.

Source: https://ars.els-cdn.com/content/image/1-s2.0-S1471489217301571-fx1.jpg

7.3.3. Importance of Adherence To Treatment

Drug compliance is a vital factor in the successful treatment of tuberculosis (TB), a disease-causing agent that continues to pose a significant public health risk at the global level. Successful treatment depends on a patient's sustained and complete compliance with medication regimens, which are typically six months in duration. Incompliance can have terrorizing outcomes, from failure of treatment to increased transmission risk and development of multidrug-resistant (MDR) TB strains. These strains that are resistant to multiple drugs do not only complicate the outcome in a given patient but are also more risky to global health and more costly and complex to treat. Poor compliance, for instance, adds to increased infectiousness, which complicates the public health issue of TB, prompting overall intervention by health systems to enhance treatment adherence by affected individuals (Elmuttalut M, 2024). A variety of complicated influences shape TB treatment adherence, and for this reason, a detailed understanding of patients' experiences is necessary. Healthcare access, mental health, and socioeconomic status all have significant effects on a patient's ability to adhere to treatment. Patients with poor education or health literacy, for example, will struggle to grasp the reasons why they need to complete their regimens. Second, those with economic hardship may not be able to afford transport to health centers or obtain drugs regularly. A review of literature indicates that the combination of strategies centered on the patient, such as Directly Observed Therapy (DOT) and community interventions, can enhance adherence through the provision of help in pragmatic terms that follow individualized patient needs. Addressing these diverse barriers, as corroborated by exhaustive evidence, highlights adopting strategies that consider the unique traits of each patient (Elmuttalut M, 2024). Furthermore, advanced technological advancements have accompanying prospects for improving compliance to TB treatment. The utilization of machine learning techniques has been shown to be effective in identifying patients at risk of loss to follow-up (LTFU), thereby making it easier to enact targeted interventions that can improve compliance rates. For example, research using models like XGBoost has identified some of the most influential predictors of LTFU to be education history and insurance for health. With the use of such predictive models, medical practitioners can actively target patients with higher risk factors, adjusting support systems according to their needs. Such technology-based interventions, in addition to enhancing treatment outcomes for individual patients, also aid in overall public health programs aimed at preventing the transmission of TB. Therefore, the use of technology in managing TB has immense potential to facilitate adherence as well as the overall efficacy of treatments.

Test Your Knowledge

1. What are the standard treatment regimens for tuberculosis?
2. What is drug-resistant tuberculosis?

7.4. Global Impact

Learning Outcome

1. Prevalence of tuberculosis worldwide
2. Socioeconomic factors influencing spread
3. Public health initiatives and their effectiveness

The global impact of tuberculosis (TB) extends beyond the health of people to influence economic and social systems within populations. With an estimated quarter of the global population infected, the disease selectively strikes low- and middle-income countries, where healthcare is typically strained. The economic burden of TB is significant; it contributes not only to healthcare costs but also to loss of productivity due to morbidity and mortality. In addition, social stigma for TB aggravates social inequality, such that it becomes challenging for people to seek necessary treatment and care. Such interlinked matters must be addressed through integrated strategies that utilize both medical and socio-economic levels, prompting the philanthropic sector to provide support for funding proposals aimed at eliminating TB and reducing its global repercussions (Kissane R, 2009). Urbanization is also a major driver of the TB burden globally, as rapidly growing urban areas become settings of high disease incidence. As cities expand, they often face overcrowding, suboptimal housing, and inadequate health infrastructure. These conditions offer a breeding ground for the transmission of TB, particularly in the presence of poor health systems that cannot keep up with increasing populations. According to research, urban living significantly influences health outcomes, with cities' complex dynamics affecting the prevalence and management of diseases like TB. Understanding how urbanization correlates with TB transmission is essential for developing targeted public health interventions that address both the immediate healthcare needs and the underlying social determinants of health. This crossing highlights the importance of unitary planning and policymaking, considering urbanization's multifaceted impact on population health (Freudenberg et al., 2005). Furthermore, international health efforts towards eliminating TB show the importance of international cooperation and dedication towards fighting this problem rooted deep in the world. Global coordination among governments, nongovernmental organizations, and international institutions has led to the establishment of programs aimed at prevention, diagnosis, and treatment. However, the successful implementation of such programs is largely reliant on long-term financing as well as political will. The charitable community, as proposed in health care funding discussions, could provide vital support for multi-decade TB programs with sustained investment (Kissane R, 2009). This forward-looking action emphasizes the need for a multi-factor approach, like holistic policies involving various stakeholders, to reduce the worldwide burden of tuberculosis effectively. While the world is struggling to cope with this perpetual public health scourge, solidarity and shared responsibility have never been more urgently needed.

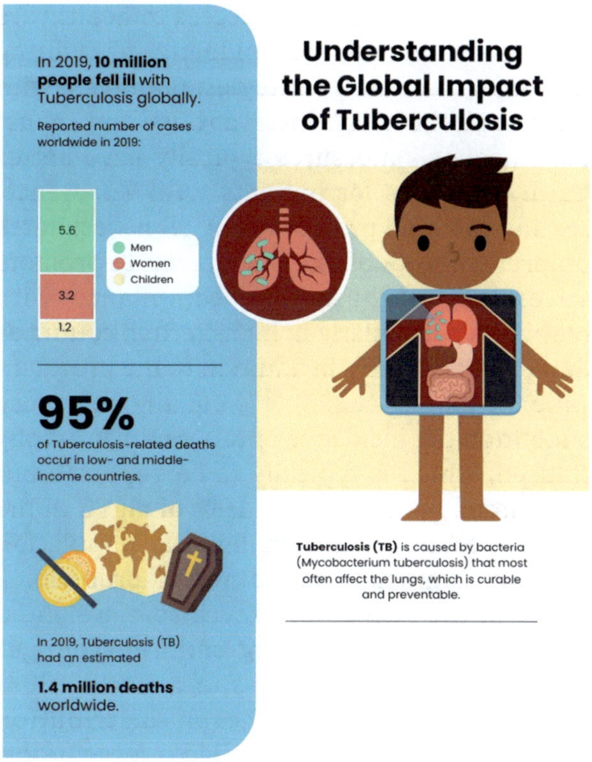

Figure 7.9. The global impact of tuberculosis (TB).

Source: https://cdn.venngage.com/template/thumbnail/full/7c6ce0ab-800e-4679-8ffd-0df9526923bb.webp

7.4.1. Prevalence of Tuberculosis Worldwide

Tuberculosis (TB) is still a primary world health concern with high incidence rates that are affecting populations in resource-poor environments. Around 630,000 new cases of infectious TB are diagnosed each year, highlighting the problem of controlling the disease in both developing and developed nations. India, for instance, is a classic example of the challenge presented by countries lacking proper public health infrastructure. Despite ongoing developments in medicine and pharmacology, infections such as multidrug-resistant tuberculosis (MDR-TB) continue to plague healthcare systems. Social determinants such as poverty and inadequate access to healthcare services exacerbate the epidemic, preventing successful treatment strategies. Countries with effective public health interventions and robust early diagnosis measures typically have better health outcomes for patients with TB. Hence, tackling the high prevalence of TB necessitates comprehensive public health reforms to promote prevention, diagnosis, and compliance with treatment, particularly in high-burden countries (Gamon et al., 2013). In addition to the prevalent epidemic among adults, it is equally necessary to mention the incidence of tuberculosis among children, which is typically underreported but substantial. Approximately 10% of all TB in the world is found in this vulnerable population and is a significant public health problem. A survey in the Philippines revealed a weighted prevalence of 6.4% among children younger than 15 years, with pockets of alarming 29% in some places. Such uneven distribution makes it a rationale for stratified interventions, particularly in geographically peripheral regions with limited healthcare access. The correlation between distance to health facilities and TB incidence indicates that increased accessibility will be paramount to effective treatment and prevention. Outreach programs must therefore be implemented to increase access to care in hard-to-reach areas, facilitating earlier detection and reduced rates of transmission among children and their respective communities (LEINING et al., 2019). TB prevalence also addresses not only short-term health service provision but long-term interventions that can consolidate health in the community. Proper monitoring and timely intervention programs are crucial in regions with high TB rates. Health literacy among community leaders and the general public can also enable people to take charge of their own health. Growing awareness around MDR-TB and its implications is essential, as the strain of the disease makes treatment more difficult and elevates transmission risks. Nations such as India need to take cue from examples of successful models in countries with lower MDR-TB rates by adapting stringent surveillance systems, effective public health policies, and culturally acceptable treatment strategies. Ultimately, a comprehensive strategy that encompasses healthcare access, community education, and policy reform is necessary to effectively curb the global burden of tuberculosis and mitigate its impact on future generations (Gamon et al., 2013).

7.4.2. Socioeconomic Factors Influencing Spread

TB transmission is strongly linked to socioeconomic determinants that enhance risk and susceptibility among populations. Poverty continues to be among the most significant TB transmission drivers, as it creates a fertile environment for conditions favorable to disease spread. Individuals in lower socioeconomic groups have poor access to quality healthcare services, thereby resulting in late identification and treatment of TB. Furthermore, unfavorable living conditions, such as crowding and inadequate ventilation, significantly increase the likelihood of airborne transmission. Health status and socioeconomic conditions paint a grim picture: poor populations are disproportionately affected by infectious diseases, such as TB. Historical data demonstrate that US declines in mortality were strongly correlated with socioeconomic improvements, making it clear that economic stability is a powerful driver of public health improvement and disease burden reduction (Cutler et al.). Education is yet another key socioeconomic factor, influencing TB transmission, awareness, and health-seeking behavior. Lower levels of education typically entail a lack of understanding of TB transmission, symptoms, and the importance of seeking healthcare early. This ignorance is responsible for delayed medical care, facilitating ongoing household and community transmission. Studies have consistently demonstrated that higher levels of education are associated with higher rates of health literacy, allowing the individuals to seek care early and complete treatment more effectively. In addition, educational disparities have a tendency to reflect greater systemic inequalities that are likely to perpetuate the inequity of poverty and ill health. By addressing educational inequality and emphasizing overall health education, interventions can be designed to interrupt the spread of TB in an effort to highlight the intersection of societal determinants of socioeconomic status and disease control interventions (Koskella et al., 2014).

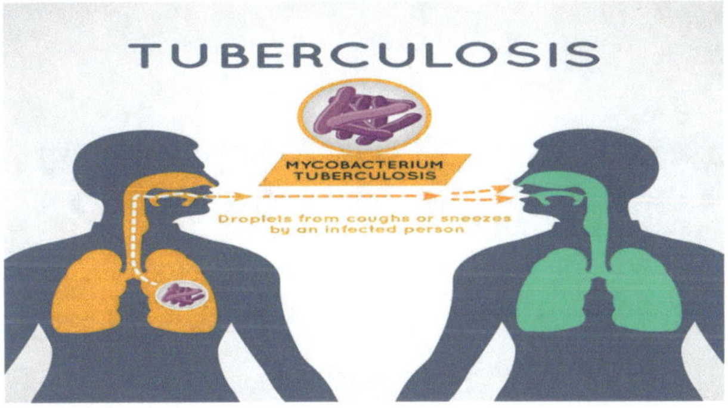

Figure 7.10. The spread of tuberculosis (TB).

Source: https://images.everydayhealth.com/images/lung-respiratory/tuberculosis/tuberculosis-risk-factors-causes-and-prevention-722x406.jpg?sfvrsn=ca8e72b1_1

Public health policy must therefore consider these socioeconomic determinants as a means to combat TB effectively. Focusing interventions on high-risk groups can also extend the impact on disease transmission. For instance, fortifying social support structures in poor communities can improve living conditions and access to healthcare, reducing rates of TB. Additionally, integrating educational programs into community healthcare services can improve awareness and facilitate Successful TB control programs. These programs will not only target the medical aspects of prevention but will also identify and address the broader socioeconomic context that determines the progression of the disease. Ultimately, a strong understanding of the socioeconomic determinants that influence TB transmission is crucial for developing effective public health interventions and reducing the disease's global burden (Cutler et al.).

7.4.3. Public Health Initiatives and Their Effectiveness

Public health interventions play an important role in combating infectious diseases, and one such disease is tuberculosis (TB), because it is found extensively across the globe. Effective interventions are often multipronged with treatment, prevention, and education. Directly observed therapy (DOT), for instance, has been proven to be highly effective in ensuring drug compliance among TB patients. Not only does this type of strategy improve specific individual health outcomes, but it also contributes to the broader goal of reducing transmission rates at the community level. The success of public health efforts relies not just on the medical treatments themselves, but on the combination of bringing people in the community together with resources. To have the most significant effect, tailoring messages and knowledge of local context are key because it makes populations concerned confident and actively engaged. Despite the achievements attributed to many programs, there are often challenges in implementation that render them overall ineffectual. For example, there may not be an adequate supply of medicines and medical supplies within public health facilities, and this has a direct impact on TB outcomes. The case of Tanzania's Prime Vendor System (PVS) is a concrete manifestation of this issue. Although the PVS was designed to enhance supply chain effectiveness, recent evaluations revealed that it was unable to meet the demand for essential drugs, with a mean availability level of only 74.8% across the facilities. In addition, health facilities reported that 80% of them experienced shortages, underscoring the urgent need for reliable and consistent supply chains to support public health programs in meeting their intended objectives. These results highlight the need to address infrastructural and logistical issues in health systems to improve the effectiveness of TB control activities for vulnerable groups. The application of digital technology in public health strategies carries promising potential for enhancing the efficiency of TB programs. As highlighted in discussions in Digital Public Health (DiPH) debates, the common language among actors is essential in breaking through the intricacies of health interventions. Clear communication facilitates interdisciplinary partnerships tailor culturally sensitive strategies that target diverse groups. For example, enhanced education regarding digital tools can improve follow-up of TB patients, enable teleconsultation, and optimize the utilization of available resources. For these opportunities to be fully harnessed, however, it is essential that regulatory standards and mechanisms keep pace with the evolving landscape of digital health. By controlling both terminological accuracy and the structural barriers in healthcare provision, public health interventions can make a significant contribution to population health outcomes for TB and other infectious conditions.

Test Your Knowledge

1. What is the prevalence of tuberculosis worldwide?
2. What are the socioeconomic factors influencing the spread of tuberculosis?

7.5. Prevention Strategies

Learning Outcome

1. Vaccination efforts (BCG vaccine)
2. Screening and early detection
3. Education and awareness campaigns

Successful prevention is the cornerstone of the fight against tuberculosis (TB) due to its global prevalence and the numerous factors that contribute to its dissemination. Multifaceted intervention comprises public health education, vaccination, and targeted interventions in high-risk groups.

Mass campaigns to increase awareness of TB transmission and presentation can significantly enhance early detection and adherence to treatment. Moreover, the BCG vaccine, while not entirely effective in preventing pulmonary TB in adults, remains a crucial tool in reducing the severity and incidence of the disease, particularly among infants and young children. The integration of these strategies ensures that communities are better equipped to combat the spread of TB, aligning with the World Health Organization's goal of eliminating the disease as a public health threat. In parallel with educational measures, the availability of medical facilities is also significant in TB prevention. Having diagnostic units and treatment facilities available throughout the population helps in regulating TB incidence. Community health workers help enhance access by providing education and support, particularly to underprivileged communities. A joint effort with local healthcare centers enhances the delivery of services, highlights the case of drug compliance, and addresses problems that have arisen for patients. From the use of evidence-based research, it is evident that solutions to socio-economic problems experienced by patients undergoing treatment, such as food insecurity and financial difficulties, are essential for building a supportive community for TB patients. By focusing on multidimensional prevention strategies that take into account the individualized challenges experienced by affected individuals, public health interventions with greater involvement and success rates in TB control are achieved, thereby improving health outcomes. New non-pharmacologic interventions have also become integral components of TB prevention. Patient-centered care has been identified by recent research as playing an essential role in ensuring maximum compliance and overall health outcomes. Engagement of patients in treatment regimens not only enhances patient empowerment but also promotes their continued participation in the healthcare process. For example, utilization of community support programs such as peer education and group therapy sessions reduces stigma associated with TB as stated in recent studies. Also, the promotion of healthy behaviors, including a good diet and the avoidance of cigarette smoking, can fortify the immune system, thereby providing another defense against TB infection. The integration of these non-pharmacologic measures with established medical treatment—like routine immunization and early diagnosis—constitutes a holistic program that acts against TB's social as well as biological determinants and ultimately leads to more effective prevention strategies (Choi JY, 2025) (Ondiro et al., 2024).

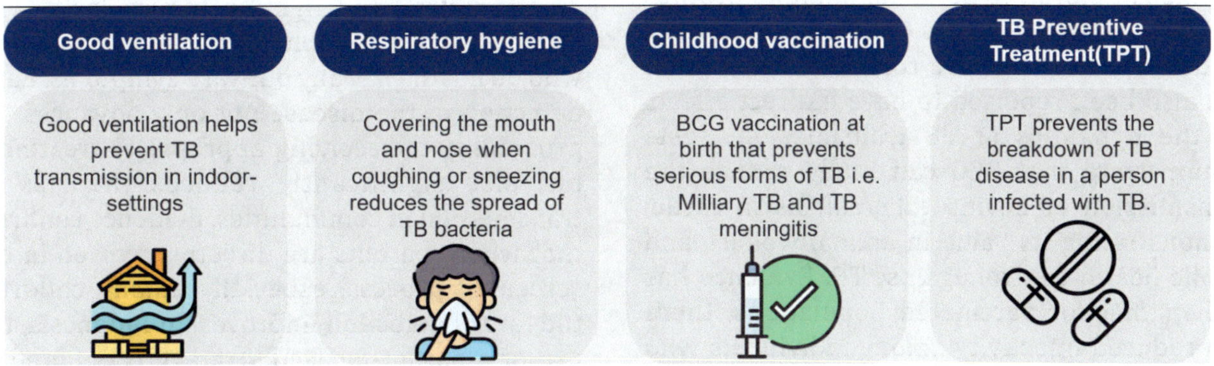

Figure 7.11. Prevention strategies for tuberculosis (TB).

Source: https://ntep.in/sites/default/files/h5p/content/14931/images/file-649bef8db33b8.png

7.5.1. Vaccination Efforts (BCG Vaccine)

The Bacillus Calmette-Guérin (BCG) vaccine has been a valuable tool in the global effort to combat tuberculosis (TB), particularly in protecting infants and young children against severe forms of the disease. Despite being utilized for centuries, since the 1920s, the vaccine's effectiveness has been the subject of intense debate and research. The primary aim of BCG vaccination is to reduce the incidence of severe TB, particularly extrapulmonary forms such as meningitis and disseminated disease in immunocompromised hosts. However, its effectiveness against pulmonary TB, the most common and infectious form of the disease, is weaker, with various studies reporting variable protection rates among different populations and geographic locations. These discrepancies emphasize the complexity of TB epidemiology when coupled with the need for ongoing evaluation of BCG's function in TB control programs, particularly in high-prevalence environments. Recent advances in TB immunology, underlying BCG vaccination, have also shed additional light on its variable impact. The. The study indicates that factors such as when administered and the neonatal immune context can significantly influence the vaccine's performance. Specifically, BCG-induced immune responses in infancy may be undermined by mechanisms such as interleukin-27 (IL-27), an immunosuppressive cytokine that is operational during early life. The implications are significant with respect to the innate memory response of the immune system following BCG vaccination and have repercussions that indicate adjustment of administration regimens may be required in order to optimize long-term protection against *Mycobacterium tuberculosis*. Future research approaches targeting these variables can potentially unlock more effective TB vaccination regimens tailored to personal immune profiles and developmental stages (Fromsa et al., 2024). Aside from its protective role, BCG vaccination has also been reported to have indirect effects on the dynamics of TB transmission. Tests demonstrate that BCG can really reduce the transmission of bovine tuberculosis in cattle, demonstrating its value in animal welfare and public health control against TB. Evidence has shown that for vaccinated populations, there is a reduced infectivity among individuals who fall ill, thus ending the chain of transmission. These results are significant in global TB control programs and particularly where bovine and human TB are found together. Attention to effective vaccination techniques, including potential development and modification of the BCG vaccine, is significant in reducing TB's burden globally. Continued quantification and understanding of these indirect effects will enhance the strategic application of BCG as well as inform future development in vaccines (Fromsa et al., 2024).

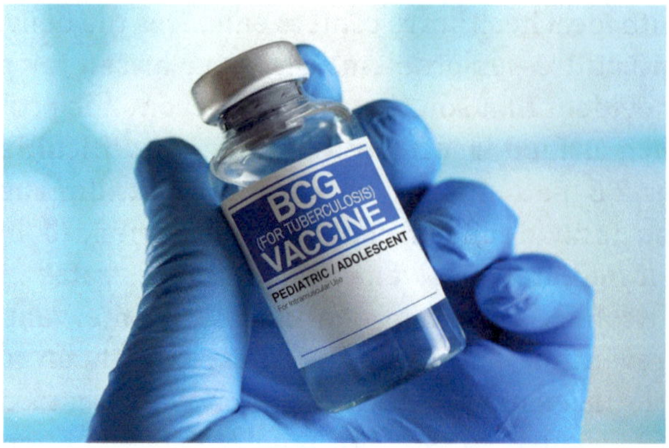

Figure 7.12. Vaccination efforts (BCG vaccine).

Source: https://www.cidrap.umn.edu/sites/default/files/styles/article_detail/public/article/BCG%20vaccine.jpg?itok=Sp98E_gJ

7.5.2. Screening and Early Detection

The screening and early detection process is most important in fighting tuberculosis (TB), especially with its rapid progression in patients who do not display any outward symptoms. Early detection of the disease not only advances the probability of receiving appropriate treatment but also significantly reduces the risk of transmission in communities. Evidence confirms that where parents are directly involved in the screening process, especially among children, the rate of detection improves. In Indonesia, the use of a parent-focused strategy was found to greatly enhance the identification of TB cases among children aged 0-14 years. Through the research, the researchers established increased knowledge and confidence among parents in TB screening, which prompted more effective early detection interventions in the community (Deswita et al., 2024). Hence, utilizing parents to the fullest extent is a key consideration for enhancing public health responses to TB. Additionally, the use of technology in screening processes provides another avenue for optimizing the early detection process. An example of such innovation is the Electronic Screening System (ESS), which offers an efficient process for assessing risk factors for TB in primary care. In private healthcare settings, researchers aimed to determine the feasibility of integrating ESS into existing electronic medical records (EMRs). ScreenMy integration into the EMR system was successful in demonstrating that an electronic device had the capability of streamlining the efficiency of screening procedures, facilitating bi-directional TB-DM assessments, and reducing the process complexity for healthcare professionals (Suryanto et al., 2024). This technology-driven approach not only allows for early detection but also enables health workers to maintain comprehensive patient histories, ultimately allowing for better-informed clinical decision-making regarding TB screening and treatment.

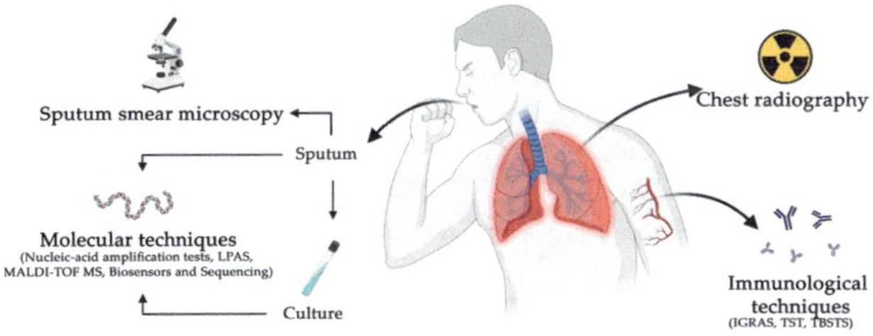

Figure 7.13. Screening and early detection for tuberculosis (TB).

Source: https://pub.mdpi-res.com/diseases/diseases-12-00202/article_deploy/html/images/diseases-12-00202-g001.png?1725351172

Beyond the level of individual cases, the significance of effective screening practices is in their ability to shift community perception of tuberculosis. When screening programs are well implemented, populations have a greater opportunity to instill a culture of awareness and active health-seeking behavior among their people. For instance, the community-based intervention studied in Indonesia demonstrated how well-educated parents could be empowered to take ownership of the screening process and instill a culture that imposes health education and preventive care (Deswita et al., 2024). This not only aids in the detection of cases earlier but can also reduce the stigma that is more commonly related to TB, and be more conducive to supporting individuals who suffer from it. Therefore, improving efforts in screening and early detection through both education and technology not only enhances individual healthcare improvements but also advances community healthcare efforts against tuberculosis.

7.5.3. Education and Awareness Campaigns

Education and awareness programs are crucial in the fight against tuberculosis (TB), as they raise awareness and encourage preventive measures among high-risk groups. They aim to disseminate critical information on TB infection, illness, and treatment, which in turn breaks down stigma barriers and leads to early medical attention. By employing diverse strategies, including public service announcements, community-level workshops, and partnerships with local health organizations, the programs aim to educate individuals about their health. Particularly in areas where there is a high incidence of misinformation, education helps to clear misconceptions surrounding TB, which ultimately leads to improved health-seeking behavior. The effectiveness of such campaigns can be observed in numerous settings, as greater awareness has led to increased levels of testing and treatment compliance, illustrating the appropriate relationship between education and health metrics in the fight against TB. The design and mode of delivery of education and awareness campaigns must be modified to respond to the cultural and social setting of the target groups. This requires a thoughtful awareness of the community's particular needs and challenges, which can be achieved through the facilitation of local stakeholders' collaboration. For instance, the use of indigenous channels of communication, such as regional leaders or community theater, can significantly increase campaign reach and worth. Additionally, the use of technology, such as social media platforms, can facilitate the wider dissemination of information and increased exposure to youth audiences. With a multi-dimensional approach, campaigns can tackle a variety of determinants of health decisions like socio-economic limitations and cultural attitudes, and thus establish an enabling environment for TB control and prevention interventions. Lessons learned from successful education programs in other aspects of public health can provide valuable guidelines for fitting TB awareness drives accordingly. Sustaining the vigor of education and awareness campaigns demands ongoing monitoring and sensitivity to new challenges. Tracking the effectiveness of these interventions is essential to determine their effectiveness and identify areas for improvement. Regular feedback from community members can inform program modification to ensure that messages are heard and remain pertinent. Moreover, eliminating participation barriers, such as limited access to healthcare resources or economic constraints, can enhance participation and effectiveness. Collaborative efforts with the health care providers and decision-makers can also broaden the scope of such campaigns, making them a concerted effort against TB eradication initiatives. As indicated in public health education research, sustained support and advocacy are also crucial for establishing long-term change and a culture of sensitization that can influence behavior towards TB control and prevention (Uniyal DJ, 2024; Debi S Fuadi et al., 2024).

Test Your Knowledge

1. What are the vaccination efforts?
2. What is screening and early detection?

7.6. Current Research and Developments

Learning Outcome

1. Advances in vaccine research
2. New diagnostic technologies
3. Innovative treatment approaches

Current research on tuberculosis (TB) is progressing rapidly, particularly in vaccine development, which is a matter of great importance in combating the disease. As advocated by (Zeng et al., 2023), novel vaccines for *Mycobacterium tuberculosis* (Mtb) are needed immediately since current options, in particular, the Bacillus Calmette-Guérin (BCG) vaccine, are few and of varied efficacy. Latest advances try to gain deeper insight into the most informative antigens, which need to be accorded top priority in vaccine trials. Scientists seek to identify correlates of protection and the important immune responses required for effective vaccination. This approach not only recognizes the demand for improved TB vaccines but also illustrates increased collaboration among international specialists towards streamlining the research process needed to attain the objectives defined in the End TB Strategy. The merging of technology and education represents another line of rigorous research, according to (Zeng et al., 2023). With the advent of new learning methods, the development of personalized learning systems has been a growing area of interest for researchers. The technology is particularly relevant in TB research, where learning complex material needs effective learning mechanisms. Combining artificial intelligence and deep learning in these learning systems has been the most significant trend to offer a personalized learning experience that suits a broad number of learning needs. Through the application of these advanced pedagogical methods, researchers are better equipped to disseminate crucial information on TB prevention, treatment, and care to healthcare workers, thereby enhancing the public's understanding of the disease.

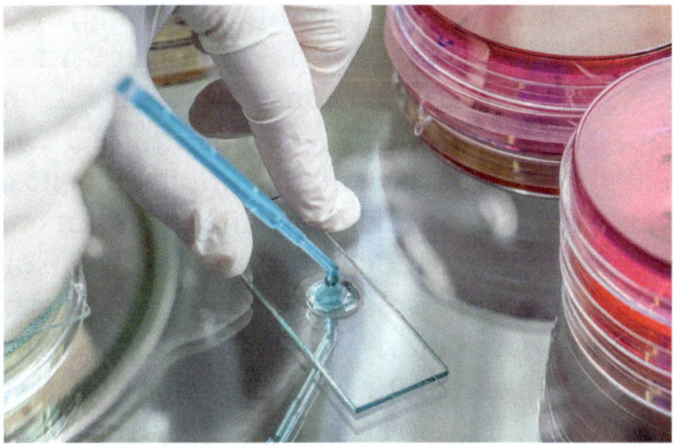

Figure 7.14. Current research and developments of tuberculosis (TB).

Source: https://www.surrey.ac.uk/sites/default/files/styles/1200xauto/public/2021-09/TB%20GettyImages-181394718.jpg?itok=YEfvKFqp

In the area of concerted action, the TB research community has undergone rapid growth. Initiatives such as the recently concluded workshop, co-sponsored by the Stop TB Partnership Working Group on New TB Vaccines (WGNV) and the National Institute of Allergy and Infectious Diseases (NIAID), demonstrate a collaborative approach to overcoming the challenges of TB vaccine development. These sessions allow for the sharing of ideas, experiences, and current information among international experts, as indicated in the workshop conclusions outlined in Young et al., (2023). By focusing on advancements as well as persistent knowledge deficits, these sessions play a crucial role in informing directions for future research, thereby enhancing the collective capability to combat TB. Along with the evolution of the TB research environment, greater collaborative efforts will be required to bridge current knowledge gaps and bring innovative solutions to the table.

7.6.1. Advances in Vaccine Research

Research on vaccines for tuberculosis (TB) has shown significant advances in the last few years, driven by the increasing disease burden and the emergence of drug-resistant strains. Traditional methods, by using the Bacille Calmette-Guérin (BCG) vaccine, have provided limited efficacy, particularly in adults. Thus, new studies should be developed to design the next generation of vaccines that induce more intense and specific immune responses. A focus on multi-antigen vaccines that incorporate a combination of proteins to elicit cellular and humoral immunity is gaining traction. This strategy aims to overcome the limitations of the BCG vaccine and develop a novel immunization paradigm that can more effectively protect diverse populations against TB. With the strength of technology and greater awareness of TB immunobiology, these breakthroughs have the potential to transform the trajectory of TB prevention and control worldwide. Furthermore, the exploration of mRNA vaccine platforms is a revolutionary step towards TB vaccine development. With the success of mRNA vaccines against COVID-19, researchers are adapting these technologies to prevent mycobacterial diseases. The flexibility and brief development period of mRNA vaccines enable a faster response to new TB strains and enhance the potential for regionalization based on local epidemiological data. As attention shifts toward optimizing delivery systems, such as lipid nanoparticles for mRNA vaccines, scientists look forward to the effect on enhanced stability and bioavailability. This groundbreaking approach might pave the way for not only a more effective TB vaccine but also potentially serve as a model for a response to other infectious illnesses, as highlighted by the review of the intersection of infectious disease approaches and novel therapeutic objectives for other pathogens (Hassan et al., 2024). In the wake of such advancements in technology, scientists are compelled to collaborate interdisciplinarily to further decipher the intricacies of TB. Even with innovative platforms of variable design, the multifaceted aspects of TB infection necessitate a comprehensive plan for vaccine development.

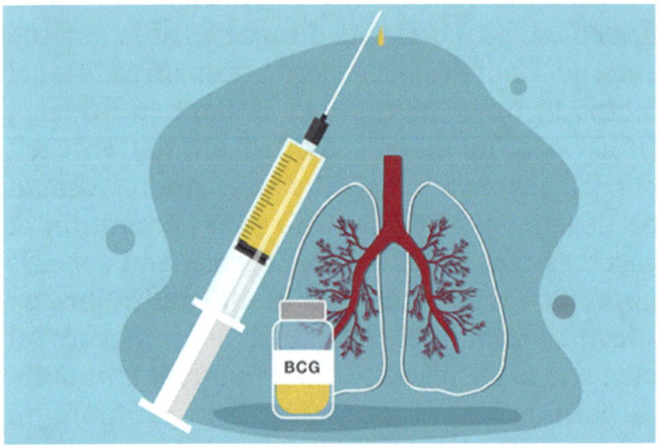

Figure 7.15. Advances in vaccine research of tuberculosis (TB).

Source: https://dug.com/wp-content/uploads/2022/07/image-6.jpg

Deciphering the problems of antigenic variability, population immunity, and the pathophysiological foundation of TB will be decisive in overcoming the constraints of current vaccines. Holistic strategies that involve assessing vaccine efficacy in heterogeneous populations, along with considerations for host-directed therapy, can provide a more effective platform for TB intervention. Such strategies demonstrate a rising awareness of gaps in existing knowledge, coupled with an unrelenting commitment to strengthening research efforts aimed at enhancing TB prevention as well as treatment outcomes (An et al., 2025).

7.6.2. New Diagnostic Technologies

New diagnostic technologies have significantly revolutionized the landscape of tuberculosis (TB) detection and treatment. Molecular tests and imaging modalities are new technologies that enable rapid and accurate diagnosis, which is necessary for timely treatment. For instance, GeneXpert, a widely used molecular diagnostic tool, can detect TB and drug-resistant TB in two hours, serving to bridge the critical time gap often associated with traditional culture-based methods. Additionally, the application of artificial intelligence (AI) in radiology offers significant opportunities for improving diagnostic accuracy. AI-powered algorithms analyze chest radiographs and scans using deep learning techniques to identify TB with great accuracy, surpassing traditional diagnosis techniques. The advanced technologies not only expedite clinical decisions but also ensure optimal utilization of resources in healthcare facilities, particularly in regions beset with rampant cases of TB. AI applications, such as convolutional neural networks (CNNs), are the technological innovations in TB diagnosis. Thousands of radiographic images are analyzed to detect patterns typical of TB using CNNs, providing physicians with a valuable tool. These deep learning algorithms effectively automate image interpretation work, which is typically reliant on skilled human judgment. According to recent literature, such AI systems offer rapid, reproducible outputs, which are especially valuable in low-resource settings where it could be challenging to have experienced radiologists. Utilizing such technologies bypasses the delay in diagnosis and enhances the public health response to TB. As the healthcare system becomes more mature and embraces AI solutions, not only does it improve human functions but also takes the industry to even better TB management and better patient outcomes, thereby shaping the future of diagnostics in infectious diseases. Despite the optimistic outlook for the application of cutting-edge diagnostic technologies, several challenges exist that must be addressed to facilitate their effective utilization. Large, diverse training datasets are needed most acutely, as AI models trained on small datasets don't necessarily transfer to all populations or even all clinical settings. Model interpretability is also important, as healthcare professionals need to be able to understand why an AI-recommended action was taken, so that they can trust and effectively utilize these technologies. Moreover, the incorporation of such advanced systems into existing clinical protocols also poses logistics concerns for medical professionals to plan and train for. As mentioned in the literature, future R&D efforts are needed to develop and enhance AI-based diagnostic systems to achieve accurate precision and reliability, particularly in cases of drug-resistant TB. By overcoming such setbacks, recent diagnostic technologies have the potential to play a crucial role in the global fight against tuberculosis, ultimately leading to healthier lives worldwide.

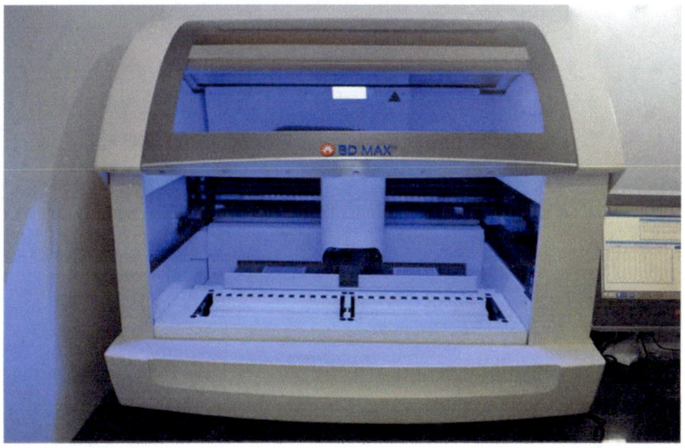

Figure 7.16. New diagnostic technologies of tuberculosis (TB).

Source: https://etimg.etb2bimg.com/photo/98093428.cms

7.6.3. Innovative Treatment Approaches

The emergence of drug-resistant tuberculosis (MDR-TB) has seen treatment policies reviewed, which had depended on a few selected antibiotics. The new treatment options have become some of the most crucial factors in controlling public health diseases. In illustration, developments in drug discovery have resulted in the availability of new drugs such as bedaquiline and delamanid. They not only increase the effectiveness of treatment in treatment-resistant patient strains but are also evidence of increased personalization of medication. The application of treatments decreases the frequency of developing additional resistance, based on the *Mycobacterium tuberculosis* genetic signature. The need for new drug delivery systems is also imperative because traditional methods are mostly inadequate in overcoming drug absorption and distribution limitations in infected tissues, particularly in the lungs, where TB activity is predominantly resident (Omoteso et al., 2025).

Adjunctive therapy added to traditional antibiotic therapy alongside new drugs is also rapidly becoming important in shaping the future of TB management. Of these, immune modulation strategies have been highly promising, particularly in enhancing the host's capacity to combat infection. Immunotherapies based on cytokine modulation can be potent inducers of immune response that enhance antibiotic activity, whereas novel vaccines are promising preventive as well as therapeutic agents. Research on mRNA vaccines, based on recent evidence, identifies a revolutionary approach in TB prevention that involves the induction of specific antigens from Mycobacterium tuberculosis to generate robust immune responses. Such cutting-edge treatments, supported by enhanced conventional antibiotics, present a comprehensive solution that is urgently needed in the evolving landscape of drug-resistant TB (Shi et al., 2024). Furthermore, the use of nanotechnology for treating tuberculosis presents promising avenues for improving therapeutic efficacy. Nanoparticle-based drug delivery systems have immense potential to enhance the bioavailability and site-specific release of anti-TB medications, thereby optimizing treatment compliance and efficacy rates. For instance, the system can be engineered to release the drug at TB-infected macrophages, the key perpetrators of TB pathogenesis, to provide a more targeted therapeutic effect. Moreover, the possibilities of inhalation drugs for anti-tb medicines show how drug delivery innovation can adapt and fulfill the anatomical and physiological constraints of tuberculosis disease. Therefore, interprofessional research activities that combine molecular biology, immunology, and nanotechnology are necessary to advance the potential innovation into practical applications for combating TB in various populations (Omoteso et al., 2025).

Test Your Knowledge

1. What are the new diagnostic technologies for tuberculosis?
2. What are the innovative treatment approaches of tuberculosis?

SUMMARY

The chronic recurrence of tuberculosis (TB) still presents a significant challenge to global health systems, with a need for complex interventions for management and prevention. Despite significant improvement in treatment options and the establishment of vaccines, the prevalence of TB is still alarmingly high, especially among vulnerable populations. The intricate relationship between tuberculosis and common mental disorders emphasizes the need to assume an integrative healthcare perspective that caters to both physical and psychological health. The evidence that links mental illness with an elevated risk of tuberculosis, as documented in studies reporting a high probability of TB in those who suffer from it, points towards the imperative of holistic care strategies that take into consideration the psychological demands as well as the physiological demands of the patients (Barreto et al., 2014). In addition, the issue of under-reporting tuberculosis cases, especially in industrialized countries like the United Kingdom, is a significant hindrance to effective disease control. The regulatory mandate for medical practitioners to report tuberculosis cases is not being significantly addressed, resulting in an inexact estimation of its actual prevalence. The estimates suggesting under-reporting to be quite variable, with the proportion in a few studies as high as 27% undernotification, highlight the importance of system-level reforms in public health infrastructure (Grove et al., 2003). Enhanced notification, through increased education and training among healthcare providers, would have a significant impact on case detection and management, leading to improved outcomes in TB control programs. Finally, the overlap of existing health disparities and tuberculosis makes it even harder to eradicate the disease. Vulnerable groups like the economically disadvantaged and minority groups have limited access to adequate healthcare and support services, thereby enhancing the impacts of TB. There is a need to craft public health interventions that are not only responsive to the clinical presentation of tuberculosis but also sensitive to social determinants, preventing it from spreading. Future research must attempt to examine the sociocultural determinants influencing the incidence and treatment of tuberculosis, particularly mental health. Enhancing our understanding of these dynamics will be crucial to the development of evidence-based interventions that effectively address the tuberculosis burden in multiplexed communities (Grove et al., 2003; Barreto et al., 2014).

One would only know the magnitude of tuberculosis (TB)'s impact on public health and social order with the knowledge of TB. TB is an infectious condition that primarily affects the lungs and is caused by the Mycobacterium tuberculosis bacterium. It thrives in low-resource environments with high crowding and poor healthcare infrastructure, making it easy to spread. TB affects socially marginalized populations disproportionately, with significant socio-economic disparities manifesting in the access to and outcomes of health care. The need to address such inequality is also highlighted by differing responses to TB outbreaks, with communities that have strong healthcare systems having lower prevalence rates compared to communities with systemic injustices. The implication is that emphasis on these social determinants is central in formulating effective TB prevention and treatment programs among affected populations. Besides socio-economic factors, the environmental context significantly influences TB transmission dynamics, as environmental factors act to amplify or mitigate TB dynamics. Ecological modifications—urbanization, mining, and agricultural encroachment—create conditions that promote or accelerate the spread of TB. For instance, rapid industrialization has the effect of increasing population densities, which can promote the spread of disease. Additionally, political instability and resource shortages may hinder government intervention in managing TB outbreaks and maintaining healthy health systems. To effectively combat TB, it is essential to understand the complex dynamics of environmental, political, and economic factors that contribute to its prevalence. Intervention in these areas could lead to initiatives that foster community resilience and healthier environments. TB research must also prioritize the integration of social and behavioral sciences to create comprehensive public health strategies. An examination of socio-cultural practices, economic determinants, and health-seeking behavior can enlighten us about barriers facing patients in acknowledging and treating TB. By taking a multidimensional approach, stakeholders are in a position to design improved health communication practices that make sense culturally across diverse groups. This aligns with research that calls for prioritization in determining the knowledge gap in social determinants and health behaviors that contribute to TB, as observed in current studies. Furthermore, creating awareness and education enables the community response in collaboration that plays a crucial role in effective TB control activity, especially in areas most impacted by morbidity as a result of neglected diseases like TB, where entrenched poverty and inequities predominate (Danso-Appiah et al., 2009; Lungu et al., 2010).

Critical Thinking Questions

1. **What is the primary mode of transmission of tuberculosis?**
   a. Fecal-oral route
   b. Droplet inhalation
   c. Direct skin contact
   d. Blood transfusion
2. **Which test is used to detect latent tuberculosis infection?**
   a. Sputum culture
   b. Tuberculin skin test (Mantoux test)
   c. Chest X-ray
   d. Acid-fast bacilli (AFB) smear
3. **Which of the following is a first-line anti-tubercular drug?**
   a. Ciprofloxacin
   b. Isoniazid
   c. Erythromycin
   d. Amphotericin B
4. **What characteristic finding is typically seen on chest X-ray in reactivation tuberculosis?**
   a. Lower lobe infiltrates
   b. Apical cavitary lesions
   c. Diffuse interstitial infiltrates
   d. Pleural thickening
5. **Which immune cell type is primarily responsible for forming granulomas in tuberculosis?**
   a. Neutrophils
   b. B lymphocytes
   c. Macrophages and T lymphocytes
   d. Eosinophils

Short Answer Questions

1. What is the causative organism of tuberculosis?
2. Which part of the lung is most commonly affected in reactivation tuberculosis?
3. Name the primary diagnostic test used for detecting latent tuberculosis infection.
4. What is the typical duration of treatment for active pulmonary tuberculosis?
5. Which drug is considered the cornerstone of tuberculosis treatment?

Answer to Critical Thinking Questions

1. (b) 2. (b) 3. (b) 4. (b) 5. (c)

REFERENCES

1. Zumla, A., Abubakar, I., Raviglione, M., Hoelscher, M., Ditiu, L., Mchugh, T. D., Squire, S. B., Cox, H., Ford, N., McNerney, R., Marais, B., Grobusch, M., Lawn, S. D., Migliori, G., Mwaba, P., O'Grady, J., Pletschette, M., Ramsay, A., Chakaya, J., . . . Atun, R. (2012). Drug-Resistant Tuberculosis—Current dilemmas, unanswered questions, challenges, and priority needs. *The Journal of Infectious Diseases, 205*(suppl_2), S228–S240. https://doi.org/10.1093/infdis/jir858An, Y., Ni, R., Li, Z., Yang, L., Ye, Z., Li, L., Parkkila, S., et al. (2025). Tuberculosis vaccines and therapeutic drug: Challenges and future directions. *Molecular Biomedicine, 6.* https://www.semanticscholar.org/paper/a615624943937b2573ef93b4f75890db24537a3d (accessed on 16th June 2025).
2. ASPHER Digital Public Health Taskforce. (2024). 3.B. Scientific session: Why do we need clear understanding of digital public health interventions? *The European Journal of Public Health, 34.* https://www.semanticscholar.org/paper/c4a50708c56db20bbe6fd3b2e199e91f96805c26 (accessed on 16th June 2025).
3. Barreto, M. L., de Araújo, G. S., dos Santos, D. N., Marinho, L. F., et al. (2014). Common mental disorders associated with tuberculosis: A matched case-control study. https://core.ac.uk/download/42631907.pdf (accessed on 16th June 2025).
4. Bartoszek, L., Kapłan, W., Kaus, M., Klepacz, D., et al. (2025). Application of artificial intelligence in radiological image analysis for pulmonary disease diagnosis: A review of current methods and challenges. https://core.ac.uk/download/636386127.pdf (accessed on 16th June 2025).
5. Bhatti, A. (2012). Optimization of rTDMH as a reagent toward improving the sensitivity of the RT-PCR based diagnosis for *Mycobacterium tuberculosis.* https://core.ac.uk/download/12210342.pdf (accessed on 16th June 2025).
6. Bradford, S. D., Ryan, K. J., Divens, A. M., Povroznik, J. M., Bonigala, S., & Robinson, C. M. (2024). IL-27 alters inflammatory cytokine expression and limits protective immunity against *Mycobacterium tuberculosis* in a neonatal BCG vaccination model. *Frontiers in Immunology, 15.* https://www.semanticscholar.org/paper/37eac21032fa7e5ea0c666f9314c89a7b7e1468a (accessed on 16th June 2025).
7. Chen, J., Jiang, Y. J., Li, Z., Zhang, M., Liu, L., Li, A., & Lu, H. (2024). Predictive machine learning models for anticipating loss to follow-up in tuberculosis patients throughout anti-TB treatment journey. *Scientific Reports, 14.* https://www.semanticscholar.org/paper/2e278034f8008f2a9e18df0849e7f11b9c48b419 (accessed on 16th June 2025).
8. Chiu, C. Y., & Miller, S. A. (2019). Clinical metagenomics. https://core.ac.uk/download/323062552.pdf (accessed on 16th June 2025).
9. Choi, J. Y. (2025). Non-pharmacologic prevention of AECOPD. *Tuberculosis and Respiratory Diseases.* https://www.semanticscholar.org/paper/d28c233e3532c4901f7498204bbb29cbc8702436 (accessed on 16th June 2025).
10. Cutler, D., & Meara, E. (2025). Changes in the age distribution of mortality over the 20th century. https://core.ac.uk/download/pdf/6587121.pdf (accessed on 16th June 2025).
11. Danso-Appiah, A., Utarini, A., Crampin, A. C., Pond, B., Paul, B. D., Babu, B. V., Braga, C., et al. (2009). Social research on neglected diseases of poverty: Continuing and emerging themes. https://core.ac.uk/download/338058.pdf (accessed on 16th June 2025).

12. Debi, U., Simran, Singh, L., Sagar, S., Sharma, V., Bhatia, V., Maralakunte, M., et al. (2020). Gastrointestinal tuberculosis: An overview. *Archives of Clinical and Medical Case Reports.* https://www.semanticscholar.org/paper/aab76f51770979c20b85719ac95bd1cdcecf5926 (accessed on 16th June 2025).

13. Denysova, O. M., Hrebeniuk, K. R., Yakimenko, T. I., Hladka, N. I., Prykhodchenko, V. O., Zhegunov, G. F., & Ugai, K. D. (2024). Veterinary transfusible in the historical context. *Veterinary Science, Technologies of Animal Husbandry and Nature Management.* https://www.semanticscholar.org/paper/19037a1750143f7df50a93f73288d3f552320dec (accessed on 16th June 2025).

14. Deswita, A., Mansur, A., & Farlina, M. (2024). Pediatric tuberculosis screening through parent involvement. *South Eastern European Journal of Public Health.* https://www.semanticscholar.org/paper/02f9151a557969c14a246a5d12e3be2fb0d48676 (accessed on 16th June 2025).

15. Egli, A., & Schulthess, B. (2024). Tuberculosis in times of war and peace. https://core.ac.uk/download/636781636.pdf (accessed on 16th June 2025).

16. Elias, L., & Mushi, L. (2024). Effectiveness of prime vendor system on availability of medicines and medical supplies in the selected public health facilities in Arusha district council. *BMC Health Services Research, 24.* https://www.semanticscholar.org/paper/5e15664fa0c812ca33682f24aee7efa9b996814a (accessed on 16th June 2025).

17. Elmuttalut, M. (2024). The key factors influencing tuberculosis treatment outcomes: A literature review. *International Journal of Recent Innovations in Medicine and Clinical Research.* https://www.semanticscholar.org/paper/f61d93a729e3ae6bce7de1cbf9498adf27ba4418 (accessed on 16th June 2025).

18. Farrugia, B. (2013). Tuberculosis in Malta: A case for sputum induction. https://core.ac.uk/download/46602348.pdf (accessed on 16th June 2025).

19. Filippova, V., Huba, M., Pronina, O., Lohachov, D., & Mykolaiets, A. (2023). Historical insights into the evolution of local self-government and state administration. *Research Journal in Advanced Humanities.* https://www.semanticscholar.org/paper/aa989857e6eebbeb60158944cecf911b5e29f97b (accessed on 16th June 2025).

20. Freudenberg, N., Galea, S., & Vlahov, D. (2005). Cities and population health. https://core.ac.uk/download/323072008.pdf (accessed on 16th June 2025).

21. Fromsa, A., Willgert, K., Srinivasan, S., Mekonnen, G., Bedada, W., Gumi, B., Lakew, M., et al. (2024). BCG vaccination reduces bovine tuberculosis transmission, improving prospects for elimination. *Science, 383.* https://www.semanticscholar.org/paper/e857931e0472d71f1a1ae33caabfbbdd59d23934 (accessed on 16th June 2025).

22. Fuadi, D. S., Hufad, A., Ismawati, D., Jaya, A., Pratama, A., Haryanto, H., & Hidayat, T. (2024). Building public awareness: Education and campaigns to prevent stunting in the next generation. *The Eurasia Proceedings of Health, Environment and Life Sciences.* https://www.semanticscholar.org/paper/8bb297c2b6b6af3dd4c497d52f0464571acbeac9 (accessed on 16th June 2025).

23. Gamon, M. (2013). Maribel Gamon - Multidrug-resistant tuberculosis in India: Solving a problem by reconstructing the public health infrastructure. https://core.ac.uk/download/67755957.pdf (accessed on 16th June 2025).

24. Gerrish, K., Ismail, M., & Naisby, A. (2025). Tackling TB together: A community participatory study of the socio-cultural factors influencing an understanding of TB within the Somali

community in Sheffield. https://core.ac.uk/download/16670096.pdf (accessed on 16th June 2025).

25. Gravlee, C. C. (2020). Systemic racism, chronic health inequities, and COVID-19: A syndemic in the making? *American Journal of Human Biology, 32.* https://doi.org/10.1002/ajhb.23482 (accessed on 16th June 2025).

26. Grove, A., Hayward, A., McCormick, A., Menon, A., Bloch, A. B., Langmuir, A. D., Clarke, A., et al. (2003). An evaluation of completeness of tuberculosis notification in the United Kingdom. https://core.ac.uk/download/pdf/3321489.pdf (accessed on 16th June 2025).

27. Hassan, Y., Dar, I. M., Uddin, J. M., Saleem, S., Rather, M. Y., & Waza, A. (2024). Tackling infectious diseases with special reference to India: Need for multidimensional approach. *Journal of Advances in Medicine and Medical Research.* https://www.semanticscholar.org/paper/da183cdb8d329647d480413246d8503f110f0942 (accessed on 16th June 2025).

28. Huang, X. H., Wang, Y., Wu, L. Y., Jiang, Y. L., Ma, L. J., Shi, X. F., Wang, X., et al. (2025). mTORC2 is crucial for regulating the recombinant *Mycobacterium tuberculosis* CFP-10 protein-induced phagocytosis in macrophages. *BMC Immunology, 26.* https://www.semanticscholar.org/paper/5f8a873abda580bb4c01ad80720b93a9637e01d5 (accessed on 16th June 2025).

29. Institute of Health. (2023). 9.L. Workshop: Mental health literacy in schools: new insights from key European studies across populations. *The European Journal of Public Health, 33.* https://www.semanticscholar.org/paper/2a9fe5ea5694bca7c5240c09aa9dd5e1ea541bf5 (accessed on 16th June 2025).

30. Ivanova, R. Y. (2025). WHO financing intervention in health-related equipment projects in Ukraine: A strategic evaluation. *Analytical and Comparative Jurisprudence.* https://www.semanticscholar.org/paper/aee14a89c7b4796217b5436329f4acb22f7c9c4d (accessed on 16th June 2025).

31. James, S. L., Abate, D., Abate, K. H., Abay, S. M., Abbafati, C., Abbasi, N., Abbastabar, H., et al. (2018). Global, regional, and national incidence, prevalence, and years lived with disability for 354 diseases and injuries for 195 countries and territories, 1990–2017: A systematic analysis for the Global Burden of Disease Study 2017. *The Lancet, 392*, 1789–1858. https://doi.org/10.1016/s0140-6736(18)32279-7 (accessed on 16th June 2025).

32. Jin, D. (2025). Gut microbiota and comprehensive analysis of drug resistance mechanisms in tuberculosis. *Journal of Medicine and Healthcare.* https://www.semanticscholar.org/paper/9a0512dfce9343c090f5936cf2e26e4d3f9dbdaa (accessed on 16th June 2025).

33. Kesehatan, F., Masyarakat, U., Agus, Z., Junadi, P., & Rusadi, R. A. (2024). Factors associated for anti-tuberculosis treatment non-adherence among tuberculosis patients: Scoping review. *Media Publikasi Promosi Kesehatan Indonesia (MPPKI).* https://www.semanticscholar.org/paper/3d966fd979a2d5eeaaf8738abca08506263088e6 (accessed on 16th June 2025).

34. Kissane, R. (2009). The future role of the philanthropy sector fighting HIV/AIDS. https://core.ac.uk/download/75779539.pdf (accessed on 16th June 2025).

35. Koskella, B., & Lin, D. (2014). Friend and foe: Factors influencing the movement of the bacterium *Helicobacter pylori* along the parasitism-mutualism continuum. https://core.ac.uk/download/323080778.pdf (accessed on 16th June 2025).

36. Leining, L. M. (2019). Geospatial analysis of pediatric tuberculosis in Bohol, Philippines: Disease clusters and access to care. https://core.ac.uk/download/212904016.pdf (accessed on 16th June 2025).

37. Lungu, K., Morse, T., & Taulo, S. (2010). Gap analysis of environmental health research in Malawi: Report to the National Commission of Science and Technology. https://core.ac.uk/download/19610167.pdf (accessed on 16th June 2025).

38. Maharani, P. I. P., Putri, B. A. C., & Rahmasita, S. A. (2021). Musculoskeletal tuberculosis. *KESANS: International Journal of Health and Science.* https://www.semanticscholar.org/paper/26e0148d2ebf0d0b4657f7e2e28ff1588aef724b (accessed on 16th June 2025).

39. Mayangsari, A. S. M., Purniti, N. P. S., Subanada, I. B., Witarini, K., & Clearesta, K. E. (2024). Prevalence and risk factors of tuberculosis infection in orphanage children in Bali, Indonesia. *Intisari Sains Medis.* https://www.semanticscholar.org/paper/0d97192b6978fcc71e3255164a673c78a28fb14b (accessed on 16th June 2025).

40. Mishra, M., Arya, A., Malik, M. Z., Mishra, A., Hasnain, S. E., Bhatnagar, R., Ahmad, S., et al. (2025). Differential genome organization revealed by comparative topological analysis of *Mycobacterium tuberculosis* strains H37Rv and H37Ra. *mSystems.* https://www.semanticscholar.org/paper/00f65ac239e1406055ac50d89f942a6a08476421 (accessed on 16th June 2025).

41. Müller, J., Tanner, R., Matsumiya, M., Snowden, M. A., Landry, B., Satti, I., Harris, S. A., et al. (2019). Cytomegalovirus infection is a risk factor for tuberculosis disease in infants. *JCI Insight, 4.* https://doi.org/10.1172/jci.insight.130090 (accessed on 16th June 2025).

42. Murray, C. J. L., Ikuta, K. S., Sharara, F., Swetschinski, L. R., Robles Aguilar, G., Gray, A. P., Han, C., et al. (2022). Global burden of bacterial antimicrobial resistance in 2019: A systematic analysis. *The Lancet, 399*, 629–655. https://doi.org/10.1016/s0140-6736(21)02724-0 (accessed on 16th June 2025).

43. Nell, A. J., & van Vugt, F. (2025). BOCI-Egypt: Brucellosis and tuberculosis control 21–25 March 2011. https://core.ac.uk/download/pdf/29235285.pdf (accessed on 16th June 2025).

44. Nijman, L. W., Cristescu, S. M., & Jansen, R. S. (2025). Broadening the diagnostic landscape of *Mycobacterium tuberculosis* infection: Analyzing exhaled breath. *Journal of Breath Research, 19.* https://www.semanticscholar.org/paper/849e40cb74f482f00fddfb1cee535ce43b3a8e4f (accessed on 16th June 2025).

45. Omoteso, O. A., Fadaka, A., Walker, R. B., & Khamanga, S. (2025). Innovative strategies for combating multidrug-resistant tuberculosis: Advances in drug delivery systems and treatment. *Microorganisms, 13.* https://www.semanticscholar.org/paper/6db61d6a1c40ea7276320c694a9e619b4af33974 (accessed on 16th June 2025).

46. Ondiro, J., Onyangore, F., Onyango, R., Muema, L., & Aduda, D. (2024). Lived experiences of persons on tuberculosis treatment in Nairobi County, Kenya: A mixed methods study. *BMC Public Health, 24.* https://www.semanticscholar.org/paper/7560e55c8631cde1a0a53e94c2f85df5f8fc72c6 (accessed on 16th June 2025).

47. Ovsyankina, E. S., Panova, L., Krushinskaya, E., & Bagirov, M. A. (2024). Short-course chemotherapy regimens for treatment of multiple and pre-extensive drug-resistant tuberculosis in combination with surgery in older children and adolescents. *Tuberculosis and Lung Diseases.* https://www.semanticscholar.org/paper/78453ef1a64df721032a31255ecba63194be7078 (accessed on 16th June 2025).

48. Ramanthan, R., & Jayapritha, M. (2025). Clinic-epidemiological profile and diagnostic procedures in suspected pediatric tuberculosis in a tertiary care center in Tamil Nadu. *International Journal of Contemporary Pediatrics.* https://www.semanticscholar.org/paper/1cee110ae8d9e77ce9a02059f3c6f8791ef6ab2b (accessed on 16th June 2025).

49. Semianiv, I., Todoriko, L., Vyklyuk, Y., & Nevinskyi, D. (2024). Application of geospatial multi-agent system for simulation of different aspects of tuberculosis transmission. *Infusion & Chemotherapy.* https://www.semanticscholar.org/paper/880d259d2e070b175c7f5ce1fdab6f9ceafe7cd9 (accessed on 16th June 2025).

50. Shi, H., Zhu, Y., Shang, K., Tian, T., Yin, Z., Shi, J., He, Y., et al. (2024). Development of innovative multi-epitope mRNA vaccine against central nervous system tuberculosis using *in silico* approaches. *PLOS ONE, 19.* https://www.semanticscholar.org/paper/334cbf14ead346d6f4069675bbcff0b6dfbe0c13 (accessed on 16th June 2025).

51. Suryanto, F., Arini, M., & Riadi, I. (2024). ScreenMy: A lightweight architecture of tuberculosis-diabetes mellitus screening system integrating with EMRs. *JUITA: Journal Informatika.* https://www.semanticscholar.org/paper/afd9a711526971afa984583267063e68bdb7560d (accessed on 16th June 2025).

52. Uniyal, J. (2024). Exploring the role of education and awareness campaigns in shaping consumer behavior towards green products. *International Journal for Multidisciplinary Research.* https://www.semanticscholar.org/paper/29d89d18937020c5d9b953c6b56445d7e78de061 (accessed on 16th June 2025).

53. Xu, X., Han, M., Li, T., Sun, W., Wang, D., Fu, B., Zhou, Y., et al. (2020). Effective treatment of severe COVID-19 patients with tocilizumab. *Proceedings of the National Academy of Sciences, 117,* 10970–10975. https://doi.org/10.1073/pnas.2005615117 (accessed on 16th June 2025).

54. Yatskevich, N., Gurevich, G. L., Skryagina, E. M., & Gurbanova, E. (2023). Evaluation of effectiveness of 9- and 6-month treatment regimens in patients with multiple drug resistant or rifampicin-resistant tuberculosis in the Republic of Belarus. *Tuberculosis and Lung Diseases.* https://www.semanticscholar.org/paper/31c2279163323c08f9750dc0cd46293c9040197c (accessed on 16th June 2025).

55. Yin, X., Zhang, Q., Wang, Y., Tao, B., Zhang, X., Shi, J., Deng, X., et al. (2024). Genomic and spatial analysis on the recent transmission of *Mycobacterium tuberculosis* in Eastern China: A 10-year retrospective population-based study. *Infection and Drug Resistance, 17,* 4257–4269. https://www.semanticscholar.org/paper/121c8c5d66341281eb922d8c9df3fd00f7ee8093 (accessed on 16th June 2025).

56. Young, C., Mkhonza, M. N., & Ogongo, P. (2023). Recognition and control of *Mycobacterium tuberculosis*-infected cells: From basics to the clinic: A NIAID/WGNV workshop report 2023. *Frontiers in Tuberculosis.* https://www.semanticscholar.org/paper/afc8d92348ba9ecb24906c56a46724b5c6dd1244 (accessed on 16th June 2025).

57. Zeng, X., Luo, W., & Li, Y. (2023). Current research on personalized teaching system based on CiteSpace visual analysis. *2023 International Conference on Computer Engineering and Distance Learning (CEDL).* https://www.semanticscholar.org/paper/c8f41e4ab6728a28f1e24bc8cf030c4d8f5119ad (accessed on 16th June 2025).

INFECTION DUE TO NONTUBERCULOUS MYCOBACTERIA

8

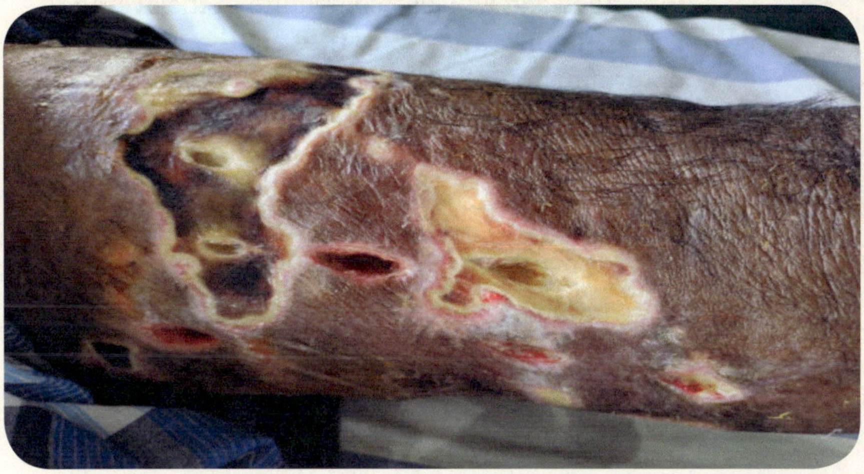

LEARNING OBJECTIVES

After studying this chapter, you will be able to:

1. Describe the classification of nontuberculous mycobacteria
2. Explain the pathogenesis of nontuberculous mycobacterial infections
3. Explore the diagnosis of nontuberculous mycobacterial infections
4. List the treatment options for nontuberculous mycobacterial infections
5. Discuss the epidemiology of nontuberculous mycobacterial infections
5. Focus on the public health implications

Introduction

The identification of nontuberculous mycobacteria (NTM) as pathogens has been a growing public health concern over time, particularly in respiratory infections. In contrast to their notorious cousin, Mycobacterium tuberculosis, NTM are usually underappreciated but can cause serious pulmonary disease, particularly in immunocompromised hosts and pre-existing pulmonary disease. Latest studies indicate a notable increase in the incidence of pulmonary NTM diseases worldwide, with an average annual growth rate of approximately 4.0% per 100,000 population (Victor Næstholt Dahl et al., 2022). The trend points to the need for clinicians to remain vigilant in terms of presentation of NTM infection signs and symptoms and to possess high indices of suspicion, particularly in vulnerable populations. Understanding the underlying causes of this increase, in terms of environmental and genetic factors, is crucial for developing effective prevention and treatment strategies. The classification of NTM infections complicates diagnosis and treatment because these pathogens are not typically included in routine diagnostic panels for mycobacterial infection. Clinicians must be able to differentiate between colonisation and true infection, far from easy with the myriad clinical presentations mimicking other pulmonary illnesses. Guidelines for the diagnosis and treatment of NTM infections emphasize the importance of a thorough clinical assessment and the application of specific criteria to distinguish between disease and asymptomatic carriage (Raghu et al., 2020).

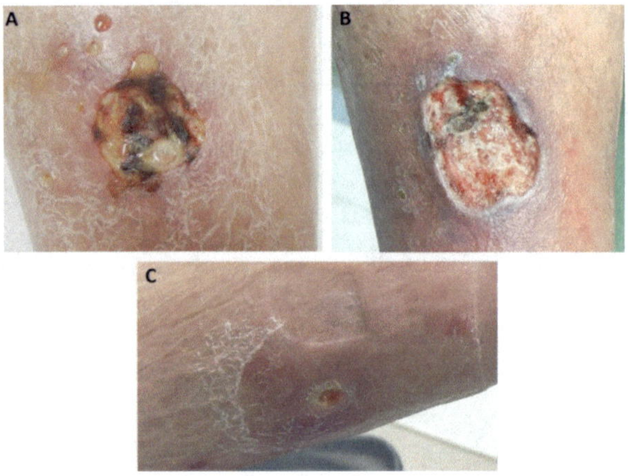

Figure 8.1. Nontuberculous mycobacterial infections.

Source: https://media.springernature.com/lw685/springer-static/image/art%3A10.1007%2Fs13671-023-00417-5/MediaObjects/13671_2023_417_Fig1_HTML.jpg

It is not only necessary for effective treatment but also for understanding the broader epidemiological context of NTM infections, particularly as they have become linked to increasing healthcare burdens associated with their chronic and complicated treatments. Moreover, the evolving protocols for treating NTM infections also illustrate an ongoing response to ever-changing disease landscapes. Many NTM species, including the Mycobacterium avium complex, are resistant to standard antitubercular agents, and hence a combination regimen tailored to patient profiles is employed. Recent data show that, despite the challenges in treatment, successful regimens can lead to significant improvements in patient outcomes. As the global burden of NTM infection continues to escalate, it is essential that healthcare practitioners remain informed about the latest clinical guidelines and research frontiers on these mycobacterial infections. This will ensure a proactive approach to treating infections and will also contribute to the overall scientific literature on the epidemiological determinants influencing the dissemination of NTM pathogens (Victor Næstholt Dahl et al., 2022).

Definition of Nontuberculous Mycobacteria (NTM)

The nontuberculous mycobacteria (NTM) category has a broad variety of non-tuberculous mycobacterial species. They are also known as atypical mycobacteria and are usually found in environmental reservoirs such as soil, water, and dust. NTM primarily results in pulmonary infections, predominantly among immunocompromised patients or those with predisposing pulmonary diseases. In contrast to Mycobacterium tuberculosis, whose pathogenesis and route of transmission are well-defined, NTM infections are likely to be the consequence of environmental exposure rather than person-to-person spread, leading to a complex clinical presentation that varies by mycobacterial species. This diversity significantly complicates diagnosis and therapy, underscoring the importance of understanding NTM in the context of clinical disease and public health relevance. More recent data indicate growing awareness of the public health effects of NTM. A six-year Nebraska study found 759 cases of NTM infection and reported that a large proportion of infections are nonpulmonary, with *Mycobacterium avium-intracellulare* being the most frequently isolated species (Hoffman et al., 2018). This finding illustrates that nonpulmonary NTM may contribute significantly to morbidity, which was previously underestimated. Furthermore, the shifting trends in isolation rates are a concern regarding geographic variation and risk factors associated with NTM infection in populations. As populations, it highlights the need for more sensitive surveillance and data collection to improve patient management and public health interventions. The clinical presentation of NTM disease can be multifaceted, typically being pulmonary disease with cough, dyspnea, and loss of weight. According to studies, older age and the presence of underlying pulmonary comorbidities make individuals particularly vulnerable to infection from NTM (Mohanty et al., 2023). Interestingly, the outcome of the treatment of NTM varies significantly, with the outcomes of approximately 47% of the patients who received antibiotic treatment being positive. However, concerns regarding spontaneous culture conversion and relapse emphasize the need for sustained monitoring and increased knowledge of the predictors of successful treatment. With NTM infection remaining a significant clinical problem, access to specific patient populations, symptomatology patterns, and outcomes will be necessary to create effective treatment regimens and reduce the disease burden in future years.

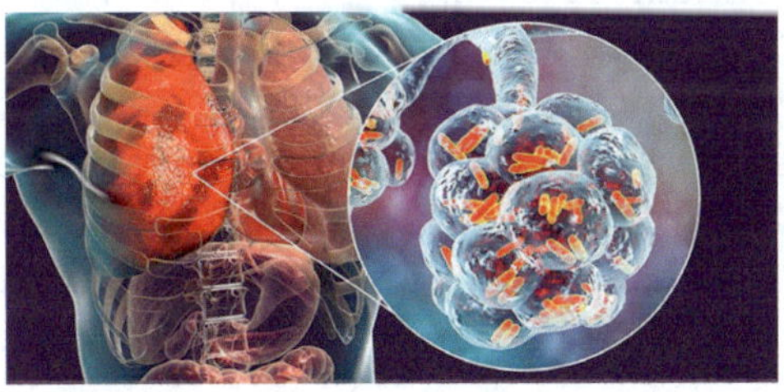

Figure 8.2. Nontuberculous mycobacteria (NTM).

Source: https://uthealtheasttexas.com/sites/default/files/styles/services_node_image/public/sub-service-images/NTMLungDisease_subservice.jpg?itok=YbcCzZYm

Importance of studying NTM infections

The increasing prevalence of nontuberculous mycobacterial (NTM) infections underscores the need for intensified research in this field. Once regarded as opportunistic pathogens, NTMs are now recognized as etiologic agents of a wide range of diseases in both immunocompetent and immunocompromised hosts. Their unique environmental reservoirs and capacity for biofilm formation significantly contribute to their pathogenicity, rendering treatment difficult. Without adequate understanding of these factors, the healthcare field will experience ineffective management of NTM-related illnesses, particularly with their rise in healthcare settings. The clinical presentation of NTM infection is noteworthy, as these varied manifestations may lead to misdiagnosis or delayed therapy, resulting in worsening of health conditions and additional healthcare costs. This highlights the critical importance of extensive research into the pathogenesis and therapeutic modalities of NTM infections (Faria et al., 2015). The economic implications of NTM infection also deserve serious investigation. Current research indicates a significant economic burden associated with hospitalization for NTM, suggesting a rising trend in treatment-related costs over the last decade. Specific data indicate that expenses incurred for pulmonary NTM treatment have increased substantially, amounting to approximately $903,767,292 for the period between 2001 and 2012. The economic cost is a compelling justification for continuing to research prevention and therapy to identify improved approaches. An understanding of the economic impact of these infections at a population level will not only define healthcare policy but also guide resource allocation and strategic planning in public health interventions. Comprehensively addressing NTM infections through research can lead to more effective interventions that alleviate both clinical and economic burdens (Allen et al., 2016).

Moreover, global health implications are not just restricted to patient morbidity and economic burden; NTM infections pose serious challenges to public health infrastructure. With rising resistance against current treatments, such pathogens can become a serious health threat to healthcare centers, especially given their environmental prevalence. As NTM infections become more widespread, they can increasingly contribute to the burden of management of respiratory disease globally and necessitate an integrated, multidisciplinary approach. Emphasizing the importance of researching these infections encourages collaboration between researchers, clinicians, and public health professionals. Increased knowledge leads to improved diagnostics, targeted therapies, and effective public health policies, ultimately resulting in better patient outcomes. Therefore, the continuation of NTM research contributes to greater infectious disease control and prevention goals, and thus the necessity to prioritize such efforts within medical and public health research.

8.1. Classification of Nontuberculous Mycobacteria

Learning Outcome

1. Major species of NTM and their characteristics
2. Environmental sources of NTM
3. Differences between NTM and Mycobacterium tuberculosis

Classification of nontuberculous mycobacteria (NTM) is a complex process, primarily due to the heterogeneity of species found in various environments. Nontuberculous mycobacteria are categorized primarily into two groups: slow-growing and fast-growing species. Slow-growing NTMs, such as *Mycobacterium avium* complex and *Mycobacterium gordonae*, tend to have longer incubation times for culture in the laboratory and are commonly implicated in pulmonary infections and other infections in immunocompromised individuals. Conversely, rapidly growing mycobacteria, such as *Mycobacterium abscessus* and *Mycobacterium fortuitum*, can grow more rapidly in culture, leading to acute infections. Identification of these species not only aids in the correct diagnosis but also in proper management and treatment since different species have different antibiotic susceptibility and pathogenicity. Environmental determinants play a critical role in the epidemiology of NTM infections and are therefore vital to be well understood in terms of their ecological niches. NTM species are ubiquitous all around in soil, water, and biofilms and can have appreciable genetic diversity there. For instance, studies have recovered the slow-growing species Mycobacterium moriokaense and Mycobacterium riyadhense, which are prevalent in different soil environments, highlighting the importance of their ecological reservoirs (Pontiroli et al., 2013). Understanding the ecological distribution of NTMs in the environment serves to pinpoint the sources of human infection as well as the precautions required to prevent exposure. Environmental NTM surveillance using molecular methods, such as PCR and sequencing, has enabled the identification of organisms and their reservoirs, leading to more effective public health interventions against potential outbreaks. The clinical relevance of the classification of NTM extends beyond epidemiological concerns to inform treatment regimens in medicine. Noteworthy is the novel research on *Mycobacterium gordonae*, which discovered that the species, although frequently observed as insignificant contamination, can periodically lead to infection, resulting in misdiagnosis or unwarranted treatments of patients (Cottarelli et al., 2016). The process of identifying the species of NTM is crucial in determining the appropriate treatment interventions, particularly given the increasing prevalence of resistant strains. Additionally, the genetic characterization of the NTM isolates enables the differentiation between pathogenic and environmental strains, thereby enhancing monitoring and management in potential outbreaks. This quiet image of NTM classification enables healthcare professionals to implement targeted treatment strategies and public health programs with enhanced effectiveness, thereby reducing the burden of infection caused by these mycobacteria.

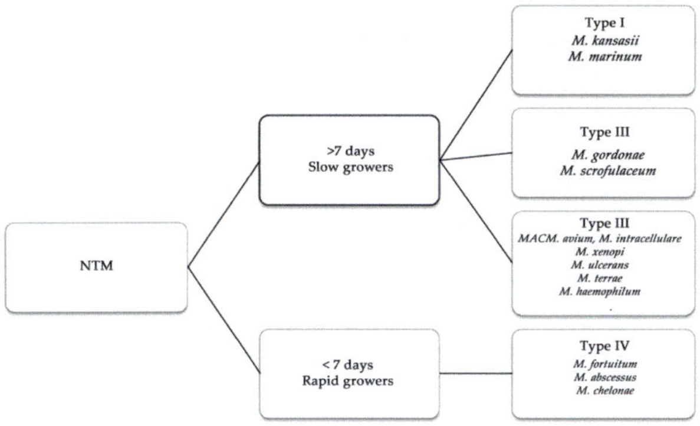

Figure 8.3. Classification of nontuberculous mycobacteria.

Source: https://www.researchgate.net/profile/Juraj-Mokry/publication/305203589/figure/fig1/AS:614118432194600@1523428652925/Classification-of-non-tuberculous-mycobacteria-NTM-Adapted-from-Runyon-1959.png

8.1.1. Major Species of Nontuberculous Mycobacteriaand Their Characteristics

Nontuberculous mycobacteria (NTM) are commonly a heterogeneous collection of mycobacterial species that are increasingly being recognized as significant human pathogens, particularly in immunocompromised individuals. *Mycobacterium avium* complex (MAC) is one of the most frequent species among these, consisting predominantly of *Mycobacterium avium* and *Mycobacterium intracellulare*. MAC is associated with pulmonary infection and often has a history of underlying lung disease, such as bronchiectasis or chronic obstructive pulmonary disease. MAC's potential for survival in certain environmental niches, particularly in water supplies, underscores its opportunistic pathogen behavior, which often creates clinical management challenges in susceptible populations. Understanding MAC's unique growth characteristics and its capacity for pathology is of utmost significance in the successful treatment and diagnosis of infections by this category of NTM, given its established association with increased morbidity in infected individuals (Ambrose et al., 2016). Another prominent member of the NTM complex is the *Mycobacterium abscessus*, which is known for its rapid growth and increasing incidence in clinical practice. Cutaneous and soft tissue infections, particularly those occurring following trauma or surgery, are commonly associated with M. abscessus. Its environmental persistence in aquatic environments further projects its infective nature, as evidenced by its isolation from various water systems (Bland et al., 1951). Patients with cystic fibrosis are also among the high-risk individuals, as they might experience serious lung infections that are notoriously difficult to eliminate due to the inherent resistance of the bacterium to a variety of antibiotics. Thus, identifying the nature of M. abscessus and its reservoirs in the environment is important for designing targeted interventions and guiding therapeutic strategies tailored to individual patient requirements. Further, Mycobacterium fortuitum, a pathogen of rapidly growing mycobacteria, is most often related to opportunistic infection in patients with compromised immune systems. *Mycobacterium fortuitum* is known for its environmental resilience and has been isolated from various sources, such as tap water and environmental samples, which shows the opportunistic pathways through which it can develop pathogenicity. *M. fortuitum* is frequently linked with soft tissue infections after injection or surgical procedures and may complicate the clinical course in immunocompromised patients. Identification of the organism is essential in the clinical scenario, since it mandates specific treatment regimens different from those against more traditional pathogens. For this reason, identification of the distinctive features and clinical relevance of *M. fortuitum* helps clinicians diagnose and treat nontuberculous mycobacterial disease correctly as part of an overall infection control strategy (Ambrose et al., 2016).

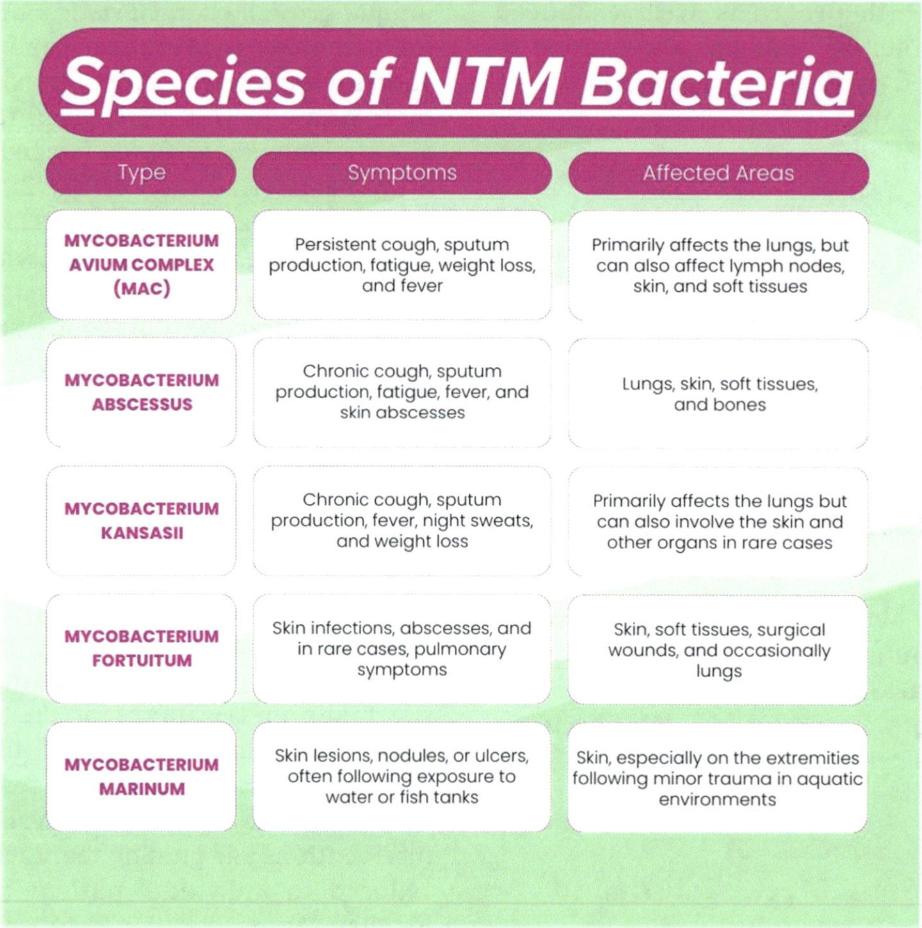

Figure 8.4. Major species of nontuberculous mycobacteriaand their characteristics.

Source: https://encrypted-tbn0.gstatic.com/images?q=tbn:ANd9GcSh3oq237g8iZhFO_aObp0i8Q7gftnoBeURIg&s

8.1.2. Environmental Sources of Nontuberculous Mycobacteria

The environmental reservoirs of nontuberculous mycobacteria (NTM) are key to their role in human infection. NTM thrive in various environments, primarily soil and freshwater habitats, as integral members of microbial communities. Their prevalence suggests that environmental reservoirs must pose an ongoing risk for potential exposure in humans. Climate, geographic location, and human activity may influence the density and distribution of NTM. For instance, water sources contaminated with pathogens, such as those used for drinking and hot tub water, have been implicated in NTM infection, particularly in high-risk populations. Furthermore, the coincidence of

NTM in such an environment can be exacerbated by environmental disturbance, which enhances aerosolization and inhalation, key routes of infection. It is therefore essential to consider these environmental factors in understanding the epidemiology of NTM infection. Research has shown that various NTM species occupy distinct ecological niches, making the understanding of their transmission even more complex. MAC, for example, is often linked with water sources and can be cultured from both drinking and non-potable water systems. The frequent isolation of these agents from environmental specimens implies a close association with clusters of humans. In Nebraska, research highlighted the predominance of Mycobacterium avium in nonpulmonary infections, especially the importance of these environmental reservoirs in the total disease burden of NTM. As more attention is given to monitoring the prevalence of NTM in public health efforts, it is crucial to recognize the individual environmental reservoirs, particularly since infection rates have been rising in certain groups, including women and elderly individuals, as indicated by more recent epidemiological studies (Hoffman et al., 2018). NTM environmental reservoirs are not limited to water. Soil is the second crucial environment for these organisms, where their survival and growth are based on climate, vegetation, and soil properties. Soil disturbances, such as construction or agriculture, further amplify the aerosolization of mycobacteria, potentially leading to inhalation exposure. It is particularly true for vulnerable individuals with prior health conditions, which render a person susceptible to NTM infections. Further, NTM infections are not only expressed as pulmonary disease, but also involve soft tissues and the skin, which complicates the clinical presentation. Hence, there needs to be an interdisciplinary effort to fully appreciate environmental sources such that ecological and health-related factors are considered to mitigate the risk of NTM infection across various demographic categories (Adcock et al., 2017).

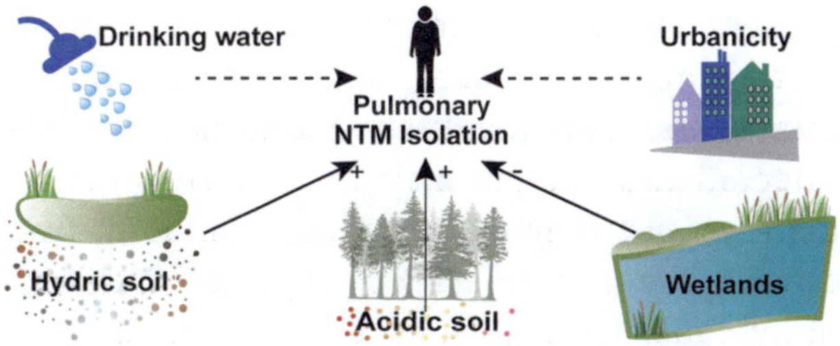

Figure 8.5. Environmental sources of nontuberculous mycobacteria.

Source: https://ars.els-cdn.com/content/image/1-s2.0-S0048969720380839-ga1.jpg

8.1.3. Differences Between Nontuberculous Mycobacteriaand Mycobacterium Tuberculosis

The distinction between nontuberculous mycobacteria (NTM) and *Mycobacterium tuberculosis* is characterized according to their pathogenicity and natural niches. NTM, a heterogeneous collection of environmental bacteria, are omnipresent in natural aquatic and terrestrial surroundings.

They are not typically transmitted between humans and cause illness only in some groups with predisposing diseases, such as bronchiectasis or immunosuppression. By contrast, *Mycobacterium tuberculosis* is an obligate pathogen that is mainly linked with tuberculosis, a communicable disease that has widespread global transmission pathways. *Mycobacterium tuberculosis*'s spread by air highlights the critical difference in epidemiological patterns between these two groups, making public health interventions for each distinctly different. In terms of disease presentation, *Mycobacterium tuberculosis*-and NTM-induced infections have essential differences. While *M. tuberculosis* typically induces granulomatous inflammation of the lungs characterized by pleural effusion alongside systemic symptoms, NTM infections usually present in local pulmonary manifestations or, in a minority of cases, skin and soft tissue infections. For instance, pulmonary NTM-infected individuals may feature respiratory distress, but they could remain symptom-free during the initial stages, especially among individuals with no lung diseases. Compared to this, the systemic effects of tuberculosis, such as the one observed in pleural tuberculosis, can lead to large effusions and lymphadenopathy, as evident in research showing preponderant T cell predominance in effusions due to TB. One needs to be aware of these differences so that there is proper diagnosis and treatment modalities. *Mycobacterium tuberculosis* and NTM exhibit differential immunologic responses upon host invasion.

Mycobacterium tuberculosis initiates the robust activation of T lymphocytes within the body, leading to the generation of various cytokines that support granuloma development, which is necessary for containing the infection. Cytokine reactions and T lymphocyte recruitment in conditions such as pleural tuberculosis are not yet fully understood, but they emphasize the unique immunological processes mobilized by *M. tuberculosis* (Adcock et al., 2017). Conversely, NTM infections that provoke a milder immune response regularly strike patients with predisposing conditions. This disparity has practical relevance in the clinical context: patients with NTM may not exhibit the same degree of immunological reaction, which will make diagnosis and treatment more difficult. In this way, understanding these disparities enhances our approach to treating infections from these two mycobacterial diseases (Adcock et al., 2017).

Test Your Knowledge

1. What are the major species of NTM and their characteristics?
2. What are the environmental sources of NTM?

8.2. Pathogenesis of Nontuberculous Mycobacterial Infections

Learning Outcome

1. Mechanisms of infection and host response
2. Risk factors for NTM infections
3. Clinical manifestations of NTM infections

The etiology of disease caused by nontuberculous mycobacteria is multifactorial, influenced predominantly by host defense mechanisms and the environmental availability of these organisms. Nontuberculous mycobacteria (NTM) are ubiquitous in soil and water, posing the greatest risk to individuals with underlying lung disorders, such as bronchiectasis, cystic fibrosis, or chronic obstructive pulmonary disease. Environmental pathogens exploit impaired pulmonary defense, leading to infection and resultant inflammation. While significant advances have been made in identifying NTM using sophisticated imaging and microbiological methods, questions persist regarding the precise immunological pathways that predispose them to pathogenesis. Furthermore, the escalating pandemic of NTM infections in certain groups underscores the need to identify the underlying immunogenetic susceptibility factors that put individuals at risk for such infections, given that most infected persons do not have overt risk factors, thereby complicating their pathogenesis (Adcock et al., 2017).

One of the key elements in the pathogenesis of NTM infection is the interaction of the mycobacteria with the host's immune system. NTM can evade detection and clearance due to their unique cell wall structures for immune evasion. The complexity of the immune response is exemplified in patients with cystic fibrosis (CF), where mutations in the CFTR gene disrupt pathogen clearance, leading to chronic bacterial persistence and inflammation. This chronic infection with NTM, or rather the complex of rapidly growing *Mycobacterium abscessus*, is highly clinically challenging because it is intrinsically resistant to most drugs. It is vital to understand how M. abscessus infection occurs in patients with CF because the compromised immune status leads to increased pulmonary pathology, ultimately exacerbating the disease burden in these patients (VongtongsaLee et al., 2019). As NTM illnesses grow more identifiable, the need to understand their pathogenesis becomes more urgent. Especially worrying is the finding that people who have lived with immunological compromise, e.g., those who have human immunodeficiency virus (HIV) infection or other immunologic disease, are at increased risk for severe NTM disease. This weakness suggests that the complex host-immunity/NTM-pathogen interaction may cause not only localized pulmonary disease but also systemic dissemination, particularly in immunocompromised hosts. Further research into the pathogenesis mechanisms of NTM will be necessary to develop more effective prevention and treatment strategies. Thus, the integration of immunogenetics and microbiological data could provide valuable insights into host-pathogen interactions and inform clinical practices in the successful treatment of NTM disease (Adcock et al., 2017).

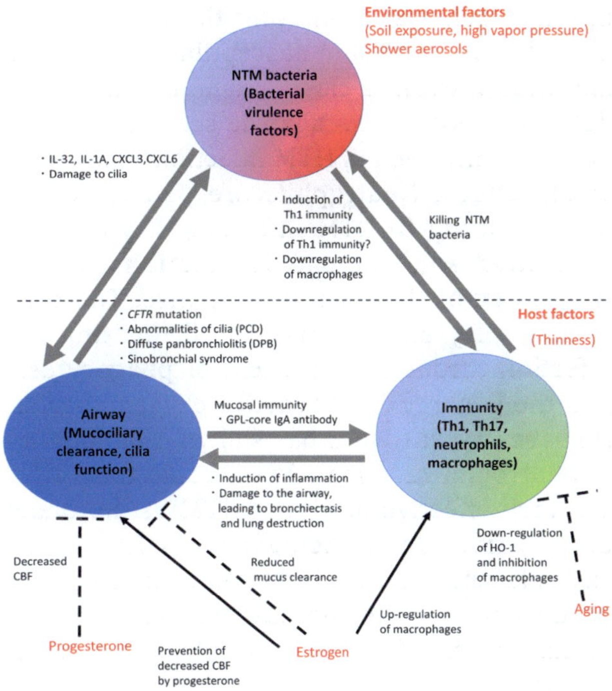

Figure 8.6. Pathogenesis of nontuberculous mycobacterial infections.

Source: https://ars.els-cdn.com/content/image/1-s2.0-S2212534522001745-gr2.jpg

8.2.1. Mechanisms of Infection and Host Response

The mechanism of infection with nontuberculous mycobacteria (NTM) is complex and multifaceted, resulting from the interaction between the host's immune system and the causative pathogen. NTM bacteria are highly virulent, being well-adapted to evade the immune system due to their well-developed cell wall structure, which makes them resistant to phagocytosis and increases their survival rate in host tissue. Upon invading the host, these pathogens are typically detected by immune cells, which initiate an inflammatory response. However, the success of such a response depends largely on various factors within the host, including genetic susceptibility and pre-existing immunological status. Diseases such as primary immune deficiencies can lead to a weakening of the immune defense, facilitating the survival and propagation of NTM in susceptible individuals, and thus warrant a closer examination of host defense mechanisms against certain immune pathways involved in NTM infections (Ambrose et al., 2016). Neutrophils are pivotal in the host response to NTM infection, playing both protective and pathogenic functions during the course of the immune response. The cells initially play an essential role in limiting the infection through the process of phagocytosis and the generation of reactive oxygen species. However, recent work has shown a bimodality in neutrophil function;. At the same time, they are very effective at killing NTM at the onset of infection; in bronchiectatic patients, for example, they can be pathogenic and result in tissue damage and disease progression. This mutual interaction reveals the intricacy of NTM-PD immunity, demonstrating that neutrophils possess the ability to create a harmful microenvironment, for example, by augmenting inflammatory responses and contributing to the causation of chronic lung infections (Alkarni et al., 2023).

One should understand this balance to create efficient therapeutic strategies. Because the growing incidence of NTM disease necessitates the identification of the interaction among various immune factors and host responses to achieve better clinical results, investigating some of these immune pathways, such as the interferon-gamma (IFNγ) and interleukin-12 (IL-12) signaling pathways, gives us great insights into how the mechanisms can fail in vulnerable populations. In addition, the implication of iatrogenic causes, such as immunosuppressive therapy, provides further complexity to the host's failure to sustain an adequate defense against NTM. Understanding these mechanisms not only improves clinicians ability to diagnose and treat NTM infection but also guides public health measures to minimize risk factors for NTM disease. A careful strategy involving in-depth study of host immunity and the mechanisms of pathogens will ultimately lead to the development of targeted therapies, as well as prevention strategies, against such challenging infections (Ambrose et al., 2016).

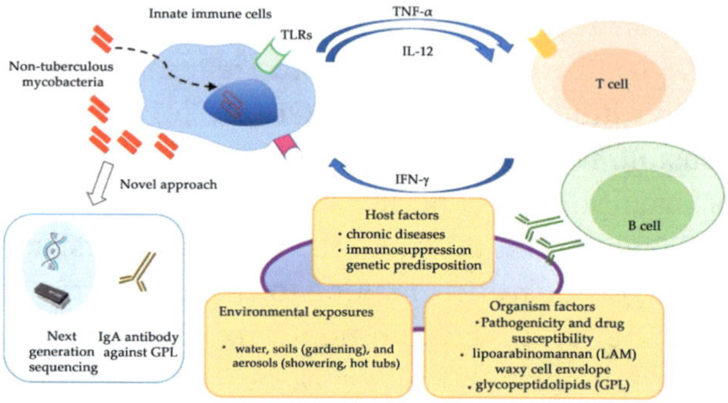

Figure 8.7. Mechanisms of infection and host response in infection with nontuberculous mycobacteria (NTM).

Source: https://www.mdpi.com/ijms/ijms-21-04351/article_deploy/html/images/ijms-21-04351-g001.png

8.2.2. Risk Factors For NTM Infections

The increasing prevalence of nontuberculous mycobacterial (NTM) infections highlights the need to determine various risk factors associated with these infections. NTMs are, in fact, environmental organisms, also found in water and soil, that may opportunistically infect patients with compromised pulmonary anatomy. Bronchiectasis, emphysema, and a history of tuberculosis highly predispose patients to NTM infections. This vulnerability primarily stems from the structural lung injury caused by these diseases, allowing colonization and eventual infection with bacteria. The technical challenge posed by NTM infections is further exacerbated by their potential to infect diverse populations, including immunocompromised patients, underscoring the importance of identifying the driving risk factors behind them in terms of prevention and treatment

(Adcock et al., 2017). Apart from structural lung abnormalities, immune deficiencies also have a critical role in susceptibility to NTM infection. Some congenital disorders, most notably those affecting the interferon-gamma and interleukin-12 axis, have been identified as significant in inducing enhanced susceptibility. Patients with primary immunodeficiencies are also found to be more susceptible to NTM due to dysfunctional cellular immunity, which is central to host defense against mycobacterial infection.

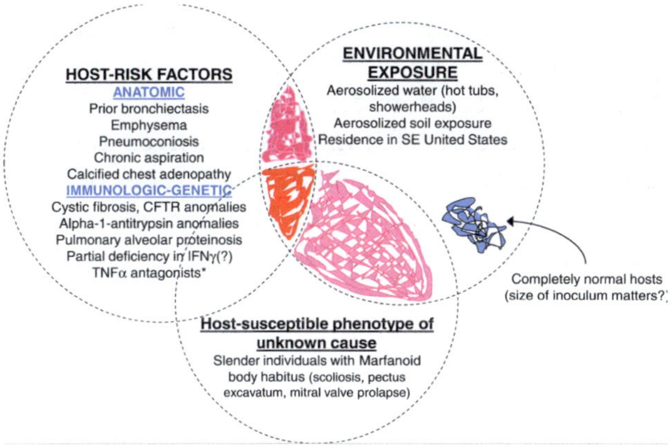

Figure 8.8. Risk factors for nontuberculous mycobacteriainfections.

Source: https://www.chestmed.theclinics.com/cms/10.1016/j.ccm.2014.10.001/asset/d9a70efb-f6da-4867-b472-091297517a0e/main.assets/gr1_lrg.jpg

Furthermore, patients on immunosuppressive therapy—either for autoimmune conditions or following procedures such as organ transplantation—are at increased risk of developing NTM disease. As the immunological processes that regulate host defense continue to be better appreciated, it is evident that an understanding of these immune processes can facilitate enhanced control and prevention of NTM infection (Ambrose et al., 2016). Some host-related factors, including age, body habitus, and some chronic conditions, also significantly contribute to the determination of risk for NTM infection. Older people typically experience a decline in immune function, making them more vulnerable. Additional weakening of the respiratory system's defense barrier is brought about by diseases like cystic fibrosis and malnutrition, which facilitate NTM colonization and infection. Lifestyle issues, such as smoking, contribute to risk because they can lead to chronic lung inflammation and tissue changes that predispose to NTM overgrowth. By exploring the diverse risk factors, clinicians will be better equipped to identify higher-risk groups, leading to targeted preventive measures and screening that can slow the progression of NTM disease among vulnerable individuals (Adcock et al., 2017).

8.2.3. Clinical Manifestations of NTM Infections

Nontuberculous mycobacterial infections present with a diverse variety of clinical manifestations that are most commonly confined to the pulmonary system. The lung is most commonly the site of primary infection in patients with underlying respiratory illness such as bronchiectasis, cystic fibrosis, and emphysema. Such patients may present with manifestations mimicking tuberculosis, including chronic cough, sputum production, hemoptysis, and chest pain. The gravity of these manifestations may vary significantly in affected individuals, emphasizing the importance of early diagnosis and intervention. In addition, infected patients with compromised immune responses, such as HIV/AIDS patients, can develop an enhanced risk of dissemination beyond the lungs, demonstrating the delicate balance between immunological host function and NTM disease (Adcock et al., 2017). As a better understanding of these clinical presentations becomes apparent, it becomes more critical to maximize diagnostic models to better diagnose NTM-related respiratory infections. In addition to pulmonary infection, NTM can occur in extrapulmonary sites, leading to a wide variety of clinical syndromes. Soft tissue infections and lymphadenitis in children are just some of the high-profile extrapulmonary manifestations associated with NTM. Such infections can present as localized infections, swelling, and tenderness at the site of inoculation and may require surgical management. Also, in an immunocompromised host, disseminated infection is highly likely. Such infections can lead to multisystem disease, with symptoms ranging from wasting and fever to gastrointestinal disturbances, making diagnosis and treatment more challenging. Recognition of these diverse clinical presentations is thus paramount, as it guides clinicians to specific therapeutic interventions and increases our understanding of the epidemiology of NTM infection (Ambrose et al., 2016). The rising incidence of NTM infections highlights the importance of ongoing investigations into the pathogenic processes involved, including host immunopathogenesis. One of the primary focuses of this research is the immunological pathways that predispose individuals to NTM susceptibility, particularly in patients with primary immunodeficiencies or those undergoing immunosuppressive therapy. Phagocytic dysfunction and deranged interferon-gamma production can lead to predisposition for NTM infection with a more virulent clinical presentation. The host variables of age, body habitus, and chronic health status continue to complicate the clinical profile of NTM infection. The patients are left asymptomatic even after colonization, while others become symptomatic and have invasive disease patterns that require costly medical interventions. As the clinical profile of NTM infection evolves, further research into these dynamics is necessary to optimize patient outcomes and inform clinical practice (Adcock et al., 2017).

Test Your Knowledge

1. What are the mechanisms of infection and host response?
2. What are the risk factors for NTM infections?

8.3. Diagnosis of Nontuberculous Mycobacterial Infections

Learning Outcome

1. Laboratory techniques for identification
2. Challenges in diagnosing NTM infections
3. Role of imaging studies in diagnosis

The diagnosis of nontuberculous mycobacterial (NTM) infection is becoming more relevant in light of its rising incidence and complex clinical profiles. Compared with well-defined tuberculosis and its identification in public health machinery, NTM infection is often not detected due to the lack of specificity of the presentation. Designating environmental exposure as a frequent implication, NTM infection presents in a manner similar to other diseases, such as fungal or viral diseases, which can provoke diagnostic uncertainty. Clinical suspicion typically arises in instances where patients have unresponsive chronic cough or skin lesions to standard treatment. Due to such difficulties, clinicians are forced to adopt a multi-modal diagnostic approach, integrating clinical history, radiological studies, and microbiological studies to establish an accurate diagnosis. Unless promptly and effectively identified, NTM infection can progress and lead to significant morbidity, increasing the need for heightened awareness among clinicians. Microbiological culture remains the primary method for diagnosing NTM infections, despite the development of newer molecular techniques. While mycobacterial cultures are time-consuming and can take several weeks to yield results, they provide valuable information about the specific mycobacterial species involved. Specifically, accelerated mycobacteria are frequently suspected in acute infection, requiring prompt identification and treatment to enhance patient outcomes. An epidemiological study of NTM infections revealed that clinically relevant cases primarily involve pulmonary and soft-tissue illnesses, underscoring the importance of accurate diagnosis in distinguishing these from other diseases. Furthermore, molecular methods such as PCR assays are helpful for providing rapid identification, but are limited in routine diagnosis due to cost factors and accessibility. Therefore, there needs to be an integration of traditional cultural techniques with novel molecular diagnostics for accurate diagnosis and management. The clinical importance of proper diagnosis is not to be underestimated, as timely intervention can significantly alter the disease course in patients with NTM infections. For instance, a delayed diagnosis can lead to a chronic disease that must be treated over many years, and this may take the form of a regimen of several drugs, such as aminoglycosides, macrolides, and fluoroquinolones. The combination therapy has been shown to enhance prognosis and minimize drug resistance, organism, highlighting the importance of early and accurate diagnosis. NTM keratitis is an example of the diagnostic challenge that clinicians face; the infection can easily be masked by its overlapping features with other forms of infections, such as herpes or fungal keratitis, thereby causing increased morbidity if not treated promptly. As NTM infection rates continue to rise, further advances in diagnostic techniques and technology are necessary to streamline patient treatment and improve outcomes in this growing public health issue (Ancona-Lezama et al., 2013; Brandli et al., 2017).

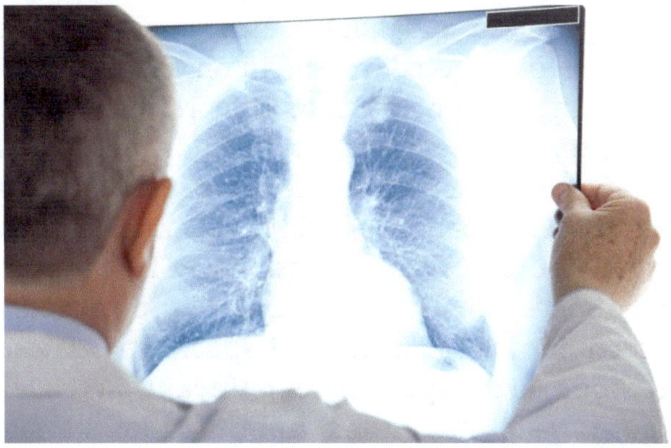

Figure 8.9. Symptoms of nontuberculous mycobacteriainfections.

Source: https://external-content.duckduckgo.com/iu/?u=https%3A%2F%2Fcrestonepharma.com%2Fwp-content%2Fuploads%2F2022%2F11%2Fx-ray-of-the-lungs-being-held-up-by-a-doctor.jpg&f=1&nofb=1&ipt=b366ba74f3651a6377a9c877a88e7d2ca385467a1c9cc6c1409f3a341f0a9f5e

8.3.1. Laboratory Techniques For Identification

Precise identification of nontuberculous mycobacteria (NTM) is crucial in diagnosing diseases caused by these organisms, particularly since they are becoming increasingly prevalent. Traditional methods, such as culture, are time-consuming and not very specific. Significant improvements have been made in laboratory technology, leading to a revolution in diagnosis. One recent method employs electrospray ionization tandem mass spectrometry, which allows mycolic acids in cell walls of various species of mycobacteria to be examined. By defining these fatty acid compositions, researchers can create unique biochemical fingerprints for every mycobacterial species, greatly enhancing the accuracy of identification. The method possesses excellent sensitivity and specificity, identifying active infection in hours or days, compared to weeks using conventional culturing techniques (Janiszewska-Drobinska et al., 2013). This paradigm revolution not only speeds up diagnosis but also enables the initiation of targeted treatment on time, thereby enhancing patient outcomes in NTM-infected patients. Furthermore, molecular diagnosis techniques have proved to be precious tools in the identification of NTM. Techniques such as polymerase chain reaction (PCR) amplify mycobacterial DNA, enabling the precise detection of NTM in clinical specimens. These methods are especially significant in cases where NTM infections mimic tuberculosis, creating diagnostic difficulties. The increasing global incidence of NTM necessitates continued refining of these molecular methods, as they have the potential to offer quicker turnaround times and greater sensitivity than traditional methods. Moreover, their integration into everyday clinical practice would help overcome many of the barriers to early diagnosis and therapy, particularly in relation to the growing immunocompromised population (Aung et al., 2018). The more that clinicians are aware of the nuances of NTM, the more sophisticated laboratory techniques will be demanded. Lastly, the role of such overall laboratory identification techniques extends not only to diagnosis but also significantly to the epidemiology and clinical aspects of NTM infections. With the help of contemporary technologies, researchers can increase our understanding about the distribution and character of various NTM strains, which is crucial for the modification of therapeutic methods. Enhanced diagnostic accuracy enables the identification of specific mycobacterial pathogens, which in turn guides treatment based on the individual susceptibility profiles of these organisms. Additionally, continued investigation into laboratory techniques may pave the way for the development of standard guidelines that can guide global management of NTM infections. Looking to the future, it will be imperative to facilitate communication between clinicians and microbiologists to optimize the laboratory facilities available, thereby enhancing our response to infections caused by high-tech pathogens.

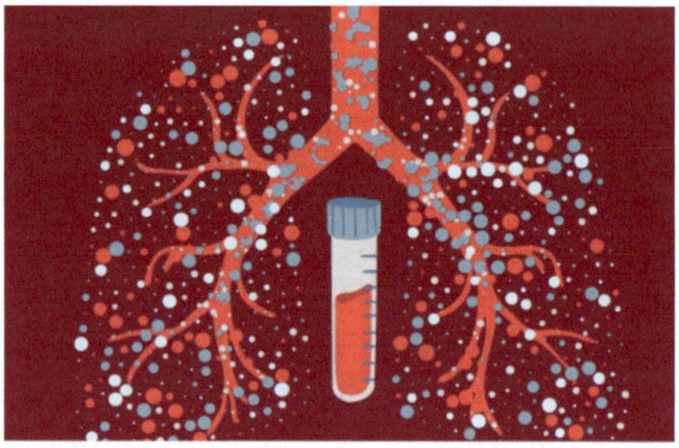

Figure 8.10. Laboratory techniques for identification of nontuberculous mycobacteriainfections.

Source: https://external-content.duckduckgo.com/iu/?u=https%3A%2F%2Fwww.biotechniques.com%2Fwp-content%2Fuploads%2F2024%2F03%2FNTM-infection-800x344.png&f=1&nofb=1&ipt=38bc46ef2c7e4a851b8baa28d1d7d6a3622aed7a4451faba677a84fc77e26d84

8.3.2. Challenges in Diagnosing nontuberculous mycobacteriaInfections

Diagnosis of NTM infection is a serious issue for clinicians. The problem primarily stems from the common overlapping clinical presentations with other pulmonary infections, particularly those caused by *Mycobacterium tuberculosis* (TB). Cough, dyspnea, and weight loss are typically misdiagnosed or diagnosed late because they are nonspecific features of most respiratory infections. Additionally, the lack of well-defined diagnostic criteria exacerbates the difficulty in identifying NTM infections. NTM may be overlooked by doctors since other, more common causes are often presumed to be involved. In this way, early intervention can be delayed, and infections can go unchecked, making it difficult to treat both the infections and the patients. This diagnostic ambiguity highlights the need for enhanced awareness and education among health workers regarding NTM, to facilitate more accurate assessments in symptomatic respiratory patients. Complexity in the diagnosis of NTM infection also stems from the diverse array of mycobacterial species. Those most frequently encountered, e.g., Mycobacterium avium complex (MAC), require specialized testing strategies that are not readily available in every healthcare setting. Variability in laboratory practice complicates the consistency of results and also leads to further mismanagement of patients. The diagnostic process itself is also time-consuming, with several weeks for culture techniques for NTM. This prolonged duration not only adds to anxiety in patients but also delays the start of possibly beneficial treatment. Additionally, diseases like underlying patient disease states, for example, pulmonary comorbidities, can obscure the clinical presentation and obscure decision-making for initiating appropriate therapy. Thus, surmounting these diagnostic challenges is crucial to better manage and treat patients with NTM infections. The economic implications of delayed or inaccurate diagnosis of NTM infection cannot be overstated. According to current studies, national hospital spending related to pulmonary NTM has risen significantly over time, corresponding to the demand for intensive healthcare services because of late presentation and undiagnosed infection complications (Allen et al., 2016). The need for extended hospital stays and NTM follow-up treatment can strain healthcare systems, resulting in substantial financial pressures on patients. Besides, the complexity of treatment regimens for NTM, often involving numerous types of antibiotics over several years, also contributes to the high healthcare costs and the risk of drug-related side effects. Ongoing research is necessary to develop efficient diagnostic tools and procedures that will help offset these economic costs, delivering improved patient outcomes and enhancing resource allocation in infection control for Nontuberculous Mycobacteria. Addressing these economic challenges reaffirms the need to improve diagnostic accuracy in NTM infection (Mohanty et al., 2023).

8.3.3. Role of Imaging Studies in Diagnosis

Imaging studies play a crucial role in the diagnosis of nontuberculous mycobacterial (NTM) infections. Computed tomography (CT) and chest X-ray, for instance, enable the visualization of pulmonary infiltrates and nodules characteristic of NTM infection. Because the diseases are insidious, imaging results can provide important information about lung involvement in terms of extent and severity. In patients, especially those with primary lung diseases such as emphysema or bronchiectasis, imaging enables physicians to differentiate NTM infection from other lung conditions and therefore direct the appropriate management modalities. Despite the significant improvements in diagnostic sensitivity brought about by recent imaging technology advancements, the correlation of radiographic findings with clinical presentation remains problematic, necessitating a multidisciplinary approach that combines imaging with microbiologic examination to define NTM infections (Adcock et al., 2017). Furthermore, the evolving architecture of imaging modalities enhances the clinician's ability to monitor disease activity and response to treatment. Imaging tests following an initial diagnosis of NTM infection are crucial for evaluating the efficacy of therapeutic measures. Regular chest CT scans can illustrate lung morphology changes and resolution of lesions, thus alerting the clinician to the patient's response to therapy. Apart from that, in suspected pseudo-outbreaks, such as the one caused by Mycobacterium gordonae, systematic imaging enables the detection of false infections and aids epidemiological surveys (Cottarelli et al., 2016). This constant surveillance through imaging not only informs the choice process in clinical practice but also enables treatment regimens that are personally tailored and specifically designed based on the patient's needs. Lastly, the use of new imaging techniques, including molecular imaging and the hybrid methods, promises exciting pathways toward an understanding of NTM disease pathophysiology. Such advanced imaging data enable the assessment of metabolic activity within lesions, thereby facilitating an early indication of treatment failure or disease progression. The use of imaging to gain biologically informative data is most beneficial to patients with complex comorbidities, such as those that coexist with HIV or who require evaluation for other opportunistic diseases (Adcock et al., 2017). As imaging continues to evolve, it holds the promise not only of enhanced diagnostic performance, but also of enhanced optimization of patient care and enabling enhanced clinical outcomes in the battle against nontuberculous mycobacterial infection.

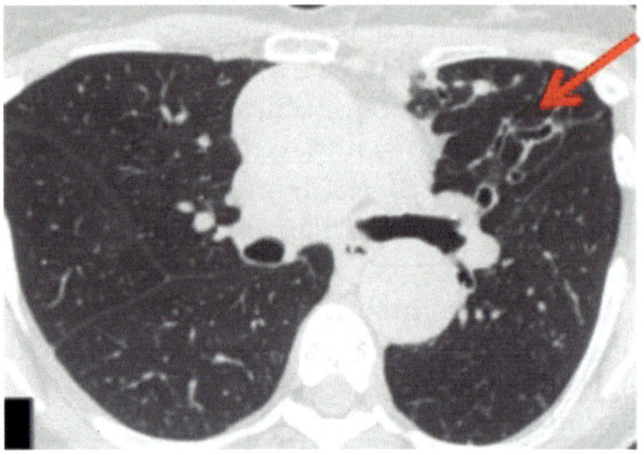

Figure 8.11. Role of imaging studies in diagnosis of nontuberculous mycobacterial infections.

Source: https://ars.els-cdn.com/content/image/1-s2.0-S2405579421000334-gr2.jpg

Test Your Knowledge

1. What are the laboratory techniques for identification?
2. What are the challenges in diagnosing NTM infections?

8.4. Treatment Options For Nontuberculous Mycobacterial Infections

Learning Outcome

1. Antibiotic regimens and their effectiveness
2. Duration of treatment and patient adherence
3. Emerging therapies and research directions

The increasing prevalence of nontuberculous mycobacterial (NTM) infection has intervened beneficial treatment modalities necessary. Contemporary treatment is typically a combination of antibiotics depending on the specific NTM species. Macrolides, such as azithromycin and clarithromycin, are regularly employed in combination therapy because they are effective against most NTM. In addition, rifamycins and ethambutol may be incorporated into the regimens to improve bacterial elimination, along with preventing drug resistance. The polycaeted character of the disease calls for the proper selection of drugs, immunocompromised patients or patients with underlying lung disease being particularly vulnerable. As the treatment of such infections becomes increasingly expensive, better treatment methods become increasingly significant in addressing not only the health but also the economic burden of these infections (Allen et al., 2016).

In addition to further enhancing patient outcomes, strict compliance with standard clinical guidelines is also required. The Infectious Diseases Society of America and the American Thoracic Society have developed comprehensive guidelines to guide clinicians in assessing and treating NTM infections (Agusti et al., 2017). However, guideline compliance is suboptimal, resulting in uneven treatment that is not suitable for patients. Multidisciplinary therapeutic approaches have been encouraging, as they provide an open channel for interaction among physicians, microbiologists, and allied health professionals, ultimately leading to a more concerted management strategy. In addition, patient education about the nature of NTM infections, as well as the importance of adhering to therapy, has been useful in achieving treatment optimization. With new studies ongoing to explore new treatment options and approaches, adherence to guidelines and multidisciplinary care become increasingly significant. The treatment of NTM diseases is evolving, with newer therapies offering improved efficacy and tolerability. New randomized controlled trials are focused on comparing the effectiveness of new antibiotics and combination therapies against various NTM species, thereby individualizing treatment regimens (Agusti et al., 2017). Additionally, the development of drug delivery systems can enhance drug tolerability, patient compliance, and overall treatment outcomes. The epidemiology of NTM infection and its risk factors remain relevant to understand; COPD and bronchiectasis predispose individuals to such an infection. Ongoing efforts to understand the pathogenesis of NTM infections will continue to reveal the nuances of this process and inform the development of targeted prevention strategies. Overall, the marriage of treatment research with vigilant adherence to current recommendations will have a radical impact on the control of these challenging infections.

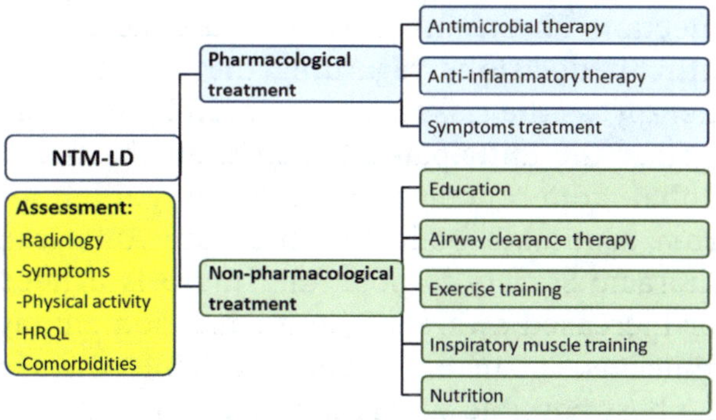

Figure 8.12. Treatment options for nontuberculous mycobacteriainfections.

Source: https://ars.els-cdn.com/content/image/1-s2.0-S0929664620302035-gr1.jpg

8.4.1. Antibiotic Regimens and Their Effectiveness

Treating infections caused by nontuberculous mycobacteria (NTM) is challenging due to the high variability and complexity of these pathogens. The antibiotic regimen of choice is typically prolonged therapy with, in most instances, a three-drug regimen for almost 18 months. Despite such prolonged treatment, the rate of culture conversion of Mycobacterium avium complex, the most frequently isolated NTM, ranges from 45% to 70% (Conyers et al., 2024). In addition, the relapse and reinfection rates are up to 60% (Conyers et al., 2024). This diminished potency is even more illustrative of the need for more effective therapeutic protocols. The unique characteristics of NTM, such as the formation of biofilms and inherent antibiotic resistance, make them challenging to treat and counterintuitive to the typical properties of antibiotics. Thus, the development of maximized therapies for NTM infection is critical to improved patient outcomes. Contemporary approaches to the treatment of NTM are largely antibiotic-based, but most patients experience side effects, intolerance, and partial responses to therapy. Side effects of the standard regimens are often significant, leading to noncompliance and even exacerbating the infection. Physicians worldwide are faced with difficult decisions regarding the initiation of therapy, as the risks must be carefully weighed against the anticipated benefits. Furthermore, global adherence to established guidelines from reputable bodies such as the American Thoracic Society is poor, and there is a need for increased awareness and education among clinicians. The management of such infections in the best possible way is through an integrated, multidisciplinary approach among physicians, microbiologists, and allied health professionals to tailor regimens based on patient needs and response. New studies highlight the need for new drugs and drug combinations to achieve optimal treatment for NTM infections. Clinical studies are in progress to evaluate new as well as established antibiotics, including drugs like Amikacin, Clofazimine, and Linezolid, which may improve treatment more optimally (Conyers et al., 2024). Moreover, targeted studies on the mechanisms of resistance and biofilm development may identify newer strategies that effectively combat such infections. The growing incidence of NTM worldwide, coupled with an aging population and increased use of immunosuppressive therapy, warrants urgent attention to this field. As the understanding of NTM-related conditions grows, the medical community needs to prioritize research focused on epidemiology, clinical evaluation, and optimization of drug regimens against these difficult-to-treat pathogens.

8.4.2. Duration of Treatment and Patient Adherence

The duration of treatment for NTM disease is one of the biggest challenges that directly influences patient adherence. Compared to more straightforward infections, NTM therapy typically includes complex drug regimens with long treatment periods that extend into several months or even years. The prolonged duration tends to cause treatment burnout in patients due to their continuous dedication to effective therapy. This fatigue can undermine adherence, leading to treatment gaps that adversely impact clinical outcomes. As highlighted in guidelines by specialist panels, such as Cystic Fibrosis Foundation findings, understanding patient motivation and barriers becomes increasingly crucial in addressing adherence to treatment regimens for NTM pulmonary disease (Bilton et al., 2015). This multifaceted approach helps personalize education and support interventions designed to stimulate patient activation throughout the entire treatment duration. Other than the inherent complexity of NTM treatment regimens, the side effects of the treatment also tend to discourage patient adherence. Patients tend to be exposed to different unwanted effects like gastrointestinal upset, fatigue, and potential drug interactions, and thus avoid taking medicines regularly as prescribed. Clinicians are therefore left with a dilemma of balancing the therapeutic benefits against the risk of side effects, which may impact patients' quality of life. Additionally, with the advancement of research, evidence suggests a pressing need for effective adherence interventions, particularly as NTM infections become increasingly prevalent (Agusti et al., 2017). Comprehensive care models must ensure that patients are provided with appropriate information regarding treatment expectations, as well as the ability to manage side effects, thereby fostering a strong partnership between patients and healthcare professionals. In order to increase patient compliance, health care systems must establish multidisciplinary care encompassing a variety of health care professionals, including physicians, pharmacists, and allied health professionals. Such collaborative efforts can help to enhance communication and provide a more holistic approach to addressing the complexity of NTM infections. Encouraging regular follow-ups and interactive discussions about treatment modalities can help in dealing with patients' anxieties, myths, and phobias. Furthermore, integrating training modules on the significance of adherence and the long-term benefits of completing therapy can help prevent treatment attrition. The multidisciplinary team's working necessity resonates with the global recognition of the needs of NTM infections, accompanied by an interlinked demand for holistic and empathetic care procedures to ensure patient adherence continues (Bilton et al., 2015; Agusti et al., 2017). Through such collaborative efforts, the outcomes of treatments for patients with NTM infections can be significantly enhanced by healthcare practitioners.

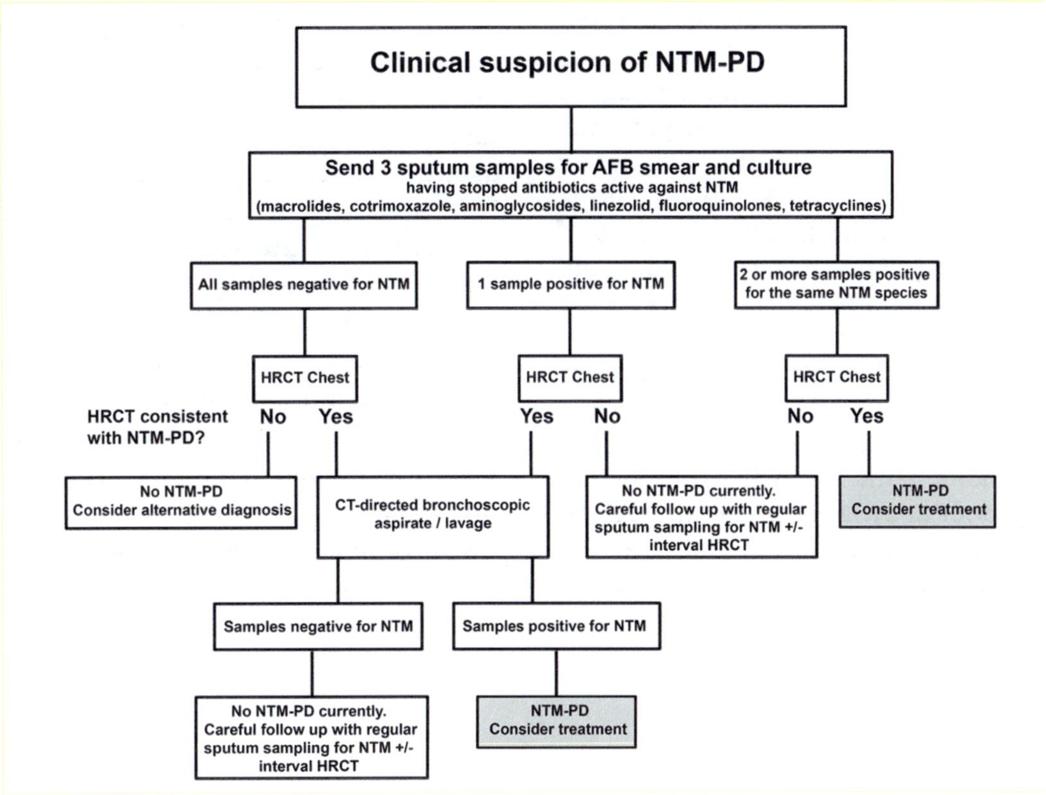

Figure 8.13. Duration of treatment and patient adherence for nontuberculous mycobacteria infections.

Source: https://www.mdpi.com/pharmacy/pharmacy-12-00126/article_deploy/html/images/pharmacy-12-00126-g001.png

8.4.3. Emerging Therapies and Research Directions

The modern understanding of non-tuberculous mycobacterial (NTM) infections is undergoing a significant shift, particularly with respect to new treatments and research avenues. New evidence suggests that NTM may have a global appearance as opportunistic disease pathogens, particularly among immunocompromised hosts, as well as those who appear to be otherwise healthy. This viewpoint requires careful monitoring and proper treatment planning. In addition, since each species of NTM possesses a unique pathogenic profile, personalized therapeutic regimens are increasingly being advocated. Increased epidemiological research efforts would undoubtedly lead to these targeted therapies because epidemiological research can delineate the interplay of various risk factors and some NTM species. As researchers continue to explore the complexities of immune responses implicated in such infections, the potential for developing targeted interventions has never seemed brighter (Alarico et al., 2016). Research has even enabled the detection of the immunological defects underpinning NTM-infected patients, unlocking the potential for novel diagnostic and therapeutic approaches. Notably, Champa Ratnatunga's work on the immune systems of different patient groups has revealed some immune dysfunctions associated with specific NTM strains. Immune response information enables the identification of biomarkers that can be applied in diagnostics, thereby facilitating easier patient management and therapy decisions. With advancing therapeutic strategies, proper knowledge of the interaction between the host's immune reaction and the infecting mycobacterial species will guide the development of novel interventions based on each patient's need, ultimately improving patient outcomes (Ratnatunga et al., 2019).

The integration of high-tech approaches, such as genomics and proteomics, into NTM research offers promising avenues for identifying new drug targets. With the advent of multi-drug resistant NTM strains, cutting-edge research assumes a critical responsibility to combat these pathogens. Utilizing high-throughput sequencing can help elucidate drug resistance and virulence factors at the genetic level, paving the way for the discovery of Next Generation Antimycobacterial agents that could potentially eradicate NTM infections. This novel school of thinking, coupled with inter-disciplinary collaboration between microbiologists, immunologists, and pharmacologists, offers a platform to initiate breakthroughs in NTM therapies. While the scientific community is still learning about the complex biology of NTM and how it interacts with the human host, the promise of novel therapies is increasingly within sight, opening the door to more effective treatment protocols and public health frameworks.

Test Your Knowledge

1. What are the antibiotic regimens and their effectiveness?
2. What is the duration of treatment and patient adherence?

8.5. Epidemiology of Nontuberculous Mycobacterial Infections

Learning Outcome

1. Global prevalence and incidence rates
2. Demographic factors influencing infection rates
3. Geographic distribution of NTM species

The epidemiology of nontuberculous mycobacterial (NTM) infection has gained increasing recognition in recent years with its rising prevalence. Even though NTMs are common in environmental reservoirs such as water and soil, their pathogenicity is mainly manifested in individuals with pre-existing health problems. The most problematic risk groups to be infected with these diseases are chronic pulmonary patients, such as those with bronchiectasis and emphysema. Fresh evidence suggests that individuals with no risk factors can also get NTM infections, highlighting the complexity of vulnerability and exposure to environmental factors. Descriptive epidemiology of out that geography, climate, and socioeconomic factors play a significant role in influencing rates of NTM disease incidence. Recognizing these trends is crucial for the development of targeted public health policies and heightened clinical suspicion for the risk of NTM infection among diverse populations (Adcock et al., 2017). Investigating further the host responses that predispose an individual to NTM infections reveals key immunological and genetic factors to be weighed. A weakened immune response due to an underlying illness can increase vulnerability; prime candidates are patients with severe primary immunodeficiency, characterized by defects in the interferon-gamma (IFNγ)-interleukin-12 (IL-12) pathway, and individuals exhibiting phagocytic defects. Such discoveries reveal vital pathways that control the body's defense against NTM organisms. Iatrogenic reasons for immunosuppressive drugs, such as those arising from cancer therapy and organ transplantation, further complicate the epidemiology by putting patients at a higher risk of NTM exposure and infection. Chronic illness, particularly human immunodeficiency virus (HIV) infection and malnutrition, also has a vital impact on this risk and reemphasizes the need for clinicians to have a broader vision of patient history when assessing infection risk (Ambrose et al., 2016). The wider implications of NTM infection epidemiology are in clinical practice and public health. As evidence mounts of a rising incidence, there is an urgent need for expanded surveillance and research setups centered on NTM ecology and man-pathogen interaction patterns. The incorporation of NTM infection awareness into clinical education and public health policy is imperative, particularly among high-risk populations. Moreover, this dynamic epidemiological information can inform the development of targeted diagnostic and therapeutic interventions, thereby diminishing the NTM disease burden in at-risk populations. As healthcare systems adapt to changes in the rates of infectious diseases, ongoing research must continue to accurately map the epidemiological trends of NTM infections and implement efficient interventions (Ambrose et al., 2016; Adcock et al., 2017).

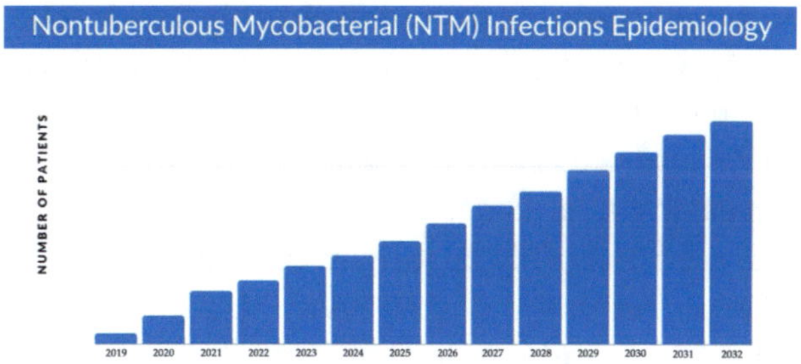

Figure 8.14. Epidemiology of nontuberculous mycobacteriainfections.

Source: https://delveinsight-images.s3.amazonaws.com/products/ck-editor/nontuberculous-mycobacterial-ntm-infections-epidemiology.png

8.5.1. Global Prevalence and Incidence Rates

The worldwide incidence and prevalence of nontuberculous mycobacterial (NTM) disease have garnered increasing attention within the medical literature due to their significant impact on public health. The NTM species, particularly the Mycobacterium avium complex (MAC), are well-recognized as etiologic agents of pulmonary infections, especially in individuals with underlying respiratory diseases. Evidence indicates a dramatic rise in NTM cases, particularly among industrialized countries, resulting from environmental exposure to contaminated land and water, which facilitates the spread of the bacteria. The increased rate may also be proof of greater sensitization and improved diagnostic methods that enable early detection and treatment. With the rising trend, epidemiological trends are of utmost significance for accommodating prevention programs and treatment strategies, which currently do not exist due to the sparse evidence on the disease burden (Mohanty et al., 2023).

Other studies reveal a shocking rising trend in hospitalization rates for NTM infections, particularly in the United States. A survey between 2001 and 2012 a staggering increase in hospitalization costs because of pulmonary NTM, to a close estimate of $904 million, versus the cost of pulmonary TB between 2001 and 2012. This disparity indicates the increasing healthcare burden of NTM. The data analyzed not only highlight the prevalence of NTM infections but also invite vast studies to determine epidemiological factors responsible for this rise. Formulation of reliable cost estimates for NTM hospitalization will be indispensable for policymakers in healthcare to prepare for resource planning and improve healthcare delivery among affected individuals (Allen et al., 2016). In addition to economic impacts, rising NTM infection rates are linked with age, comorbidities, and geographical variation. Patient demographics analysis reveals that individuals over the age of 65 years and individuals with pulmonary comorbidities are at higher risk of developing NTM infection, a revealing point where population aging and chronic lung illnesses overlap. Where access to and availability of healthcare are both low, the rates may be systematically underreported, making the problem of estimating the true reach of NTM infection rates around the world even more difficult. Notably, determining populations at risk is crucial for guiding targeted prevention measures and developing effective treatment regimens that can ultimately lower patient morbidity. A multi-pronged approach involving awareness, correct diagnostics, and economic considerations will be essential in addressing the rising global prevalence of nontuberculous mycobacterial diseases (Mohanty et al., 2023).

8.5.2. Demographic Factors Influencing Infection Rates

Knowledge about demographic determinants of rates of infection with nontuberculous mycobacteria (NTM) is crucial for the development of effective public health interventions. Age is a significant demographic determinant, as corroborated by the fact that approximately 70% of NTM pulmonary patients are over the age of 65 years. This population is more susceptible to infections due to a combination of immune function decline related to aging and the general prevalence of respiratory comorbidities, which increase vulnerability to such infections. In addition, socioeconomic status, i.e., access to healthcare, directly influences the capacity of older populations to obtain timely diagnosis and treatment, thus compounding disparities in infection outcomes. The trends observed between 2000 and 2019 indicate the need to prioritize older people in public health interventions for NTM, considering their higher risk and the corresponding strain on healthcare resources (Mohanty et al., 2023). Gender further plays a significant role in NTM infection rates, with incidences indicating variations in susceptibility and clinical presentation among men and women. Historically, research has shown a greater incidence of male patients with NTM pulmonary infections that can be partially explained by lifestyle factors, including the prevalence of smoking and work exposures that vary according to sex. Cultural and sociodemographic characteristics, including the availability of medical care and health-seeking behavior, may also make a contribution to differences noted between men and women in the experience and management of NTM infection. Knowledge of these gender differences is crucial for effectively targeting education and prevention efforts. With ongoing commitment of healthcare resources to NTM care, the recognition and resolution of these demographic conditions are more likely to provide an equitable public health response (Allen et al., 2016).

Geographic distribution further influences NTM infection rates, with some regions bearing far higher incidences. This variation can be attributed to environmental factors such as climate, soil, and exposure to particular mycobacterial strains common in specific environments.

Regions with higher humidity or those with certain industrial activities may experience more severe NTM infection rates due to increased exposure to contaminated water or aerosols. Urbanization could also be a factor favoring the transmission of NTM, as dense population centers often have a higher incidence of respiratory diseases. As healthcare systems become increasingly desperate to combat NTM, local epidemiological studies are essential. Through consideration of geographic variables, health policymakers can develop region-specific interventions that account for environmental conditions present in a given location, thereby reducing the incidence of NTM infection (Mohanty et al., 2023).

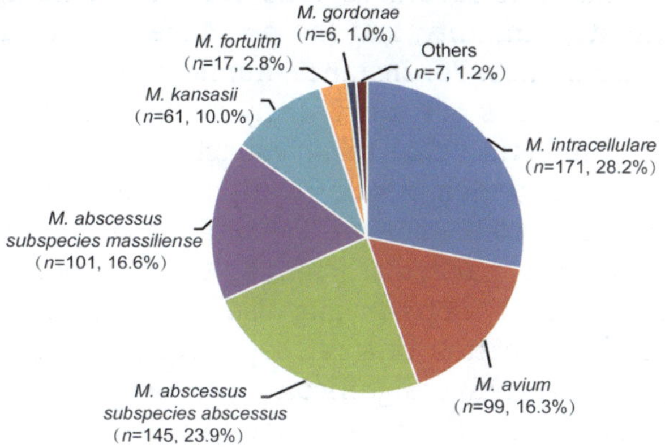

Figure 8.15. Demographic factors influencing infection rates.

Source: https://media.springernature.com/lw1200/springer-static/image/art%3A10.1186%2Fs12890-018-0728-z/MediaObjects/12890_2018_728_Fig1_HTML.png

8.5.3. Geographic Distribution of NTM Species

The geographical distribution of nontuberculous mycobacterial (NTM) species is incredibly diverse from region to region and influenced by a multitude of environmental and socio-economic determinants. In the developed world, i.e., Europe and North America, the rising incidence of NTM infections has become a public health concern. This transformation is particularly observed in urban areas, where alterations in human activity and environmental conditions can create favorable conditions for the growth of these organisms. Additionally, increased awareness and diagnostic capacity for NTM have contributed to its achievement of higher reported rates, as clinical practitioners become more skilled at identifying such infections. The evolving epidemiological situation of microbial infections highlights the necessity of more rigorous surveillance to understand the reservoirs in the environment and the routes of transmission of NTM species among these populations more clearly. The prevalence of disease caused by NTM can be attributed to several regional factors, including climate, humidity, and the presence of natural water bodies. For instance, humid and warmer temperatures are more likely to be at risk of NTM infection due to mycobacteria in water and soil, which result in higher case rates. According to the study, NTM lung infections are on the rise, particularly among the elderly and individuals with prior lung disease. Switzerland was the location of a retrospective study that demonstrated a significant increase in NTM isolation rates, further solidifying the observation that while tuberculosis cases were trending downwards, mycobacterial infection cases were rising, most notably in patients aged 41-50 years. This population shift further underscores the importance of acquiring knowledge about the geographic distribution of NTM species, as specifically tailored interventions can be formulated to reduce risk based on regional patterns and patient populations (Brandli et al., 2017). Moreover, the prevalence of particular NTM species is correlated with both local environmental factors and human factors, rendering treatment challenging. For example, areas characterized by widespread industrial and agricultural activities would be expected to exhibit distinctive NTM species profiles that reflect the impact of anthropogenic modification of the microbial environment. MAC and *Mycobacterium abscessus* infections have been noted in contaminated urban cities where risk populations habitually expose themselves to sources of contaminated water. This raises critical questions about infection control and environmental management practices among risk groups. The emerging appreciation of these organisms as significant human pathogens has led to a study of the geographic epidemiology of NTM, further emphasizing the need for ongoing surveillance and investigation of the interrelationships between environment, geography, and NTM infection dynamics (Braunstein et al., 2009).

Test Your Knowledge

1. What are the demographic factors influencing infection rates?
2. Illustrate the geographic distribution of NTM species.

8.6. Public Health Implications

Learning Outcome

1. Impact of NTM infections on healthcare systems
2. Prevention strategies for at-risk populations
3. Importance of awareness and education

The rise in the public health burden of nontuberculous mycobacteria (NTM) emphasizes the importance of intensified surveillance and infection control procedures. Research has shown that in clinical settings, NTM can most often be misidentified, leading to unnecessary treatments and distress to patients. For instance, one study reported a pseudo-outbreak of Mycobacterium gordonae, where isolates were cultured from clinical specimens of patients who had undergone bronchoscopy, and environmental contamination was raised as a question. The study identified that no patients met the diagnostic criteria for NTM lung disease, which underscores the necessity of averting mismanagement of such infections through correct detection and surveillance (Cottarelli et al., 2016). Public health measures must be directed at improving communication between healthcare providers and laboratories, enabling the early identification of NTM in both clinical and environmental samples, and thereby preventing potential outbreaks. In addition, the and ecological pathogens that cause NTM infections pose a public health challenge. Tap water and hospital equipment be contaminated with NTM organisms, as evidenced by the recovery of *M. gordonae* from water supply channeling in environmental surveys. This necessitates the inclusion of routine environmental sampling in infection control procedures in health facilities (Cottarelli et al., 2016). These preventive interventions may identify sources of contamination before they create clinical cases, safeguarding patient health. Environmental health strategies must take center stage in public health programs, combining epidemiological research with robust water quality testing. Broader screening practices can substantially reduce the exposure risk of NTM, ultimately leading to improved patient outcomes and more general community health. The therapeutic setting for NTM infections must be carefully considered to develop therapeutic options with far-reaching public health implications. Bedaquiline (BDQ), initially used in drug-resistant tuberculosis, has been shown to have promising activity against NTM in initial reports. BDQ's growth inhibition activity against several strains of NTM suggests repurposing potential; however, variations in minimal bactericidal concentrations suggest that additional studies are required. Most effective application of such new treatments could lead to improved treatment protocols, lowering the disease burden and death rate due to NTM infection. Public health interventions must incorporate ongoing investigations into the effectiveness and resistance of drugs to keep treatment recommendations current and efficacious, thereby establishing trust and compliance among patients in the management of NTM infections.

8.6.1. Impact of NTM Infections On Healthcare Systems

The rise in the occurrence of nontuberculous mycobacterial (NTM) disease presents a challenge to healthcare systems worldwide. As the pathophysiology of the infections becomes better known, its implications on patient care are better appreciated. NTM disease, which was previously thought to primarily affect immunocompromised patients, is increasingly recognized in immunocompetent hosts. The challenge demands a reassessment of prevention and treatment strategies within the healthcare environment. Additionally, the multifactorial etiology of susceptibility to NTM, encompassing both genetic and environmental factors, further complicates clinical management (Ambrose et al., 2016). As healthcare systems grapple with these emerging trends, increased awareness among healthcare providers regarding risk factors and management strategies is essential for an effective response. The impact of NTM infection extends to morbidity at the patient level, significantly affecting resource planning and models of healthcare delivery. Diagnosis and treatment of NTM require complex laboratory tests and long courses of antibiotics, which can strain healthcare resources, especially in already strained systems due to high patient volumes. Hospitals need to invest in advanced diagnostic machinery and training of health workers so that cases are correctly identified and referred, otherwise leading to mismanagement and wasteful healthcare spending. Furthermore, the chronic nature of the majority of NTM infections is likely to require repeated hospitalizations and longer hospital stays, thus placing increased burdens on healthcare systems (Faria et al., 2015). Such a growing burden helps advocate for integrative approaches to improving patient outcomes and optimal utilization of resources.

With the rising number of NTM infections, healthcare systems should implement multi-faceted approaches that emphasize prevention, early detection, and specific treatment. Strengthened surveillance systems can help detect emerging NTM strains and track rates of community transmission, which is essential since they have environmental reservoirs and the ability to form biofilms (Faria et al., 2015). Besides this, government-driven education can provide patients and healthcare workers with awareness about the risks of NTM, leading to earlier treatment and diagnosis. With these early interventions and research into novel drugs as well as vaccine development, the burden of NTM infection can be significantly reduced on the healthcare system. Ultimately, an interagency, coordinated approach from clinical, public health, and research perspectives is required to tackle the complexities of NTM infection effectively.

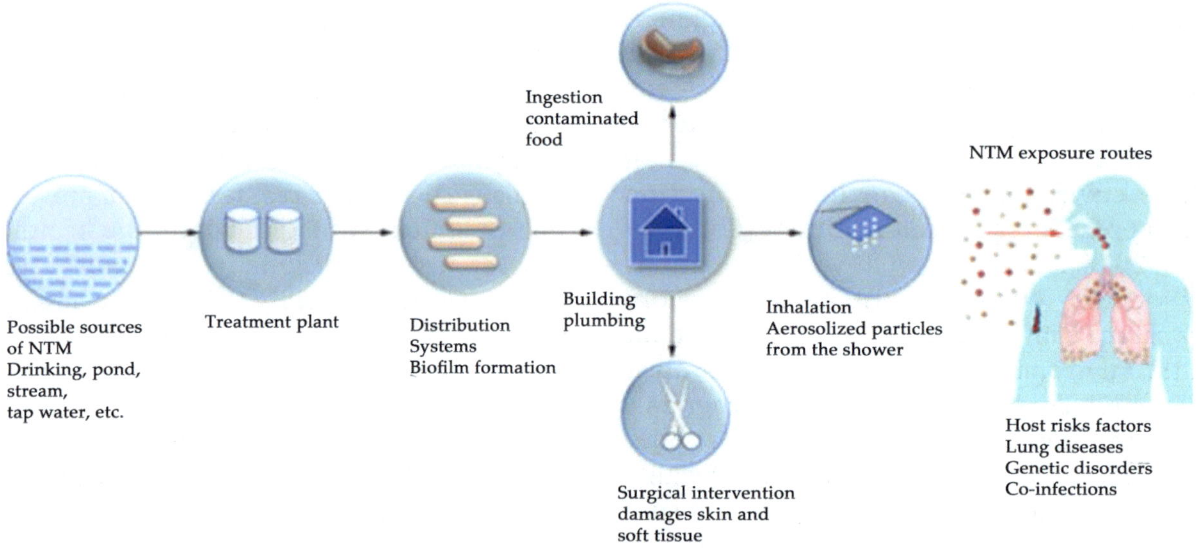

Figure 8.16. Impact of nontuberculous mycobacteria infections on healthcare systems.

Source: https://www.tandfonline.com/cms/asset/d624220e-4eee-4021-b16b-5820a2789c67/ifmb_a_2339763_f0005_c.jpg

8.6.2. Prevention Strategies For At-Risk Populations

Prevention among high-risk populations is crucial in controlling nontuberculous mycobacteria (NTM) infections. High-risk groups, including high-risk women and older age groups, are disproportionately affected by NTM, necessitating focal public health action. Public education must be used to alert these groups to the necessity of identifying early warning signs, such as persistent cough and fatigue, which are predictors of infection. Through increased awareness of the symptoms, medical practitioners can cause timely visits to healthcare centers. Preventive interventions also take into account the following environmental factors, as NTM are commonly found in water and soil. Accordingly, safe maintenance of clean water supply and practicing hygiene in some environments can significantly lower exposure to potential NTM reservoirs, ultimately decreasing the rate of infection among vulnerable members of society. Pre-existing health issues that increase the risk for NTM infection are another crucial prevention element. These patients have weakened immune function, chronic respiratory disease, or previous pulmonary history and are at risk, and therefore, certain healthcare for these patients becomes a must. Patients with cystic fibrosis or bronchiectasis, for example, need regular NTM tests. Regular monitoring facilitates the early detection and control of disease, hence limiting its impact on health. Furthermore, healthcare systems should integrate comprehensive patient and caregiver education about lifestyle modification that can potentially minimize infection risk. They include the avoidance of factors likely to worsen pulmonary disease, such as cigarette smoking, and undergoing evaluation for possible harmful environmental exposure. By emphasizing proactive management of health and the prevention of disease, we can help at-risk populations protect themselves from NTM infection. Furthermore, collaboration between local health authorities and community organizations is also essential in formulating effective prevention measures.

A multifaceted effort will strengthen disease surveillance and facilitate support responses. For instance, health surveillance system data integration is applied to determine trends and areas with heightened risk that can guide resource allocation and response plans. In Nebraska, due to the particular trends in NTM infections in the area, demographic analysis simplified the understanding of the disease extent (Hoffman et al., 2018). Similarly, further research on NTM trends is also required, as mentioned, hospitalization costs for treating NTM in the United States are increasingly placing a burden on healthcare systems (Allen et al., 2016). Broadening the scope of involvement by engaging community leaders in public health initiatives can also ensure culturally sensitive solutions that will be more readily accepted by community members. Thus, constructing public health infrastructure and forging community partnerships are essential building blocks of an effective plan to prevent the burden of NTM infections among high-risk groups.

8.6.3. Importance of Awareness and Education

Awareness and education regarding nontuberculous mycobacterial (NTM) infections are crucial pillars in the battle against the rise in these infections. The increase in clinical detection of NTM isolates signifies a severe public health concern, a sign of the need for adequate communication regarding risk factors, symptoms, and potential prevention measures. To solve such problems, there is an imperative need to enhance both public and healthcare provider knowledge. Increased awareness has the potential for better identification of risk groups and can lead to lifestyle and environmental determinants of NTM pathology being modified. Secondarily, patient education about the complications of NTM is key to ensuring active participation in the healthcare process, thereby improving clinical outcomes and quality of life in the involved patients. This emphasis on education can be a genesis for more effective public health interventions against NTM infections and also for better control of disease in general. Education is critical, particularly in having medical professionals capable of providing the best possible care to patients afflicted with NTM infections. Because treatment for nontuberculous mycobacterial pulmonary disease (NTM-PD) is often complex and requires multidisciplinary care, healthcare professionals should be aware of the disease's complexity. Standardizing training and establishing accepted nursing treatment protocols for NTM could aid in accurate diagnoses and more effective therapy. Physicians, microbiologists, pulmonologists, and allied health clinicians participating in joint training programs are essential because they provide a method for establishing common best practices in managing NTM-PD. By improving the skills of healthcare professionals in this area, patients will receive treatment in a timely and adequate manner, alleviating some of the pressure associated with these complex infections. Actually, an educated healthcare workforce lies at the center of resolving the intricacies of NTM infections and improving patient outcomes. Secondarily, developing supportive groups and facilitating collaborative research among healthcare stakeholders can significantly enhance the understanding of NTM infections. The creation of clinical networks enables experts to share their experiences, data, and treatment protocols effectively, leading to improved patient care and better overall NTM epidemiology. Further research can also offer valuable information regarding the diseases' complexity, motivating new approaches to treatment and diagnosis development. There is a proven need for greater participation in clinical trials and research programs to bridge the existing knowledge gap and improve compliance with guidelines set by international health agencies. This common focus on education and awareness can not only enhance the medical education but also provide patients with access to support groups and resources that can benefit them, ultimately providing a better quality of life as well as full engagement in their own health care (Agusti et al., 2017; Cleverley et al., 2020).

Test Your Knowledge

1. What is the impact of NTM infections on healthcare systems?
2. What are the prevention strategies for at-risk populations?

SUMMARY

In researching the rising prevalence and importance of nontuberculous mycobacteria (NTM)-induced infections, it is clear that a collaborative approach would be vital to understanding their roles in public health. Their ecological reservoirs, particularly in water, highlight the importance of monitoring their presence in various bodies of water. Experiments have demonstrated that NTM can thrive in various environments, including surface and potable water, indicating their potential to cause opportunistic infections, particularly in vulnerable individuals (Pontiroli et al., 2013). As NTM infections are increasingly recognized in immunocompromised patients, ongoing investigation into transmission dynamics and environmental reservoirs will be vital to formulating effective prevention strategies. Additionally, improvements in molecular technologies have significantly clarified NTM biodiversity, including information on their ecological functions and epidemiological trends. With techniques such as PCR-DGGE and tag-encoded pyrosequencing, scientists can definitively determine the diversity of nontuberculous mycobacteria in environmental samples (Pontiroli et al., 2013). This scientific development not only informs us about the abundance and diversity of these microbes in nature but also highlights the need for continued research efforts. The report reveals a wealth of new, previously unknown species, some of which may be causing opportunistic infection, reaffirming the need for expanded diagnostic capability and public health surveillance. Overall, the solution to the problem of infection caused by nontuberculous mycobacteria requires a multifaceted strategy that includes environmental monitoring, improved diagnostic techniques, and education on infection risk. The intricate relationship between NTM, their aquatic habitat, and human health should never be overestimated. It is necessary to indicate the role that water has been shown to play as a key reservoir of these microorganisms, particularly in light of its relevance to populations at greater risk (Bland et al., 1951). Future studies will need to emphasize longitudinal studies to monitor NTM in various conditions and reach out to marginalized populations to stop the effects of these infections effectively. This integrated approach will be the key to safeguarding public health against the threat posed by nontuberculous mycobacteria.

The NTM infection has been increasingly recognized as a significant public health concern, particularly among susceptible populations. Key findings indicate that NTM infection is most commonly observed in individuals with a potentially compromised immune system, although it is also increasingly being noted in older individuals without underlying immunodeficiency. Susceptibility heterogeneity suggests a variety of genes and environmental factors influencing the risk of NTM infection. Understanding these dynamics is crucial for developing effective prevention and treatment practices, particularly since hospitalization rates for pulmonary NTM have shown a statistically significant increase over the years, indicating an urgent need for enhanced clinical guidelines and public health interventions for these infections, especially in the United States (Allen et al., 2016). Various environmental reservoirs facilitate the spread of NTM, contributing to the complexity of the infection. Research has implicated sources such as hospital plumbing, family showers, and soil as potential carriers of NTM pathogens. Clinical and epidemiological research has established associations between clinical NTM isolates and their environmental counterparts, indicating that strains can sometimes be traced to local environmental reservoirs. However, considerable knowledge gaps exist regarding how bacteria interact with human hosts in diverse environments and climates, particularly in developing countries where data are lacking. This is a stark reminder of the need for in-depth environmental studies to track and chart the channels of NTM transmission (Halstrom et al., 2015). The effects of increasing NTM infection rates have implications that extend beyond the treatment of individual patients, affecting healthcare spending and resource utilization. Hospitalization trends are found to provide evidence that the burden of NTM rose substantially with total related hospital charges over $903 million for a twelve-year study interval. This shift places a greater emphasis on the need for health systems to adapt to the rising burden of NTM infection through enhanced prevention strategies and timely intervention efforts. Furthermore, as the epidemiology of NTMs becomes better understood, there is a need to invest resources in research studies that not only elucidate modes of transmission but also develop targeted treatment regimens aimed at curbing the growing prevalence of nontuberculous mycobacterial disease (Allen et al., 2016).

KEY TERMS FROM THIS CHAPTER

- Nontuberculous mycobacteria (NTM)
- Mycobacterium kansasii
- Environmental reservoirs
- Pulmonary NTM disease
- Bronchiectasis
- Sputum culture
- Immunocompromised host
- Disseminated NTM infection
- Macrolide antibiotics
- Mycobacterium avium complex (MAC)
- Mycobacterium abscessus
- Opportunistic infection
- Chronic cough
- Nodular infiltrates
- Acid-fast bacilli (AFB)
- Skin and soft tissue infection
- Treatment regimens
- Antimicrobial susceptibility testing

CRITICAL THINKING QUESTIONS

1. **Which of the following is true about nontuberculous mycobacteria (NTM)?**
   a. They are obligate human pathogens like Mycobacterium tuberculosis
   b. They are environmental organisms found in soil and water
   c. They are exclusively transmitted person-to-person
   d. They do not cause pulmonary disease
2. **The most common clinical presentation of pulmonary NTM infection resembles which disease?**
   a. Lung cancer
   b. Tuberculosis
   c. Asthma
   d. Pneumothorax
3. **Which of the following species is a common cause of pulmonary NTM infections?**
   a. Mycobacterium leprae
   b. Mycobacterium avium complex (MAC)
   c. Mycobacterium tuberculosis
   d. Mycobacterium bovis
4. **What is the typical method to diagnose NTM infections?**
   a. Blood culture
   b. Acid-fast bacilli (AFB) staining and culture of respiratory samples
   c. Urine antigen test
   d. PCR for HIV
5. **Which of the following is a key challenge in treating NTM infections?**
   a. Rapid resistance to all antibiotics
   b. Lack of effective antimicrobial therapy
   c. Prolonged treatment duration and complex drug regimens
   d. Inability to isolate the organism in the laboratory

Short Answer Questions

1. What are nontuberculous mycobacteria (NTM)?
2. Name two common species of NTM that cause pulmonary infections.
3. How do NTM infections differ from tuberculosis in terms of transmission?
4. What are common risk factors for developing pulmonary NTM infections?
5. Which patient population is most at risk for NTM lung disease?

Answer to Critical Thinking Questions

1. (b) 2. (b) 3. (b) 4. (b) 5. (c)

REFERENCES

1. Adcock, I. M., Garssen, J., Kazempour Dizagie, M., Mirsaeidi, M., et al. (2017). What immunological defects predispose to non-tuberculosis mycobacterial infections? https://core.ac.uk/download/157859147.pdf (accessed on 16th June 2025).
2. Aguilar-Ayala, D. A., Cnockaert, M., André, E., Andries, K., Gonzalez-Y-Merchand, J. A., Vandamme, P., Palomino, J. C., & Martin, A. (2017). *In vitro* activity of bedaquiline against rapidly growing nontuberculous mycobacteria. *Journal of Medical Microbiology*, *66*(8), 1140–1143. https://doi.org/10.1099/jmm.0.000537Agusti, A., Ahn, J., Aksamit, T., Albert, R., Albrecht, D., Aliberti, S., et al. (2017). Non-tuberculous mycobacterial pulmonary infections. https://core.ac.uk/download/195289768.pdf (accessed on 16th June 2025).
3. Alarico, S., Costa, D. N., Dalcolmo, M. P., Empadinhas, N., et al. (2016). The looming tide of nontuberculous mycobacterial infections in Portugal and Brazil. https://core.ac.uk/download/84348495.pdf (accessed on 16th June 2025).
4. Alkarni, M., Lipman, M., & Lowe, D. M. (2023). The roles of neutrophils in non-tuberculous mycobacterial pulmonary disease. https://core.ac.uk/download/554845259.pdf (accessed on 16th June 2025).
5. Allen, M. B. W. (2016). Cost of care for hospitalized patients with pulmonary mycobacterial diseases in the United States. https://core.ac.uk/download/143833879.pdf (accessed on 16th June 2025).
6. Ambrose, L. R., Lake, M. A., Lipman, M. C. I., Lowe, D., et al. (2016). "Why me, why now?" Using clinical immunology and epidemiology to explain who gets nontuberculous mycobacterial infection. https://core.ac.uk/download/77017188.pdf (accessed on 16th June 2025).
7. Ancona-Lezama, D. A., Gutiérrez-Sánchez, L., Pérez-Balbuena, A. L., Vanzzini-Zago, M., et al. (2013). Nontuberculous mycobacterial keratitis. https://core.ac.uk/download/322421622.pdf (accessed on 16th June 2025).
8. Aung, T. T., & Beuerman, R. W. (2018). Nontuberculous mycobacterial infections: Negligent and emerging pathogens. https://core.ac.uk/download/322438998.pdf (accessed on 16th June 2025).
9. Bilton, D., Corris, P., Daley, C. L., Floto, A., et al. (2015). US Cystic Fibrosis Foundation and European Cystic Fibrosis Society consensus recommendations for the management of non-tuberculous mycobacteria in individuals with cystic fibrosis. https://core.ac.uk/download/33575703.pdf (accessed on 16th June 2025).
10. Bland, M., Covert, T. C., Dailloux, M., Eaton, T., Falkinham, J. O. III, et al. (1951). Occurrence of nontuberculous mycobacteria in aquatic sources of Sri Lanka. https://core.ac.uk/download/pdf/82073793.pdf (accessed on 16th June 2025).
11. Brandli, O., Debrunner, M., Salfinger, M., von Graevenitz, A., et al. (2017). Epidemiology and clinical significance of nontuberculous mycobacteria in patients negative for human immunodeficiency virus in Switzerland. https://core.ac.uk/download/85216859.pdf (accessed on 16th June 2025).
12. Braunstein, M., Carruthers, M., Viboud, C., Centers for Disease Control and Prevention, Steiner, C., Conger, N. G., Covert, T. C., et al. (2009). Nontuberculous mycobacteria–associated lung disease in hospitalized persons, United States, 1998–2005. https://core.ac.uk/download/pdf/8406344.pdf (accessed on 16th June 2025).

13. Chen, J., Chen, L., Ernst, J., Fan, J., et al. (2012). Induction of CCL8/MCP-2 by mycobacteria through the activation of TLR2/PI3K/Akt signaling pathway. https://core.ac.uk/download/287623858.pdf (accessed on 16th June 2025).

14. Cleverley, J., Fardon, T., Lipman, M., Musaddaq, B., et al. (2020). Current and future management of non-tuberculous mycobacterial pulmonary disease (NTM-PD) in the UK. https://core.ac.uk/download/326517944.pdf (accessed on 16th June 2025).

15. Conyers, L. E., & Saunders, B. M. (2024). Treatment for non-tuberculous mycobacteria: Challenges and prospects. https://core.ac.uk/download/622645280.pdf (accessed on 16th June 2025).

16. Cottarelli, A., Mastroianni, C. M., Cirillo, D. M., Mengoni, F., Fattorini, L., Scorzolini, L., Marinelli, L., et al. (2016). Pseudo-outbreak of *Mycobacterium gordonae* in a teaching hospital: Importance of strictly following decontamination procedures and emerging issues concerning sterilization. https://core.ac.uk/download/54531524.pdf (accessed on 16th June 2025).

17. Dahl, V. N., Mølhave, M., Fløe, A., van Ingen, J., Schön, T., Lillebæk, T., Andersen, A. B., et al. (2022). Global trends of pulmonary infections with nontuberculous mycobacteria: A systematic review. *International Journal of Infectious Diseases, 125*, 120–131. https://doi.org/10.1016/j.ijid.2022.10.013 (accessed on 16th June 2025).

18. Faria, S., Jordao, L., & João, I. (2015). General overview on nontuberculous mycobacteria, biofilms, and human infection. https://core.ac.uk/download/70642066.pdf (accessed on 16th June 2025).

19. Halstrom, S., Price, P., & Thomson, R. (2015). Review: Environmental mycobacteria as a cause of human infection. https://core.ac.uk/download/195658086.pdf (accessed on 16th June 2025).

20. Hoffman, M. (2018). An assessment of nontuberculous mycobacteria in Nebraska. https://core.ac.uk/download/268252751.pdf (accessed on 16th June 2025).

21. Janiszewska-Drobinska, B., Behr, M. A., Beukes, M., Brennan, P. J., Butler, W. R., Centers for Disease Control and Prevention (CDC), Chang, A., et al. (2013). Rapid method for *Mycobacterium tuberculosis* identification using electrospray ionization tandem mass spectrometry analysis of mycolic acids. https://core.ac.uk/download/71976389.pdf (accessed on 16th June 2025).

22. Mohanty, B. K. (2023). Trends of non-tuberculous mycobacterial pulmonary disease in a low-tuberculosis prevalence setting. https://core.ac.uk/download/588769996.pdf (accessed on 16th June 2025).

23. Pontiroli, A., Aseffa, A., Pontiroli, A., Amend, A. S., Haas, B. J., Oakley, B. B., Le Dantec, C., et al. (2013). Prospecting environmental mycobacteria: Combined molecular approaches reveal unprecedented diversity. https://core.ac.uk/download/16664133.pdf (accessed on 16th June 2025).

24. Raghu, G., Rémy-Jardin, M., Ryerson, C. J., Myers, J. L., Kreuter, M., Vašáková, M., Bargagli, E., et al. (2020). Diagnosis of hypersensitivity pneumonitis in adults: An official ATS/JRS/ALAT clinical practice guideline. *American Journal of Respiratory and Critical Care Medicine, 202*, e36–e69. https://doi.org/10.1164/rccm.202005-2032st (accessed on 16th June 2025).

25. Ratnatunga, C. N. (2019). Deconstructing the immunopathogenesis of lung infections. https://core.ac.uk/download/399588010.pdf (accessed on 16th June 2025).

FUNGAL INFECTIONS OF THE LUNG AND PARASITIC LUNG DISEASES

9

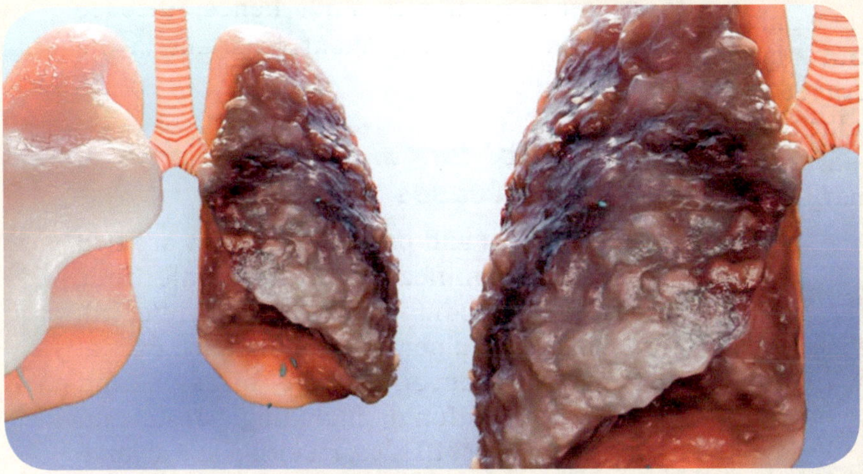

LEARNING OBJECTIVES

After studying this chapter, you will be able to:

1. Give an overview of fungal infections
2. Explain the pathophysiology of fungal infections
3. Explore the diagnosis of fungal lung infections
4. List the treatment options for fungal infections
5. Give an overview of parasitic lung diseases
6. Understand the diagnosis and treatment of parasitic lung diseases

Introduction

The respiratory system, being a part of human physiology, is susceptible to infectious damage from various pathogens, primarily fungal pathogens and parasites. Fungal infections of the lung are significant health problems, and these occur most prominently among immunocompromised hosts. These diseases, ranging from histoplasmosis to aspergillosis, are often underestimated in terms of incidence and severity. Given the increasing incidence of such lung diseases, it is crucial to enhance awareness and knowledge levels among both the medical community and the general population. The multifactorial etiology of lung infections caused by fungi necessitates ongoing research on their pathogenesis and optimal treatment protocols. Furthermore, with the transformation of farming, the risk of zoonotic infections and parasitic diseases affecting the lung function also rises, which emphasizes the need for an extensive analysis of these interrelated notions in respiratory pathology. Simultaneously, parasitic pulmonary disease raises another issue, particularly in regions where environmental conditions facilitate the transmission of such infections. Conditions such as eosinophilic bronchopneumopathy illustrate the complex interplay between host immune response and parasitic infection. Eosinophilic lung disease, eosinophilic inflammation, can cause severe morbidity in infected individuals, particularly in dogs, with a variable range of clinical presentation obscuring conventional diagnostic procedures (Dear et al., 2019). Understandings of these interactions not only augment our medical knowledge but also assists in developing personalized therapeutic interventions for the infected populations, illuminating the interaction between parasitic infections and lung function in veterinary and human medicine.

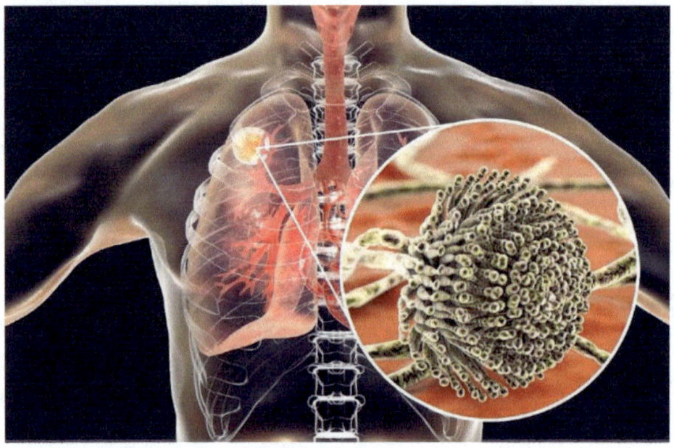

Figure 9.1. Fungal infections of the lung and parasitic lung diseases.

Source: https://www.ddw-online.com/wp-content/uploads/2021/05/pulmonary-Aspergillosis.jpg

The inclusion of agricultural life and its implications for health is also vital in comprehending the broader picture of fungal and parasitic lung diseases. The organic livestock production sector, for instance, as much as it promotes sustainable practices, also faces parasitic infestation challenges and their consequent health impacts on animals and humans. From the facts, conventional agriculture could expose livestock to fewer burdens of infection, but the assumption that organic processes yield better health outcomes remains unsubstantiated (Eijck et al., 2003). Thus, interdisciplinary research will be required to evaluate the influence of farming practices on the incidence of pathogens and zoonotic transmission rates. This collaborative strategy will give a better understanding of how fungal and parasitic infections collectively contribute to respiratory health and, hence, disease prevention and management programs in the future.

Definition of fungal infections and parasitic diseases

Fungal diseases and parasitic diseases are two distinct but significant classes of infectious diseases that compromise human health, particularly in vulnerable populations. Fungal diseases are caused by the invasion and proliferation of fungi, including yeasts and molds, within host tissues, resulting in a diverse range of disease presentations. The diseases may manifest as superficial conditions, such as athlete's foot, to systemic conditions, such as invasive aspergillosis, and this is especially sinister in immunocompromised patients. On the other hand, parasitic illnesses are caused by organisms that obtain food and shelter from their hosts. They may be unicellular (protozoa) or multicellular (helminths) and can infect any organ system, including the respiratory one. These need to be defined because they provide the fundamental understanding of more complex interactions in a specific disease, particularly in diseases involving the respiratory system. Fungal infection and lung illness have particularly become significant in the context of the modern era of medicine, when patients with impaired immune responses, such as those with malignancies involving the blood system, are at heightened risk. In one analysis of patients presenting with acute respiratory failure (ARF), many etiologies, such as fungal infection, accounted significantly for morbidity and mortality. Specifically, invasive pulmonary aspergillosis was associated with a significantly increased risk of mortality, illustrating the serious ramifications of fungal infections in immunocompromised hosts (Azoulay et al., 2016).

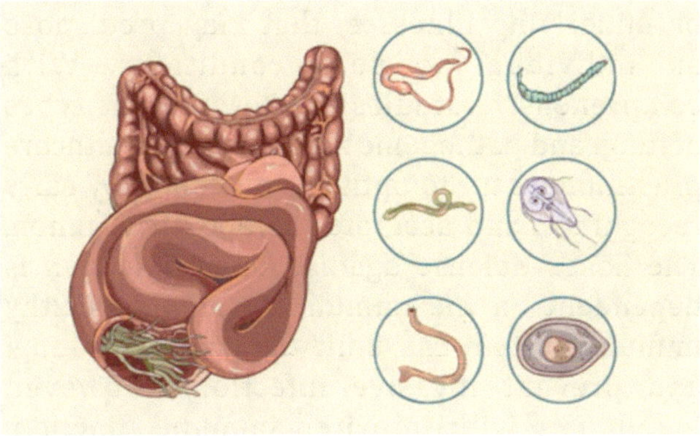

Figure 9.2. Fungal infections and parasitic diseases.

Source: https://knyamed.com/cdn/shop/files/parasitic-and-fungal-infections-708x364.jpg?v=1718798230&width=600

The fine line between background disease and the virulence of the fungal organism highlights the importance of accurate diagnostic techniques in the early identification of such infections, which is of direct consequence to therapeutic efficacy and improved patient outcomes. Parasitic infections also present a severe problem in lung health, particularly in endemic regions where there is frequent exposure to various pathogens. Conditions like eosinophilic lung disease, which can result from parasitic infections, demonstrate how such parasites can lead to significant inflammatory responses, ultimately resulting in respiratory illnesses. Eosinophilic lung disease has been studied to explain differences in presentation based on diagnostic classification like eosinophilic bronchitis and eosinophilic bronchopneumopathy and hence the need for certain therapeutic approaches (Dear et al., 2019). The diversity presents another factor in achieving lung health, as relevant evidence demonstrates that eosinophilic lung disease can have enduring effects unless properly managed. In general, precise definitions of fungal infections and parasitic diseases must be utilized in defining their roles in respiratory pathology.

Importance of studying lung infections

The significance of studying lung infections cannot be overstated, particularly in the settings of fungal disease and parasitic pulmonary illness. Lung infection remains among the leading causes of morbidity and mortality throughout the world, and its pathophysiologies and etiologies should be elucidated. Fungi such as *Aspergillus* and Candida species are the causative agents for serious pulmonary complications, particularly among immunocompromised individuals. This vulnerability highlights the importance of conducting in-depth research on diagnostic tools, treatment protocols, and preventive measures that may mitigate the severity of such infections. Furthermore, the examination of lung infections across various populations reveals disparities in health outcomes, which can inform public health programs aimed at reducing morbidity for these diseases. Parasitic infections are also a significant burden on lung pathology, with parasites like Ascaris suum causing severe respiratory responses. The interaction between the parasitic infection and the host's immune system presents the pathology of lung disease. The elucidation of how these parasites evade the immune system and lead to inflammation can contribute to more effective therapeutic approaches. New evidence in host-pathogen interaction research with animal models, as reported in Agnone et al. (2017), has yielded some fascinating discoveries to open up improved vaccine and treatment strategy development with antigen-specific immunity at its heart. It is essential to reveal these pathways to aid the battle against parasitic infection respiratory comorbidities, ultimately resulting in improved patient care and public health protocols. Furthermore, learning about lung infections in various cultures and geographic regions highlights the need for tailored public health interventions. For instance, Adams et al. (2010) identify that Africa is characterized by a diverse array of diseases, which demand localized disease control approaches. Fungal and parasitic lung infections are overlooked in overall health programs, yet have significant impacts on marginalized populations. It is essential to understand the socioeconomic and environmental determinants of these infections to devise effective and practical strategies that work towards prevention as well as treatment. By synthesizing research evidence and community-level action, health systems can make evidence-based priority setting decisions regarding the most urgent respiratory diseases, thereby strengthening the resilience of at-risk populations. This multidisciplinary approach highlights the importance of examining lung infections within the broader context of global health.

9.1. Overview of Fungal Infections

Learning Outcome

1. Common types of fungal infections affecting the lungs
2. Risk factors for developing fungal lung infections
3. Symptoms and clinical presentation

Fungal diseases are a significant public health issue due to the capacity of the fungi to infect a wide range of host organisms, such as plants, animals, and humans. Infections can be caused by opportunistic pathogens or saprophytic fungi that occur naturally in the environment. The diversity of fungal organisms contributes to the challenge of treatment and diagnosis since it may manifest in various ways, ranging from superficial dermatological infections to incapacitating systemic infections. The most critical aspect of knowledge about fungal infections is the ability to identify risk factors, such as immunocompromised status or underlying illnesses, that may predispose an individual to such conditions. With comprehensive studies of the different types of fungi and pathogenic mechanisms, healthcare practitioners try to optimize outcomes by early recognition and accurate therapeutic regimen. The host's defense against fungal infection is dependent on the immune system. A healthy immune system can limit the growth of fungi and prevent invasive infections; however, individuals with impaired immune function, such as those undergoing chemotherapy or those with HIV/AIDS, are more susceptible to fungal invasion. In addition, environmental factors, such as exposure to some fungal spores, have a significant impact on infection rates, particularly in patients with lung disease. For instance, eosinophilic lung disease can be caused by exposure to fungi, indicating an intricate interaction between environmental and immunologic factors in the development of fungal disease. Understanding these dynamics is paramount in developing targeted interventions and promoting strategies that enhance resistance and reduce risks of fungal disease (Dear et al., 2019). Recent research indicates a disturbing trend of antifungal resistance development, further complicating the treatment of fungal infections. Fungi such as *Aspergillus* species and *Candida* species have developed resistance to the antifungals used conventionally, further complicating treatment with conventional methods and necessitating the investigation of novel therapeutic compounds. This increase is exacerbated by excessive use of antifungal medications in clinical and agricultural settings and has created a desperate demand for surveillance and stewardship programs. Paying attention to the treatment of existing infections while avoiding resistance calls for the experts to place emphasis on research to determine the root mechanisms of resistance and public health concerns. These findings are crucial for the development of effective guidelines that address this new challenge and for promoting further education on the importance of prudent use of antifungals in all contexts (Eijck et al., 2003).

9.1.1. Common Types of Fungal Infections Affecting the Lungs

Fungal pneumonia is becoming a growing concern due to its increasing incidence, particularly in immunocompromised patients. The most common of these is Aspergillosis caused by the *Aspergillus* fungi, which are ubiquitous in soil and decaying organic material. People with weakened immunity or chronic pulmonary disease may have trouble with an invasive type of this infection, invasive pulmonary aspergillosis. This is a very morbid condition and may be fatal if not treated. Clinically, it can present as cough, fever, and chest pain, similar to bacterial pneumonia, making diagnosis difficult. Effective treatment requires addressing the multifactorial disease with antifungal therapy and treating any underlying diseases that predispose patients to infection. Another common fungal lung infection is Histoplasmosis, caused by Histoplasma capsulatum, which is typically found in areas with high concentrations of bird and bat droppings. The inhalation of spores can lead to asymptomatic infections or result in respiratory diseases, particularly among individuals with compromised immune systems. Most healthy individuals clear the asymptomatic infections without treatment, but others develop chronic pulmonary histoplasmosis, which resembles tuberculosis, and is both a diagnostic and therapeutic challenge. Chronic infections may lead to progressive lung damage, necessitating antifungal treatment or even surgery in severe situations. The environmental distribution of *Histoplasma* becomes significant for prevention and early detection, especially in regions of high endemicity, underscoring the need for public health interventions and education aimed at minimizing exposure risks, particularly in high-risk groups. Coccidioidomycosis, caused by *Coccidioides* species, is another significant fungal lung disease that affects the southwestern region of the United States. Inhalation of its aerial spores can cause a variety of illnesses, ranging from mild flu-like symptoms to severe lung infections. The condition can resolve as primary pulmonary coccidioidomycosis, which may spontaneously clear in healthy individuals but can progress to become chronic or disseminate, especially in immunocompromised individuals. Complications of this infection can necessitate extended antifungal treatment, with some cases requiring surgery. It is essential for medical professionals to be aware of the geographic prevalence and clinical manifestations of coccidioidomycosis, as early diagnosis and treatment are crucial in improving patient outcomes and reducing the burden of fungal infection-induced lung diseases.

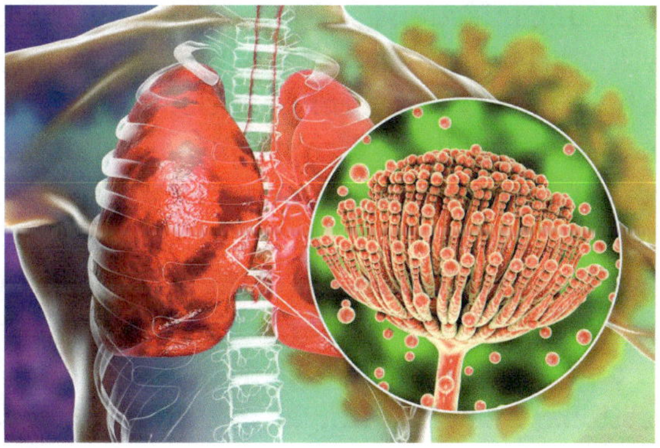

Figure 9.3. Fungal infections of lungs.

Source: https://external-content.duckduckgo.com/iu/?u=https%3A%2F%2Fcdn.mdedge.com%2Ffiles%2Fs3fs-public%2FPulmonary_aspergillosis_web.jpg&f=1&nofb=1&ipt=171d6c457cffe0f572fd48bad5f5a2ef7f56fd7afb8a0916ee194a8c033cad03

9.1.2. Risk Factors For Developing Fungal Lung Infections

Fungal pneumonia infections are increasingly being recognized as significant health threats, particularly for specific populations with higher susceptibility to certain risk factors. Immunocompromise is a risk factor, which can be caused by underlying health conditions such as HIV/AIDS, diabetes, or cancer, and therapies such as chemotherapy and corticosteroid therapy. Individuals with compromised immune systems are compelled to fight against opportunistic pathogens, such as fungi that normally inhabit soil and decomposing organic matter. Secondly, exposure is also important; individuals who reside in environments with excessively disturbed soil or dust are at a higher risk of inhaling spore-form fungi that inhabit such environments.

As the soil is home to a diverse population of microorganisms, including potential pathogens, the interaction of these factors significantly increases the risk of infection in vulnerable populations (Lee et al., 2011). A second important risk factor for acquiring a fungal lung infection is underlying lung diseases, particularly chronic obstructive pulmonary disease (COPD) and asthma. Patients with such illnesses often have compromised pulmonary structure and ciliary mucociliary clearance that predispose them to fungal colonization and eventual infection. Smoking also increases lung disease, with further compromise in the immune state and increased susceptibility to infections, including fungal infections. Present evidence suggests that patients with asthma may have altered immune reactions, making them susceptible to specific fungal pathogens, such as *Aspergillus* spp., which are notorious for triggering allergic bronchopulmonary aspergillosis in predisposed individuals. The interaction of such predisposing factors with environmental exposures adequately depicts the integrative nature of risk factors for fungal lung infections (Firkins et al., 2015). Moreover, socioeconomic factors cannot be overlooked when assessing the risk environment for fungal lung infection. Individuals of low socioeconomic status are likely to come with issues such as limited access to healthcare, malnutrition, and unsanitary living conditions that are conducive to fungi growth and exposure. For instance, overcrowded living conditions may lead to humidity and mold growth, creating a conducive habitat for air-borne fungi. Moreover, populations engaged in specific occupational environments, such as farm laborers or construction workers, may be exposed to a greater intensity of fungal spore exposure. Addressing these socioeconomic disparities is crucial for formulating successful public health interventions to mitigate the impact of fungal disease. Together, it is evident that a general understanding of these diverse risk factors is crucial in developing targeted prevention and management policies for fungal lung infections (Lee et al., 2011).

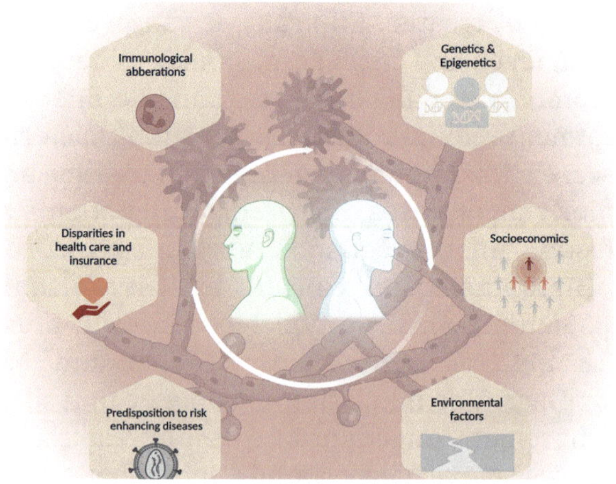

Figure 9.4. Risk factors for developing fungal lung infections.

Source: https://journals.plos.org/plospathogens/article/figure/image?size=medium&id=10.1371/journal.ppat.1011025.g001

9.1.3. Symptoms and Clinical Presentation

A comprehensive understanding of the signs and clinical presentation of fungal lung infections and parasitic lung diseases is essential for accurate diagnosis and early management. Patients present with respiratory symptoms, which can initially mimic other more common illnesses, such as viral infections or bacterial pneumonia. Usually, patients have a chronic cough, dyspnea (dyspnea is shortness of breath), chest pain, and systemic signs and symptoms such as fever and malaise. In deep fungal infections, the patient can also present with hemoptysis, a sign of cavitating lung lesions. Because these are often mimicked by other illnesses, a heightened index of suspicion on the part of clinicians, particularly in immunocompromised hosts who are most likely to develop serious disease, is necessary. Hence, early clinical evaluation and appropriate diagnostic workup are essential in the differential diagnosis of these infections from other pulmonary illnesses. In specific environments, especially those with restricted resources, health professionals may rely on clinical presentation to guide their provisional diagnostic plan. This leads to diagnostic mistakes, as shown by studies documenting the clinical diagnosis of tuberculosis (TB) among individuals with lymphadenopathy. Research has shown that, despite presenting symptoms paradigmatic for TB, many of these patients were diagnosed with other diseases, including malignant processes and fungal infections. Not only does misdiagnosis lead to delay in treatment, but it also propagates poor patient outcomes, which makes the imperative for comprehensive diagnostic workups encompassing the entire spectrum of potential etiologies even greater. Doctors should be aware that, although fungal infections typically present in acute worsening, simulating bacterial pneumonia, chronic and less severe forms can also be present in endemic regions. Therefore, histological analysis and imaging studies should be part of a comprehensive assessment (Abba et al., 2017).

Parasitic lung infections, while less commonly diagnosed, have their own clinical presentations that should not be overlooked in differential diagnosis. Their presentation is generally characterized by cough, wheezing, and eosinophilia, an indicator that reflects an immune reaction to parasitic antigens. For instance, *Strongyloides stercoralis* and *Ascaris lumbricoides* both present with respiratory and gastrointestinal manifestations that complicate their symptomatology. Similar to fungal infections, inappropriate treatment methods can result from the misidentification of these symptoms, particularly in groups with limited access to healthcare. Furthermore, new evidence suggests a correlation between environmental exposure and soil-borne pathogen-associated respiratory clinic profiles, implying that environmental exposure is a significant factor in the prevalence of disease (Lee et al., 2011). Clinicians thus must include patient history, travel exposure, and environmental exposures in their evaluations for proper diagnosis and treatment of parasitic lung disease.

Test Your Knowledge

1. What are the common types of fungal infections affecting the lungs?
2. What are the risk factors for developing fungal lung infections?

9.2. Pathophysiology of Fungal Infections

Learning Outcome

1. Mechanisms of fungal invasion in lung tissue
2. Immune response to fungal infections
3. Consequences of untreated fungal infections

The pathophysiology of fungal infection, with a focus on infection in the lungs, is a complex interaction between the infectious pathogen and the host's immune system. Fungal pathogens are known to enter the respiratory tract through inhalation, whereupon they can evade the host's defense mechanism through exploitation of multiple virulence factors. These include adhesins that promote colonization and toxins that can potentially kill host tissue, which can be culpable for the establishment of infection. When they arrive at the lungs, fungi can cause an inflammatory response that leads to tissue damage and granuloma formation, areas where immune cells clump to encapsulate the fungi. Ongoing stimulation of the immune system by fungal antigens can lead to chronic inflammation, further complicating the disease process and resulting in impaired or complete respiratory function, as well as tissue necrosis. Of fungal lung infections, certain species are of particular note, including Aspergillus, Cryptococcus, and Histoplasma. All of these pathogens possess certain mechanisms for pathogenicity that influence both disease severity and clinical picture of the host. Aspergillus, for example, can cause invasive aspergillosis most often in immunocompromised hosts. The pathophysiology involves not only direct invasion of tissues by the organism, but also secondary manifestations, such as hemoptysis and lung cavitation. Cryptococcal infections are most commonly manifested with respiratory symptoms as well as systemic dissemination, usually in immunocompromised hosts. Identification of these pathogens and their pathogenesis is crucial to determining effective treatment and improving patient outcomes. Therapy for fungal pneumonia is complicated by the potential for coinfection with other pathogens, such as parasites and bacteria. For example, in cases of mixed fungal pneumonia and standard bacterial pneumonia, a combined diagnostic approach is necessary to guide appropriate treatment.

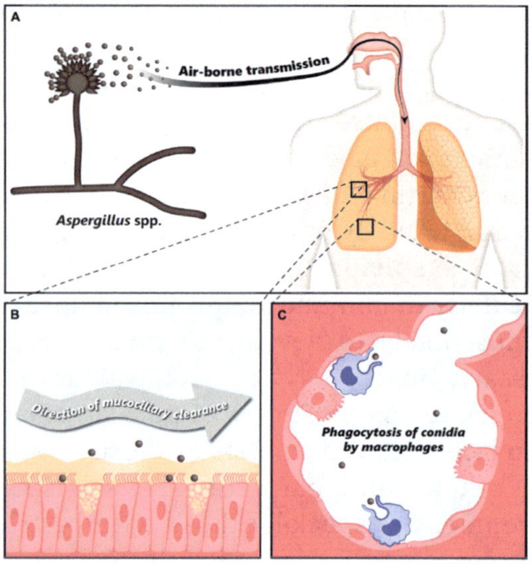

Figure 9.5. Pathophysiology of fungal infections lung infections.

Source: https://www.frontiersin.org/files/Articles/832510/fmed-09-832510-HTML/image_m/fmed-09-832510-g001.jpg

The clinical significance of such infections is that they are likely to complicate the intrinsic pulmonary illnesses and convalescence from other pulmonary diseases. In the context of parasitic lung infections, co-infection of fungal and parasitic factors adds another layer of complexity to patient care, as with parasitic infestations complicated by eosinophilic pneumonia. Recognition of interactions between parasitic and fungal pathogens can influence therapeutic strategy and population-based prevention measures among populations at risk (Thamsborg et al., 2004; Dear et al., 2020).

9.2.1. Mechanisms of Fungal Invasion in Lung Tissue

Fungal lung tissue infections are a complex interplay between pathogens and host defenses, and central to disease progression is the mechanism of invasion. When inhaled, fungal spores such as those from *Aspergillus* penetrate the respiratory epithelium, exploiting compromised mucosal barriers. The initial point of contact with lung tissue is critical, involving adherence to epithelial cells through heterogeneous surface receptors, which facilitates attachment. This interaction is not just passive; it triggers the host immune response and can alter the microenvironment to favor fungal growth. Pathogens have evolved various mechanisms to bypass host defense, including the production of proteolytic enzymes that degrade connective tissue and disrupt immune signaling pathways. Recognition of the mechanisms by which fungi gain entry can explain the process of disease and reinforce the necessity for targeted therapeutic regimens capable of breaking the invasive capacity of fungi and re-establishing pulmonary health. The immune system is equally crucial in defending against fungal invasion in lung tissue. A key component of such a defense involves cytokines, such as interleukin-17 (IL-17), that are pivotal in coordinating an effective immune response against fungal pathogens. The induction of IL-17A and IL-17F, for example, enhances the release of pro-inflammatory molecules that facilitate the recruitment and activation of neutrophils and other immune cells to the site of infection. (Das et al., 2017) highlights the dual-edged nature of IL-17's action, establishing that while it is protective in nature, excessive IL-17 responses can also result in tissue damage and chronic inflammation. This association highlights the delicate balance that the immune system must maintain to combat fungal infections without causing collateral damage to the lung tissue itself, underscoring the complexity of the immune response to fungal penetration. Furthermore, the respiratory mucosal barrier is a crucial defense against fungal penetration, representing not only a physical barrier but also an active participant in immune surveillance. The lung mucosal surface houses specific immune cells that come into contact with inhaled pathogens and thus trigger protective mechanisms. Recent studies have brought to light the role of inflammasomes and other immune components within the mucosa in detecting fungal threats and triggering an appropriate defense response. (Upadhyay et al., 2023) further emphasizes the importance of innate immune signaling as well as coordination between various mucosal sites, which individually enhance the host's capacity to fight infection. Through understanding how these mucosal barriers function and how they interact coordinately, researchers can identify potential targets that can enhance and strengthen immunity and improve prognosis in patients with lung fungal infection, enabling new mechanisms to manage the diseases.

9.2.2. Immune Response To Fungal Infections

The immune response against fungal infections, particularly in the lung, is a complex synergy of innate and adaptive mechanisms. As the innate immune system initially comes into contact with fungal pathogens, it acts as the first line of defense, comprising phagocytes such as macrophages and neutrophils. They identify fungal organisms, e.g., beta-glucans present in the cell wall, through pattern recognition receptors (PRRs). Activation of such immune cells leads to the production of pro-inflammatory cytokines that attract other constituents of the immune system to the site of infection. Cytokine action is exemplified through the function of interleukin-17 (IL-17), which coordinates inflammation and enhances neutrophils' capacity for combating fungal infections. However, this response must be carefully regulated to avoid triggering excessive inflammation, which can cause tissue damage and lead to lung pathologies associated with fungal infection (Das et al., 2017). As the immune response progresses, the adaptive immune system assumes a more significant role, particularly through the activation of T cells. CD4+ T helper cells differentiate into several subsets, and Th17 cells produce IL-17, which further enhances the response to fungal pathogens. This adaptive immune response is essential for the induction of immunological memory, which provides for a quicker and more effective response to subsequent exposure to infection. Additionally, antibody production, primarily by B cells, complements T cell immunity by inactivating fungal components and opsonizing the pathogens for better phagocytosis. The delicate balance between protective immune defense and potential tissue damage remains a challenge because overabundant IL-17 responses can drive inflammatory lung disease. The dual role of IL-17 highlights the complexity of the immune response to fungal infections, as well as its implications for therapeutic interventions (Alcazar-Fuoli et al., 2014). The consequence of an abnormal or excessive immune response can manifest in various clinical presentations, including some chronic pulmonary conditions, such as allergic fungal sinusitis and allergic bronchopulmonary aspergillosis. Dissection of the immune mechanisms underlying fungal lung infections significant implications for the development of targeted therapies. As such, current research aims at immunomodulatory treatment that is able to increase protective function without concomitant harm to lung tissue. Targeting key players of immune response, such as IL-17 and its signaling mechanisms, is a promising strategy to maximize effective anti-fungal immunity with minimal inflammatory complications. Ultimately, understanding these immune dynamics not only provides a deeper insight into fungal infections but also has broader implications for lung health management in parasitic diseases and other pulmonary infections (Das et al., 2017).

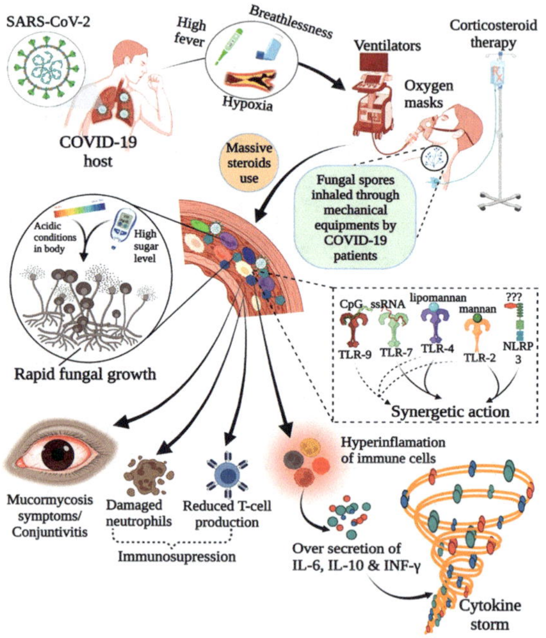

Figure 9.6. Immune response to fungal infections in lung.

Source: https://www.researchgate.net/publication/361015886/figure/fig3/AS:11431281081512482@1661825273576/Mechanism-of-immune-response-in-COVID-19-and-co-fungal-infection-image-created-by.png

9.2.3. Consequences of Untreated Fungal Infections

The consequences of uncontrolled fungal infections, particularly in the respiratory system, are serious and multifaceted. Fungal infections such as aspergillosis and cryptococcosis often present in individuals with compromised immune systems, leading to sequelae that may evolve into chronic respiratory arrest. Uncontrolled infections can result in tissue necrosis, as the fungus colonizes and destroys lung tissue, leading to symptoms such as chronic cough, hemoptysis, and worsening dyspnea. The ongoing damage can compromise respiratory function, resulting in chronic complications that may require lobectomy surgery. Secondly, unresolved fungal infections

might exacerbate underlying lung conditions, predisposing the patient to an enhanced risk for secondary infections that could even result in life-threatening situations. The severity of the effects underscores the importance of early diagnosis and treatment to prevent the hazards of fungal pathogens within the lungs. Apart from respiratory issues, untreatable fungal infections can also significantly add to morbidity and mortality among vulnerable groups such as individuals with comorbid disease states. An incomplete intervention can allow for extrapulmonary spread of the fungi to lead to invasive infection with organ dissemination, such as the brain, liver, or kidneys. These issues are of particular relevance in the cases of immunocompromised patients, e.g., HIV/AIDS or chemotherapy patients, who have weakened defensive mechanisms against pathogens. Findings suggest that it is crucial to screen immunocompromised patients for signs of fungal infection, as early treatment and diagnosis are essential in preventing systemic spread and resulting complications. The ripple effects of untreated fungal infections could then propagate from individual health to influence healthcare systems, contributing to care burdens and expenses to address late stages of disease and complications, exacerbating public health concerns. Additionally, the effect of untreated fungal infections is also linked to other diseases caused by pathogens, and it is likely to create complex health issues. As suggested by studies, the existence of fungal infection has been associated with increased risk of developing other respiratory illnesses, such as bacterial pneumonia, particularly in patients with existing chronic pulmonary disease. Furthermore, the interactivity of most pathogens—e.g., those in the TORCH acronym, which identifies major infectious pathogens that target fetal development—shows the potential for fungal infections to impact maternal and fetal health during pregnancy adversely. Interacting infections complicate treatment scenarios, as they require elaborate management plans that consider the dual burden of fungal and other infections affecting patients. This intricate dynamic asserts the significance of addressing untreated fungal infections not just for the preservation of individual health but also for improving overall public health status in many populations, as suggested by ongoing research on preventive measures and treatment protocols, particularly to combat such illnesses.

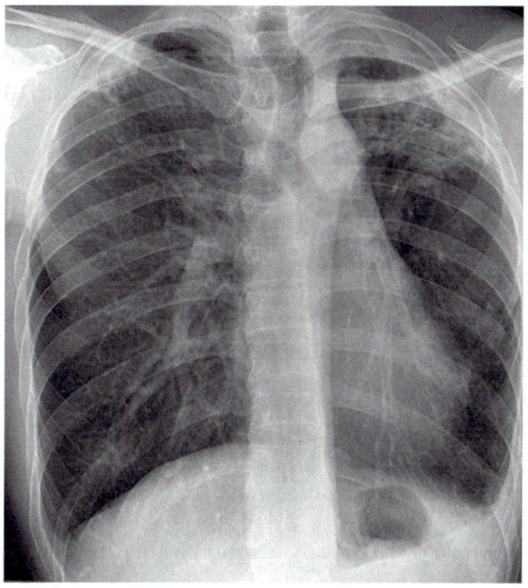

Figure 9.7. The consequences of untreated fungal infections in lung.

Source: https://gaffi.org/wp-content/uploads/Patient-with-early-bilateral-upper-lobe-CPA-from-Hanoi.png

Test Your Knowledge

1. What are the mechanisms of fungal invasion in lung tissue?
2. What is the immune response to fungal infections?

9.3. Diagnosis of Fungal Lung Infections

Learning Outcome

1. Diagnostic imaging techniques
2. Laboratory tests and cultures
3. Differential diagnosis

Fungal lung infections are diagnosed in a unique manner by clinicians due to the vast range of causative pathogens and intricate clinical profiles. The initial set of diagnostic tests is most likely to include a thorough patient history and physical exam, which may yield clues regarding risk factors such as immunocompromised status or environmental exposures to high-fungal-spore environments. Non-surgical diagnostic measures, such as imaging tests —particularly chest X-rays and computed tomography (CT) scans —play an important role in detecting unusual changes in the lungs related to infections like aspergillosis or histoplasmosis. These are, nonetheless, insensitive and nonspecific in nature, leading to the need for more direct and definite methods like bronchoscopy and bronchoalveolar lavage that are capable of producing specimens for microbiological culture and histological examination, leading further to the diagnosis of lung fungal infections. Despite advancements in diagnostic tests, most patients continue presenting with an etiologically undetermined acute respiratory failure etiology even after intensive testing. In a multicenter cohort study of patients in a critical illness, about 12.9% were diagnosed with an unknown etiology of ARF, highlighting the complexities involved in diagnosing fungal infection. Such undetermined cases are of concern because they come with high hospital mortality, which goes to drive the importance of increasing diagnostic methods for ARF, especially among patients with hematological malignancy and who are likely to have opportunistic infections. This complex interplay between clinical presentation and the limitations of available diagnostic methodologies underscores the necessity for continuous research to improve and expand second-line diagnostic approaches that aim to identify evasive fungal pathogens, which could significantly alter management and outcomes in infected patients (Azoulay et al., 2016). Against the backdrop of shifting populations and increasing incidences of fungal infections, it is essential to situate lung infection diagnosis within the context of epidemiological trends.

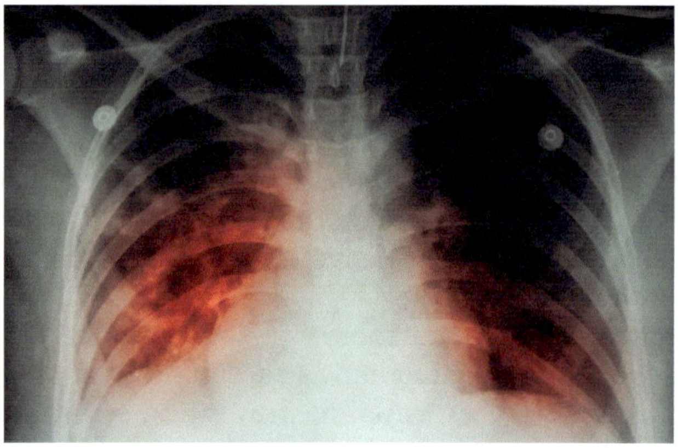

Figure 9.8. Diagnosis of fungal lung infections.

Source: https://www.belmarrahealth.com/wp-content/uploads/2016/01/New-imaging-technique-aids-earlier-diagnosis-of-fungal-lung-infection.jpg

Societal transitions, such as urbanization and environmental shifts, have been the forces behind the re-emergence and emergence of fungal infection, particularly among immunocompromised individuals. Advanced laboratory tests, including antigen detection, polymerase chain reaction (PCR), and serology, are now available to identify individual fungal pathogens at an earlier and more specific level. The case of the finding of gender and geographic predispositions of diseases such as coccidioidomycosis gives an illustration of the impact of socioeconomic status on the prevalence of certain infections. Therefore, understanding the social and historical contexts of these infections is crucial for formulating effective treatment and diagnostic approaches that are sensitive to the evolving patterns of fungal lung diseases (Homei et al., 2020).

9.3.1. Diagnostic Imaging Techniques

The diagnosis of parasitic infections and fungal diseases in the lungs has been much enhanced through the use of diagnostic imaging techniques. Tests such as magnetic resonance imaging (MRI), computed tomography (CT), and chest X-rays yield valuable information on the degree and presence of pulmonary diseases. Chest X-rays are often the first line of investigation, providing a rapid assessment of lung abnormalities, such as nodules or infiltrates characteristic of infection. However, the resolution and pathology differentiation limits of X-rays lead most practitioners to favor CT scans, which provide accurate cross-sectional images of lung anatomy. CT imaging is also optimal for identifying the mild manifestations of lung disease, such as the cavitary form of fungal infections, and is a valuable diagnostic tool for differential diagnosis and treatment planning (Reeve et al., 2018).

Combination of advanced imaging modalities plays a vital role in the management of parasitic lung disease, where ascariasis can mimic more frequent respiratory disorders. HRCT scans enable visualization of parasitic infections, and thus clinicians are able to diagnose if respiratory symptoms are a consequence of helminths or secondary infection. As soil-transmitted helminthiasis, including Ascaris lumbricoides, can lead to pulmonary symptoms and may produce chronic cough or wheezing, imaging investigations are essential to establish a proper diagnosis. Visualization of the presence of larvae or an inflammatory response also aids in making a final diagnosis. This is particularly relevant, as parasitic illnesses often present with nonspecific respiratory findings, highlighting the need for the most recent imaging modalities to assist in differentiating such illnesses from other etiologies of lung disease (Jourdan et al., 2015). In addition to CT and MRI, more recent molecular imaging techniques like positron emission tomography (PET) are increasingly enhancing diagnosis for both fungal and parasitic lung infections. These imaging modalities capitalize on the metabolic activity of the pathogens, providing information regarding the viability and spread of infection. These techniques enable a deeper understanding of disease progression, which is crucial for developing effective treatment plans. In addition, advances in imaging have led to the study of hybrid modalities that combine anatomical and functional imaging for enhanced diagnostic accuracy. As these technologies continue to improve through research, the affordability of high-level imaging remains a challenge, and with it, the relevance of access to enable all patients to benefit from these advances in diagnosis (Jourdan et al., 2015; Reeve et al., 2018).

9.3.2. Laboratory Tests and Cultures

Diagnosis of fungal infections in the lungs involves the synthesis of laboratory tests and culture, which are vital in providing accurate and timely diagnosis. The laboratory tests enable the detection of targeted pathogens present in respiratory specimens, such as sputum, bronchoalveolar lavage (BAL), or lung biopsy. Histopathological examination is particularly vital, as it provides initial evidence of potential fungal causes. Morphological findings observed in tissues can guide clinicians in initiating provisional treatments, especially before receiving final culture results. But exclusive use of histopathology can lead to misinterpretation because of overlapping morphological features, which confound accurate identification (Sabino et al., 2022). Thus, a multidisciplinary approach that combines both histopathological reports and extensive laboratory analysis is paramount in determining the overall picture of the causative organism. Outside of histopathology, cultures are at the forefront of diagnosis in fungal infection. Organism culture of respiratory specimens enables the definitive detection and susceptibility testing. Although cultures take time to yield results, they remain the "gold standard" in identifying the specific fungal pathogen responsible for the infection. For instance, a fungus may appear similar when examined under the microscope but differ considerably in terms of its responsiveness to treatment. This distinction is permitted by culture methods, thus effective antifungal treatment. Effective culture, however, depends on other factors such as utilization of the best growth medium and conditions tailored towards the likely pathogens. The need for an appropriate culture not only demonstrates the concern for single patients but also provides epidemiological information significant for the understanding of fungal infection in specific populations (Dear et al., 2020). Moreover, advances in molecular techniques have also increasingly diversified the character of laboratory tests for the detection of fungi. A few of these techniques include PCR assays, which offer quick and sensitive detection of fungal DNA in clinical samples directly. These molecular diagnostic tests can shorten the time needed for diagnosis in a very short time compared to traditional culture methods. Nonetheless, despite such improvements in diagnostic performance, these must be interpreted in the context of both phenotypic and genotypic factors to avoid errors such as false negatives or positives. The alignment of culture, histopathology, and molecular diagnostics is particularly intended to emphasize the importance of a multifaceted approach in lung fungal infection treatment. This overall approach, besides optimizing the therapeutic effect, eventually enhances the understanding of fungal pathogenesis and host interaction (Sabino et al., 2022).

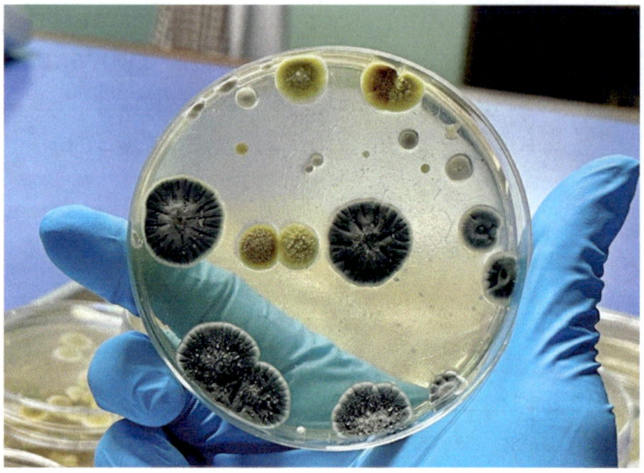

Figure 9.9. Laboratory tests and cultures of fungal lung infections.

Source: https://pathologytestsexplained.org.au/content/summaryimages/Fungi.jpg

9.3.3. Differential Diagnosis

Differential diagnosis is crucial in distinguishing between various lung infections, particularly in the evaluation of patients with suspected fungal or parasitic lung infections. Fungal infections such as aspergillosis or histoplasmosis can present clinically like bacterial pneumonia and are therefore challenging. Clinical practitioners must therefore conduct a comprehensive patient history examination, imaging, and laboratory investigations to identify the causative pathogen involved. For instance, bacterial pneumonia is common in veterinary practice and can be caused by factors such as viral infection or aspiration trauma, necessitating careful consideration of potential underlying causes to maximize treatment (Dear et al., 2020). Differential diagnosis not only plays a pivotal role in ensuring appropriate treatment but also in preventing complications resulting from an incorrect diagnosis. Apart from the use of clinical history and imaging tests, BAL fluid examination can be beneficial in separating eosinophilic lung disease from fungal or parasitic infections. Specific cytological features are necessary for conditions such as eosinophilic bronchitis or eosinophilic granuloma to establish a correct diagnosis, as illustrated by studies of several canine lung diseases. Research has demonstrated that BAL fluid can quantify significant variations in eosinophil counts, which may help distinguish between infection and inflammatory diseases (Dear et al., 2019). Understanding cellular response such as this not only assists with diagnosis but also improves treatment by making targeted therapies available for the underlying cause. Lastly, the differential diagnosis of lung infections is based on a multidimensional method that incorporates clinical, cytological, and radiological information. Clinicians must pay close attention to superimposed signs and symptoms of parasitic, fungal, and eosinophilic illnesses because they can lead to high morbidity if not well addressed. This complex diagnostic dilemma highlights the importance of comprehensive evaluation protocols that incorporate both traditional and innovative diagnostic techniques. By enhancing the precision of differential diagnoses, physicians can minimize diagnostic delays and implement timely interventions, thereby improving patient outcomes within the domain of respiratory health.

Test Your Knowledge

1. What are the diagnostic imaging techniques?
2. What are the laboratory tests and cultures?

9.4. Treatment Options For Fungal Infections

Learning Outcome

1. Antifungal medications
2. Supportive care and management strategies
3. Role of surgery in severe cases

The treatment options for fungal lung infections primarily depend on the specific type of fungus, the severity of the infection, and the patient's immune status. Antifungal medications are the cornerstone of treatment, with azoles, echinocandins, and polyenes being among the most commonly prescribed classes. Azoles, such as fluconazole and itraconazole, are typically used for their effectiveness against a variety of fungal pathogens, including *Candida* and *Aspergillus* species. Echinocandins, such as caspofungin, are a newer class of antifungal agents that possess significant effectiveness against resistant strains. In cases of serious or resistant infections to typical therapy, amphotericin B, a polyene antifungal, may be utilized despite potential side effects. A precise workup is required to assess the efficacy of such therapies and quantify patient outcomes, particularly among high-risk groups, such as patients with hematological malignancies, where acute respiratory failure makes treatment significantly more challenging (Azoulay et al., 2016).

Besides pharmacological therapy, supportive care also plays a crucial role in managing fungal lung infections. Those patients whose immunity is impaired, i.e., patients undergoing chemotherapy or AIDS/HIV in its latter stages, are most susceptible to such pathogens and may require hospitalization. Supplemental oxygenation therapy, respiratory therapy, and strict monitoring are capable of minimizing the possibility of developing the associated complication of acute respiratory distress syndrome.

Also, optimal nutritional integrity and comorbidity control are incredibly crucial in such situations as these enhance the overall resistive capacity of the patient against infection. Therapeutic management with antifungal therapy, combined with supportive care strategies, can significantly improve patient outcomes and mortality related to lung fungal infections, especially in groups with multifactorial risk factors for the development of aggressive disease (Azoulay et al., 2016). However, increased rates of antifungal resistance necessitate reevaluating treatment strategies. The emergence of resistant fungal strains underscores the importance of developing not only potent antifungal therapy but also other complementary treatments. Researchers are exploring non-chemotherapeutic methods, such as those that integrate ecological and organic farming, which can be highly beneficial in addressing parasitic lung disease and associated fungal infections. Non-chemotherapeutic treatments may involve enhancing host immunity, applying probiotics to maintain intestinal integrity, and preserving a balanced microbiome to counter opportunistic infections. By opening up treatment avenues to both conventional antifungal treatments and novel, non-traditional approaches, clinicians are better equipped to address the complexities of lung fungal infections and improve overall patient outcomes.

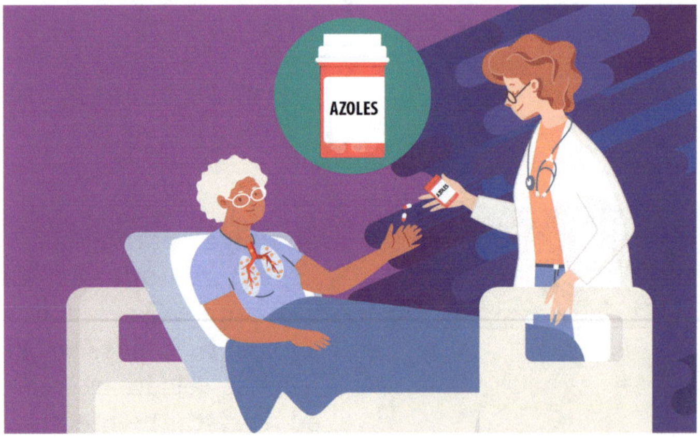

Figure 9.10. The treatment options for fungal infections of the lung.

Source: https://www.cdc.gov/fungal/media/images/2024/04/23_342632-A_Galluzzo_Aspergillus_fumigatus_STILL_TW_no_text_03_azoles.jpg

9.4.1. Antifungal Medications

Therapy of fungal infections, particularly pulmonary infections, relies primarily on antifungal agents that exploit the unique characteristics and features of fungi. The antifungal agents are broadly classified into three groups: polyenes, azoles, and echinocandins. Polyenes such as amphotericin B interfere with the fungal cell membrane by binding with ergosterol, increasing membrane permeability and ultimately leading to cell death. Azoles, including fluconazole and itraconazole, bind to the lanosterol 14α-demethylase enzyme, which is critical to ergosterol biosynthesis, thereby stopping fungal growth. Echinocandins, like caspofungin, disrupt the synthesis of glucan, a vital cell wall component of the fungus. The antifungal drug selected will often depend on factors such as the type of fungal pathogen, the patient's overall health, and whether drug interactions are likely. Therefore, understanding the pharmacodynamics of such drugs is crucial to optimizing therapy in patients suffering from fungal lung infection. Antifungal pharmacotherapy still has challenges despite advancements in the treatment, and among them, drug resistance and side effects of drugs upon long-term usage are significant problems. Candidiasis, a fungal infection, has become increasingly resistant to fluconazole, adding complexity to the treatment regimen and potentially leading to therapeutic failure. In addition, antifungal drug toxicities, especially involving polyene drugs, need careful observation and dose adjustment, particularly in immunocompromised individuals who usually experience pulmonary fungal infections. Antifungal therapy analysis confirms that while significant progress has been achieved, an ever-evolving strategy must be employed to overcome resistance. Increased surveillance of antifungal resistance patterns and more intensive clinical guidelines comprise the pillars of managing likely complications effectively, thus ensuring that patient outcomes are desirable in the event of complicated pulmonary fungal infections (Calvet et al., 2017). In combating the raging epidemic of fungal lung infections, the role played by antifungal medications cannot be downplayed; however, the role of simultaneous preventive strategies and multidisciplinary treatment is of critical significance. Antimicrobial stewardship is optimized in the context of tertiary care to ensure the safe use of antifungal agents, thereby limiting the risk of resistance (Olowe et al., 2023). Also, prevention strategies like vaccination studies and enhanced environmental controls significantly assist in reducing the risk of exposure to individuals in vulnerable populations. Immunocompromised patients, for instance, are most susceptible to infection from organisms like Aspergillus. Thus, with an effective antifungal treatment combined with supportive care interventions—such as advising the patient to avoid exposure and maintaining a robust immune system—both acute and chronic management of fungal lung infections can be enhanced. Thus, a multidisciplinary strategy is essential to eradicate the occurrence and severity of these challenging diseases.

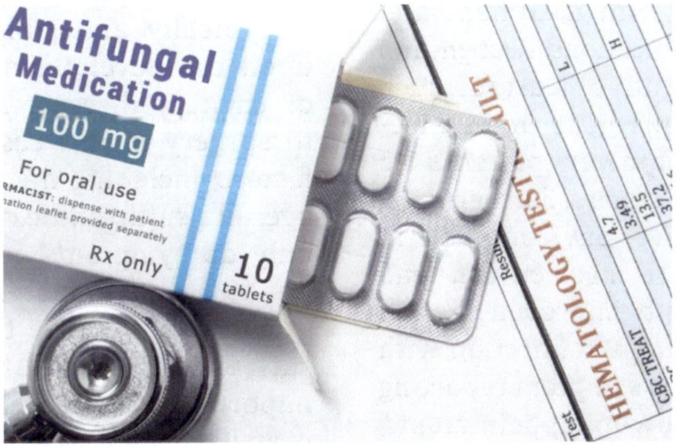

Figure 9.11. Antifungal medications for lung infections.

Source: https://images.theconversation.com/files/238436/original/file-20180928-48647-12ud27s.jpg?ixlib=rb-4.1.0&q=45&auto=format&w=926&fit=clip

9.4.2. Supportive Care and Management Strategies

Effective therapy of pulmonary fungal infections and parasitic lung disease involves an integrated strategy that incorporates supportive care interventions. Improved general comfort and immune function and resolution of the disease cause are among the essential goals of supportive care. Improved hydration and nutrition may be part of this, as both are essential for sustaining immune processes. Moreover, supplemental oxygen may be used for respiratory distress, as oxygen therapy increases tissue oxygenation and alleviates symptoms of hypoxia. Routine monitoring, including clinical examination and diagnostic imaging, is also crucial for tracking the disease progression and adjusting treatment protocols accordingly. This dynamic monitoring system guarantees that possible complications are detected early to enable timely interventions that would reduce the risk of additional lung damage. Apart from primary medical interventions, patient education is an important factor in the management of pulmonary fungal infections and parasitic diseases. Healthcare providers need to inform patients about their illnesses, with special attention to compliance with treatment and potential side effects of medications. Recognition of the importance of preventive measures, such as avoiding recognized allergens or disease-causing agents, can empower patients to become active treatment partners. Furthermore, establishing a supportive environment in which family members are involved can lead to greater compliance and improved mental well-being. Since developing a connection with care providers can enhance symptom reporting and compliance with follow-up appointments, incorporating psychosocial support into the care plan can significantly improve patient outcomes for treating complicated pulmonary illnesses. Multidisciplinary approaches must be contained in tackling the complex issues related to fungal infections and parasitic lung disease. As with pulmonary hypertension, diagnosis of underlying diseases such as respiratory disease and parasitic infection is key to establishing an effective treatment plan. This involves collaboration among experts, such as pulmonologists, infectious disease specialists, and veterinarians, to address all aspects of the patient's condition. Additionally, the application of innovative strategies, such as exploring biological or phytotherapeutic adjuncts, although at an initial stage, may present viable avenues for add-on therapy. Exploration of patient-specific treatment protocols, particularly among comorbid patients, remains crucial as they hold the key to altering the success of management programs and ultimately improving the quality of life in individuals affected (Eijck et al., 2003; Abbott et al., 2020)).

9.4.3. Role of Surgery in Severe Cases

In the field of acute pulmonary infections with fungi and parasites, the role of surgery presents itself as a relevant question, particularly when conservative medical treatment fails. *Aspergillus* infection has been known to lead to invasive pulmonary aspergillosis, which is typically amenable to surgical resection upon the development of extensive necrosis or cavitary disease. The decision to proceed to surgery in this case rests on a number of factors, including the patient's immune status, overall health, and extent of lung damage. Not only do symptoms get alleviated by surgery, but it also eliminates the infectious burden that may jeopardize the patient's recovery. In such extreme circumstances, this is particularly important when the integrity of lung function is at stake. By removing the source of infection, surgical intervention can immensely significantly enhance long-term prognosis in patients with aggressive fungal disease. Besides, the surgery of parasitic lung disease demonstrates the intricacies in dealing with serious diseases. One of the best examples is alveolar echinococcosis that occurs as a consequence of the growth of *Echinococcus multilocularis* parasites. When the condition is diagnosed in its advanced form, it most often manifests as malignancy and, in the absence of treatment, has a high mortality rate. Surgical procedures, such as the removal of infected lung tissue, play a pivotal role in cases that are advanced in nature, especially if infection leads to complications such as failure of the lungs or spread of the disease beyond the lungs. Surgical therapy not only stops the immediate threat of infection but can also be crucial in preventing the potential for extension into the systemic circulation, underscoring the inter-special solution that combines the dual realms of surgical and medical expertise in the treatment of parasitic pulmonary infections. Secondary to this is the association of underlying immunological states and the requirement for surgical intervention to be considered in the context of widespread pulmonary infection. Hypersplenic conditions such as autosomal dominant hyperimmunoglobulin E syndrome (AD-HIES) are associated with heightened susceptibility to a range of infections, such as recurrent chronic pneumonia and atypical parasitic infestations. Surgical intervention in these patients can be supplemented with comprehensive medical management to enhance immunity and manage episodes of infection. For instance, while the initial management may be antimicrobial therapy, an underlying chronic pulmonary disease might necessitate surgery as a strategy of preventing further complications, again highlighting the importance of long-term observation of the patient. The subtleties revealed in situations such as those caused by STAT3-LOF mutations illustrate how modern medicine is driven to adapt and expand its armamentarium, effectively incorporating surgery as part of its comprehensive arsenal in managing virulent lung infections.

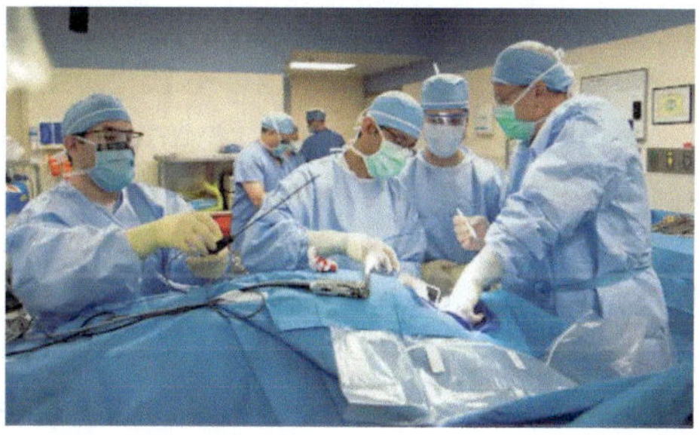

Figure 9.12. Role of surgery in severe lung infections.

Source: https://stgaccinwbsdevlrs01.blob.core.windows.net/newcorporatewbsite/blogs/April2024/TaKCH7htHj4KIhORoI71.webp?w=828&q=75

Test Your Knowledge

1. What are the antifungal medications?
2. What is the role of surgery in severe cases?

9.5. Overview of Parasitic Lung Diseases

Learning Outcome

1. Common parasites that affect the lungs
2. Transmission routes of parasitic infections
3. Symptoms and clinical presentation

Parasitic lung diseases are a heterogeneous collection of respiratory conditions caused by infection with various helminths and protozoa that infect the pulmonary system. Among these, parasitic diseases caused by Ascaris lumbricoides and Strongyloides stercoralis are of significance due to their global prevalence and significant health impacts. The parasites may become infected with eggs or penetrate the skinand make the larvae , allowing the larvae to develop and travel via the circulatory system to the lungs. Once they enter the pulmonary system, the parasites can potentially trigger severe immune responses, leading to clinical symptoms such as cough, dyspnea, and wheezing. The pathology of such infections is likely to be multicentric, with eosinophilic inflammation and often involves replicating other respiratory infections, making diagnosis and treatment difficult. Comprehensive knowledge of parasitic lung infections is crucial for effective management in clinical situations. Additionally, certain organisms are linked to specific pathophysiological responses in the lungs. For instance, eosinophilic lung diseases like eosinophilic bronchitis and eosinophilic granuloma are presented clinically differently based on their underlying etiology. Veterinary patient examinations, particularly those involving dogs, have been enlightening in this aspect, and bronchoscopic assessment and analysis of bronchoalveolar lavage fluid are vital for accurate diagnosis (Dear et al., 2019). These methods have demonstrated that while eosinophilic bronchitis is typically characterized by variable levels of mucus production and inflammation, eosinophilic granuloma exhibits more focal infiltrates and may demonstrate prolonged survival in treated patients. Knowledge of these distinctions is valuable within the broader context of parasitic lung diseases because it guides the selection of proper therapeutic alternatives. Moreover, the interaction of parasitic infections with environmental determinants is another essential aspect of understanding parasitic lung diseases. The impact of climate, land use, and cattle husbandry on parasitic transmission and burden cannot be overstated. Organic livestock farming, for example, has been described as having a complex interaction with health outcomes, including potentially increased parasitic infestations (Eijck et al., 2003). Clinical evidence suggests that management methods, such as stocking density and disinfection regimes, can influence the occurrence of such infections. In addition, zoonotic disease transmission caused by organic agriculture raises new challenges for public health and calls for broad research concerning the causative agents of parasitic lung infections and preventive and therapeutic measures in different ecological regimes.

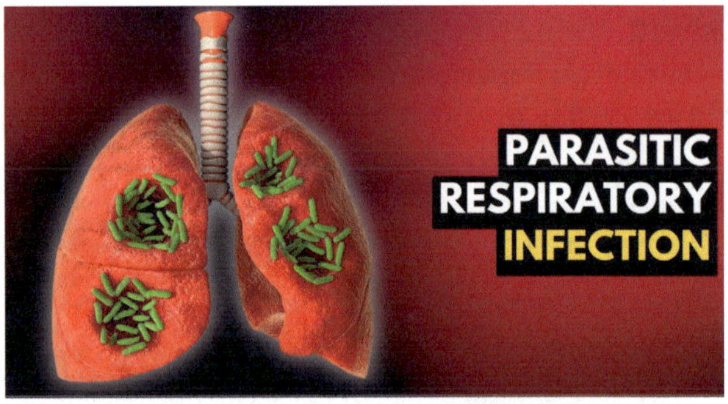

Figure 9.13. Parasitic lung diseases.

Source: https://i.ytimg.com/vi/Ov8SnxBx640/maxresdefault.jpg

9.5.1. Common Parasites That Affect the Lungs

The lung is also a critical location of numerous parasitic infestations that have the capacity to lead to severe morbidity in infected subjects. One of the most notable parasites is *Strongyloides stercoralis*, which can infest individuals who may develop a condition known as strongyloidiasis. The helminth is capable of evading the host's immune system, allowing it to migrate from the lungs and other organs, where respiratory symptoms are typically presented as cough and wheezing. Infection can arise from contact with soiled objects and soil on the skin, entering through the respiratory tract, or spread by mother-to-child transmission, highlighting the importance of maintaining sanitation, hygiene behavior, and practicing appropriate disinfection to limit transmission. Due to its capability for autoinfection, *S. stercoralis* is an exception in terms of treatment and control, especially for immunocompromised patients who develop life-threatening disseminated disease. The growing incidence of strongyloidiasis highlights existing public health concerns, particularly in populations with reduced access to care and awareness of parasitic infection. Another significant lung-infecting parasite is Ascaris lumbricoides, which causes ascariasis, a prevalent infection that is typically presented by asymptomatic carriers.

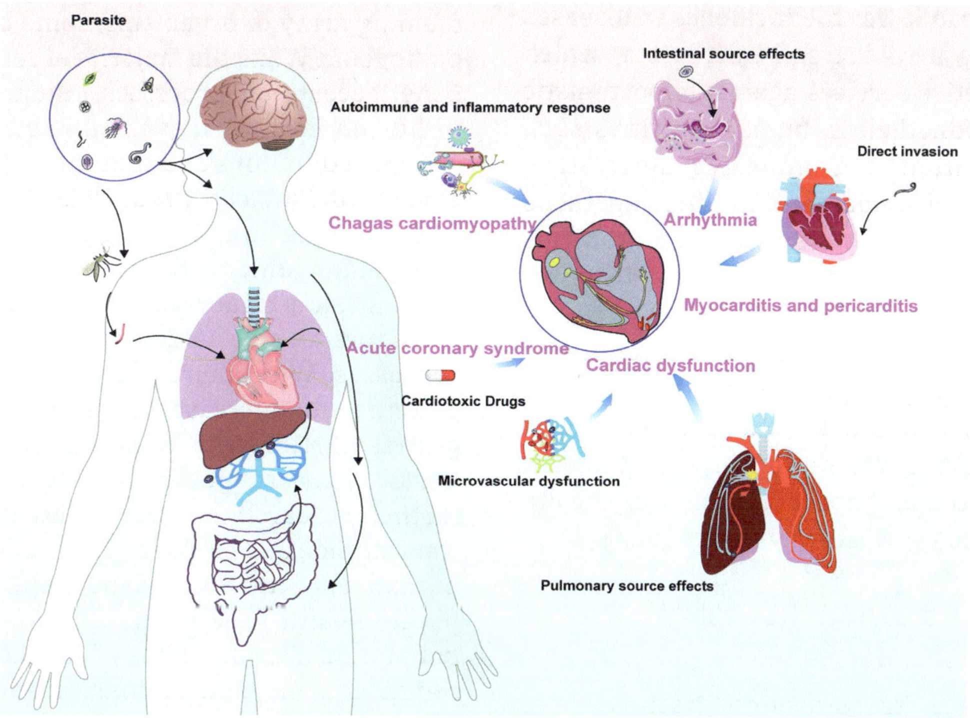

Figure 9.14. Common parasites that affect the lungs.

Source: https://html.scirp.org/file/8-2151700x2.png?20220617093452065

The eggs, upon ingestion, hatch within the intestine, and the larvae travel through the lungs during their life cycle. The migration stage can present with acute respiratory symptoms, such as cough and dyspnea, which are often mistaken for other respiratory illnesses. In certain cases, heavy infection can lead to more severe complications, such as bronchial obstruction and pneumonia. Additionally, the synergism between the mechanisms of parasitic adaptation and the host immune response makes the infection difficult to treat. Information about these interactions is crucial for strategy development in terms of prevention, considering the widespread environmental transmission of this parasite by fecal contamination of water supplies and soil in most endemic regions. Lastly, the health effects of parasitic infections are compounded by the environmental nature of their causes. Helminth parasites and other soil-transmitted pathogens contribute not only to the acute health issues but also to the extensive effects on community health infrastructure and ecosystems in general. The complicated interplay between soil biodiversity and parasitic life cycles is a characteristic example of the holistic nature of human disease and environmental health. As recent studies have pointed out, healthy ecosystems can lower the incidence of diseases by imparting a robust soil microbiota, which offers protective services against opportunistic infections. Nonetheless, human activities such as deforestation and intensive agriculture are capable of fundamentally altering these ecosystems, thereby leaving communities vulnerable to parasitic pulmonary diseases, including those caused by *S. stercoralis* and *A. lumbricoides*. All these factors require a multidisciplinary approach involving public health, environmental management, and education to mitigate the upsurge of parasitic infections and their impact on respiratory health (Lee et al., 2011; Upadhyay et al., 2023).

9.5.2. Transmission Routes of Parasitic Infections

The intricate transmission pathways of parasitic infections are crucial in revealing the transmission and maintenance of such infections. The parasites possess intricate life cycles that involve multiple hosts and interactions with the environment. For instance, the transmission modes involve vertical and horizontal pathways, and studies indicate that genes control these pathways. As highlighted in research, evolutionary adaptations are typically accompanied by alterations in transmission patterns, indicating their importance in disease epidemiology and control. Insights into evolutionary mechanisms are pivotal in shaping effective public health interventions used to control infections among vulnerable populations. Strategies that incorporate this understanding could enhance preventive interventions against parasitic infections, especially in areas where transmission dynamics are constantly changing due to environmental conditions and host behaviors (Wilson et al., 2017). Besides direct contact between hosts, ecological conditions also make a significant contribution towards facilitating parasitic transmission. Soil, for example, hosts a teeming array of organisms, some of which are pathogenic. While the majority of soil microbiota benefit ecosystem processes, others are harmful to human health. They can inhabit the soil for extended durations and thus impact people who come into contact with unclean environments. The association between soil integrity, land management processes, and parasite transmission underscores the importance of a comprehensive understanding of infection processes. With altered land-use patterns, the potential for increased exposure to parasites grows, particularly in immunocompromised hosts. This suggests an urgent need for further research to understand the mode of transmission and propagation of soil-transmitted parasites, with significant implications for public health (Lee et al., 2011). The ironing out of transmission routes of parasitic infections requires a multidisciplinary framework that unites epidemiology, environmental science, and clinical sciences. The diverse strategies that parasites use to invade hosts demand advanced diagnostic and surveillance practices to monitor and control outbreaks effectively. As the health risks associated with parasitic diseases are on a global decline, identifying the evolutionary basis of transmission modes becomes increasingly relevant. Research efforts must target the identification of factors influencing host-parasite relationships, including the effects of environmental fluctuations on the likelihood of zoonotic diseases and other patterns of transmission. This holistic method not only enhances the study of parasitic infections but also provides insight for targeted interventions that can curb their distribution, ultimately guaranteeing public health on a broader level (Wilson et al., 2017).

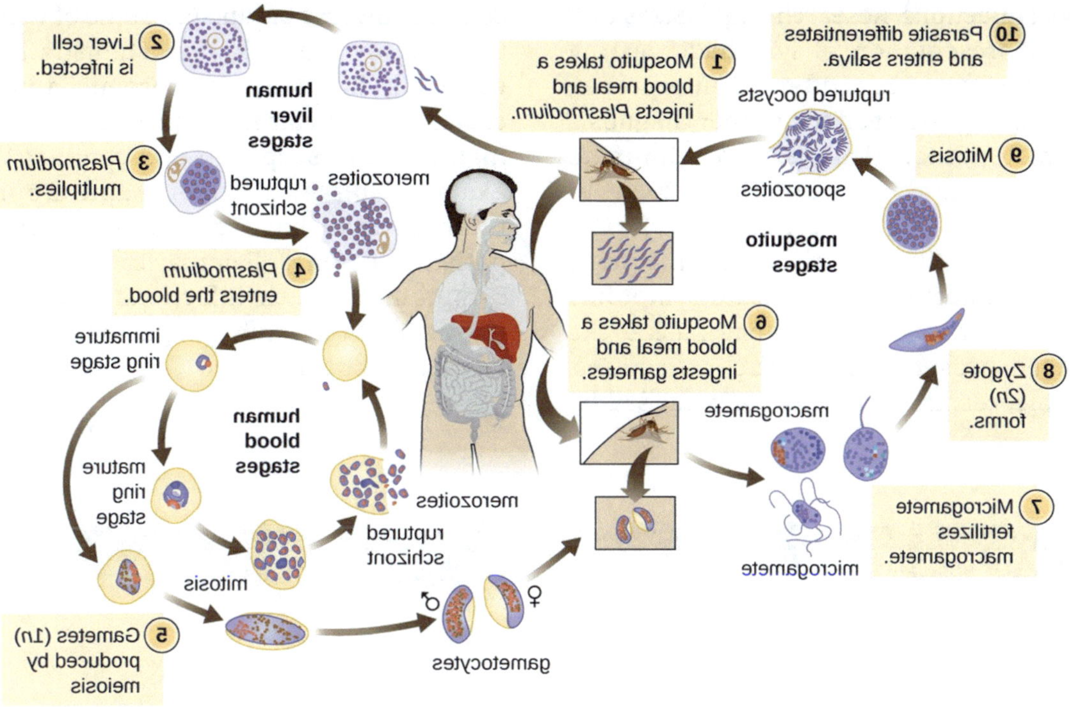

Figure 9.15. Transmission routes of parasitic infections the lungs.

Source: https://s3-us-west-2.amazonaws.com/courses-images/wp-content/uploads/sites/1094/2016/11/03175823/OSC_Microbio_25_04_Malaria.jpg

9.5.3. Symptoms and Clinical Presentation

Clinical manifestation of lung fungal infection tends to have a broad spectrum of symptoms, which is mainly related to the causative fungus. The majority of patients present with respiratory impairment, characterized by chronic cough, wheezing, and chest discomfort. Systemic manifestations such as fever, night sweats, fatigue, and weight loss can also present, complicating the clinical scenario. In immunocompromised individuals, such as those with HIV/AIDS or those receiving immunosuppressive therapy, the presentation can be more acute and severe. This is best exemplified by research that showed that HIV-positive patients reported fever and gastrointestinal complaints more commonly than HIV-negative patients, implying a significant threat to fungal pneumonia infection leading to misdiagnosis and unnecessary delay in treatment among susceptible groups (Abba et al., 2017). Thus, clinicians must be vigilant to rule out fungal infections from other respiratory diseases. For parasitic lung infections, too, in the case of parasites, there is a mixing of symptoms with those of fungal infections, as well as diagnostic challenges. Respiratory complaints, such as cough, dyspnea, and wheezing, can occur, as can systemic presentations, including fever and profound malaise. Also, parasitic diseases caused by parasites such as *Strongyloides stercoralis* or *Ascaris lumbricoides* can result in eosinophilia and can lead to widespread pulmonary pathology. The clinical presentation requires a thorough investigation, particularly as eosinophilia can aid in differentiating parasitic from fungal infections. Research emphasizes that the clinical presentation of lymphadenopathy due to infectious causes is often misinterpreted, thus highlighting the need for proper diagnosis through histopathological tests to eliminate misdiagnosis that can potentially lead to injurious delays in treatment (Abba et al., 2017). Moreover, the ability of both fungal infections and parasitic infections to replicate symptoms of diseases further serves to emphasize the multifaceted presentation of such infections. For example, respiratory syndromes caused by soil fungi can be triggered by environmental exposure, whereas parasitic infections can remain asymptomatic until they reach the lung stage. Research has established that the soil contains diverse organisms, some of which infect the lung by inducing opportunistic infections, especially in immunocompromised hosts. It is crucial that healthcare providers maintain a high index of suspicion and conduct thorough examinations, as timely and appropriate interventions have a significant impact on patient outcomes. Familiarity with the diverse symptoms of such infections remains crucial for achieving timely diagnosis and effective treatment strategies.

Test Your Knowledge

1. What are the common parasites that affect the lungs?
2. What are the transmission routes of parasitic infections?

9.6. Diagnosis and Treatment of Parasitic Lung Diseases

Learning Outcome

1. Diagnostic methods for identifying parasitic infections
2. Treatment options and medications
3. Prevention strategies for parasitic lung diseases

Diagnosis of parasitic lung infections is a multifaceted process that, in most cases, begins with a thorough clinical examination. Physicians must be able to identify the common signs of these infections, such as cough, hemoptysis, chest pain, and dyspnea. Proper identification is achieved by conducting a detailed interview with the patient, including exposure to potential sources of parasitic infection. Diagnostic approaches typically involve imaging tests, such as chest X-rays or computed tomography scans, which can reveal distinctive patterns of parasitic lung infections. Laboratory tests, including serological assays and sputum tests, can also yield critical information regarding the etiologic pathogens involved. Notably, eosinophilia in peripheral blood is a common laboratory finding in most parasitic infections, which in turn prompts a further search for a potential helminthic or protozoan etiology. Early and accurate diagnosis is essential as it significantly impacts the outcome of treatment and patient care. Following confirmation of a parasitic lung infection, a treatment plan tailored to the individual becomes imperative. Treatment tends to take a different course based on the kind of parasite found, the severity of infection, and the overall condition of the patient. Antiparasitic medications are typically the first line of treatment, with albendazole or ivermectin being employed in helminthic infection. For protozoan infections, pentamidine or trimethoprim-sulfamethoxazole may be used. Supportive therapy is also essential, along with drug treatment, in complicated cases with associated respiratory failure or widespread pulmonary involvement. Additionally, treatment may require managing underlying risk factors, such as immunosuppression, which can complicate the clinical course of the disease. Therefore, an integrated strategy should be pursued to enhance recovery and prevent potential complications.

Such intricacies of diagnosis and therapy of parasitic lung disease extend also to the prognosis of patients with these infections. It has been proven through studies that delayed diagnosis results in increased morbidity and mortality associated with complications such as acute respiratory failure. More specifically, hematological malignancy patients tend to have increased difficulties, since their immunocompromised state can mask simple diagnostic pathways. In a critically ill population, up to 13% of the conditions can remain unresolved following aggressive diagnostic workups, with an increased risk of hospital mortality. Healthcare providers must recognize such dynamics because prompt identification and effective management of parasitic infections will have a significant impact on clinical outcomes. With advancing practice, continuous studies on effective diagnostic and treatment strategies will be crucial for improving care for patients with parasitic lung disease (Azoulay et al., 2016) and enhancing patient survival (Dear et al., 2020).

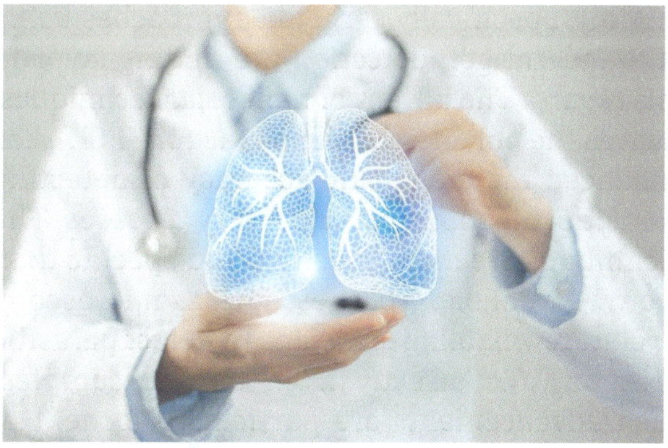

Figure 9.16. Treatment of parasitic lung diseases.

Source: https://external-content.duckduckgo.com/iu/?u=https%3A%2F%2Fsa1s3optim.patientpop.com%2Fassets%2Fimages%2Fprovider%2Fphotos%2F2583312.jpg&f=1&nofb=1&ipt=c421eac84e76910b193517fa561433c1dc244a3ebdc998771725cff3556999f6

9.6.1. Diagnostic Methods For Identifying Parasitic Infections

Diagnosis of parasitic infections, particularly in the context of lung disease, necessitates a multimodal diagnostic approach involving both clinical evaluation and laboratory testing. Initial testing typically involves a patient's history, symptoms, and physical examination findings, all directed towards identifying probable parasitic disease. Respiratory symptoms are present in most of the parasitic infections, e.g., those caused by protozoa or helminths, and can mimic other pulmonary conditions. As such, correct diagnosis is essential to prevent mismanagement. Laboratory methods are indispensable in verifying suspicion, with stool studies and serology tests being typical examples. Nevertheless, when respiratory manifestations are present, BAL fluid analysis has proven to be a valuable tool for isolating parasitic etiology, highlighting the need for focused diagnostic approaches to maximize patient outcomes and avoid delays in the application of proper therapy. Specifically, targeted approaches using PCR and antigen detection are finding favor in this regard. The advent of molecular techniques, such as the polymerase chain reaction (PCR), has enhanced the diagnostic accuracy of detecting parasitic infections in respiratory diseases. The techniques are more sensitive and specific than the traditional approaches, such as microscopy or culture, enabling clinicians to detect parasitic DNA or RNA directly from clinical samples. Such advancements are particularly beneficial in identifying organisms that are likely to exist in small quantities and therefore cannot be isolated through standard methods. Further, PCR with analysis of bronchoalveolar lavage fluid allows for the simultaneous identification of multiple pathogens, like fungi and parasites, and thus makes diagnosis easier. The validity of such tests relies on the capability of specimen handling and processing, thus highlighting the importance of standardized protocols in the clinical laboratory to achieve meaningful results that can guide therapeutic interventions accordingly. In brief, the diagnosis and detection of parasitic infections, which are implicated in lung diseases, is an ever-evolving field, filling the gap between traditional methods and emerging technologies to achieve maximum clinical accuracy. While classical procedures, such as microscopy and serology, provide valuable information, the uniqueness of each case underscores the relevance of an integrated process that incorporates molecular diagnostics, such as PCR. Such technologies not only enhance our understanding of parasitic infection but also inform treatment regimens for the specific requirements of individual patients. As with increased research in this field, there remains a critical need for more efficient diagnostic methods, thereby reducing the rate of undiagnosed infections. Heightened awareness of the importance of BAL fluid analysis and application of sensitive diagnostics will be instrumental in the battle against the complexities of fungal and parasitic lung disease in the clinic (Hage et al., 2005; Hemalatha et al., 2011).

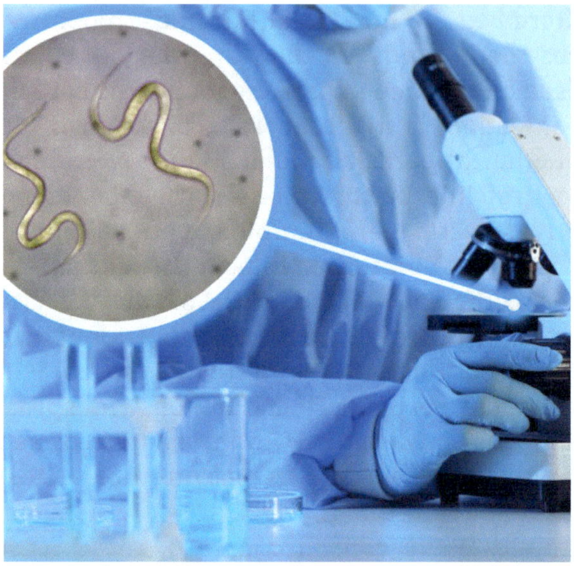

Figure 9.17. Diagnostic methods for identifying parasitic infections.

Source: https://www.cor-ntd.org//sites/default/files/styles/landscape_4_3_small/public/content/news-roundup/files/2024-04/stool%20sample.png.jpeg?itok=LRQOuSqp

9.6.2. Treatment Options and Medications

Therapeutic interventions for pulmonary fungal infections and parasitic infections differ significantly, primarily focusing on the application of antifungal and antiparasitic medications. Fungal lung infections, among them histoplasmosis and aspergillosis, are generally treated under normal conditions with azole compounds itraconazole and voriconazole, inhibitors of ergosterol synthesis—a critical component of fungal cell membranes. The choice of drug generally depends on the severity of the disease, the etiological fungal pathogen, and the patient's health status, particularly their immunity. Additionally, in systemic or invasive fungal infections, amphotericin B can be used due to its broad spectrum of antifungal activity, despite the nephrotoxicity it carries. Therefore, proper treatment choice is paramount, as it can have an impact on patient results and overall quality of life. In the case of parasitic lung disease, treatment approaches are often based on the organism causing the infection. For example, Chagas disease, which is a parasitic disease caused by *Trypanosoma cruzi*, is very challenging to treat due to the drugs like nifurtimox and benznidazole that are available at present, since their efficacy is variable and so is their side-effect potential. Recent advances in the inhibition of CYP51, the key enzyme involved in sterol biosynthesis, have opened research into new inhibitors with the ability to make treatment more efficient against fungal and parasitic diseases. Notably, drugs tested experimentally have proved to manifest encouraging impacts on reducing parasitemia and mitigating concomitant tissue damage in animal models, but long-term sterile cures are not forthcoming. This underscores the necessity for continued research and the periodic re-evaluation of treatment regimens to allow for the evolution of therapeutic wisdom (Calvet et al., 2017). In addition, the interaction between parasitic and fungal infections is particularly applicable in immunocompromised individuals, for instance, HIV/AIDS patients. Both opportunistic infections and side effects of drugs are significant problems in these patients. Active therapy of such infections typically requires a combined, multidisciplinary approach, involving a combination of antiretroviral therapy and pathogen-specific treatment. Although AIDS enteropathy represents a unique diagnostic and therapeutic problem, symptomatic management through nutritional support and intensive medical therapy remains a critical component of care. The trajectory of anti-infective treatment can profoundly improve the quality of life in patients and reduce morbidity. The dynamic nature of these infections necessitates ongoing research studies and clinical vigilance to enhance therapeutic options and maximize patient outcomes (Cello et al., 2009).

9.6.3. Prevention Strategies For Parasitic Lung Diseases

Effective prevention interventions of parasitic lung infections are pivotal in lessening morbidity and mortality due to such infections. Health education and awareness campaigns are vital within high-risk populations, highlighting the modes of transmission of parasites such as those causing Chagas disease, which is caused by the protozoan parasite *Trypanosoma cruzi*. Prevention measures include limiting exposure to vectors, such as triatomine insects that carry the parasite, and improving living conditions in a manner that minimizes infestations. Public health can also employ vector control strategies, including insecticide application and environmental management, to lower infection risks in vulnerable populations. These multifaceted approaches are applied not only to interrupt the lifecycle of the parasites but also to increase awareness of how socio-economic factors may influence parasitic disease and prevention. In addition to education, outreach, and vector control, the availability and provision of effective medications can become an integral part of prevention. For instance, studies have shown the efficacy of novel CYP51 inhibitors against *T. cruzi*, showing potential for improved therapeutic approaches against Chagas disease (Calvet et al., 2017). The challenge lies in the availability of safe and effective access to them, particularly in areas where healthcare systems are affected by endemicity. Prophylactic treatment and periodic screening among high-risk groups can prevent infection before it develops into a full-blown disease. Furthermore, integrating such pharmaceutical interventions into broader healthcare schemes, such as immunization and routine surveillance, can significantly enhance community immunity against parasitic lung diseases. Finally, to facilitate overall prevention, the comorbidities that otherwise compound the impact of parasitic infections have to be treated. Chronic diseases, like lung diseases, can be exacerbated by parasitic infections, leading to complications like pneumonia (Dear et al., 2020). By promoting overall wellness through improved diets, immunization against other respiratory pathogens, and management of underlying health conditions, communities can become resistant to parasitic lung diseases overall. It requires collaboration among medical professionals, public health experts, and community groups to create synergistic programs that address both direct prevention and the broader context of health. Such integrative strategies will ultimately enable an improved fight against parasitic lung disease, thereby enhancing health benefits within affected communities.

Test Your Knowledge

1. What are the diagnostic methods for identifying parasitic infections?
2. What are the prevention strategies for parasitic lung diseases?

SUMMARY

The research on fungal lung infections and parasitic lung diseases is worth mentioning, as it highlights the significant public health issues created by these diseases. Fungal infections, particularly those caused by endemic mycoses such as coccidioidomycosis and histoplasmosis, pose a unique challenge in that they often present in a hidden way and can cause severe respiratory distress. In addition, the increasing prevalence of co-infections, particularly among immunocompromised individuals, necessitates an interdisciplinary approach of early diagnosis, surveillance, and specifically tailored treatment approaches. Intimate relationships between environmental etiologies and the epidemiology of these infections necessitate public health interventions among high-risk groups to prevent outbreaks and enhance disease management. Lastly, the complex interaction between fungal pathogens and the host immune system has a significant impact on clinical outcomes. Recent comparisons have been made between the respiratory microbiomes of cetaceans and humans, and studies have suggested that both share microbial communities that may include disease-causing organisms, such as *Aspergillus* spp. and *Cryptococcus* spp. (Seepaulsingh et al., 2014). This information is significant since it suggests that changes in lung microbiota may predispose an individual to infection, particularly in individuals with underlying immunological weaknesses. This relationship is used to demarcate the need for continued research into the microbiota of the respiratory tract that, in turn, can guide better prevention and treatment interventions in susceptible individuals. And finally, attention to the rising incidence of inborn errors of immunity (IEI) further complicates the clinical landscape for respiratory infections, as these disorders also increase the risk of fungal and parasitic lung infections. The recent phenotypic classification of IEIs has led to better clinical detection and treatment of the disorders that can manifest as episodic respiratory infections (Ailal et al., 2020). Similar to fungal pathogens, the diagnosis and treatment of parasitic infection involve a multi-disciplinary approach that includes laboratory diagnosis and an understanding of host susceptibility. Later research must continue to examine the relationships among them, as learning more will enhance our personal and overall capacity to combat the burdens of lung disease caused by fungal diseases and parasitic pathogens.

The complexities of pulmonary fungal infection reflect a significant area of research in respiratory medicine. Fungal infections, typically opportunistic, have the potential to yield severe outcomes in immunocompromised hosts. Certain of the issues that are being addressed in the literature include the requirement for implementation of comprehensive treatment regimens that include the utilization of antifungal therapy as well as adjunctive supportive interventions. The European Respiratory Society has addressed this need by developing a syllabus for postgraduate education in respiratory infections, enabling healthcare professionals to be adequately educated to tackle such challenges (Farr et al., 2018). Such educational paradigms are intended to enhance diagnostic capabilities and treatment strategies, which would ultimately lead to improved patient outcomes in terms of fungal lung infections. Parasitic lung illnesses, particularly helminthic ones, are another condition of respiratory pathology that cannot be overlooked, however. The widespread prevalence of such infections, particularly in tropical and subtropical regions, poses a severe public health problem. In terms of numbers, an estimated 1.5 billion infected individuals exist globally, which underscores the need for both preventive and therapeutic measures (Alhallaf et al., 2018). An understanding of the immunomodulatory mechanisms employed by helminths becomes critical when envisioning a potential vaccine, as noted in existing research. Research has emphasized the inflammasome's role in mediating immunity against parasites and how the NLRP3 and NLRP1 inflammasome signaling pathways are of utmost relevance in innate immune reactions to helminth infections. The concomitant occurrence of parasitic and fungal infections in the lung underscores the importance of a cohesive patient care and research approach. To dissect such diseases holistically requires not only insight into the pathogen's biology but also the host's immune response. Research has demonstrated that insight into host defense mechanisms against helminthic infections can inform the development of new vaccines, a crucial goal given the significant impact of these infections on vulnerable populations. Ongoing research into immune regulation via inflammasomes is providing profound insights, potentially opening a gateway to new therapies (Alhallaf et al., 2018). As intervention strategies in public health are developed and refined, it is critical that health practitioners keep pace with these advancements to reduce the impact of both parasitic and fungal infections on lung function.

KEY TERMS FROM THIS CHAPTER

- Aspergillosis
- Coccidioidomycosis
- Cryptococcosis
- Allergic bronchopulmonary aspergillosis (ABPA)
- Granulomatous inflammation
- Hydatid cyst
- Löffler's syndrome
- Schistosomiasis
- Bronchiectasis (parasitic cause)
- Antifungal therapy
- Histoplasmosis
- Blastomycosis
- Pneumocystis jirovecii pneumonia (PJP)
- Fungal spores
- Eosinophilia
- Paragonimiasis
- Strongyloidiasis
- Parasitic lung infiltrates
- Serological tests
- Immunocompromised host

CRITICAL THINKING QUESTIONS

1. **Which fungal infection commonly causes lung disease in immunocompromised patients and is diagnosed by detecting the "halo sign" on a CT scan?**
   a. Coccidioidomycosis
   b. Aspergillosis
   c. Histoplasmosis
   d. Cryptococcosis
2. **Which of the following is the most common parasitic cause of lung cysts (hydatid disease)?**
   a. Ascaris lumbricoides
   b. Echinococcus granulosus
   c. Paragonimus westermani
   d. Strongyloides stercoralis
3. **Paragonimus westermani infection primarily affects which organ system?**
   a. Gastrointestinal tract
   b. Central nervous system
   c. Lungs
   d. Skin
4. **Which of the following fungal infections is endemic to the Ohio and Mississippi River valleys and can cause granulomatous lung disease?**
   a. Histoplasmosis
   b. Blastomycosis
   c. Coccidioidomycosis
   d. Aspergillosis
5. **Which diagnostic test is commonly used to identify pulmonary fungal infections?**
   a. Sputum Gram stain
   b. Acid-fast bacilli stain
   c. Fungal culture and serology
   d. Chest X-ray alone

Short Answer Questions

1. What is the characteristic radiologic finding in pulmonary aspergillosis?
2. What is the typical mode of transmission for histoplasmosis?
3. Which diagnostic test is most helpful in identifying fungal infections of the lung?
4. Name two parasitic infections that can involve the lungs.
5. Name three common fungi that cause pulmonary infections in immunocompromised patients.

Answer to Critical Thinking Questions

1. (b) 2. (b) 3. (c) 4. (a) 5. (c)

REFERENCES

1. Abba, A., Al Kadah, Albasri, Carlton, A. E., Evans, C. A., Ugarte-Gil, C., Chau, D. E., Kirwan, D. E., et al. (2017). Histological examination in obtaining a diagnosis in patients with lymphadenopathy in Lima, Peru. https://core.ac.uk/download/187116216.pdf (accessed on 16th June 2025).
2. Reinero, C., Visser, L. C., Kellihan, H. B., Masseau, I., Rozanski, E., Clercx, C., Williams, K., Abbott, J., Borgarelli, M., & Scansen, B. A. (2020). ACVIM consensus statement guidelines for the diagnosis, classification, treatment, and monitoring of pulmonary hypertension in dogs. *Journal of Veterinary Internal Medicine*, *34*(2), 549–573. https://doi.org/10.1111/jvim.15725Adams, H., Araujo, A., Araujo, M., Asmah, R., Breman, J., Brugman, P., Butler, C., et al. (2010). Allergic disorders in Africa and Africans: Is it primarily a priority? https://core.ac.uk/download/pdf/18410775.pdf (accessed on 16th June 2025).
3. Agnone, F., Araújo, R., Bacher, M., Bacher, T., Bacher, P., Bacher, L., Bacher, H., et al. (2017). Pathogen-reactive T helper cell analysis in the pig. https://core.ac.uk/download/84594831.pdf (accessed on 16th June 2025).
4. Ailal, F., Al-Herz, W., Bousfiha, A., Casanova, J. L., et al. (2020). Human inborn errors of immunity: 2019 update of the IUIS phenotypical classification. https://core.ac.uk/download/323074666.pdf (accessed on 16th June 2025).
5. Alcazar-Fuoli, L., Armstrong-James, D., Bertuzzi, M., Bignell, E., et al. (2014). The pH-responsive PacC transcription factor of *Aspergillus fumigatus* governs epithelial entry and tissue invasion during pulmonary aspergillosis. https://core.ac.uk/download/30435716.pdf (accessed on 16th June 2025).
6. Alhallaf, R. A. (2018). Regulation of immunity and inflammation during parasitic helminth infection by inflammasomes. https://core.ac.uk/download/303788921.pdf (accessed on 16th June 2025).
7. Azoulay, E., Benoit, D., Bruneel, F., Contejean, A., et al. (2016). Increased mortality in hematological malignancy patients with acute respiratory failure from undetermined etiology: A Groupe de Recherche en Réanimation Respiratoire en Onco-Hématologique (Grrr-OH) study. https://core.ac.uk/download/84044246.pdf (accessed on 16th June 2025).
8. Calvet, C. M., Choi, J. Y., de Mesquita, L. B., de Souza Pereira, T., et al. (2017). 4-aminopyridyl-based lead compounds targeting CYP51 prevent spontaneous parasite relapse in a chronic model and improve cardiac pathology in an acute model of *Trypanosoma cruzi* infection. https://core.ac.uk/download/323066331.pdf (accessed on 16th June 2025).
9. Cello, J. P., & Day, L. (2009). Idiopathic AIDS enteropathy and treatment of gastrointestinal opportunistic pathogens. https://core.ac.uk/download/323073564.pdf (accessed on 16th June 2025).
10. Das, S., & Khader, S. (2017). Yin and yang of interleukin-17 in host immunity to infection [version 1; referees: 2 approved]. https://core.ac.uk/download/84911322.pdf (accessed on 16th June 2025).
11. Dear, J. D. (2020). Bacterial pneumonia in dogs and cats: An update. https://core.ac.uk/download/286361309.pdf (accessed on 16th June 2025).

12. Dear, J. D., Hulsebosch, S. E., Johnson, E. G., Johnson, M., et al. (2019). Eosinophilic bronchitis, eosinophilic granuloma, and eosinophilic broncho pneumopathy in 75 dogs (2006–2016). https://core.ac.uk/download/286361756.pdf (accessed on 16th June 2025).

13. Dhanya, M. S., Anandhi, D., Roy, D. D., Alex, R. B., Karthick, S., Joseph, B., Renjith, K. R., et al. (2024). The influence of maternal infections on congenital heart defect. https://core.ac.uk/download/603897437.pdf (accessed on 16th June 2025).

14. Eijck, I., Groot, M., Kasteel, D., Kijlstra, A., et al. (2003). Analysis of black holes in our knowledge concerning animal health in the organic food production chain. https://core.ac.uk/download/10919416.pdf (accessed on 16th June 2025).

15. Farr, A., Torres, A., Ringshausen, F. C., Blasi, F., Dimopoulos, G., Rohde, G., Migliori, G. B., et al. (2018). *ERS Syllabus for Postgraduate Training in Respiratory Infections: A Guide for Comprehensive Training.* https://core.ac.uk/download/195292060.pdf (accessed on 16th June 2025).

16. Firkins, M. P. (2015). Prevalence and distribution of Rana virus, chytrid fungus, and helminths in North Dakota amphibians. https://core.ac.uk/download/235078269.pdf (accessed on 16th June 2025).

17. Hage, C. A., Knox, K. S., & Sarosi, G. A. (2005). Endemic mycosis. https://core.ac.uk/download/333956976.pdf (accessed on 16th June 2025).

18. Hemalatha, S. (2011). A study on aerobic bacterial and fungal isolates in bronchoalveolar lavage in patients with lower respiratory tract infection in a tertiary care hospital. https://core.ac.uk/download/322550552.pdf (accessed on 16th June 2025).

19. Homei, A., & Worboys, M. (2020). Chapter bibliography. https://core.ac.uk/download/478137736.pdf (accessed on 16th June 2025).

20. Ikinciogullari, A., Altun, D., Ciftci, E., Dogu, F., Bahadır, G. G., Kologlu, M., Akyuzluer, S., et al. (2020). An unexpected infection in loss-of-function mutations in STAT3: Malignant alveolar echinococcosis in liver. https://core.ac.uk/download/492893215.pdf (accessed on 16th June 2025).

21. Jourdan, P. M., & Lamberton, P. H. L. (2015). Human ascariasis: Diagnostics update. https://core.ac.uk/download/46559165.pdf (accessed on 16th June 2025).

22. Lee, J. S., & Van der Putten, W. (2011). Soil borne human diseases. https://core.ac.uk/download/38621779.pdf (accessed on 16th June 2025).

23. Olowe, A., Olowe, R. A., & Otutu, O. (2023). Microbial and parasitic infections in tertiary care: Diagnosis, treatment, and prevention strategies. https://core.ac.uk/download/591219458.pdf (accessed on 16th June 2025).

24. Reeve, J. (2018). The diagnostic approach to coughing in dogs and cats. https://core.ac.uk/download/616484685.pdf (accessed on 16th June 2025).

25. Sabino, R., & Wiederhold, N. (2022). Diagnosis from tissue: Histology and identification. https://core.ac.uk/download/553619747.pdf (accessed on 16th June 2025).

26. Stellick Seepaulsingh, S. H. (2014). *Using Comparative Metagenomics to Determine the Role of Atlantic Bottlenose Dolphins (Tursiops truncatus) as Sentinels for Human Respiratory Health.* https://core.ac.uk/download/217669418.pdf (accessed on 16th June 2025).

27. Thamsborg, S. M., & Waller, P. J. (2004). Nematode control in 'green' ruminant production systems. https://core.ac.uk/download/10921653.pdf (accessed on 16th June 2025).

28. Upadhyay, R. K. (2023). Mucosal membranes, their interactions to microbial infections and immune susceptibility in human hosts. https://core.ac.uk/download/558839684.pdf (accessed on 16th June 2025).

29. Wilson, A. J., Longdon, B., Okamura, B., Brem, D., Centers for Disease Control, Kallio, E. R., Ewald, P. W., et al. (2017). The evolution of transmission mode. https://core.ac.uk/download/74236453.pdf (accessed on 16th June 2025).

BRONCHIAL ASTHMA

10

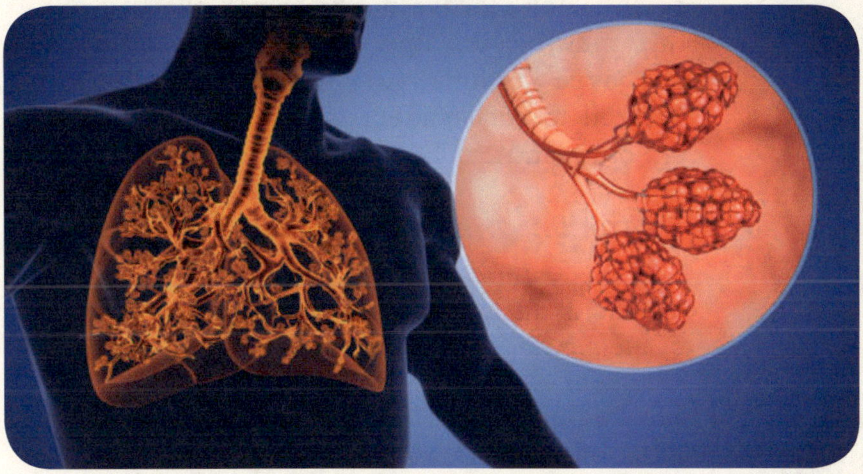

LEARNING OBJECTIVES

After studying this chapter, you will be able to:

1. List the causes of bronchial asthma
2. Describe the symptoms of bronchial asthma
3. Understand the diagnosis of bronchial asthma
4. Explore the treatment options for bronchial asthma
5. Explain the management strategies for bronchial asthma
6. Focus on the impact of bronchial asthma

Introduction

Bronchial asthma is a global, serious public health problem with many patients involved from different populations. The chronic airway disease is characterized by recurrent wheezing, shortness of breath, and chest tightness. It results from a multifactorial interaction between genetic, environmental, and immunologic determinants. The pathophysiologic mechanism of the disease involves hyperreactivity and remodeling of airways, which enhance symptoms and compromise respiratory function on the long term. As a multifactorial disease, asthma can be triggered by various factors, including allergens, air pollution, and respiratory infections, making a comprehensive understanding and control essential. Increasingly, though, studies have examined the part that modern technology can play in managing bronchial asthma through advances in wearable technology and digital health interventions. New technologies in wearable devices hold promise for real-time monitoring and management of bronchial asthma, as well as improved patient outcomes and quality of life. These devices can monitor physiological parameters such as respiratory rate and peak flow measurement, providing individuals and care providers with valuable information in decision-making. Furthermore, as highlighted by today's medical talks, wearable medical devices have considerable potential for incorporation into chronic disease treatment plans. By actively monitoring and examining health parameters, such developments not only aid in the real-time alleviation of symptoms but also provide insight into longer-term health monitoring initiatives.

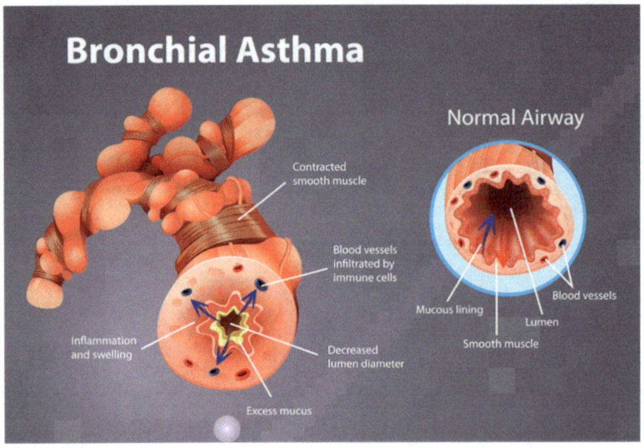

Figure 10.1. Bronchial asthma.

Source: https://drsyedarshadhusainpulmonologist.com/wp-content/uploads/2024/01/bronchial-asthma.webp

Additionally, as the field continues to grow, critical research is essential for studying the general applications of these technologies in asthma management, making them more effective and accessible. Second, the fact that the condition is chronic necessitates increased understanding of its pathophysiological mechanisms, particularly airway remodeling, which is long-term airway structural changes resulting from ongoing inflammation. These structural changes, resulting from multifaceted cellular responses, can lead to chronic symptoms and impaired lung function, underscoring the importance of early treatment and effective control. As outlined by the most recent studies, environmental exposures more often than not are the precipitating factor for airway remodeling, exacerbating an already vulnerable state of lung health. Control of the environmental determinants of asthma and the application of advanced technology, therefore, are not only therapeutic and preventive strategies but also essential for effective management. Collectively, this multifaceted approach could result in improved asthma care recommendations tailored to each patient in the ever-evolving era of respiratory health.

Definition of bronchial asthma

Bronchial asthma, a chronic inflammatory airway disease, is characterized by hyperresponsiveness of the airways to a variety of stimuli. It causes recurrent episodes of wheezing, breathlessness, chest tightness, and cough, particularly at night or in the early morning. Pathological processes are inflammation of the bronchus, increased mucus secretion, and bronchoconstriction, leading to airflow obstruction. The relevance of an appropriate definition of bronchial asthma lies in its treatment and management, which, to a large extent, rely on an understanding of such pathophysiological mechanisms. The epidemiology of the condition is also characterized by a high prevalence in numerous populations, with significant implications for quality of life and healthcare burden, underscoring the importance of effective public health planning. Diagnostic standards for bronchial asthma are essential for effective treatment planning and management. In most cases, a thorough clinical history is obtained, including the frequency and relationship of symptoms to potential precipitating events. Objective spirometric testing is necessary to ensure the diagnosis of airway obstruction and reversibility. Distinguishing between asthma and other respiratory illnesses, such as chronic obstructive pulmonary disease (COPD), is critical because the treatment approach differs vastly. Furthermore, the recognition of the role of occupational exposures is significant in understanding certain asthma subtypes, such as the prevalence of occupational asthma across various industries. The recognition of bronchial asthma causes and variations enables medical professionals to tailor treatment procedures for individual patients, thereby enhancing patient outcomes and reducing the long-term cost of the disease (EJ et al., 2000). Comorbidities play a significant role in the clinical management of bronchial asthma and have a substantial impact on the overall health and well-being of the patient. Among the several comorbidities that worsen asthma symptoms and make treatment more complex, allergic rhinitis, gastroesophageal reflux disease (GERD), and obesity are prominent. Their control is crucial for managing asthma effectively. Lastly, the socioeconomic aspects of bronchial asthma imply that integrated strategy must be employed to deliver fair access to care. For example, the variability in access to healthcare is associated with the prevalence and severity of asthma symptoms, as noted in research assessing the prevalence rates of asthma among diverse groups. Further research on the non-repeatable and repeatable sampling processes in asthma epidemiology is crucial for prevention and an understanding of the asthma epidemic among different populations (Kozhyna et al., 2019).

Importance of understanding asthma

It is not only essential to know about asthma because it allows for maximal management and quality of life in those with this chronic respiratory illness, but also because asthma is often associated with airway narrowing and inflammation that may lead to respiratory distress and increased risk of life-threatening asthma attacks. By comprehensively knowing the mechanisms and stimuli of asthma, patients and clinicians can design individualized management plans. This includes identifying environmental allergens, such as pollen or dust mites, and their impact on asthma symptoms. Without a full understanding of these factors, patients may struggle to control their symptoms effectively, exposing them to unwanted dangers and complications of poorly controlled asthma, such as hospitalization for exacerbations and loss of overall health status. Most notably, as an integral part of asthma education, it is one thing that has a profoundly positive effect on the lives of children and their families. As indicated by research, children with bronchial asthma encounter significant adversity in addition to physical symptoms; such adversity includes significantly impaired quality of life in terms of physical activity, emotional health, and school functioning. Parents and guardians themselves must play an essential part in this situation, managing the complexities of asthma control while addressing their children's needs. Research shows that ideal control in asthma is not only associated with better symptom control but also with improved psychosocial outcomes for participating children. By empowering individuals with knowledge of such associations, healthcare workers can equip families with the necessary information and competencies to manage asthma issues in their daily lives, thereby maximizing overall well-being and functionality (Theofilou et al., 2023). Aside from its impact on the quality of individual life, it is crucial to understand asthma in order to develop effective public health programs for reducing the prevalence and burden of the disease. Asthma not only affects those who have been diagnosed but also places an economic burden on the healthcare system through related medical costs and lost productivity. Increased education and awareness of asthma management can lead to enhanced preventive and self-management practices among patients, thereby reducing hospitalizations and acute exacerbations. Education and community-based programs that provide education and materials on managing asthma can empower individuals and families and lead to an active way of controlling asthma, which depletes the population burden of asthma. Lastly, a holistic model of asthma can support improved health outcomes grounded in evidence-based approaches and facilitative interventions that resonate with patients' actual experiences (Boda et al., 2024).

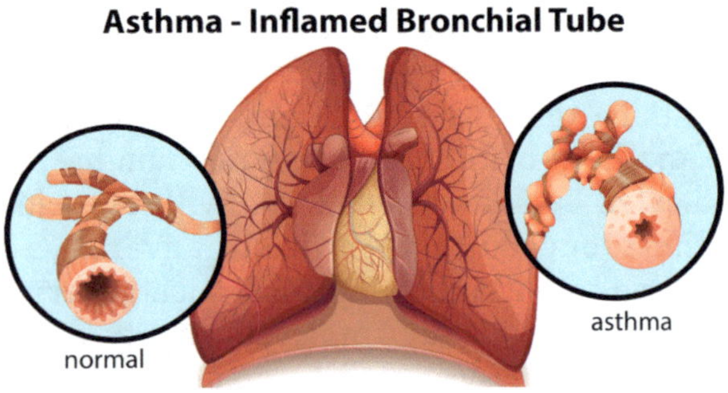

Figure 10.2. Understanding asthma.

Source: https://totalcarefc.com/wp-content/uploads/2025/05/Understanding-Asthma-and-Its-Impact-on-Breathing.png

10.1. Causes of Bronchial Asthma

Learning Outcome

1. Genetic factors
2. Environmental triggers
3. Occupational exposures

The interplay of genetic, environmental, and immunological factors emphasizes the complex etiology of bronchial asthma. Genetics plays a significant role in asthma susceptibility, with patients with genetic predispositions by family history of allergy or asthma having a higher risk of developing the condition. Such genetic predisposition is usually accompanied by precipitating factors from the environment, such as allergens from dust mites, pet dander, and pollen. These environmental stimuli elicit an immune response in predisposed individuals, leading to the inflammation characteristic of asthma. Prenatal and early childhood exposure to cigarette smoke is also a proven risk factor that promotes the accelerated onset of asthma in genetically predisposed populations. It has been affirmed in scientific studies that the associations between such environmental exposures and these genetic predispositions basically determine the course of the disease, proving the difficulty in explaining asthma's etiology (Головко et al., 2024).

The second significant etiologic factor for the onset and aggravation of bronchial asthma includes the presence of various allergens and irritants, which can trigger allergic reactions in susceptible individuals. In children, viral respiratory infections are becoming frequent precipitants, with a tendency to cause acute exacerbations. On clinical grounds, in children below the age of six years, foods, indoor dust, and exercise are also found to be significant precipitants of asthma exacerbation. With increasing age, the list of potential precipitants also gets extended to include emotional stress and exposure to animals, thereby further complicating the asthmatic course. These triggers play a role in causing bronchial hyperresponsiveness, perpetuating an inflammatory-obstructive cycle that makes treatment challenging. A sensitive awareness of these triggers is crucial for effectively managing and preventing asthma exacerbations, especially among children (Головко et al., 2024). Moreover, the discovery of COVID-19 has added new aspects to the etiology and treatment of bronchial asthma. While the interaction between asthma and COVID-19 is complex, the studies have shown that the trajectory of the disease in patients with asthma remains unclear during the pandemic, with a pattern either of severe disease or a better course of illness. The relationship between SARS-CoV-2 infection and exacerbation of asthma has raised concerns regarding viral contributions to the course of the disease. Moreover, demands for particular treatment during viral pandemics have highlighted the need for maintaining therapeutic regimens consistently, such as the infusion of omalizumab, which was reported as safe and possibly therapeutic for patients with severe asthma during COVID-19. Ultimately, knowledge about the evolving variables related to bronchial asthma is crucial for developing effective management strategies in a rapidly evolving medical environment.

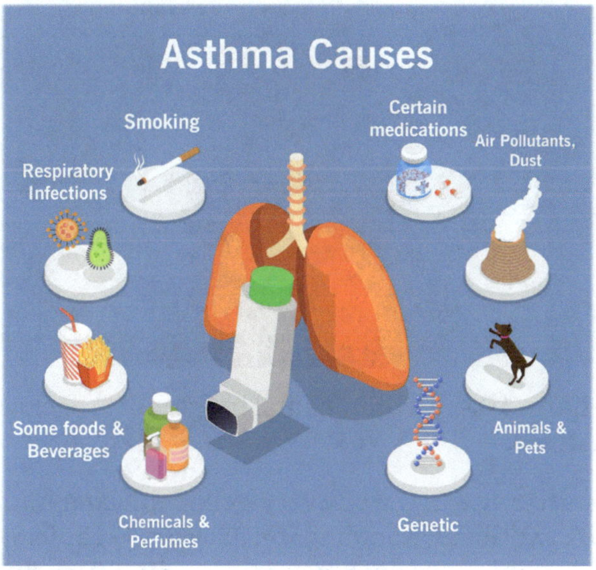

Figure 10.3. Causes of bronchial asthma.

Source: https://lirp.cdn-website.com/69c0b277/dms3rep/multi/opt/Asthma+causes-+causes+of+bronchial+asthma-640w.jpg

10.1.1. Genetic Factors

Genetic factors form the core of the pathophysiology of asthma bronchiale, influencing susceptibility and severity of illness. The literature suggests that an intricate interplay between environmental exposures and a genetic predisposition underlies the development of asthma. Some alleles that influence inflammation, immune response, and lung function can increase susceptibility to asthma development, but concomitant exposure to precipitants, such as allergens or pollutants, further enhances the risk. For instance, individuals with specific polymorphisms in cytokine-related genes may experience more severe asthmatic manifestations. Understanding genetic susceptibilities identifies risk groups and guides personalized treatment approaches to alleviate asthma symptoms and improve quality of life (Hufnagl et al., 2020).

Immune dysregulation is closely linked to genetic factors in the pathogenesis of asthma. The key actors in this process are several cytokines and growth factors, notably transforming growth factor-beta (TGF-β). TGF-β plays a crucial role in lung organogenesis, as well as in maintaining lung homeostasis, and is also involved in the induction of airway remodeling and epithelial-mesenchymal transition in asthma patients. Genetic polymorphisms can influence the activation and signaling pathway expression of TGF-β, thereby modulating patient responses to asthma stimuli and therapies. A modified TGF-β function was also associated with increased airway hyperresponsiveness and inflammation in patients with asthma, emphasizing the importance of genetic determinants in controlling the underlying pathomechanisms of the disease (Saito et al., 2018). The multifactorial pathogenesis of asthma necessitates a comprehensive approach that considers both genetic and environmental factors. Genetic differences associated with the lung microbiome also contribute to asthma susceptibility and potentially influence the inflammatory phenotype of patients. For instance, disruptions in the benign microbial community—regardless of the responsible agent, ranging from antibiotics to diet—can create an asthma predisposition by suppressing the immune system's regulatory properties. This example of genetic susceptibility combined with microbial dysbiosis illustrates the complex network of factors that affect asthma development. With the increasing prevalence of asthma worldwide, there is a growing need for future studies to identify the genetic markers of asthma, providing prospects for more effective diagnostic and therapeutic measures tailored to individuals' genetic backgrounds (Hufnagl et al., 2020).

10.1.2. Environmental Triggers

The initiation of bronchial asthma usually closely related to certain environmental factors that individuals may come into contact with in their daily lives. These range from common allergens like pollen, dust mites, and dander from pets, which are highly contributory to the induction of asthma attacks since they tend to induce inflammatory responses in predisposed individuals. Most prominently in regions like Al-Baha City, where environmental conditions are characterized by elevated levels of dust, such triggers significantly contribute to the disease burden of asthma patients. The relationship between environmental conditions and respiratory wellness is highlighted by evidence that many individuals experience exacerbated symptoms from exposure to certain allergens, hence the need for interventions that consider localized environmental conditions (Alzahrani et al., 2024). Identifying the nature of these environmental triggers is crucial to the development of successful public health interventions and education initiatives aimed at minimizing exposure and optimizing asthma control. Another challenge to controlling asthma are additional environmental irritants, such as cigarette smoke and air pollution. In Al-Baha, where the population supposedly finds itself annoyed by cigarette smoke and environmental dust, consideration of these omnipresent triggers is a priority. Health-related quality of life among patients with asthma is highly influenced by exposure to these irritants, and the majority experience activity limitation due to worsening asthma. In addition, an alarming number of individuals may not feel confident to deal with or avoid these environmental irritants, highlighting a significant gap in asthma awareness and education (Alzahrani et al., 2024). With public health initiatives adapting to rising prevalence rates for asthma, environmental triggers must be a focus as a means to enhance overall quality of life for those afflicted with this chronic condition.

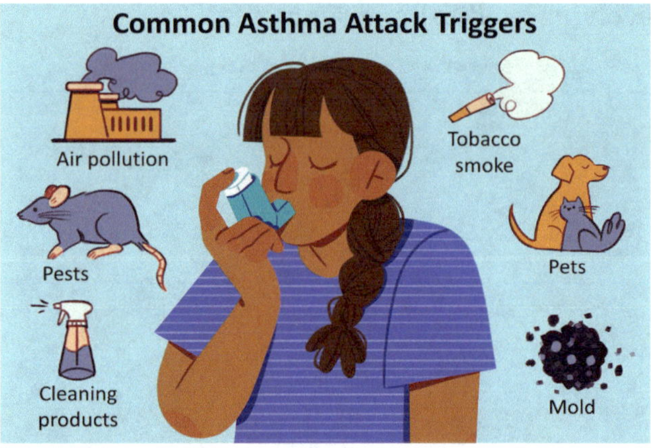

Figure 10.4. Environmental triggers of bronchial asthma.

Source: https://www.verywellhealth.com/thmb/0sXtJGbaitQK5nMmg5U4OSaRBiU=/1500x0/filters:no_upscale():max_bytes(150000):strip_icc()/VWH_Illustration_Common-Asthma-Attack-Triggers_Illustrator_Theresa-Chiechi_Final-1c387bbd03424e4988f03e2b442a10e5.jpg.

Moreover, the contribution of environmental triggers extends beyond individual exposure, with entities such as climate change receiving increased attention for their impact on asthma prevalence and severity. Fluctuations in weather patterns can potentially lead to increased allergen levels, such as higher pollen counts in warmer months. This change in environmental conditions can potentially exacerbate existing asthma and further the disease burden, particularly for susceptible populations, i.e., children and the elderly. In studies conducted among children with acute asthmatic attacks, environmental exposures have been revealed to play a pivotal role in their health status. It is thus paramount that healthcare professionals and policymakers remain vigilant in learning how environmental exposures continually affect asthma control prevalence. Solving these problems that are interlinked could realize improved health outcomes among populations with asthma.

10.1.3. Occupational Exposures

The relationship between occupational exposures and bronchial asthma is best seen in occupations where workers are frequently exposed to toxic chemicals. Diisocyanates are among the groups of chemicals that are most concerning, and they are widely used in construction, automotive, and manufacturing sectors. Evidence has indicated that exposure to diisocyanates can result in sensitization, occupational asthma, and BHR, thus pointing out the necessity of monitoring and controlling such exposures in the workplace. In Finland, studies conducted on MDI- and TDI-exposed industries show that, although with similarly low mean exposure levels, the risk of developing severe BHR remains, particularly in certain industries such as construction and car repair. Evidence places special importance on implementing effective prevention practices and conducting health impact assessments to mitigate occupational asthma risk from diisocyanate exposure (Huuskonen et al., 2023). In non-ferrous metallurgy, exposure to various occupational hazards significantly contributes to respiratory diseases, such as bronchial asthma. Industrial workers are exposed to a blend of excessive physical exertion, high levels of noise, and toxic dust and gas mixtures. Effects include a range of medical diseases, with the most prevalent of these being bronchial asthma among aerosol-exposed industrial workers and those exposed to harmful chemicals. The complex combination of these factors not only exacerbates respiratory illnesses but also leads to a decline in overall health conditions among employees. Due to the unique chemical exposures in such a setup, identifying and removing the specific health risks are essential. Minimizing such exposures through sound health assessments plays an important role in ensuring worker health and reducing the incidence of asthma (Shur et al., 2023). Understanding the dynamics of occupational exposures is crucial, as it can help in effectively evading and controlling bronchial asthma. Several industries have reported that chronic exposure to certain irritants can significantly increase the risk of developing respiratory diseases. Thus, immediate enforcement of firm regulatory standards and company policies regarding occupational health is necessary. Increased awareness among employers and employees about the risks associated with harmful substances is necessary. Additionally, provision for periodic health checks and exposure monitoring will enable the early detection of asthma symptoms, allowing for more targeted interventions. By adopting a precautionary approach to controlling occupational exposures, industries can enhance worker protection and significantly reduce the incidence of bronchial asthma (Huuskonen et al., 2023; Shur et al., 2023).

Test Your Knowledge

1. What are the genetic factors?
2. What are the occupational exposures?

10.2. Symptoms of Bronchial Asthma

Learning Outcome

1. Shortness of breath
2. Wheezing
3. Chest tightness

Bronchial asthma is characterized by a variety of signs and symptoms that can lead to significant alterations in one's daily life and overall health. One of the most frequent symptoms is wheezing, or a heard whistling noise during breathing, particularly with exertion or nocturnal wheezing. The other symptom is shortness of breath, which occurs with some effort or when lying down, reflecting airway obstruction. Coughing, especially morning or nocturnal coughing, is another frequent symptom and may be associated with increased mucus secretion. Such symptoms are often variable in intensity, typically worsening during asthma exacerbation episodes, where patients may struggle to perform daily activities. Both patients and health care professionals should be aware of these symptoms because they can lead to early detection that results in timely intervention and consequently improve the care strategy for bronchial asthma. In addition to the typical symptoms, the occurrence of comorbid conditions makes management of bronchial asthma challenging. For instance, bronchiectasis is common with asthma, leading to increased airway inflammation and frequency of exacerbations. This contact highlights the high prevalence of respiratory disease and the need for careful assessment to identify underlying conditions that may influence asthma control. More severe exacerbations, more frequent exacerbations, and overall increased severity of the disease in patients with asthma and bronchiectasis suggest that these patients require a special therapeutic approach. Identification of such comorbidities is essential since the lack of recognition of their occurrence may result in ineffective treatment strategies, further deteriorating the patients' health. The coincidence of bronchiectasis and asthma characterizes the complex nature of respiratory system diseases and shows the importance of thorough patient' assessments for effective treatment in practice (Crimi et al., 2020). Current research also reveals that the physiological effects of bronchial asthma extend beyond acute symptoms and touch long-term health consequences.

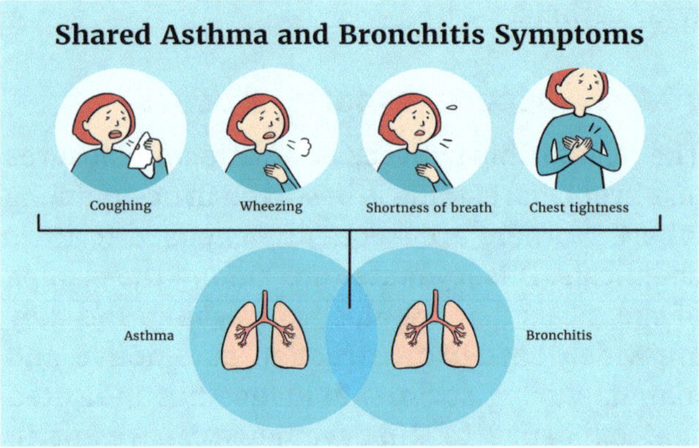

Figure 10.5. Symptoms of bronchial asthma.

Source: https://www.verywellhealth.com/thmb/VY0Yfr1GSmydhwv_Y1AR95BQdfI=/1500x0/filters:no_upscale():max_bytes(150000):strip_icc()/bronchitis-asthma-types-symptoms-200548_FINAL-b2e446c4e3584f54acc6ec526c5c9446.gif

Asthma, especially if poorly controlled, can lead to significant long-term impairment of lung function. In children, the disease can restrict normal airway growth, resulting in permanent deficits in lung volumes that persist into adulthood. In adults, uncontrolled asthma has the potential to cause accelerated decline in lung function and increase the risk of fixed airflow limitation. This association calls for early management, not merely offering symptomatic relief but also preventing chronic respiratory disease in the long run. Environmental determinants and genetic susceptibility must be considered when classifying asthma phenotypes accurately. By so doing, clinicians can develop more personalized treatment strategies, resulting in better outcomes and lower overall health impacts associated with bronchial asthma (Dharmage et al., 2019).

10.2.1. Shortness of Breath

The shortness of breath symptom, or in medical terms, dyspnea, is a key condition in the life of patients with bronchial asthma. The sensation is attributed to bronchial obstruction caused by inflammation, which limits airflow during respiration. Patients usually come with this painful symptom in the form of a feeling of chest tightness, which contributes to anxiety and reduced quality of life. The assorted external stimuli that trigger shortness of breath include environmental stimuli such as allergens, respiratory infections, and physical activity. Thus, the engagement of these external stimuli with internal vulnerability has the potential to create a pattern of recurring dyspnea, which can significantly impact daily life and global health. Treatment of the severity and prevalence of shortness of breath is also most important in the treatment of asthma, since both are directly linked to the success of treatment policies and the patients' ability to maintain physical and social activities. Additionally, understanding the causes and impact of shortness of breath on asthma sufferers requires a holistic approach to treatment. Pharmacological interventions, including bronchodilators and corticosteroids, play a crucial role in managing symptoms and regulating inflammation. Non-pharmacological methods, however, such as lifestyle modification and breathing exercises, also play their role in the management of patients. Engaging in activities that contribute to respiratory health, such as swimming, has been suggested to be beneficial in industrial settings, precisely outlining its positive impact on lung function and alleviation of asthma symptoms. In the context of established risks associated with certain physical exercises, general stimulation of regular, controlled exercise still plays a vital role in improving patients' lung function and tolerance, thereby reducing the frequency of dyspnea episodes (Ptak et al., 2024). Moreover, the Ayurvedic philosophy of asthma treatment offers fascinating information on the causative factors of shortness of breath. The philosophy emphasizes a balance of body humor and holds the belief that excessive intake of kapha-promoting foods can cause respiratory suffocation.

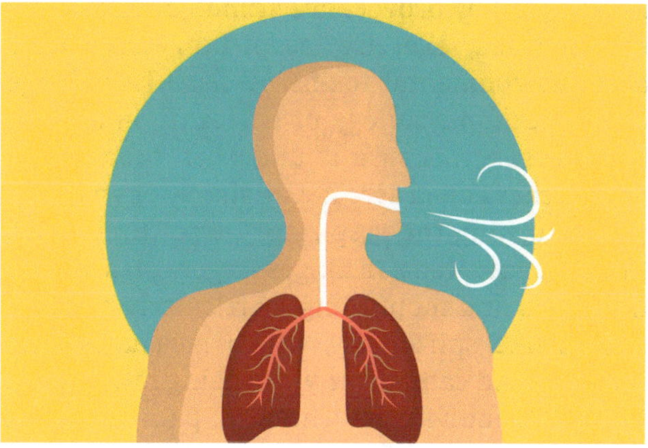

Figure 10.6. Shortness of breath.

Source: https://roshahealth.com/en/wp-content/uploads/2022/12/short-of-breath-causes-scaled.jpg

For this purpose, bronchial asthma treatment is broader than allopathic medicine, advocating food and lifestyle changes to manage symptoms effectively. Some regimens involving avoidance of known precipitants, such as environmental toxins, constitute an integral part of the preventive approach to shortness of breath caused by asthma. Prioritizing holistic care, such as environmental control and dietary optimization, is consistent with maintaining overall health and reducing the risk of acute asthma attacks (Dr. K. Bhat et al., 2025). Thus, managing shortness of breath according to polyfactorial approaches can enhance the quality of life in patients with bronchial asthma.

10.2.2. Wheezing

Wheezing is a common symptom of bronchial asthma and is potentially a significant indication of airway obstruction. Wheezing, also known as a high-pitched whistling sound both on breathing in and out, is a consequence of the narrowing of the air tubes of the lungs. Numerous reasons, like inflammation, mucus secretions, and bronchoconstriction can bring it about. In asthmatic children, wheezing is often potentiated by provocative stimuli or exposures to allergens, exercise, respiratory infection, and environmental toxins. A clear knowledge of the pathophysiology of wheezing in asthma is necessary because it underlies therapeutic approaches aimed at reducing airway obstruction and returning the respiratory tract to normal. Effective intervention hinges largely on accurate diagnosis and monitoring, particularly through means like spirometry, which measures lung function and can quantify wheezing intensity in asthmatic individuals. The local pain effects of wheezing are only secondary to the impact of wheezing that reflect the chronic, inflammatory, and persistent nature of asthma. Remodeling of the airway, characterized by structural changes in bronchial walls, can lead to chronic wheezing and reduced lung function in the long term if asthma is not well-controlled. Ideal control can require both pharmacologic interventions and behavioral changes. As postulated in recent publications, the preexercise administration of short-acting beta-agonists (SABA) can help prevent exercise-induced bronchoconstriction (EIB) and wheezing attacks, emphasizing the importance of individualized treatment recommendations. Furthermore, cautionary actions such as warming up before exercising and avoiding known environmental stimuli can supplement orthodox therapy, improving general asthma control as well as reducing wheeze attack frequency in bronchial asthma patients. The linkage between wheezing and asthma also relates to treatment alternatives considerations. While several studies have examined the efficacy of complementary treatments, including reflexology and homeopathy, current evidence suggests that these methods may have no significant impact on asthma control or quality of life when incorporated into usual care. Specifically, research has established that combining homeopathy or reflexology does not yield statistically significant improvements in asthma quality of life compared with usual care alone. Hence, focus on evidence-based practices that focus on established medical therapy is essential. Understanding wheezing mechanisms of bronchial asthma with appropriate management and treatment remains essential to achieve optimal patient outcomes as well as enhancing respiratory health in patients with the disease.

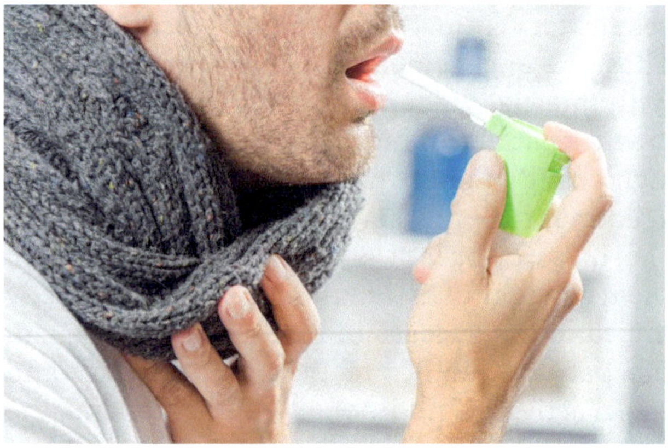

Figure 10.7. Wheezing.

Source: https://www.metropolisindia.com/upgrade/blog/upload/2023/04/ezgif.com-gif-maker-25.jpg

10.2.3. Chest Tightness

Tightness in the chest is a familiar, uncomfortable symptom associated with bronchial asthma, typically described as a sensation of being enveloped around the thorax. It may be minimal or severe, and its variability can complicate diagnosis, particularly in atypical presentations such as the chest tightness variant asthma (CTVA). In such situations, chest tightness is the dominant clinical presentation that overshadows other classic asthma symptoms, including wheezing and dyspnea. As a result, patients may experience significant delays in diagnosis, which can hinder the timely initiation of effective treatment modalities. This condition highlights the need for a thorough assessment, including a detailed medical history and appropriate diagnostic tests, to differentiate chest tightness from other causes of discomfort. In interpreting the correlation between chest tightness and bronchial asthma, consideration should be given to the underlying mechanisms of this symptom. Exercise-induced bronchoconstriction (EIB) is a demonstration of how exercise can reveal airway reactivity, causing impaired airflow and subsequent chest tightness. EIB is characterized by airway obstruction that frequently occurs post-exercise, with presenting symptoms including cough, dyspnea, wheezing, and chest tightness. The etiology of EIB remains to be fully understood, although theories such as osmotic and heat mechanisms have been proposed. Because some patients present with an abnormally increased respiratory response to exercise, clinicians must use some work-up measures like spirometry and exercise challenge tests not only to confirm a diagnosis of asthma but to determine the severity and impact of chest tightness on patients' lives. To effectively treat chest tightness in bronchial asthma, a multimodal treatment strategy that combines pharmacological and behavioral therapies is necessary. Traditional interventions typically include short-acting beta-agonists (SABA) for acute relief and inhaled corticosteroids (ICS) for chronic management. In cases where patients experience symptoms that are entirely localized to chest tightness, such as CTVA, professionals must consider an individualized treatment approach in accordance with the most recent guidelines. Patient education and self-management have recently been emphasized as key elements that can enhance both the quality of the patient experience and treatment compliance. The application of warm-up maneuvers, controlled breathing exercises, and avoidance of environmental pollutants will significantly decrease the frequency of chest tightness events and improve both physical activity levels and quality of life for individuals with bronchial asthma.

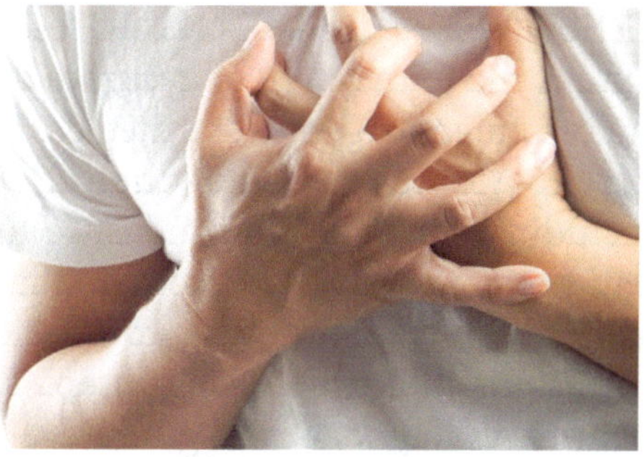

Figure 10.8. Chest tightness.

Source: https://www.liebscher-bracht.com/en/wp-content/uploads/2021/08/tight-chest-remedy-featured-image-08272021-liebscherbracht.jpg

Test Your Knowledge

1. Define the term shortness of breath.
2. What is wheezing?

10.3. Diagnosis of Bronchial Asthma

Learning Outcome

1. Medical history assessment
2. Physical examination
3. Diagnostic tests (e.g., spirometry)

Diagnosis of bronchial asthma involves a comprehensive examination that includes clinical history, physical examination, and innumerable investigative procedures. Clinicians take a clear history from the patient first, emphasizing symptoms such as wheezing, breathlessness, chest tightness, and cough, particularly if these symptoms vary over time or are provoked by a specific trigger. Physical examination is relevant and typically detects wheezing or other signs of airflow obstruction. Careful assessment of this kind is the foundation of accurate diagnosis and successful management strategies. The following diagnostic tests could then be employed, including spirometry to measure lung function and responsiveness to bronchodilators, as well as peak flow monitoring to check day-to-day variations in airflow. These steps can lead to a definitive diagnosis and guide the next choices of therapy, which are crucial for asthma control. In addition to clinical evaluation, reliance on objective tests in asthma diagnosis cannot be overstressed. One significant advancement is the proposal that fractional exhaled nitric oxide (FeNO) be employed as an objective test for assessing airway inflammation. It is an indirect marker of eosinophilic inflammation, a condition that often accompanies asthma. FeNO application is beneficial where the diagnosis of asthma is questionable, and it provides valuable information regarding the inflammatory profile that can assist clinicians in tailoring therapy. The revisions to guidelines further emphasize that while FeNO may be used for diagnosis and monitoring, it cannot be the sole basis for asthma diagnosis. This subtle tactic emphasizes the importance of employing multiple diagnostic approaches to enhance accuracy in identifying bronchial asthma and addressing the unique needs of individual patients (Cloutier et al., 2020). There are instances where differential diagnosis of bronchial asthma is indicated, especially when clinical presentations overlap with other illnesses, for example, COPD or other respiratory illnesses. According to the latest evidence, individuals with chronic respiratory diseases can have elevated serum levels of biomarkers, such as hypoxia-inducible factor 1-alpha (HIF-1α), which complicates the diagnosis. In particular, patients with a definite diagnosis of bronchial asthma can have elevated HIF-1α levels, potentially leading to confusion within the typical clinical presentation. Clinicians thus need to systematically exclude other respiratory illnesses through extensive evaluation, i.e., thorough pulmonary function testing and polysomnography as required, to differentiate asthma from the remaining potential etiologies of respiratory symptomatology (Gabryelska et al., 2019). This meticulous process ultimately results in more effective management strategies tailored to the unique patient profile.

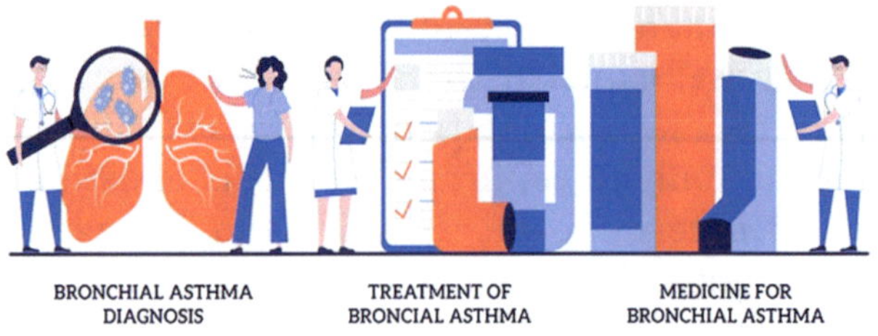

Figure 10.9. Diagnosis of bronchial asthma.

Source: https://img.freepik.com/premium-vector/bronchial-asthma-diagnosis-treatment-medicine-set-respiratory-illness-shortness-breath_269730-844.jpg

10.3.1. Medical History Assessment

The assessment of history is an essential component of learning about bronchial asthma because it provides details regarding patient-specific factors responsible for disease development and exacerbation. Good history must begin with a question regarding the patient's symptoms, i.e., wheezing, breathlessness, and chest tightness, which are typical features of asthma. Additionally, it is essential to distinguish between allergic and non-allergic stimuli that are responsible for symptoms. Factors such as a family history of allergic diseases, exposure to aeroallergens in the environment, and respiratory tract infections during early childhood are highly relevant to the etiology and severity of bronchial asthma. For instance, viral infections, particularly in early life, have been linked with increased asthma risk, and their timing and nature would thus be a high priority in the asthma patient's medical history taking. Medical history taking must also encompass a review of the patient's history before treatment and drug responsiveness. Information on which drugs, including inhaled corticosteroids and bronchodilators, have been utilized previously and how effective they were would be essential for decision-making now. Drugs affect different patients based on genetic or environmental influences, making this information particularly valuable. Additionally, measuring the frequency and severity of asthma symptoms can provide a baseline, allowing clinicians to identify patterns over time. Integration of a patient's history of medication compliance can also detect barriers to effective asthma care, whether they are misperceptions about medication use or access-related (Jin et al., 2020). Lastly, the contribution of environmental and lifestyle determinants cannot be overstated in the history of medical bronchial asthma. Exposure data on tobacco smoke, air pollution, occupational hazards, and home environments provide more background information regarding factors precipitating asthma. Such factors may contribute to the severity of symptoms and impact the long-term prognosis. The interaction between genetically predisposed vulnerabilities and environmental exposures is complex; accordingly, intensive assessments should also include aspects such as the frequency of acute exacerbations, any concomitant emergency room visits, and the resultant necessity for hospitalization. There has been an effective control of bronchial asthma through a multidimensional approach, utilizing extensive medical histories to guide prevention as well as individualized treatment options (Jin et al., 2020).

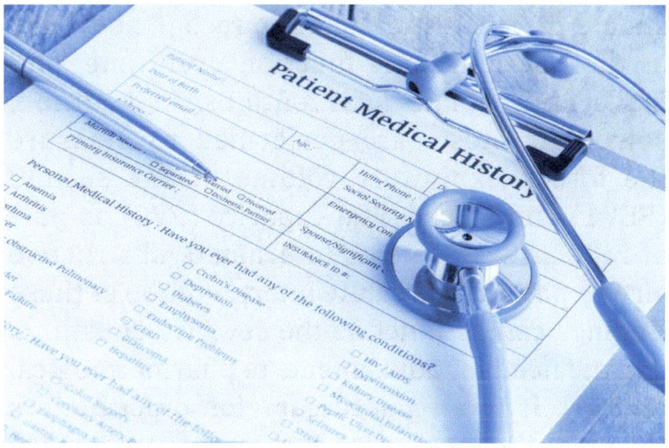

Figure 10.10. Medical history assessment.

Source: https://onlinenursingdegrees.wilkes.edu/sites/default/files/2024-05/wilkes-health-assessment-1-1200x800-compressed.jpg

10.3.2. Physical Examination

Physical examination of patients with bronchial asthma is a crucial aspect of their clinical evaluation, primarily aimed at determining the severity of the disease and identifying potential precipitating factors. During the examination, physicians typically begin by assessing the patient's effort and rate of breathing, as well as the use of accessory muscles, which may indicate increased work of breathing. Auscultation of respiratory sounds typically reveals wheezing, a characteristic sign of bronchial obstruction. The presence and intensity of wheezes can provide information about the degree of airway narrowing and can influence treatment strategies. Additionally, a review of the patient's history is also carried out, determining symptom patterns and exacerbation inducers, thereby helping in formulating a unique management plan. This integrative strategy is crucial to developing an effective strategy in managing asthma symptoms and improving the quality of life of the patients. Along with the clinical history, specific objective measurements obtained during physical examination are vital for quantifying the level of asthma control. Peak expiratory flow (PEF) readings, taken with a peak flow meter, enable the healthcare team to recognize trends in the patient's lung function over time, and make appropriate interventions. In addition, spirometry tests are performed to measure the forced expiratory volume in one second (FEV1) and forced vital capacity (FVC) as part of regular assessments to evaluate obstructive airway patterns. Accurate interpretation of these findings can help define the severity of asthma and the need for adjustments to pharmacological therapy. It is also necessary for practitioners to integrate these data into a comprehensive management plan, particularly in patients with variations in lung function. To this extent, this amount of detail enhances patient outcomes through the ability to exert control over asthma proactively. The complete physical examination also considers any underlying conditions and complications of bronchial asthma that may complicate treatment and diagnosis. For instance, conditions such as allergic rhinitis or gastroesophageal reflux disease are common comorbidities that make asthma symptoms worse and thus need to be identified during examination. Health professionals also need to consider environmental factors, such as exposure to irritants or allergens, which can be identified through the intensity of inspection, including close questioning and observation during the physical examination. This level of examination aligns with recommendations aimed at avoiding overprescription of antibiotics for conditions that can be effectively managed through proper education and intervention techniques (Bartlett et al., 2001). Understanding these interdependent factors allows for the development of a more effective and coordinated treatment plan, emphasizing patient education and self-management strategies that have the potential to lead to improvements in overall health outcomes.

10.3.3. Diagnostic Tests (e.g., Spirometry)

Accurate diagnosis of bronchial asthma is crucial for effective management and treatment, and procedures such as spirometry play a vital role in this regard. Spirometry is a test of lung function that measures the volume of air a subject can maximally inhale and then exhale forcefully. The procedure is significant in that it provides essential information about the presence of airway obstruction, a key feature of asthma. By assessing baseline values of forced expiratory volume in one second (FEV1) and forced vital capacity (FVC) through spirometry, asthma is differentiated from other respiratory diseases. Furthermore, reversibility of airway obstruction, which is determined by post-bronchodilator spirometry, is central to the diagnosis of asthma. As highlighted by studies, clinicians apply these parameters not only to diagnose asthma but also to determine the severity of the disease and monitor therapeutic response in the long term, again emphasizing the significance of spirometry in asthma management. In addition to spirometry, FeNO testing has gained popularity as a non-invasive diagnostic test for asthma. FeNO measures the amount of exhaled nitric oxide, a marker for eosinophilic airway inflammation, a condition most commonly seen in asthma patients. Its application lies in its ability to provide immediate evidence of airway inflammation, thus enabling precise treatment strategies. Research has proven that high FeNO levels can assist clinicians in modulating anti-inflammatory therapy, particularly in patients with potential asthma exacerbations, and in reducing reliance on high-dose inhaled corticosteroids when inflammation is well-controlled (Fuhlbrigge et al., 2013). This new approach complements traditional diagnostic procedures by providing additional insights into the pathophysiology of asthma, enabling a more responsive and meaningful management plan. Despite improvement in the diagnosis of asthma, misdiagnosis is a true concern that needs to be dealt with. Research indicates that a significant percentage of patients diagnosed with asthma according to clinical history may not actually have this disease on close assessment (Sumner et al., 2011). Misdiagnosis can lead to inappropriate treatment modalities, unnecessary drug costs, and possible side effects from unwarranted therapy. Implementing an organized secondary screening regimen to examine patients with asthma diagnosed by doctors accurately can offset such issues. Not only does a program like this conserve healthcare resources, but it also optimizes patient outcomes through accurate diagnosis and management. Thus, an integration of rigorous diagnostic protocols, along with continuous evaluation of their efficacy, is necessary in enhancing asthma care and avoiding the healthcare consequences of misdiagnosis.

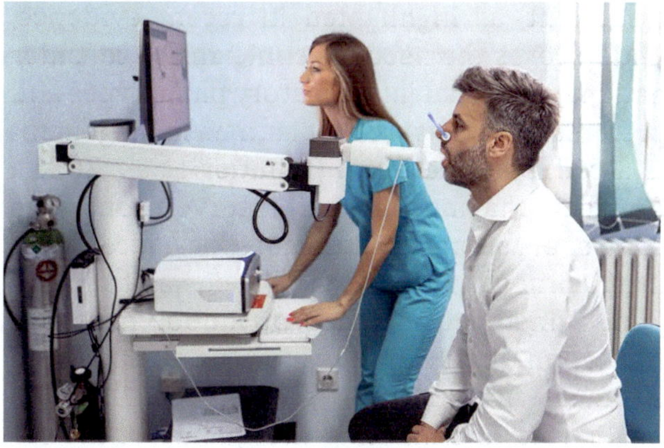

Figure 10.11. Diagnostic tests.

Source: https://img.lb.wbmdstatic.com/vim/live/webmd/consumer_assets/site_images/article_thumbnails/reference_guide/tests_that_determine_COPD_progression_ref_guide/1800x1200_tests_that_determine_COPD_progression_ref_guide.jpg?resize=750px:*&output-quality=75

Test Your Knowledge

1. What is a medical history assessment?
2. What is physical examination?

10.4. Treatment Options For Bronchial Asthma

Learning Outcome

1. Medications (e.g., inhalers)
2. Lifestyle modifications
3. Allergy management

Effective treatment of bronchial asthma requires a thorough understanding of the various treatment options, tailored to the unique needs of each patient. The 2020 Focused Updates to the Asthma Management Guidelines emphasize the importance of combining inhaled corticosteroids (ICS) with long-acting β2-agonists (LABAs) in achieving optimal asthma control, particularly in children and adolescents. These combinations not only enhance bronchodilation but also significantly reduce the frequency of exacerbations. Moreover, intermittent ICS therapy with short-acting β2-agonists (SABAs) has an effective quick-relief option that meets the immediate needs of patients when symptomatic. Emphasis on individualized treatment, as highlighted in recent evidence, underscores the need for clinicians to consider patients' personal inflammatory phenotypes and preferences to ensure that asthma management is a collaborative effort (Cloutier et al., 2021). Besides pharmacological interventions, the control of asthma involves non-pharmacological interventions. Some of the proposals from the panels included a series of indoor allergen-reduction interventions designed to reduce contact with common triggers that play a major role in enhancing the quality of life for asthmatics. These include, for instance, air filtration devices, daily cleaning routines, and the application of hypoallergenic materials within the household setting. Moreover, the role of immunotherapy, including subcutaneous (SCIT) and sublingual (SLIT) approaches, is now an extended therapeutic strategy for allergic asthmatic patients who are sensitized. The therapy can alter the intrinsic allergic process and lead to long-term improvements in asthma control. Both non-pharmacologic and pharmacologic approaches need to be used in conjunction with each other to achieve the optimal results in asthma management, ultimately meeting the unmet patient needs (Caminati et al., 2021). New treatment paradigms and new technology are providing a gateway to novel asthma management approaches. Telemedicine and e-health technologies have revolutionized patient involvement, allowing more frequent monitoring and evaluation of asthma control. These new technologies enable clinicians to assess symptoms in real-time, providing them with actionable insights to adjust treatment protocols accordingly. They also allow empowerment of patients by providing them with the education and tools needed to own their condition. Personalized medicine is also emphasized with these technologies because these instruments enable the capture of individual patient profiles, including their own unique inflammation phenotypes and treatment protocols. With the advancement of asthma treatment, it is also crucial that medical professionals stay updated on these developments so that they can provide their patients with the most effective treatment options (Caminati et al., 2021).

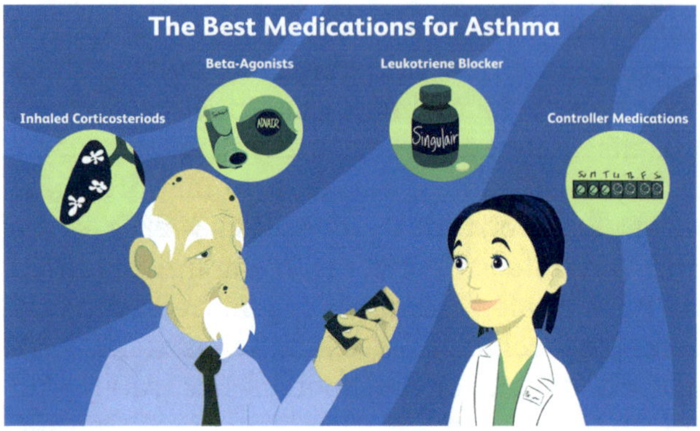

Figure 10.12. Treatment options for bronchial asthma.

Source: https://www.verywellhealth.com/thmb/V-YOtf48y6XYMCk85khY-wJVi-0=/1500x0/filters:no_upscale():max_bytes(150000):strip_icc()/what-is-the-best-medicine-for-asthma-82807_FINAL-adf48d6c4b5c4a95981e3e0201198583.png

10.4.1. Medications (e.g., Inhalers)

Medication management is the cornerstone of asthma management, involving the administration of inhalers that deliver bronchodilators and anti-inflammatory medications directly to the lungs. Inhaled corticosteroids (ICS) are the primary treatment for asthma, owing to their strong efficacy in reducing airway inflammation and preventing exacerbations. Long-acting beta-agonists (LABAs) are combined with ICS therapy to provide sustained bronchodilation, maximizing asthma control. However, many patients are not maximally controlled with ICS and LABAs, so the search for other therapies is pursued. This has led more recent guidelines to support the addition of long-acting muscarinic antagonists (LAMAs) as add-on therapy. The evidence suggests that LAMAs improve lung function and provide enhanced symptom control, particularly in those whose asthma is still poorly controlled on available treatment, thus establishing their role in a comprehensive asthma management plan (Casale et al., 2022).

The Global Initiative for Asthma (GINA) 2021 guidelines represent the ongoing evolution of asthma medication regimens, with a stepwise strategy tailored to individual patient factors. The inclusion of LAMAs in therapy reflects the need to tailor treatment regimens to meet the challenges of asthma's complex pathophysiology. Most striking is the recommendation for the use of LAMAs in addition to ICS and LABA therapy in patients aged 12 years or older. This will not only augment bronchodilation but also decrease reliance on high-dose ICS, thereby preventing the side effects associated with long-term corticosteroid use. As literature attests to the efficacy of LAMA use in improving asthma control, healthcare practitioners are increasingly mandated to consider these medications in cases where the ongoing treatment fails, promoting adherence and enhancing quality of life (Reddel et al., 2021). Moreover, the utilization of inhalers to enable dual or triple therapy enhances convenience and promotes drug adherence among patients. Single inhalers that combine ICS, LABA, and LAMA in a fixed regimen can increase patient compliance by rendering the treatment less cumbersome. These advances not only enable improved, streamlined patient care but also provide measurable benefits in reducing exacerbation frequency and asthma-related hospitalizations. Continued technological development in inhalers remains crucial in addressing the challenges faced by patients with bronchial asthma regularly. The overall aim is to achieve better asthma control and enhance patient outcomes with effective medication regimens, while curbing the health care expenditure of uncontrolled asthma (Casale et al., 2022).

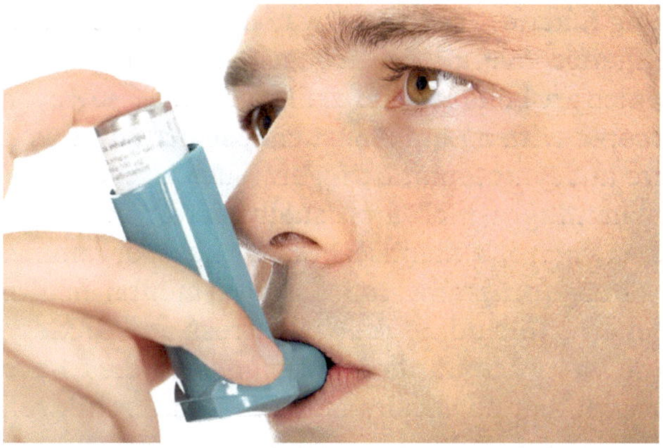

Figure 10.13. Medications for bronchial asthma.

Source: https://www.drugoffice.gov.hk/eps/do/en/images/subtitle/consumer/news_informations/dm_15/canstockphoto7949963.jpg

10.4.2. Lifestyle Modifications

Lifestyle modification forms a significant component of asthma management, offering an opportunity to reduce the severity and frequency of the disease. Perhaps above all else, dietary changes have the potential to play a significant role in reducing inflammation, a key element in asthma pathology. The incorporation of anti-inflammatory foods with high phenolic content can be added alongside standard treatment protocols. Research indicates that phenolic compounds possess protective effects against inflammation and oxidative stress, thereby warranting their consideration in the treatment of asthma. By emphasizing a balanced diet rich in fruits, vegetables, and whole grains, patients can improve their respiratory health while potentially reducing the risk of drug addiction (Md. Rahman et al., 2021). Thus, assuming a diet of nutrients is not simply an additive measure; it is part of the broader paradigm of asthma management, centered on relieving symptoms and promoting overall health. In addition to modifying one's diet, regular exercise is essential to individuals who have bronchial asthma. Engaging in moderate exercise can improve lung function, reduce airway inflammation, and enhance overall cardiovascular health, all of which are beneficial for asthma control. However, people with asthma must choose activities that are not symptomatic triggers, such as cycling or swimming, which are usually better tolerated than vigorous exercise. Furthermore, organized exercise programs can improve mental health benefits, including reduced stress and anxiety, known precipitants for asthma. Studies have shown that physically active asthmatic children are not only able to experience an improvement in their condition, but also a decrease in the frequency of hospital admissions for asthma (Dharmage et al., 2019). Thus, the inclusion of a regular exercise routine most conducive to the abilities and limitations of people is of paramount significance to enhance the quality of life and health. Lastly, environmental sensitivity and control are necessary lifestyle modifications for asthma management. Minimizing identified asthma triggers, such as pollen, dust mites, animals, and cigarette smoke, can help prevent most asthma attacks. Creating an asthma-free home environment requires practical yet easy steps, such as using air purifiers, maintaining a clean home, and reducing allergens wherever possible. Furthermore, patients should be encouraged to monitor air quality forecasts and limit outdoor activity on days with elevated pollution or pollen levels. Recognition of the patient's individual triggers will most likely empower the patient and promote active management of the disease, thereby enhancing respiratory function and reducing the total asthmatic burden significantly (Dharmage et al., 2019). In conclusion, adopting complete lifestyle modifications not only enables individuals to manage their asthma better but also promotes an active and healthier way of living.

10.4.3. Allergy Management

Effective control of allergy is a cornerstone of the holistic approach to the management of bronchial asthma, since allergic reactions have the potential to augment respiratory symptoms and increase morbidity. Pathophysiology of asthma often involves an allergic mechanism, where environmental allergens trigger inflammation and airway hyperresponsiveness. Current data highlight the crucial role of allergen-specific immunotherapy (AIT) in modulating the allergic response and enhancing disease control. Such treatment not only alleviates symptoms but also addresses the underlying causes of the disease, as attested to by recent guidelines that acknowledge the value of AIT in asthma treatment.

These recommendations focus on specialist therapies aimed at addressing the underlying allergic mechanisms, thereby reducing both the chronicity and severity of asthma exacerbations and improving the quality of life in patients affected in both clinical and community settings (Kurbacheva et al., 2025). The updated asthma therapy guidelines emphasize the importance of a standardized approach in diagnosing and managing bronchial asthma, particularly with regard to allergies. Appreciation for the heterogeneity of the clinical presentation of asthma necessitates treatment guidelines that consider the status of atopy, eosinophilic inflammation, and other factors secondary to allergens.

The efficacy of sublingual immunotherapy is emphasized explicitly in those sensitized to single allergens, such as the house dust mite. Treatment can lead to improved management of asthma and a reduced reliance on inhaled corticosteroids for symptom control. The proactive approach not only prevents acute exacerbations but may also prevent asthma worsening over time, aligning with the goals of modern asthma care, which aim to achieve long-term well-being in patients (N/A, 2025). Allergy management requires a multidimensional strategy that combines pharmacologic and non-pharmacologic therapies. Prevention of known allergens is recommended for the patients, and it is a key component of symptom control in asthmatic patients with allergy. Environmental control measures, such as the use of HEPA air purifiers and reducing indoor humidity, are effective in reducing exposure to irritants like dust mites and molds. Follow-up appointments and education are also critical in maintaining adherence to asthma management regimens. These evaluations enable adjustment in treatment plans based on the evolving status of patients and the effectiveness of allergen avoidance techniques. Ultimately, a collaborative approach involving healthcare workers, patients, and their families is required to achieve optimal management of asthma and improve long-term outcomes (Kurbacheva et al., 2025).

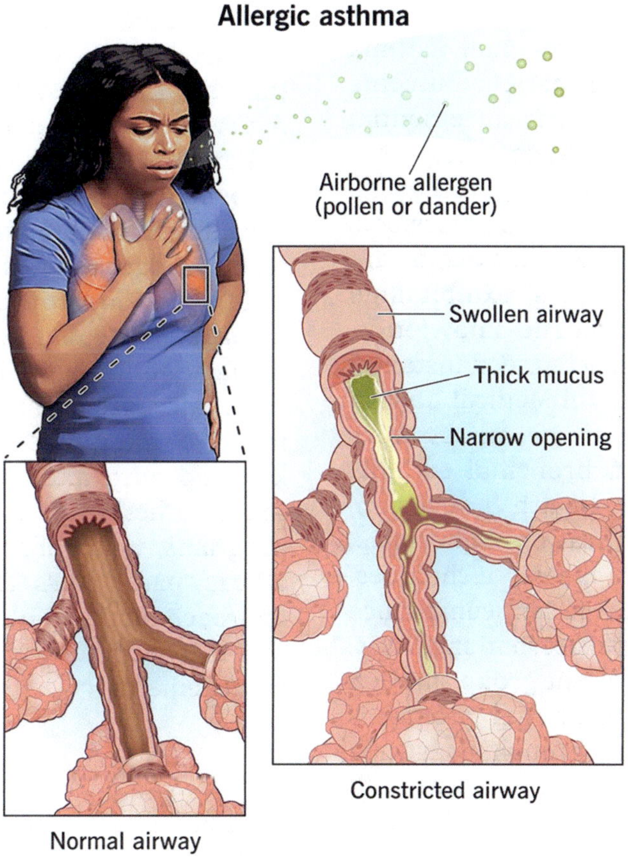

Figure 10.14. Allergic asthma.

Source: https://my.clevelandclinic.org/-/scassets/images/org/health/articles/allergic-asthma

Test Your Knowledge

1. What are the lifestyle modifications?
2. What is allergy management?

10.5. Management Strategies For Bronchial Asthma

Learning Outcome

1. Asthma action plans
2. Monitoring symptoms
3. Avoiding triggers

Adequate management of bronchial asthma is vital to achieve optimum patient outcome and quality of life. Education is an essential aspect of asthma management that helps the patient acquire information regarding his disease and adhere to treatment as prescribed. Studies have corroborated that when healthcare professionals, including nurses, exhibit high levels of asthma management knowledge, patients are positively impacted. For instance, a study conducted at Rajshahi Medical College Hospital noted that 96% of the nurses were aware of incident-related bronchial asthma. These nurses provided health education, encouraged regular medication adherence, and demonstrated correct inhaler techniques, which resulted in improved patient compliance and a reduction in asthma exacerbations. Thus, developing an educated patient group through effective nurse-based educational programs can be vital to managing bronchial asthma sustainably (Islam et al., 2024). In addition to education, pharmacologic treatment forms a second pillar in asthma management. Chronic control drugs, such as inhaled corticosteroids, reduce airway inflammation and prevent asthma attacks. Drugs are often coupled with rapid-relief inhalers for immediate relief of acute events. Nonetheless, treatment programs must be individualized by clinicians based on individual-specific asthma triggers, symptoms, and patient desires. This individualized approach can optimize the effectiveness of treatment regimens and adherence. Furthermore, home monitoring devices, such as peak flow meters, also enable patients to track their lung function, thereby facilitating early intervention by healthcare professionals and adjustments in therapy as needed. Maximized pharmacological interventions, along with ongoing surveillance, are therefore key components of successful asthma control (Islam et al., 2024). Complementary and alternative medicines are also being introduced in the management of bronchial asthma. Ayurvedic intervention, for example, has proven helpful in enhancing the quality of life in patients with this chronic illness. Research also indicates that Ayurvedic management, such as Vamana Karma, a therapy of induced vomiting with the purpose of toxin expulsion, can potentially provide more advantages in asthmatic patients. These findings would suggest that a synthesis of alternative treatments and conventional pharmacological management could bring richness to the total management regimen for bronchial asthma. With increased patients looking into other forms of therapies, health workers need to keep up with alternative methods and apply them judiciously in complete asthma care programs, while properly weighing safety and efficacy parameters. Therefore, a multi-pronged approach blending old and novel methods may prove to be the answer to improved asthma management.

10.5.1. Asthma Action Plans

Asthma action plans (AAPs) are practical tools in the effective management of bronchial asthma, particularly by enabling customized care strategies for patients. AAPs provide brief, written guidelines that inform patients and caregivers about managing asthma symptoms, indicate when to seek emergency medical services, and detail medication use. Individualized AAP implementation has been observed to enhance parental satisfaction with asthma management in children by up to 80% of parents reporting satisfaction and trust that AAPs improve their level of understanding about asthma severity and treatment (Mackle et al., 2024). These plans not only enable patients to control their asthma but also improve patient-practitioner communication, facilitating a collaborative approach to asthma management. Furthermore, empirical evidence on the efficacy of AAPs is robust, and they are shown to play a crucial role in maximizing health outcomes among patients with asthma. A randomized controlled trial revealed that asthmatic patients adhering to AAPs experienced a significant reduction in hospital and emergency department admissions due to their capacity to self-regulate early signs (Farag et al., 2018). The results indicated structured AAPs facilitated improved patient-provider communication that allowed for tailored modifications of treatment plans based on real-time patient feedback.

This visionary management not only facilitates patient empowerment but also alleviates the burden on healthcare resources, underscoring the significance of integrating AAPs into standard asthma care regimes. Apart from achieving a higher quality clinical outcome, integrating technology into AAPs may also make them more user-friendly. Most patients and caregivers prefer to utilize digital versions of asthma action plans, and a large majority report that color-coded versions would be easier to use and understand (Mackle et al., 2024). Digitalization of AAPs also offers faster access and revisions, but can utilize reminders and alerts to maintain timely medication taking and triggering avoidance behaviors. Furthermore, the inclusion of telemedicine elements in AAPs has the potential to facilitate continuous interaction with healthcare professionals, enabling constant decision-making and treatment. With changing strategies for asthma care, personalization and innovation through technology in AAPs are the keys to progressively important roles in total bronchial asthma management.

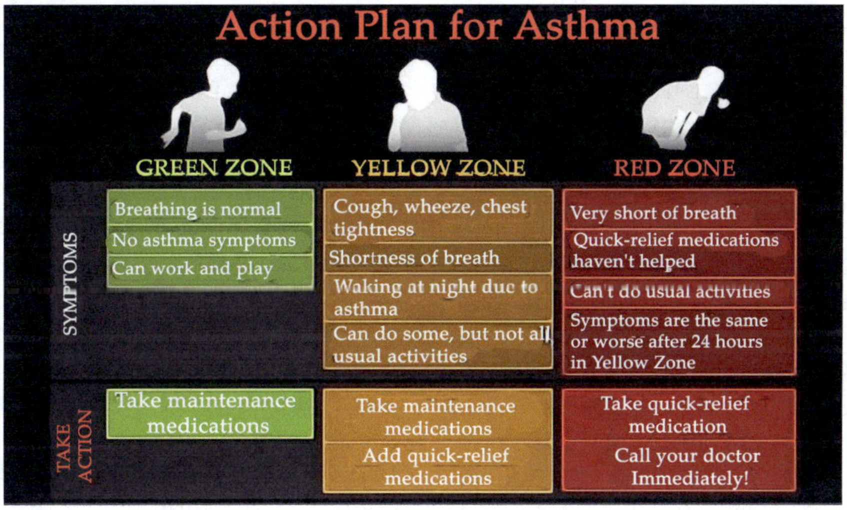

Figure 10.15. Asthma action plan.

Source: https://cdn.storymd.com/optimized/rA31y9c4dM/original.jpg

10.5.2. Monitoring Symptoms

Bronchial asthma symptom monitoring is an essential element of effective management and improvement of patient outcomes. Regular monitoring enables patients and physicians to identify the causes of exacerbations, adjust treatment approaches, and improve overall disease control. The use of telemonitoring technologies, such as the "ASTMATEST" software, represents a novel approach to symptom monitoring and adherence to medication regimens. In a study evaluating the efficacy of such an online tool, it was found that adding remote monitoring resulted in a considerable decrease in the severity of asthma in children whose parents engaged with the technology, demonstrating the potential for improved healthcare through organized symptom monitoring (Fayzullina et al., 2024). This strategy not only results in a more personalized health experience but also encourages active engagement by patients and families. Furthermore, continuous monitoring of signs and symptoms can directly influence compliance with drugs, an essential aspect of the management of bronchial asthma. Appropriate inhaler technique and adherence to therapy are pillars in achieving control of the disease. Unfortunately, inadequate inhalation technique commonly negates drug delivery, leading to ineffective control of symptoms. A clinical case characterized a child suffering from mild asthma as having a severe exacerbation by virtue of poor inhalation habits, thus highlighting the importance of proper patient education and monitoring (Ilyenkova et al., 2024). The inclusion of feedback mechanisms and training within monitoring programs enables clinicians to promote the proper use of inhalers and address potential adherence issues, ultimately leading to improved disease outcomes. With technical advances, psychological aspects of symptom tracking cannot be overlooked. Psychological states such as anxiety or stress can exacerbate asthma symptoms, and thus, mental health assistance must be incorporated with the physical tracking of the disease. By providing a comprehensive process that encompasses both symptom tracking and counseling, medical practitioners can foster patient adherence to treatment protocols. Engaging patients in the management of their health through symptom diaries, mobile applications, or web-based software like "ASTMATEST" not only empowers patients but also fosters a heightened sense of responsibility for their condition. The inclusion of symptom tracking as part of a comprehensive asthma management plan ultimately enhances patients' quality of life and reduces healthcare expenditure associated with exacerbations and emergency interventions.

10.5.3. Avoiding Triggers

Avoidance of precipitating factors is a critical management strategy in bronchial asthma because exposure to some irritants would precipitate deteriorating symptoms and increased morbidity. Asthmatic individuals develop heightened sensitivity to various allergens and irritants, such as pollen, pet dander, dust mites, and cigarette smoke. The use of effective avoidance measures not only prevents symptom development but also reduces dependence on pharmacological therapies, such as inhaled corticosteroids and bronchodilators. Such preemptive management is crucial as it enables the patient to take charge of their condition and reduces the risk of acute asthma exacerbations, which can be life-threatening. In addition, education on household trigger identification can significantly improve the asthmatic patients' and their families' quality of life, as it emphasizes the importance of creating a safe place that promotes respiratory health. Moreover, it should be understood that environmental avoidance is not only indoor but also environmental ones outside the home that can be a significant contribution in asthma control. Daily monitoring of pollen counts, air pollution levels, and weather conditions is recommended, as these factors can contribute to increased airway inflammation. Patients are advised to stay indoors during high-pollution or pollen days and wear masks if they must go outdoors. Along with this, physical exercise cannot be overlooked; while exercise is healthy for the body, it could be an inciting factor for asthmatics if not done with caution. Thus, modifying sessions for exercise to include warm-ups as well as respiratory exercises can help maintain the condition under control. By incorporating these steps, asthmatic patients can enjoy physical exercise with reduced exposure to these inciting factors, thereby allowing for a healthier lifestyle. In addition to avoiding known precipitants, patients can help create an environment that supports asthma control by having a thorough understanding of comorbid conditions that may complicate their asthma. These include allergies, gastroesophageal reflux disease, and chronic sinusitis, and these conditions, if not treated, will result in exacerbations of asthma. By managing these comorbid conditions appropriately, patients can further minimize the frequency and severity of asthmatic symptoms. Research indicates that the asthma burden, as reported in the Global Burden of Diseases, Injuries, and Risk Factors (GBD) study, underscores the importance of targeted avoidance strategies and overall management strategies (Soriano et al., 2017). On the same note, an emphasis on measures to reduce airway inflammation, coupled with avoidance of precipitants, is a holistic strategy for treatment (O'Reilly et al., 2018). Through the marriage of trigger avoidance and management of comorbidities, patients can better take charge of their asthma, leading to improved quality of life.

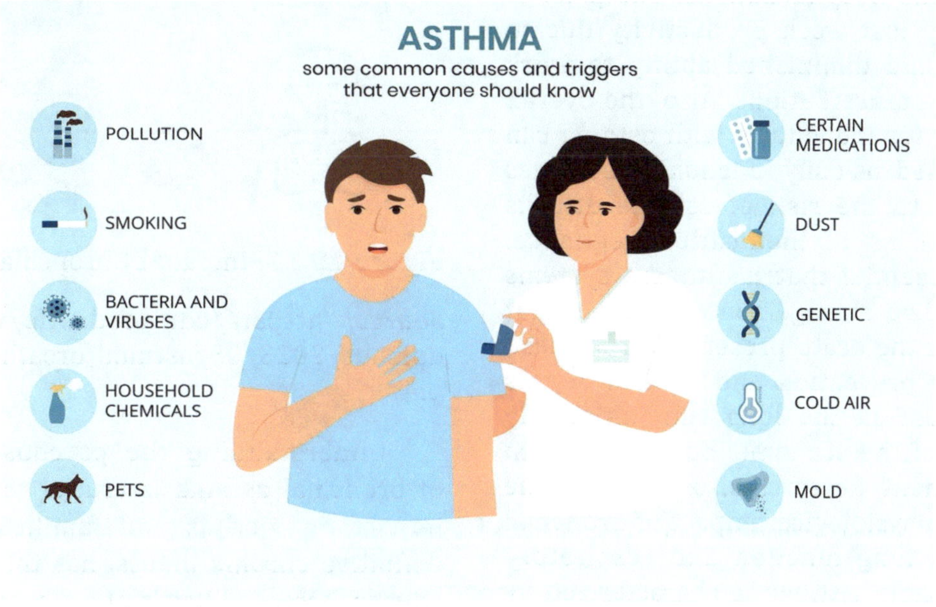

Figure 10.16. Avoiding triggers in bronchial asthma.

Source: https://www.sparshhospital.com/wp-content/uploads/2024/12/blogimg.jpg

Test Your Knowledge

1. What are the asthma action plans?
2. What are the monitoring symptoms?

10.6. Impact of Bronchial Asthma

Learning Outcome

1. Effects on daily life
2. Economic burden
3. Psychological implications

The impact of bronchial asthma extends far beyond individual well-being, as it has significant implications for healthcare systems and economies. Asthma is a common chronic disease that affects millions of individuals across the globe, bringing additional health care costs due to repeated physician visits, emergency room visits, and hospitalizations. The price is augmented by lost work productivity due to absenteeism and diminished ability to work during asthma exacerbations. Also, the overall quality of life for individuals with asthma can be compromised, as daily functioning becomes strained due to the risk of asthma attacks or the strictness of medication regimens. Thus, it is essential that healthcare systems develop effective management strategies that not only treat the acute presentation but also prioritize the prevention and control of this chronic disease in the long run, ultimately easing some of the economic burdens of such a chronic ailment. Research also highlights the considerable physiological impact of bronchial asthma upon lung function and respiratory health as a whole. Asthma is characterized by airway obstruction and inflammation, which can lead to increased symptoms such as wheezing, shortness of breath, and coughing, as well as decreased lung function. Notably, the detection of androgen receptors in bronchial tissues has been correlated with better lung function test results, suggesting that hormones and genetics might play essential roles in how individuals respond to asthma drugs and disease severity (Zein et al., 2021). Also, asthma worsening can be due to extrinsic environmental factors, i.e., air pollution, which has been correlated with higher respiratory morbidity. Particulates and other impurities may intensify the effects of asthma, leading to a cycle of inflammation and airway constriction that can profoundly impact a patient's quality of life (Manisalidis et al., 2020).

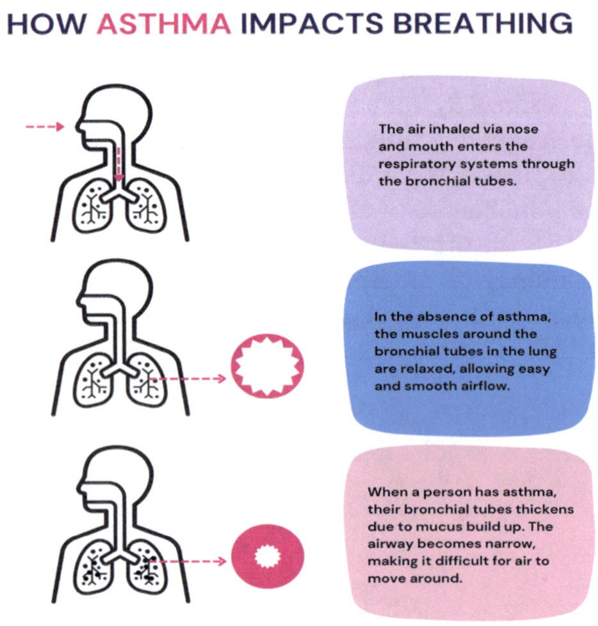

Figure 10.17. Impact of bronchial asthma.

Source: https://cdn.xcode.life/wp-content/uploads/2023/05/asthma_breathing_genetics.png

Understanding the psychosocial effects of bronchial asthma is crucial to knowing its impact on victims and families. Asthma, a definitive chronic illness, has the potential to trigger increased levels of concern and anxiety, influencing one's emotional health. Families may struggle with all aspects, from titrating medication regimens to accommodating lifestyle changes to minimize triggers. Children with asthma, especially, may be stigmatized socially or have limits placed on physical activities that predispose to social isolation and frustration. Therefore, well-functioning support and educational systems are necessary to enhance patients' and their families' resilience. Educating patients with information about asthma management and involving families in treatment can potentially enhance medication adherence, improve self-efficacy, and ultimately improve quality of life among those who are battling the disease.

10.6.1. Effects On Daily Life

The daily living of asthma patients is significantly impacted by the conditions, symptoms, and restrictions, which could hinder various aspects of their daily routine. Asthma exacerbations can lead to disruption of daily activities like work, school, and recreation. Children particularly can suffer from their involvement in sports being restricted due to exercise-induced bronchoconstriction (EIB), a common phenomenon in asthmatics. This limitation affects not only their physical growth but also causes social isolation, as they are missing out on sports and playing with friends. Also, the psychological impact of these restrictions, such as anxiety and frustration, further contributes to the effects of asthma on daily functioning. With an understanding of the multifaceted problems in asthma management, physicians are capable of administering targeted interventions that enhance patients' quality of life and mitigate the disease's adverse effects (Vera S Hengeveld et al., 2022). Apart from physical limitations, managing bronchial asthma also requires relentless vigilance that can consume a significant amount of time and effort. Patients are required to continually monitor their symptoms, adhere to their treatment regimen, and identify triggers to prevent flare-ups. Ongoing need to be vigilant can leave a patient with a sense of persistent stress, particularly caregivers for pediatric asthma patients. Moreover, the financial burden of medication, such as the potential utilization of rescue inhalers and long-term upkeep therapies, can strain family finances. The economic implications of asthma management are substantial, affecting lifestyle and, in some cases, even leading households to make difficult decisions about prioritizing healthcare. Effective management of asthma, therefore, is not just about pharmacological management, but also about the importance of patient and family education and support to effectively address these matters (Pelaia et al., 2018). New avenues of treatment, such as omalizumab, have introduced new hope to the severely allergic asthmatic by significantly improving their quality of life. In its effect on IgE, omalizumab prevents symptoms and exacerbations, saving patients' visits to the emergency room and hospitalization. These positive effects not only enhance patients' physical well-being but also reduce apprehension regarding future asthma attacks. Consequently, the patients can be more active without the background anxiety of nasty attacks. The psychological benefits of improved asthma control are realized, with patients reporting an improved quality of life and regaining confidence in participating in social events and sports. Therefore, the emergence of targeted biological therapy represents a considerable stride in the treatment of asthma, as it enables individuals to lead their day-to-day lives with a significantly reduced impact from their illness (Pelaia et al., 2018).

10.6.2. Economic Burden

The financial burden of bronchial asthma extends beyond immediate medical costs, encompassing a broad spectrum of indirect expenses that affect individuals and the healthcare system. Those who have severe asthma are particularly vulnerable, with multiple exacerbations that often lead to hospitalization and extended medical management. Not only does this strain healthcare resources, but it also imposes significant financial charges on hospitals and payers. The economic impact is even greater when one factors in missed days from work, decreased productivity, and emotional distress on patients and their families. To overcome these obstacles, there must be a multifaceted plan, which might involve augmenting access to preventative treatment and instituting comprehensive health education campaigns to help manage asthma better. This can ultimately reduce the frequency of severe exacerbations and associated economic costs on patients and the health system as well (Benlala et al., 2025).

When assessing the economic cost of bronchial asthma, it is also important to consider the role of biomarkers and non-invasive tests, including T2-weighted (T2w) magnetic resonance imaging (MRI). Modern imaging techniques can transform the management of asthma by being able to differentiate between severe and non-severe asthma, and thus, more targeted treatments may be implemented. Quantification of bronchial wall signals in patients with severe asthma can enhance clinical decision-making, leading to the most effective utilization of resources and improved cost-effectiveness in healthcare systems. Additionally, the inclusion of such technologies has the potential to make the observation of asthma exacerbations and reactions to medications more accurate, thereby reducing unnecessary hospitalizations and their associated financial burden. Because healthcare systems aim to reduce costs, these technologies can prove instrumental in addressing the financial burden posed by severe asthma (Benlala et al., 2025). In addition, the economic burden of bronchial asthma extends beyond the cost of healthcare; it has broader implications at the societal level. The consequences of asthma have far-reaching implications that extend to other sectors, such as education and the labor market. Asthma-stricken children and adults suffer from limited physical activity, recurrent school absenteeism, and impaired performance at work due to acute exacerbations. These interruptions not only affect the quality of life of those concerned but also contribute to the overall economic loss incurred by communities and reduced employer productivity. To counter these effects, an entire understanding of asthma's societal consequences is needed, along with a commitment to implementing effective interventions, for instance, public health measures focusing on environmental controls and education. These measures can alleviate the burden of asthma and thereby reduce the economic burden on individuals and society as a whole.

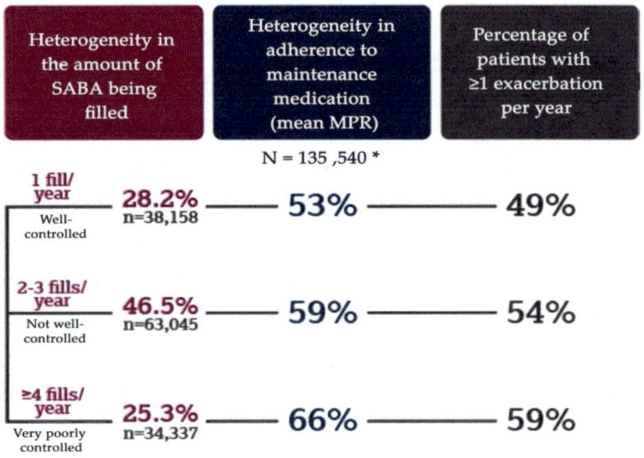

Figure 10.18. The economic burden of bronchial asthma.

Source: https://www.airsuprapayer.com/content/dam/intelligentcontent/brands/airsupra-payer/us/en/images/mobile/phase-two/burden-of-asthma/asthma-patient-chart.png

10.6.3. Psychological Implications

The psychological effects of bronchial asthma well exceed the physical symptoms of the condition. Patients with asthma are more anxious and stressed than individuals with other illnesses, mainly because of the unpredictable nature of asthma attacks. The vigilance required at all times to manage one's condition gives rise to a prevailing sense of anxiety that has negative repercussions on one's overall mental health. Moreover, social interactions can be overwhelming; individuals fear the onset of an attack when they are out in public, and they will avoid parties or interactions that could trigger their anxiety. With time, this can lead to long-term psychological consequences in the form of depression or loss of self-worth, hence impacting the quality of life profoundly. The interplay between these psychosocial factors and asthma underscores the importance of mental health to be addressed along with physical symptoms in patient treatment plans, as this could potentially raise overall well-being and coping mechanisms. Caregiver burden is also an consideration of the psychological burden of bronchial asthma, particularly among asthmatic parents. Parents will also experience a significant amount of stress since they have to constantly monitor their child's condition and intervene beforehand to avoid likely triggers. The psychological effect can be far-reaching, with symptoms that resemble caregiver burnout, such as chronic fatigue, anxiety, and helplessness. Studies show that the burden placed on parents can make them lose their mental health, hindering their ability to provide the needed care to their children. Parental stress can even increase further that parents are convinced that their child's asthma can't be managed by them, a development which can drain family life. Therefore, education and prevention of caregiver burden are significant, as it can promote parental health along with the development of a more conducive environment for the asthmatic child (Mathiazhakan et al., 2023). In addition to the direct effects of asthma upon patients and caregivers, there are broader societal psychological impacts which require attention. Stigmatization of conditions like bronchial asthma can render the patient isolated or stigmatized. Alienation is compounded if the attack occurs in public settings, and the individual is embarrassed and exposed. Adolescents, in particular, may find it difficult to accept because they feel compelled to conform to peer norms while dealing with the condition. The long-term consequences of such social stigmata can be varied, like greater anxiety and reluctance to engage in physical exercise, which can trigger a bronchial asthma attack. Therefore, mental health professionals need to encourage social awareness and support groups that can foster understanding and promote acceptance of individuals with bronchial asthma, ultimately creating a more empathetic society (Pitcho-Prelorentzos et al., 2021).

Test Your Knowledge

1. What are the effects of bronchial asthma on daily life?
2. What are the psychological implications of bronchial asthma?

SUMMARY

The polyfacial nature of bronchial asthma also highlights its complexity as a public health issue. As has come to light through many studies, asthma has far-reaching implications for people of all ages, particularly with the explosion of global prevalence. Even though asthma in children is seen more in boys, in adults, the trend is reversed, which suggests that the effects of hormones can play an essential role in disease manifestation and development (Dharmage et al., 2019). This gender disparity in asthma incidence highlights the necessity for personalized management regimens that account for developmental and hormonal factors. Furthermore, it is essential to recognize the role of environmental and genetic factors in influencing asthma. Investigating the interplay between these factors may illuminate the path to more promising prevention and treatment regimens, ultimately leading to better outcomes. Lastly, asthma is not confined to its impact on respiratory function alone; its effects extend to quality of life and overall health. Chronic asthma control requires a comprehensive approach focused on both the immediate control of symptoms and the long-term protection of lung health. It has been demonstrated that asthma that remains undiagnosed or poorly controlled can lead to significant morbidity, including impaired lung growth during childhood and accelerated loss of lung function in adults (Dharmage et al., 2019). Therefore, proactive interventions must be installed, which look not only after acute attacks but also at the long-term paths of asthma diseases. Improved education and awareness of variability in asthma experiences among patients can facilitate the implementation of a more individualized treatment strategy, resulting in improved compliance and outcomes. Ultimately, collaboration among healthcare providers, patients, and researchers will improve the management of bronchial asthma. Interdisciplinary collaboration can foster innovative treatment techniques, for example, novel pharmacologic agents based on existing evidence-based practice recommendations. Uniform care techniques and the inclusion of patient experience in studies enable the medical community to enhance the quality of care and outcomes for those who must live with asthma. Further investigations into the contribution of environmental exposures and vigilant observation of disease phenotypes and endotypes can refine asthma management. As the prevalence of bronchial asthma continues to grow, a collaborative response will be the key to effective and sustainable management of this chronic disease.

In trying to understand the multiplicity of bronchial asthma, one can that it is essential that it be considered in a multidisciplinary framework in order to grasp its multifaceted character. The new guidelines reflect the recent advances in the identification and classification of asthma phenotypes and endotypes, and asthma is not a monolithic disease but a heterogeneous group of disorders with different precipitating factors and drug responses. For instance, chronic cough has been linked to cough variant asthma (CVA) and eosinophilic bronchitis, where anti-inflammatory treatment is effective. Awareness of the varying presentations and sensitivities, such as cough hypersensitivity, allows practitioners to tailor their management strategies more effectively. Secondarily, research on personal responses to neuromodulation and low-dose opioid administration for chronic cough precedes the new treatments being studied in asthma management paradigms, which align with the need for ongoing investigation in personalized therapeutic interventions (Morice et al., 2019).

Asthma epidemiology reveals significant variability across groups, underscoring the importance of targeted public health interventions. Children have a higher rate of asthma incidence compared to adults; however, morbidity and mortality rates caused by the disease are largely more severe in adults. Surprisingly, there is a significant gender difference wherein child asthma occurs more frequently in males, whereas asthma among adults has a high increase among females. This shift may suggest the involvement of sex hormones in the pathogenesis and expression of the disease across different life stages. Through an in-depth analysis of such patterns, experts can inform measures to limit asthma's rising global burden, particularly in low- to middle-income countries, where the condition continues to increase (Dharmage et al., 2019). Apart from ascertaining demographic variation, investigating environmental determinants is crucial to understanding why asthma disparities persist. By establishing associations between environmental exposures, such as allergens and pollutants, and the exacerbation of asthma symptoms, preventive measures could be developed. Additionally, ongoing investigations into gene-by-environment interactions have the potential to unravel the complex interactions that underlie the etiology of asthma. All these studies must be conducted, particularly for kids whose development of the airway can be compromised by chronic asthma, with chronic losses in pulmonary function. It is therefore essential to address both short-term alleviation of symptoms and long-term health results to improve the overall prognosis of patients with bronchial asthma (Dharmage et al., 2019).

KEY TERMS FROM THIS CHAPTER

- Airway hyperresponsiveness
- Inflammation
- IgE-mediated hypersensitivity
- Eosinophils
- Cytokines
- Dyspnea
- Cough
- Spirometry
- Bronchodilators
- Status asthmaticus
- Bronchoconstriction
- Mucus hypersecretion
- Allergens
- Mast cells
- Wheezing
- Chest tightness
- Peak expiratory flow rate (PEFR)
- Reversible airway obstruction
- Inhaled corticosteroids
- Asthma trigger

CRITICAL THINKING QUESTIONS

1. **Which of the following is the primary pathophysiological feature of bronchial asthma?**
   a. Alveolar destruction
   b. Airway inflammation and hyperresponsiveness
   c. Pulmonary fibrosis
   d. Pulmonary edema
2. **Which type of hypersensitivity reaction is most commonly involved in allergic asthma?**
   a. Type I (IgE-mediated)
   b. Type II (cytotoxic)
   c. Type III (immune complex)
   d. Type IV (delayed)
3. **What is the typical finding in spirometry during an asthma attack?**
   a. Increased FEV_1/FVC ratio
   b. Decreased FEV_1 and reduced FEV_1/FVC ratio
   c. Normal FEV_1/FVC ratio
   d. Increased residual volume only
4. **Which of the following drugs is a short-acting beta-2 agonist used as a rescue medication in asthma?**
   a. Salmeterol
   b. Formoterol
   c. Albuterol (Salbutamol)
   d. Ipratropium
5. **Which inflammatory cells are primarily involved in the pathogenesis of asthma?**
   a. Neutrophils
   b. Eosinophils
   c. Basophils
   d. Macrophages

Short Answer Questions

1. What is the pathophysiological hallmark of bronchial asthma?
2. Name two common triggers that can precipitate an asthma attack.
3. What type of hypersensitivity reaction is typically involved in allergic asthma?
4. Which cells play a key role in the inflammation seen in asthma?
5. What are the characteristic findings on pulmonary function tests (PFTs) in asthma?

Answer to Critical Thinking Questions

1. (b) 2. (a) 3. (b) 4. (c) 5. (b)

REFERENCES

1. Alzahrani, S. J. M., Alzahrani, H. a. K., Alghamdi, S. M. M., & Alzahrani, A. N. A. (2024). Health-Related quality of life of asthmatic patients in Al-Baha City, Saudi Arabia. *Cureus.* https://doi.org/10.7759/cureus.53601Axon, E. J., Balmes, J. R., Frew, A., Gannon, P. F., Gannon, P. F. G., Balmes, J. R., Jajosky, R. A., et al. (2000). Occupational asthma: A review. https://core.ac.uk/download/323081929.pdf (accessed on 16th June 2025).
2. Bartlett, J. G., Besser, R. E., Centers for Disease Control and Prevention, Cooper, R. J., et al. (2001). Principles of appropriate antibiotic use for treatment of uncomplicated acute bronchitis: Background. https://core.ac.uk/download/323078929.pdf (accessed on 16th June 2025).
3. Benlala, I., Dournes, G., Girodet, P., Laurent, F., Ben Hassen, W., Baldacci, F., de Senneville, B. D., et al. (2025). Bronchial wall T2w MRI signal as a new imaging biomarker of severe asthma. *Insights into Imaging, 16.* https://www.semanticscholar.org/paper/7942f7bc06af69c6600d93fa40e5d14255f2eb34 (accessed on 16th June 2025).
4. Bhat, K. R., Banu, W., & Krishnan, P. (2025). A single case study on Ayurvedic approach to Thamaka Shwasa (bronchial asthma). *International Journal for Multidisciplinary Research.* https://www.semanticscholar.org/paper/2909b56867a52d4cba7b31d834a528df67e6ca21 (accessed on 16th June 2025).
5. Boda, S., Badipatla, V. N., Divya, E. N., Dutta, P., & Ganduboina, R. (2024). Navigating the complexity of Churg-Strauss syndrome presenting as acute abdomen: A comprehensive review and case report. *Annals of Medicine and Surgery, 86*, 2200–2203. https://www.semanticscholar.org/paper/553a4caaf4251194b07e84022355edd4497ef320 (accessed on 16th June 2025).
6. Caminati, M., Vaia, R., Furci, F., Guarnieri, G., & Senna, G. (2021). Uncontrolled asthma: Unmet needs in the management of patients. *Journal of Asthma and Allergy, 14*, 457–466. https://doi.org/10.2147/jaa.s260604 (accessed on 16th June 2025).
7. Casale, T. B., Foggs, M. B., & Balkissoon, R. (2022). Optimizing asthma management: Role of long-acting muscarinic antagonists. *Journal of Allergy and Clinical Immunology, 150*, 557–568. https://doi.org/10.1016/j.jaci.2022.06.015 (accessed on 16th June 2025).
8. Cloutier, M. M., Dixon, A. E., Krishnan, J. A., Lemanske, R. F., Pace, W., & Schätz, M. (2020). Managing asthma in adolescents and adults. *JAMA, 324*, 2301. https://doi.org/10.1001/jama.2020.21974 (accessed on 16th June 2025).
9. Cloutier, M. M., Teach, S. J., Lemanske, R. F., & Blake, K. (2021). The 2020 focused updates to the NIH asthma management guidelines: Key points for pediatricians. *Pediatrics, 147.* https://doi.org/10.1542/peds.2021-050286 (accessed on 16th June 2025).
10. Crimi, C., Ferri, S., Campisi, R., & Crimi, N. (2020). The link between asthma and bronchiectasis: State of the art. *Respiration, 99*, 463–476. https://doi.org/10.1159/000507228 (accessed on 16th June 2025).
11. Dharmage, S. C., Perret, J. L., & Ćustović, A. (2019). Epidemiology of asthma in children and adults. *Frontiers in Pediatrics, 7.* https://doi.org/10.3389/fped.2019.00246 (accessed on 16th June 2025).
12. Farag, H., Abd El-Wahab, E. A., El-Nimr, N., & Saad El-Din, H. A. (2018). Asthma action plan for proactive bronchial asthma self-management in adults: A randomized controlled trial.

International Health, 10(6), 502–516. https://www.semanticscholar.org/paper/793315eab9183854f1128b48e5ba657bdeb46bc1 (accessed on 16th June 2025).

13. Fayzullina, R. M., Gafurova, R., & Bogomolova, E. A. (2024). Remote monitoring of the course of bronchial asthma in children. *Clinical Medicine (Russian Journal).* https://www.semanticscholar.org/paper/d9fc7b823f3ae607f3d33b95cad79d6b68046fcd (accessed on 16th June 2025).
14. Fuhlbrigge, A., Zacharasiewicz, A., Smith, A. D., Smith, A. D., Smith, A. D., Gelb, A. F., American Thoracic Society / European Respiratory Society, et al. (2013). Using fractional exhaled nitric oxide (FeNO) to diagnose steroid-responsive disease and guide asthma management in routine care. https://core.ac.uk/download/25497481.pdf (accessed on 16th June 2025).
15. Gabryelska, A., Szmyd, B., Panek, M., Szemraj, J., Kuna, P., & Białasiewicz, P. (2019). Serum hypoxia-inducible factor-1α protein level as a diagnostic marker of obstructive sleep apnea. *Polskie Archiwum Medycyny Wewnętrznej.* https://doi.org/10.20452/pamw.15104 (accessed on 16th June 2025).
16. Grandinetti, R., Mussi, N., Rossi, A., Zambelli, G., Masetti, M., Giudice, A., Pilloni, S., et al. (2024). Exercise-induced bronchoconstriction in children: State of the art from diagnosis to treatment. *Journal of Clinical Medicine, 13.* https://www.semanticscholar.org/paper/ebc7720b73e24e125bef36e82e15d8f0c062a9af (accessed on 16th June 2025).
17. Hengeveld, V. S., Keijzer, P., Diamant, Z., & Thio, B. (2022). An algorithm for strategic continuation or restriction of asthma medication prior to exercise challenge testing in childhood exercise induced bronchoconstriction. *Frontiers in Pediatrics, 10.* https://www.semanticscholar.org/paper/f8113e9e38174518994e7b2e356c8a8fbdec48e8 (accessed on 16th June 2025).
18. Hough, K. P., Curtiss, M. L., Blain, T. J., Liu, R. M., Trevor, J., Deshane, J. S., & Thannickal, V. J. (2020). Airway remodeling in asthma. *Frontiers in Medicine, 7.* https://doi.org/10.3389/fmed.2020.00191 (accessed on 16th June 2025).
19. Huang, J., Li, C., Liu, Y., Li, E., & Lei, M. (2024). Bibliometric analysis of traditional Chinese medicine in the treatment of asthma from 2005 to 2024. *Journal of Clinical Medicine Research.* https://www.semanticscholar.org/paper/18e34fe9752f0653c8c086d81fd0679a5473fee4 (accessed on 16th June 2025).
20. Hufnagl, K., Pali-Schöll, I., Roth-Walter, F., & Jensen-Jarolim, E. (2020). Dysbiosis of the gut and lung microbiome has a role in asthma. *Seminars in Immunopathology, 42*, 75–93. https://doi.org/10.1007/s00281-019-00775-y (accessed on 16th June 2025).
21. Huuskonen, P., Porras, S. P., Scholten, B., Portengen, L., Uuksulainen, S., Ylinen, K., & Santonen, T. (2023). Occupational exposure and health impact assessment of diisocyanatos in Finland. *Toxics, 11.* https://www.semanticscholar.org/paper/ca5c6b2292d60aea02747ea0cac1e3bd84bc3f72 (accessed on 16th June 2025).
22. Ilyenkova, N. A., Sergienko, D., Stepanova, L. V., Pastukhova, S. Y., & Dvoryanskaya, S. S. (2024). Asthmatic status in pediatric practice in patients with mild bronchial asthma. *Astrakhan Medical Journal.* https://www.semanticscholar.org/paper/2e902d2c5efb0d65a40e538033ff88ff194154d1 (accessed on 16th June 2025).
23. Islam, M., Akter, L., Rana, S., Suborna, S., Khatun, S., & Islam, T. (2024). Nurses' knowledge on management of bronchial asthma disease at Rajshahi Medical College Hospital. *Middle East Research Journal of Nursing.* https://www.semanticscholar.org/paper/d3a4f0ebde61fcf9dfcf2435a828d08efb2863dd (accessed on 16th June 2025).

24. Jartti, T., & Gern, J. E. (2017). Role of viral infections in the development and exacerbation of asthma in children. *Journal of Allergy and Clinical Immunology, 140*, 895–906. https://doi.org/10.1016/j.jaci.2017.08.003 (accessed on 16th June 2025).

25. Jin, Y., Cai, L., Cheng, Z., Cheng, H., Deng, T., Fan, Y., Fang, C., et al. (2020). A rapid advice guideline for the diagnosis and treatment of 2019 novel coronavirus (2019-nCoV) infected pneumonia (standard version). *Military Medical Research, 7*. https://doi.org/10.1186/s40779-020-0233-6 (accessed on 16th June 2025).

26. Kozhyna, O. S., & Pihnastyi, O. M. (2019). On determining the volume of repeated and non-repeated sampling in the preparation of clinical studies. https://core.ac.uk/download/187298459.pdf (accessed on 16th June 2025).

27. Kurbacheva, O., Ilyina, N., Namazova-Baranova, L. S., Nenasheva, N., Fedenko, E., & Kleiner, D. (2025). Current aspects of the use of allergen-specific immunotherapy in patients with bronchial asthma: Review of GINA 2024 updates and results of the EfficAPSI study. *Russian Journal of Allergy*. https://www.semanticscholar.org/paper/ef039e886a3053992ed224d6da8b3eabb58f87e8 (accessed on 16th June 2025).

28. Lahmann, C., Loew, T., Nickel, M., & Noll-Hussong, M., et al. (2009). Functional relaxation and guided imagery as complementary therapy in asthma: A randomized controlled clinical trial. https://core.ac.uk/download/16432267.pdf (accessed on 16th June 2025).

29. Lu, L., Zhang, J., Xie, Y., Gao, F., Xu, S., Wu, X., & Ye, Z. (2020). Wearable health devices in health care: Narrative systematic review. *JMIR mHealth and uHealth, 8*, e18907. https://doi.org/10.2196/18907 (accessed on 16th June 2025).

30. Mackle, R., Chan, M., Lay, M., Purcell, M., Campbell, N., Jaffé, A., Owens, L., et al. (2024). Parental perceptions and knowledge toward asthma action plans. *Journal of Asthma, 62*, 435–444. https://www.semanticscholar.org/paper/cab3a06cec8143fdbc616b88b460c26e78ef69f2 (accessed on 16th June 2025).

31. Manisalidis, I., Stavropoulou, E., Stavropoulos, A., & Bezirtzoglou, E. (2020). Environmental and health impacts of air pollution: A review. *Frontiers in Public Health, 8*. https://doi.org/10.3389/fpubh.2020.00014 (accessed on 16th June 2025).

32. Mathiazhakan, U., & Abirami, P. (2023). Impact of caregiver's burden of children with asthma: A systematic review. *International Journal of Nutrition, Pharmacology, Neurological Diseases, 13*, 89–95. https://www.semanticscholar.org/paper/7548ea0b5c5fdf18c6474e21b825b545e5834c21 (accessed on 16th June 2025).

33. Morice, A. H., Millqvist, E., Biekšienė, K., Birring, S. S., Dicpinigaitis, P. V., Domingo, C., Hilton Boon, M., et al. (2019). ERS guidelines on the diagnosis and treatment of chronic cough in adults and children. *European Respiratory Journal, 55*, 1901136. https://doi.org/10.1183/13993003.01136-2019 (accessed on 16th June 2025).

34. O'Reilly, A., & Lane, S. J. (2018). What is the role of bronchial thermoplasty in the management of severe asthma? *Therapeutic Advances in Respiratory Disease, 12*. https://doi.org/10.1177/1753466618792410 (accessed on 16th June 2025).

35. Parwe, S., Nisargandha, M., Wanjari, A., & Nakade, M. (2024). The management of bronchial asthma (Tamak Shwasa) through Panchakarma procedure with Ishvaku (*Lagenaria siceraria*) Vamana: A case report. *Journal of Pharmacology and Pharmacotherapeutics, 15*, 355–361.

https://www.semanticscholar.org/paper/2092dc6e1318bc9b904474fd0c77b7b1108fcf4c (accessed on 16th June 2025).

36. Pelaia, C., Calabrese, C., Terracciano, R., De Blasio, F., Vatrella, A., & Pelaia, G. (2018). Omalizumab, the first available antibody for biological treatment of severe asthma: More than a decade of real-life effectiveness. *Therapeutic Advances in Respiratory Disease, 12*. https://www.semanticscholar.org/paper/d5e7c851f89d5a90a5c12863b3acc5361c0bb9fa (accessed on 16th June 2025).

37. Pitcho-Prelorentzos, S., Leshem, E., & Mahat-Shamir, M. (2021). Shattered voices: Daughters' meaning reconstruction in loss of a mother to intimate partner homicide. *Journal of Interpersonal Violence, 37*, NP15800–NP15825. https://www.semanticscholar.org/paper/3a4f335db5887c474a3866b57107f5ebea4eba17 (accessed on 16th June 2025).

38. Polverino, E., Goeminne, P., McDonnell, M. J., Aliberti, S., Marshall, S. E., Loebinger, M. R., Murris, M., et al. (2017). European Respiratory Society guidelines for the management of adult bronchiectasis. *European Respiratory Journal, 50*, 1700629. https://doi.org/10.1183/13993003.00629-2017 (accessed on 16th June 2025).

39. Ptak, A., & Szyc, M. (2024). Impact of swimming training on the course and symptoms of bronchial asthma and respiratory system function: A literature review. *Quality in Sport*. https://www.semanticscholar.org/paper/d15b596c623f587f04cb1be7da47cba8fb2787af (accessed on 16th June 2025).

40. Rahman, M. M., Rahaman, M. S., Islam, M. R., Rahman, F., Mithi, F. M., Alqahtani, T., Almikhlafi, M. A., et al. (2021). Role of phenolic compounds in human disease: Current knowledge and future prospects. *Molecules, 27*, 233. https://doi.org/10.3390/molecules27010233 (accessed on 16th June 2025).

41. Reddel, H. K., Bacharier, L. B., Bateman, E. D., Brightling, C. E., Brusselle, G., Buhl, R., Cruz, Á. A., et al. (2021). Global Initiative for Asthma Strategy 2021: Executive summary and rationale for key changes. *European Respiratory Journal, 59*, 2102730. https://doi.org/10.1183/13993003.02730-2021 (accessed on 16th June 2025).

42. Saito, A., Horie, M., & Nagase, T. (2018). TGF-β signaling in lung health and disease. *International Journal of Molecular Sciences, 19*, 2460. https://doi.org/10.3390/ijms19082460 (accessed on 16th June 2025).

43. Shur, P., Redko, S., Fadeev, A. G., Goryaev, D. V., & Fokin, V. (2023). Assessment of working conditions and health conditions of employees of non-ferrous metallurgy enterprises. *Russian Journal of Occupational Health and Industrial Ecology*. https://www.semanticscholar.org/paper/a58f0e50b99256b5db4e0942a6bd02380d210f93 (accessed on 16th June 2025).

44. Soriano, J. B., Abajobir, A. A., Abate, K. H., Abera, S. F., Agrawal, A., Ahmed, M. B., Aichour, A. N., et al. (2017). Global, regional, and national deaths, prevalence, disability-adjusted life years, and years lived with disability for chronic obstructive pulmonary disease and asthma, 1990–2015: A systematic analysis for the Global Burden of Disease Study 2015. *The Lancet Respiratory Medicine, 5*, 691–706. https://doi.org/10.1016/s2213-2600(17)30293-x (accessed on 16th June 2025).

45. Starshinova, A., Borozinets, A. A., Kulpina, A., Sereda, V., Rubinstein, A., Kudryavtsev, I., & Kudlay, D. (2024). Bronchial asthma and COVID-19: Etiology, pathological triggers, and therapeutic considerations. *Pathophysiology, 31*, 269–287. https://www.semanticscholar.org/paper/6fdb536a67ff50fc78c75154c3014099f167b8b5 (accessed on 16th June 2025).

46. Sumner, A., Awadh, B. N., Coyle, D., Sharpe, H. M., Bahadori, K., Vandemheen, K., Weiss, K. B., et al. (2011). (Correcting) misdiagnoses of asthma: A cost effectiveness analysis. https://core.ac.uk/download/29140469.pdf (accessed on 16th June 2025).

47. Theofilou, P., & Vlastos, D. D. (2023). Investigating the quality-of-life level in children with bronchial asthma: An updated systematic review of the literature. *Nursing Communications.* https://www.semanticscholar.org/paper/5ef7258228ac73a1cb7148522a2b110e2b2cdf3f (accessed on 16th June 2025).

48. Topçu, A., Løkke, A., Eriksen, L., Nielsen, L., & Dahl, R. (2020). Evaluating the effect on asthma quality of life of added reflexology or homeopathy to conventional asthma management – an investigator-blinded, randomized, controlled parallel group study. *European Clinical Respiratory Journal, 7.* https://www.semanticscholar.org/paper/dc18a2466766eb93be30067cd2e8423c9126d5c2 (accessed on 16th June 2025).

49. Yadav, A., Gupta, S., Chhabra, K., Chaurasiya, O., & Shastri, M. (2022). Efficacy of inhaled salbutamol therapy through nebulizer versus MDI with spacer in children with acute asthmatic attack and short-term course. *Indian Journal of Child Health.* https://www.semanticscholar.org/paper/1e750ac300f1a2b5e065bb766eadd15eff6ead43 (accessed on 16th June 2025).

50. Zein, J., McManus, J. M., Sharifi, N., Erzurum, S. C., Marozkina, N., Lahm, T., Giddings, O., et al. (2021). Benefits of airway androgen receptor expression in human asthma. *American Journal of Respiratory and Critical Care Medicine, 204*, 285–293. https://doi.org/10.1164/rccm.202009-3720oc (accessed on 16th June 2025).

51. Головко, В. А., Тепляков, А. А., & Мещеряков, В. В. (2024). Analysis of clinical and functional features of bronchial asthma in children of early and preschool age. *Vestnik SurGU. Meditsina.* https://www.semanticscholar.org/paper/43b722d3ddb26ced7251d289116d98a09fd0012e (accessed on 16th June 2025).

CHRONIC OBSTRUCTIVE PULMONARY DISEASES

11

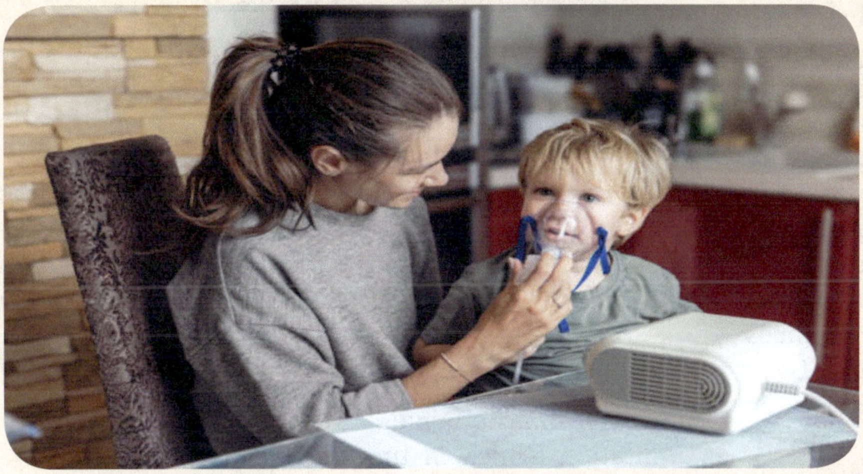

Introduction

Chronic Obstructive Pulmonary Disease (COPD) represents a significant public health issue, characterized by irreversible airway inflammation and progressive airflow obstruction. The illness encompasses a variety of pathologies, primarily emphysema and chronic bronchitis, which collectively compromise the respiratory function and decrease the quality of life. According to the Global Burden of Diseases, Injuries, and Risk Factors Study 2017, the common effects of such respiratory illnesses have led to a notable rise in global non-fatal health losses, reflecting a significant burden on healthcare systems and society at large. Because COPD remains one of the leading causes of morbidity and mortality worldwide, understanding its pathogenetic mechanisms, risk factors, and treatment options is critical for prevention and management. The initial section of this article aims to describe the heterogeneity of COPD and highlight its complex nature in patients with the condition and among physicians.

LEARNING OBJECTIVES

After studying this chapter, you will be able to:

1. Understand the causes of chronic obstructive pulmonary disease
2. List the symptoms and diagnosis
3. Explain pathophysiology of COPD
4. Focus on the treatment options
5. Discuss the management of COPD
6. Explore the impact of COPD on quality of life

The epidemiology of COPD has ominous tendencies since it is not only a disease confined to older adults. Youth exposed to tobacco smoke, occupational and environmental toxicants, and work-related risk factors are increasingly falling prey to the condition. The implications of such trends necessitate strategic health interventions to mitigate risk factors for COPD. With the increase in life expectancy, particularly in the developing world, the disease burden of conditions such as COPD has transformed. This is evident in the increased prevalence of chronic diseases, which often accompany increased life expectancy (van der Leest et al., 2018). Furthermore, the interplay between environmental exposures and genetic susceptibilities increases the complexity of COPD's clinical picture, necessitating a multidimensional approach that incorporates public health interventions, early screening, and education on lifestyle modification for risk reduction. The most recent treatment advances hold promise for patients living with COPD, particularly regarding new approaches such as high-intensity non-invasive ventilation (HI-NIV). Recent evidence appears that HI-NIV is likely to improve the physiological and clinical state of chronic hypercapnic respiratory failure patients who have a common complication of terminal COPD (van der Leest et al., 2018). This introduces a unique aspect of disease management that goes beyond traditional medications by seeking to enhance the quality of life of patients through new treatment modalities. With advancing science, it is essential to assess and implement promising treatments into clinical practice to keep up with the growing complexity of managing COPD. Ultimately, an integrated understanding of COPD, encompassing its epidemiology, risk factors, and emerging treatments, is essential to optimize patient outcomes and address the broader implications of chronic respiratory disease.

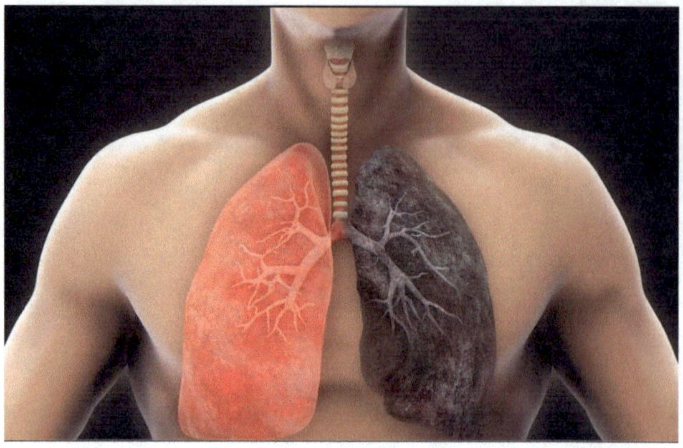

Figure 11.1. Chronic obstructive pulmonary disease.

Source: https://medtour.help/wp-content/uploads/2023/06/hobl.jpg

Definition of Chronic Obstructive Pulmonary Disease (COPD)

Chronic Obstructive Pulmonary Disease (COPD) is a complex respiratory disease that is characterized by chronic airflow limitation, which in the majority of instances is progressive and accompanied by heightened chronic inflammatory airway and lung reaction. The primary pathophysiological features are emphysema and chronic bronchitis, which contribute to airflow obstruction. Chronic bronchitis is defined as a chronic productive cough lasting three months or more in two consecutive years, while emphysema is characterized by alveolar destruction and impaired gas exchange. Recent advances in the disease have shown heterogeneity in inflammation mechanisms, suggesting the mechanisms propelling COPD to be highly varied among patients. This complexity necessitates personalized therapeutic interventions to effectively manage the disease and improve patient outcomes, underscoring the importance of research into customized treatment options (IMsci, 2024). Furthermore, it should be acknowledged that COPD is more than a smoker's disease; there is evidence to suggest a significant prevalence in never-smokers as well. New studies have identified that individuals who have never smoked but express symptoms of COPD are likely to have multifactorial risk factors such as environmental exposures and genetic factors. An example of this is a population-based study that shed light on the challenge in recruiting and diagnosing never-smokers with COPD due to the stringent criteria that need to be achieved for adequate spirometry testing. 154 never-smokers with COPD were noted in this study, which indicates the heterogeneity of the patient group and underscores the necessity for identifying different populations among COPD patients. This expands the spectrum of the condition and necessitates liberal diagnosis criteria to capture non-traditional cases (Sönnerfors et al., 2024).

Up to now, treatment of COPD is still progressive, aiming both for pharmacologic and non-pharmacologic interventions. Pharmacologic management is typically achieved through the administration of bronchodilators and corticosteroids to alleviate symptoms and reduce exacerbations. Additionally, new biological therapies targeting individual inflammatory pathways are now emerging, leading to new avenues of treatment, particularly for those with Type 2 inflammation. Effective management also involves lifestyle modification, such as smoking cessation, pulmonary rehabilitation, and exercise therapy. These combined strategies aim not only to improve respiratory function but also to optimize the quality of life in people with COPD. A correct understanding of the definitions and nuances of COPD is critical as it guides clinical practice and informs future research, eventually leading to more effective treatment models (IMsci, 2024).

Importance of studying COPD

The study on Chronic Obstructive Pulmonary Disease (COPD) is paramount due to its high prevalence and vast impact on public health. Since COPD ranks as the third leading cause of death in the United States, understanding more about its complexities becomes vital for creating appropriate management programs. The cost of treating the condition cannot be disregarded; the costs of healthcare for COPD patients are typically high, and by extension, their costs to patients and the healthcare system are also high. Moreover, as indicated in recent studies, the comorbidities of COPD patients complicate the provision of treatment and also tend to skew healthcare results, so it is critical to take into account the impacts of such elements on treatment pathways and hospital readmission (Chukmaitov et al., 2020).

Thus, increasing our understanding of COPD not only aids in the management of individual cases but also in optimizing healthcare policy and procedures for this common disease. Ultimately, the importance of rehabilitative management for patients with COPD remains a crucial area of research. Pulmonary rehabilitation has emerged as a key intervention, effectively increasing exercise capacity, decreasing respiratory symptoms, and enhancing the health-related quality of life in people suffering from this disabling illness. Evidence indicates that attendees of formal rehabilitation programs experience significant improvements in functional measures, such as walking distance and muscle strength—gains that are long-standing (Jörres et al., 2012). This highlights the need to integrate rehabilitative care into standard treatment protocols for COPD. Through further investigation into the effectiveness and administration of these programs, researchers can create interventions that target the specific needs of diverse patient groups, thereby optimizing healthcare outcomes and reducing the burden on healthcare systems.

Ultimately, the utility of studying COPD lies in its relevance to healthcare services and policy. The significant proportion of rehospitalization that comes with COPD identifies the need for targeted interventions within the healthcare system to prevent unnecessary re-hospitalizations. There is evidence that comorbid patients may have reduced rates of readmission, challenging traditional assumptions about the case management of COPD patients with multiple medical conditions (Chukmaitov et al., 2020). To address these problems through focused research is to enable healthcare practitioners to gain a deeper understanding of COPD's complexity and develop comprehensive approaches to care. Additionally, policy forums informed by well-reasoned research can influence resource investment in improving COPD care globally, with effective treatment available to all patients. Ultimately, the study of COPD provides the essential foundation upon which both patient-level care and broader systemic changes in healthcare provision can be developed.

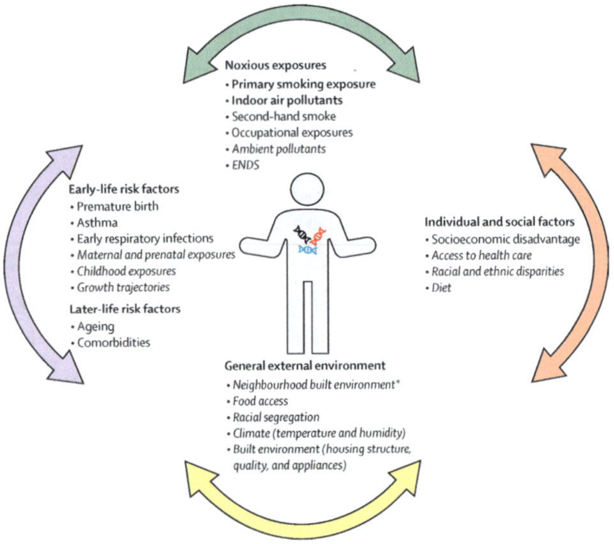

Figure 11.2. Importance of studying COPD.

Source: https://www.thelancet.com/cms/10.1016/S0140-6736(22)00470-6/asset/fb5c8161-c4e8-479f-8653-b4087c0aae06/main.assets/gr1_lrg.jpg

11.1. Causes of Chronic Obstructive Pulmonary Diseases

Learning Outcome

1. Smoking is the primary risk factor for COPD
2. Environmental pollutants and occupational hazards
3. Genetic factors and alpha-1 antitrypsin deficiency

Chronic Obstructive Pulmonary Disease (COPD) is an unremittingly progressive illness that is primarily characterized by airflow limitation, which is caused by significant risk factors. The most universally accepted cause of COPD is chronic exposure to tobacco smoke, which not only causes lung damage but also maintains ongoing inflammatory processes. Environmental exposure, including air pollution, occupational dust, and chemicals, as well as smoking, also significantly contributes to the development and onset of the disease. These risk factors interact with genetic risk factors, resulting in increased susceptibility in certain groups of individuals. The Global Burden of Diseases study reveals that incidence rates of chronic respiratory diseases, such as COPD, have exhibited fluctuating trends in various populations, underscoring the importance of targeted public health interventions aimed at addressing the multifaceted etiology of COPD, particularly in susceptible individuals (Choi et al., 2022). Another crucial aspect in the pathogenesis of COPD is the interaction between chronic inflammation and structural changes in the lungs. Chronic stimulation by pathogens and irritants results in immune reactions that produce inflammation and tissue remodeling, characteristics common in COPD. The inflammation results in lung tissue destruction and constricts the airways, causing an excessive blockade of airflow. Besides, those with a history of childhood respiratory infections or frequent bronchitis are at risk of developing COPD in adulthood. The presence of comorbid conditions, such as cardiovascular disease and diabetes, may complicate the clinical picture with worse outcomes. The interaction between these elements necessitates an integrative management strategy for not just COPD but even its associated health complications (Choi et al., 2022).

The population variables influencing the incidence of COPD also matter. Age, gender, and socio-economic status all play essential roles in the causation of the disease. Epidemiologic data support a higher prevalence of COPD in older people, considering declining lung function with advancing age. It is also significant that, historically, men have had greater rates of COPD, but at present, trends suggest rising numbers of cases in women as smoking prevalence increases. Additionally, lower socioeconomic strata are more likely to be exposed to risk factors, hence resulting in compounded health disparities. These results highlight the importance of addressing social determinants of health in the prevention and management of COPD. As the world continues to grapple with chronic respiratory diseases, understanding the etiology of COPD from a multifaceted perspective becomes essential for effective public health interventions and actions (Xie et al., 2020).

11.1.1. Smoking As the Primary Risk Factor

The overwhelming majority of evidence indicates that smoking is the prime risk factor for the development of Chronic Obstructive Pulmonary Disease (COPD). Aside from initiating a cascade of deleterious inflammatory mechanisms in the lungs, smoking also gradually compromises lung function. The harmful chemicals found in tobacco smoke ravage the respiratory tract, resulting in chronic bronchitis and emphysema, the two pathologies that define COPD. Moreover, more recent evidence suggests a staggering burden of airflow limitation among smokers and those with related cardiovascular disorders, and approximately 27% of them can have undiagnosed COPD (Hagan et al., 2014). This indicates an immediate need for interventions, particularly intended to reduce the prevalence of smoking and thereby reduce COPD cases and improve public health overall. In the clinical context, the effect of smoking extends beyond the immediate impact on lung function because it also intersects with cardiovascular disease risk. Smokers are at risk of developing respiratory complications that exacerbate underlying cardiovascular conditions, promoting a cycle of worsening health. Moreover, this association emphasizes the need for careful screening for COPD in smoking patients with previous heart problems, as many could remain undiagnosed even with a presentation of airflow limitation (Hagan et al., 2014).

Early detection, via standard lung function tests, can enable timely intervention strategies and potentially improve patient outcomes within a population known for high rates of comorbidities. Consequently, healthcare systems must prioritize education and screening, addressing the multifaceted challenges posed by smoking-related diseases. Despite the established connection between smoking and COPD, the shift towards using biomarkers for early diagnosis and prognosis holds promise in mitigating disease impact. Traditional diagnostic approaches often rely heavily on patient history and spirometry, which can be limited by variability in patients' emotional and physiological responses.

A new study suggests that biological markers detecting inflammatory responses may be better predictors of the severity and progression of COPD. This technique would pave the way for less invasive testing methods that enable timely and effective treatment strategies.

By applying the findings of biomarkers to daily clinical use, healthcare professionals could enhance diagnostic accuracy, thereby treating smoking as the primary causative factor in the instance of COPD and improving overall control of this disease in general.

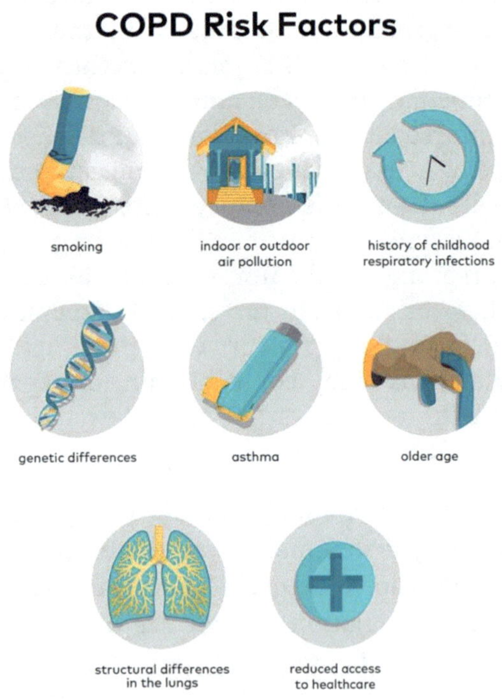

Figure 11.3. COPD Risk Factors.

Source: https://dims.healthgrades.com/dims3/MMH/ad9ab9b/2147483647/strip/true/crop/794x1024+0+0/resize/794x1024!/quality/75/?url=https%3A%2F%2Fucmscdn.healthgrades.com%2F37%2Fb6%2F377f7adb6a0b32d336f26d42216f%2F362727-chronic-obstructive-pulmonary-disease-COPD-risk-factors-1296x1672-body-794x1024.jpg

11.1.2. Environmental Pollutants and Occupational Hazards

Environmental pollutants are a significant cause of the development and exacerbation of Chronic Obstructive Pulmonary Diseases (COPD). The lung is one of the central interfaces between the body and the environment; therefore, numerous environmental factors have a profound impact on lung function. Air pollution, particularly particulate matter and ozone exposure, has been linked to increased respiratory symptoms and exacerbations of underlying lung diseases. Individuals with high levels of exposure to these pollutants report symptoms such as cough, breathlessness, and general respiratory distress. Epidemiological studies have consistently demonstrated that air pollution exacerbates chronic respiratory tract diseases, including asthma and COPD, underscoring the need for effective public health interventions to mitigate airborne pollutants in urban settings (Cacciottolo et al., 2013). Workers in certain occupations are at a higher risk of occupational exposures that cause COPD development. Professions in construction, mining, and manufacturing frequently come into contact with hazardous substances, including dust, fumes, and chemicals. The gradual loss of lung function, resulting from the cumulative effect of inhaling these harmful substances, leads to chronic inflammation. Additionally, employees in inadequately ventilated or equipped workplaces are at a higher risk, as their exposure to harmful agents is not adequately monitored. Such occupational risks are augmented by environmental exposures and the outcome is a double burden that can negatively impact respiratory health. It is a priority to identify the intricate interface between occupational hazards and environmental pollutants in order to define targeted prevention strategies for protecting workers' health and preventing chronic diseases, such as COPD (Cacciottolo et al., 2013). Additionally, the interface between occupational hazards and environmental pollutants raises critical public health and policy concerns. Good health education and imposition of effective legislative measures are required in order to counteract the undesirable effects of pollution on lung function. It is more than enhancing workers' knowledge of occupational hazards, however. It also means pushing for tighter emission limits and occupational health standards. Multi-stakeholder collaboration among occupational health professionals, government agencies, and community organizations is essential in mitigating air pollution and averting exposure of vulnerable populations to occupational and environmental pollutants. To this end, both the sources of pollutants and their reduction are necessary to stem the prevalence of COPD and improve overall respiratory health outcomes.

11.1.3. Genetic Factors and Alpha-1 Antitrypsin Deficiency

The genetic basis of chronic obstructive pulmonary disease (COPD) comprises a multitude of hereditary etiologies, with alpha-1 antitrypsin deficiency (AATD) being the most significant. AATD arises from mutations within the SERPINA1 gene, resulting in defective synthesis or the production of aberrant forms of alpha-1 antitrypsin protein. This deficiency has direct consequences for lung function, as reduced levels of this protein impair the body's ability to inhibit proteolytic enzymes such as neutrophil elastase, leading to uncontrolled tissue destruction and increased emphysema severity. Given its crucial importance, the genetic basis of AATD should be familiar for risk assessment of individuals at risk of severe phenotypes of COPD, thereby emphasizing the importance of early genetic screening and intervention strategies to manage progressive lung damage and improve the course of the disease in affected groups.

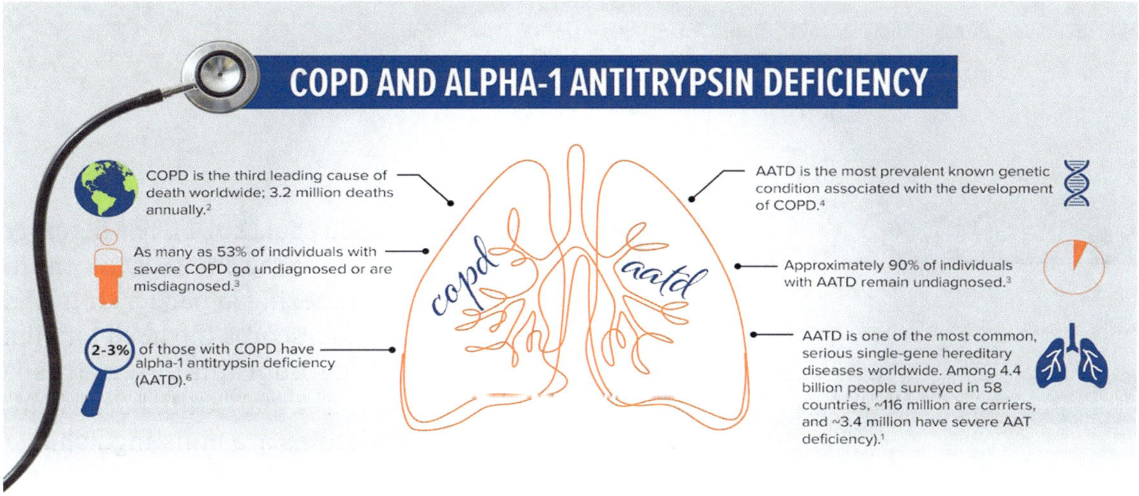

Figure 11.4. Genetic factors and alpha-1 antitrypsin deficiency of COPD.

Source: https://www.COPDfoundation.org/portals/0/images/GeneticCOPD/Genetic-COPD-101-Basic-2.jpg

Further, the implications of AATD extend to pulmonary manifestations, as the disease is linked with other systemic health disorders, including cardiovascular illnesses. There is evidence that patients with AATD are not only at risk for lung damage but also are at increased risk for vascular-related issues such as aneurysms, thus pointing toward the systemic nature of the disorder. Current case reports indicate evidence of aneurysms of the aortic and splenic artery in patients with AATD, pointing toward the importance of cardiovascular assessment in these patients (Gordon et al., 2025).

This aspect highlights the multifaceted influence of AATD on health, which must be carefully monitored and managed in conjunction with comorbidities, thereby ensuring an integrated treatment strategy for patients with both pulmonary and vascular AATD complications. In addition, the interaction between AATD and cardiovascular disease comorbidity is complex and emphasizes the need for vigilant clinical evaluation. Studies of large groups of AATD patients with COPD have shown a reduced frequency of cardiovascular disease among the AATD patients compared to non-AATD patients, suggesting unique pathophysiologic mechanisms (Zöller et al., 2024). Despite this, the presence of AATD in COPD patients highlights the recommendation for routine monitoring of cardiovascular disease, given the potential for heightened susceptibility to further systemic complications. By understanding these correlations, clinicians can more effectively tailor interventions and promote preventive strategies to reduce morbidity and mortality rates in this specialized population, ultimately improving quality of life for AATD and secondary chronic obstructive pulmonary disease sufferers.

Test Your Knowledge

1. Define smoking as the primary risk factor?
2. What are the genetic factors and alpha-1 antitrypsin deficiency?

11.2. Symptoms and Diagnosis

Learning Outcome

1. Common symptoms of COPD
2. Diagnostic methods used in identifying COPD
3. Importance of early diagnosis

Symptoms of Chronic Obstructive Pulmonary Disease (COPD) are primarily respiratory in character, which either develop slowly or abruptly. The frequently reported symptoms include chronic cough, increased sputum production, dyspnea, and wheezing. Interestingly, the patients can also have exacerbations and respiratory infections, indicating the progressive nature of the illness. One study found that younger COPD patients bemoaned a heavy load of such symptoms without receiving medical attention, indicating a lack of early detection and treatment (Gogou et al., 2021). The heterogeneity of symptom presentation, such as the higher prevalence of wheezing in participants under 55 years of age, underscores the need for clinicians to consider demographic features when diagnosing and treating COPD. Because in many cases, the symptoms are indistinguishable from those of other respiratory illnesses, advanced knowledge is required to establish an accurate diagnosis. Diagnosis of COPD is generally made through a careful assessment of clinical history, physical examination, and specific lung function tests. Among the tests used, spirometry, which measures the volume and flow of air during breathing in and out, is a key component. Still, in situations of heightened community transmission of respiratory viruses, diagnostic measures like spirometry must be employed judiciously to avoid health risks (Halpin et al., 2020). The diagnosis of COPD is initiated mainly from primary care centers, particularly in patients with significant smoking history. Proper assessment of patients, taking into account their symptom profile and any prior diagnosis of respiratory disorders, is essential for effective management. Additionally, early diagnosis will prevent disease progression and enhance patient outcomes, supporting the validity of community health interventions. Due to recent health crises, including the COVID-19 pandemic, it has been more challenging for medical practitioners to differentiate between COPD symptoms and viral infection symptoms. COVID-19 has various respiratory symptoms that overlap with those of COPD, making diagnosis and treatment procedures even more challenging (Halpin et al., 2020). As the health community is dealing with such complexities, maintaining a high index of suspicion for COVID-19 in patients of COPD becomes increasingly critical. Clinicians are best advised to remain on guard, with increased screening criteria to differentiate between stable COPD exacerbations and suspect cases of COVID-19. Furthermore, patients with COPD are recommended to adhere to proper infection control measures, including vaccination, social distancing, and the use of masks. The progressive nature of COPD diagnosis in relation to other lung disorders calls for ongoing education for healthcare providers and patients as a means of encouraging early detection and effective management of chronic obstructive pulmonary diseases.

11.2.1. Common Symptoms of COPD

The presentation of chronic obstructive pulmonary disease (COPD) is predominantly one of a constellation of characteristic symptoms that significantly affect patients' quality of life. Headed at the top of this list is chronic cough, which is a repeated instance of disabling coughing. The symptom is prone to emerging as a response to irritants in the lungs, triggering the production of sputum and exacerbation of respiratory difficulty. Also, the presence of a chronic cough is invariably accompanied by a compromised physical tolerance. Because COPD patients are more short of breath when they perform everyday activities, the disabling impact of chronic cough falls hard on them and contributes to their global respiratory impairment. Another disabling symptom characteristic of COPD is dyspnea, or shortness of breath. This sensation typically worsens with exertion, and even daily activities become unfeasible. Dyspnea is a consequence of the obstructive nature of the disease, which hinders airflow in and out of the lungs and thereby leads to a lack of sufficient oxygen supply. Patients often complain of feeling frustrated and anxious because their activities are severely hindered by the symptom. It has been noted through studies that the prevalence of dyspnea is associated with diminished health-related quality of life as patients suffer from physical as well as psychological impacts of the disease (Bobowicz et al., 2009). Effective management interventions to alleviate dyspnea are extremely crucial in enhancing the health status of patients with COPD (Bobowicz et al., 2009). During an acute exacerbation, patients experience a worsening of typical symptoms, significantly impacting their health status. During these attacks, exacerbations can lead to an increase in sputum and coloration, indicating possible respiratory infection. Exacerbations may also increase dyspnea and cough, which lead more often to patients seeking medical attention. The combination of exacerbations with other comorbid illnesses, such as cardiovascular diseases, complicates the respiratory disease even further, which is why treating these acute phases simultaneously in COPD is crucial (Bobowicz et al., 2009). As the prognosis of such patients with severe COPD may be no better than that of lung cancer patients, the understanding and effective management of these common symptoms are essential to maximizing clinical results and enhancing the quality of life in patients (Bobowicz et al., 2009).

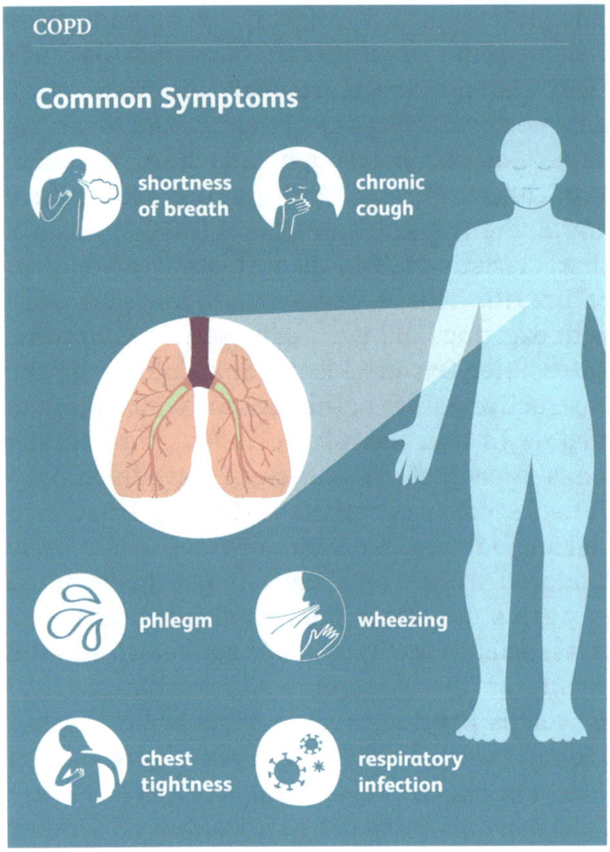

Figure 11.5. Symptoms of COPD.

Source: https://www.verywellhealth.com/thmb/ZHMqUtkGQAeUHfHSIXrBaqwWNQQ=/1500x0/filters:no_upscale():max_bytes(150000):strip_icc()/COPD-symptoms-5aeca0cb875db90037400ac1.png

11.2.2. Diagnostic Methods Used in Identifying COPD

Correct diagnosis of Chronic Obstructive Pulmonary Disease (COPD) is crucial to ensure right management and treatment. Clinical assessment and spirometry are the primary tools of diagnosis, which measure obstruction in airflow by quantifying lung function. The American Thoracic Society recommends spirometry as a gold standard in diagnosing COPD, where reduced forced expiratory volume in one second (FEV1) and a decreased FEV1/FVC ratio confirm the presence of airflow limitation. These practices not only assist in diagnosis but also define its severity, enabling specific therapeutic interventions. Additional tests of these protocols can enhance diagnostic accuracy, and tools such as Electronic Health Record (EHR) databases become crucial for streamlining patient identification and categorization (Kwok et al., 2024). In addition to spirometry, imaging techniques such as chest X-rays and computed tomography (CT) scans are used as ancillary tools in the diagnosis of COPD. While X-rays are used to rule out other illnesses responsible for respiratory symptoms, CT scans provide high-resolution images that can measure the extent of emphysema as well as other changes in lung anatomy. Both modalities assist not only with COPD diagnosis but also with information about comorbid disease. Moreover, a thorough clinical examination of patient histories emphasizes signs such as chronic cough or sputum production, thereby supplementing the diagnostic process. A combination of these imaging techniques with clinical assessment is particularly valuable in complex cases where multifactorial respiratory issues present challenges (Zhang et al., 2024). New technologies, such as machine learning algorithms and large language models (LLMs) such as GPT-4, are also being explored for their potential to enhance COPD diagnosis. Previous studies indicate that these tools can analyze vast amounts of EHR data with comparable, if not superior, performance compared to traditional disease-specific models to identify cases of COPD. The application of these models has the potential to facilitate more sophisticated data analysis, which can lead to better patient stratification and earlier treatment. The ethical dilemmas of data protection and confidence in predictions by algorithms must be addressed to fully incorporate these state-of-the-art diagnostic methods into clinical practice. With further research emerging, the harmonization of traditional practices and new technologies may redesign the diagnosis and treatment of COPD (Zhang et al., 2024).

11.2.3. Importance of Early Diagnosis

The importance of early diagnosis for Chronic Obstructive Pulmonary Disease (COPD) cannot be overemphasized since it is essential in arresting the progress of the disease and enhancing the quality of life for patients. Patients can receive appropriate intervention after being diagnosed early, as not only does it arrest the advance of the disease, but also delays the delay of its severe symptoms. Early diagnosis allows timely access to essential treatments and lifestyle changes, which are significant as exacerbations can lead to chronic long-term injury to lung function. Moreover, establishing an accurate diagnosis enables medical care providers to develop individualized treatment regimens, with medical and therapeutic interventions coordinated in concert with patients' unique needs, thereby ensuring their adherence to the regimen and the quality of health outcomes. The influence of early diagnosis extends beyond the individual patient to impact public health outcomes and also the management of the health system. By identifying COPD in its early stages, health systems can implement population-based interventions that can reduce the burden of this disease. Early detection schemes can facilitate preventive interventions, awareness, and screening programs, thereby reducing the rate of hospitalization and healthcare costs associated with complicated COPD cases. Additionally, as with the rising rates of pulmonary nodules and lung diseases in clinical accounts, incorporating lung health screening into routine health check-ups becomes imperative. The importance of recognizing conditions like pulmonary nodules—particularly if they can signal malignancies—is emphasized in current research, which demonstrates how optimal treatment can lead to more favorable patient prognoses (Peter J. Mazzone et al., 2022). Beyond treating current health issues, early COPD diagnosis can promote a vigilant approach to managing comorbidities that so often accompany chronic respiratory illness. For instance, COPD patients typically end up with cardiovascular comorbidities, which are easier to treat if respiratory disease is diagnosed early on. It is highly desirable to motivate patients to participate in a structured rehabilitation program, particularly at the onset, when interventions can be tailored to maximize lung function as well as overall fitness (Rutkowski, 2021). Not only are these kinds of interventions beneficial in retarding the progression of COPD, but they are also in educating patients about their disease. Through promoting health consciousness and preventive measures, early detection is a critical component of the comprehensive management of COPD, ultimately leading to improved patient outcomes and community health.

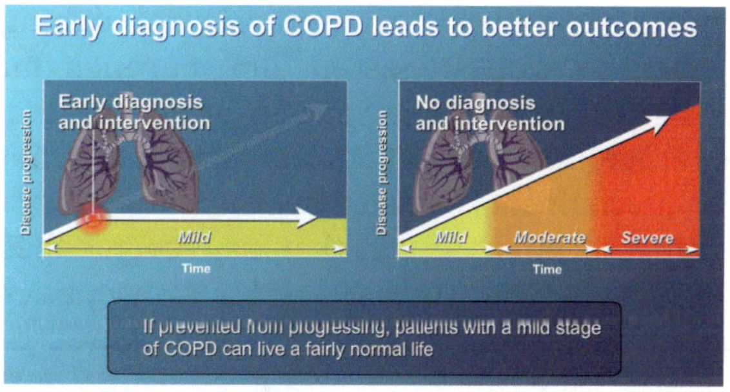

Figure 11.6. The importance of early diagnosis in Chronic Obstructive Pulmonary Diseases (COPD).

Source: https://www.animatedCOPDpatient.com/en-COPD/content.ashx?file=COPD02/slides/m2_slide_03.jpg

Test Your Knowledge

1. What are the common symptoms of COPD?
2. What are the diagnostic methods used in identifying COPD?

11.3. Pathophysiology of COPD

Learning Outcome

1. Mechanisms of airflow limitation
2. Inflammatory processes involved in COPD
3. Impact on lung function and overall health

The pathophysiology of Chronic Obstructive Pulmonary Disease (COPD) is a complex interplay between inflammation, airway obstruction, and structural changes in lung tissues. The disease is primarily attributed to long-term exposure to injurious particles, notably cigarette smoke, leading to chronic airway inflammation. The inflammation initiates the influx of inflammatory cells, including neutrophils and macrophages, which release pro-inflammatory cytokines and chemokines. Over time, the persistent inflammatory response leads to irreversible airway remodeling, characterized by increased goblet cell hyperplasia and smooth muscle hypertrophy. In addition, persistent damage to alveolar walls leads to lung parenchymal destruction and the formation of emphysema, a characteristic of COPD. It is critical to know such mechanisms in order to formulate effective therapeutic interventions that may reverse these processes of these diseases and improve patient outcomes. Recent studies have highlighted the exacerbating roles of certain environmental pollutants, such as copper oxide nanoparticles (CuONPs), in the pathophysiology of COPD. Not only do these particles trigger an inflammatory response, but they can also exacerbate the underlying disease pathophysiological processes. CuONPs exposure has been reported by studies to result in increased expression of thioredoxin-interacting protein (TXNIP), which is an essential mediator of the inflammatory reaction through activation of the NOD-like receptor protein 3 (NLRP3) inflammasome. Activation of this signaling pathway leads to the further release of the inflammatory cytokine interleukin-1β (IL-1β), which exacerbates the existing inflammation within the respiratory tract. This response highlights the need for further studies on the interactions between inflammatory processes and environmental agents that contribute to lung function deterioration in COPD patients (Kim W-I et al., 2024).

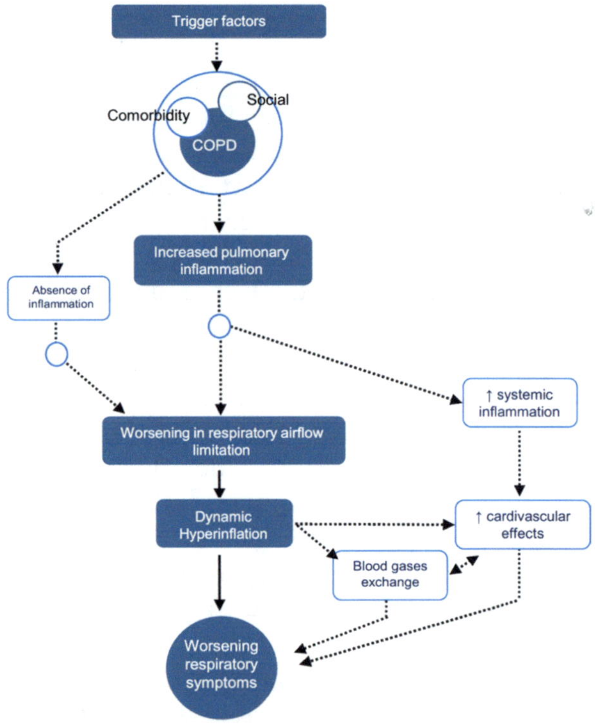

Figure 11.7. Pathophysiology of COPD.

Source: https://www.researchgate.net/publication/366668408/figure/fig1/AS:1143128111046810 5@1672578374114/Pathophysiology-of-COPD-exacerbation-syndrome-Reproduced-with-permission-from.png

COPD therapies have also been explored in the recent past through natural products acting against intrinsic inflammatory pathways. For instance, the combination of icariin and nobiletin has been found to enhance the inflammatory mechanisms that form the basis of COPD. Network pharmacology studies show that the drugs target tissue-specific inflammatory pathways such as the mitogen-activated protein kinase (MAPK) and phosphatidylinositol 3-kinase (PI3K)-protein kinase B (AKT) pathways. Experimental validation in animal models of COPD has demonstrated that the administration of icariin and nobiletin may improve lung function and reduce levels of pro-inflammatory cytokines, such as IL-1β and tumor necrosis factor-alpha (TNF-α). These findings suggest that modulating inflammation through selective molecular pathways is a promising avenue for treating COPD and improving quality of life in patients affected by this debilitating disease (Lu et al., 2022).

11.3.1. Mechanisms of Airflow Limitation

The pathophysiology of airflow limitation in COPD is multifactorial, resulting from the interaction of inflammatory events with airway structural remodeling. The mainstay of the process is chronic inflammation, resulting from long-standing exposure to inhaled irritants such as tobacco smoke and ambient pollutants. Chronic inflammation leads to airway obstruction through a cascade of mechanisms, including mucus hypersecretion, airway remodeling, and destruction of alveolar structures. Taken as a whole, these alterations culminate in constricted airways, making it challenging for patients to breathe, particularly with exertion. The role of these mechanisms highlights the importance of understanding COPD pathophysiology in developing effective treatment modalities that address the underlying causes of airflow limitation, ultimately aiming to improve patient quality of life and respiratory function (Wang et al., 2023). Dysregulation of autophagy is also a key mechanism in the development of airflow limitation in COPD. Autophagy, a cellular process that breaks down damaged organelles and proteins, promotes cellular homeostasis. The mechanism in patients with COPD is impaired mainly, leading to the accumulation of dysfunctional cellular constituents that enhance inflammation and tissue damage. In particular, macroautophagy dysfunction has been linked to an increased susceptibility to emphysema and lung inflammation, both of which contribute to airflow obstruction. Research assessing the interaction of autophagy with COPD suggests that augmenting autophagic processes can offer novel therapeutic options, potentially leading to symptom relief due to airflow limitation, as well as slowing the progression of the disease (Wang et al., 2023). Second, oxidative stress plays a central role in the pathomechanism of airflow limitation. Chronic exposure to environmental oxidative stress triggers harmful changes in lung tissue that can destabilize the equilibrium between antioxidant defense mechanisms. The Nrf2-antioxidant response element (ARE) pathway is an adaptive mechanism that counteracts oxidative damage. However, in the majority of COPD patients, this regulatory process is dysregulated, which initiates the chronic airway inflammation and structural disease remodeling. Since this pathway is strongly linked with the severity of COPD, it provides an opportunity for biomarkers to measure disease progression and response to treatment. Additionally, suppression of the Nrf2-ARE pathway may offer therapeutic benefits in the treatment of airflow limitation by restoring the body's antioxidant status and reducing inflammatory responses.

11.3.2. Inflammatory Processes Involved in COPD

The inflammatory processes in Chronic Obstructive Pulmonary Disease (COPD) are multifaceted and complex, primarily consisting of an unchecked immune response in the respiratory tract. Smoking deleterious inhalants, such as cigarette smoke or atmospheric air toxins, triggers an inflammatory reaction characterized by the influx of immune cells, such as neutrophils and macrophages, into the lungs. These immune cells release a broad variety of inflammatory mediators, including cytokines and chemokines, which perpetuate inflammation and are also implicated in airway remodeling and oxidative stress. The activation of transcription factors themselves, subsequently induced by these cytokines, further enhances inflammation, leading to an irreversible decline in lung function. As a result, COPD patients experience persistent airway obstruction and chronic respiratory signs, reflecting that the inflammatory response is not only characteristic but also a driver of disease activity. Oxidative stress plays a vital role in COPD's inflammatory processes. The inflammation produces high concentrations of reactive oxygen species (ROS) that induce damage to cellular architecture, including lipid membranes and proteins, thereby maintaining the inflammatory process. ROS are responsible for activating various signaling pathways that lead to enhanced inflammatory reactions and the recruitment and activation of immune effector cells within the lungs. Excess production of oxidative stress over antioxidant defense mechanisms in COPD patients heightens tissue damage and inflammation, thereby aggravating clinical manifestations. Significantly, therapies aimed at reestablishing such balance, such as antioxidant therapies, may have a role in enhancing the inflammatory processes of COPD and consequently patient outcomes and quality of life (Ismailov et al., 2024). In addition to traditional inflammatory markers, exhaled breath condensate (EBC) has been recognized as a promising way of monitoring the inflammatory processes of COPD. EBC contains volatile and non-volatile biomarkers that reflect the pathophysiological state of the lungs, such as various cytokines and indicators of oxidative stress. Analysis of EBC can provide non-invasive data on the inflammatory status of the respiratory tract, allowing for better discrimination between COPD and other respiratory conditions, such as asthma. By examining the EBC composition, researchers highlighted the persistence of chronic inflammation in COPD, as well as the reaction to therapeutic interventions. In addition to providing insight into the inflammatory processes underlying the disease, it also lays the groundwork for a more personalized approach to monitoring and managing COPD, as well as for future advances in the treatment of chronic respiratory diseases (Kita et al., 2024).

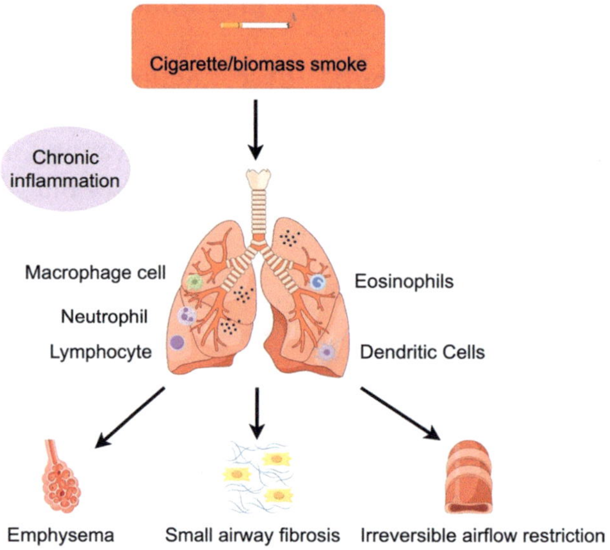

Figure 11.8. Inflammatory processes involved in COPD.

Source: https://www.frontiersin.org/files/Articles/1404615/fimmu-15-1404615-HTML/image_m/fimmu-15-1404615-g001.jpg

11.3.3. Impact On Lung Function and Overall Health

The impact of chronic obstructive pulmonary disease (COPD) on lung function is dramatic and pervasive, leading to a compromise of overall health. The advancement of COPD results in the loss of the lungs' capacity to exchange gases, leading to decreased oxygenation of the blood and increased carbon dioxide levels. Impairment of these domains is typically noted by shortness of breath (dyspnea), chronic cough, and an abnormal lung sound, all of which can severely restrict activities of daily living and decrease quality of life. Furthermore, patients with COPD frequently experience exacerbations—acute worsening of symptoms—that necessitate hospitalization and result in loss of lung function. Evidence suggests a clear correlation between disease burden and acute exacerbations, highlighting the unique importance of accurate disease management in preserving lung function and promoting patient health (Sep Wúlveda-Loyola et al., 2020). Of particular concern regarding COPD is that it is comorbid with sarcopenia, which involves progressive muscle mass loss and power. Research indicates that sarcopenia in COPD patients is associated with significantly worse lung function, reduced exercise capacity, and poorer quality of life (Sep Wúlveda-Loyola et al., 2020). Sarcopenia is most prevalent in patients with severe COPD, appearing in around 37.6% of such patients. When the two conditions coincide, they can form a cycle of deterioration: reduced physical capacity resulting from diminished lung capacity further contributes to muscle loss, which in turn restricts physical activity and leads to further decline. Therefore, muscle health as an area becomes imperative when managing COPD, as it can support lung function and lead to improved overall health. The general health of individuals suffering from COPD is also compromised by the psychological stresses arising from this chronic disease. Emotions and psychiatric illness, including depression and anxiety, are also common in patients as a consequence of limitations in activities of daily living from impaired lung function. Psychological distress can be central to dictating the disease course, hence making treatment guidelines adherence complicated. Also, individuals with substance use disorders, such as smoking, are more likely to experience severe complications on contracting respiratory illnesses like COVID-19, further complicating their health status and outcomes. All these factors collectively summarize the necessity for an overall holistic treatment strategy, addressing not just lung function, but also muscle strength, psychological well-being, and the management of co-morbid conditions to improve overall health in COPD patients.

Test Your Knowledge

1. What are the mechanisms of airflow limitation?
2. What are the inflammatory processes involved in COPD?

11.4. Treatment Options

Learning Outcome

1. Pharmacological treatments (bronchodilators, steroids)
2. Non-pharmacological interventions (pulmonary rehabilitation)
3. Surgical options (lung volume reduction surgery, transplantation)

The management of Chronic Obstructive Pulmonary Disease (COPD) is multidimensional in scope and involves both pharmacological and non-pharmacological therapy. Pharmacological treatment typically involves the use of bronchodilators, corticosteroids, and antibiotics, in some cases, to alleviate symptoms and control exacerbations. These medications act by causing dilation of the airways and inhibiting inflammation, which can significantly reduce impairment of lung function and overall enhance the quality of life for the patient. In addition to pharmacologic management of the disease, follow-up and adherence to treatment regimens can ensure the optimal use of such pharmacologic agents, which are integral elements in the management of COPD. Continuous education of healthcare providers as well as patients cannot be overlooked, as this is exceedingly important for optimum therapy and the outcome of the patient. In addition to drug therapies, non-pharmacological interventions also contribute significantly to COPD management. Such a non-pharmacological intervention is pulmonary rehabilitation, which consists of a multi-component program that includes exercise, education, and psychosocial assessment and support, tailored to the patient's needs. Several studies have shown consistently that participatory rehabilitation programs enhance patients' physical tolerance and mental state, as well as reduce hospital admissions and all-cause mortality (Marks G).

The addition of exercise in pulmonary rehabilitation is particularly effective as it enhances not only physical capacity but also motivates patients to engage in daily life activities regularly. Nevertheless, it is essential to recognize that these rehabilitation services are often underutilized, underscoring the need for increased awareness and accessibility of these vital programs within the healthcare system. Long-term oxygen therapy (LTOT) is also another essential non-pharmacological management, suggested more so in patients with severe COPD with reduced oxygen saturation levels. The administration of supplemental oxygen over extended periods, preferably greater than 15 hours a day, has been demonstrated to improve quality of life and survival in patients with chronic respiratory failure (Marks G). Nonetheless, as with pulmonary rehabilitation, the utilization of LTOT is also underrepresented in current clinical practice and may thus be perceived as implying access and utilization hurdles that need to be bridged. Underutilization will suggest an imperative for augmented observation and evaluation of such therapies within the context of comprehensive COPD management. By filling the gaps in therapy utilization, healthcare practitioners can significantly improve patient outcomes and quality of life in patients with COPD.

11.4.1. Pharmacological Treatments (Bronchodilators, Steroids)

Pharmacotherapies are a critical component in the management of Chronic Obstructive Pulmonary Disease (COPD) and are directed primarily for symptom relief and deceleration of the frequency of exacerbations. One of the primary classes of drugs utilized is bronchodilators, which function by relaxing the airway surrounding muscles, thereby improving airflow and making it easier for the patient to breathe. These medications fall into two categories: short-acting and long-acting bronchodilators, both of which are constructed with specific therapeutic capabilities. Short-acting bronchodilators are often used to achieve quick relief in acute exacerbations, whereas long-acting preparations facilitate sustained management of the symptoms. The efficiency of such medications, however, is apt to be variable from individual to individual, and thus individualized treatment is crucial. Moreover, bronchodilators in combination with other classes of medication, such as inhaled corticosteroids, have been shown to be more effective in controlling symptoms of COPD, indicating that a multidisciplinary approach is necessary (Hanania et al., 2024). Inhaled corticosteroids, in conjunction with bronchodilators, are an integral part of COPD pharmacological management, particularly for patients with recurrent exacerbations. These medications are effective in reducing airway inflammation, a feature of COPD, and can become a significant factor in improved lung function, along with the general condition of health. The cautious use of inhaled corticosteroids typically suggests the potential for such side effects as pneumonia and other systemic effects, with prudent judgment by treating physicians.

Treatment regimen innovation shows that the administration of inhaled corticosteroids with long-acting bronchodilators enhances therapeutic outcomes, presenting synergistic advantages to ensure optimal lung function while minimizing risks of exacerbation. The combination therapy has gained traction through evidence-based guidance, with the latter now advocating for its adoption as a standard practice among patients with moderate to severe COPD (Hanania et al., 2024). Further, newer research has extended the pharmacologic profile of COPD treatment, particularly with new agents that act on a multitude of pathways of the pathophysiology of the disease.

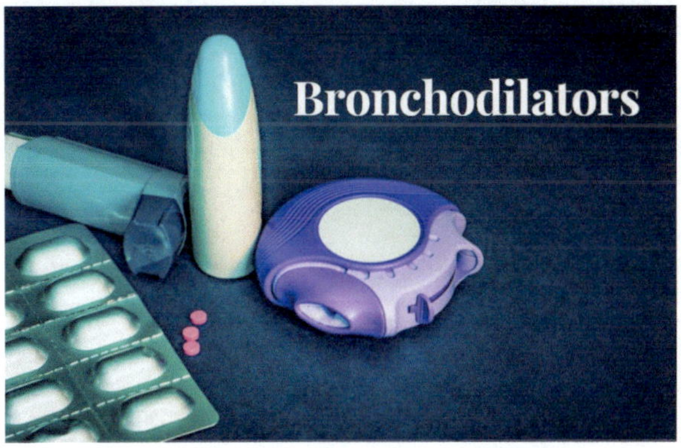

Figure 11.19. Pharmacological treatments.

Source: https://bibo.health/cdn/shop/articles/WhatsApp_Image_2023-05-29_at_2.47.35_PM.jpg?v=1685353292

The introduction of dual-acting phosphodiesterase inhibitors, for instance, which inhibit both PDE3 and PDE4, has been an exciting new alternative in management strategies. These compounds appear to deliver not just bronchodilator but also powerful anti-inflammatory effects, acting against significant aspects of COPD pathology in a multiplex manner. These technologies introduce a new vision to therapy, especially in patients with poor control using conventional bronchodilators and corticosteroids. Further, it is essential to investigate the interaction between COPD and cardiovascular comorbidities because studies have proven the effect of beta-blockers on mortality and the rate of exacerbations in this patient population. Therefore, an integrated pharmacologic treatment strategy encompassing multiple therapeutic methods is of prime importance in optimizing patient outcomes in COPD.

11.4.2. Non-Pharmacological Interventions (Pulmonary Rehabilitation)

Non-pharmacological interventions, particularly pulmonary rehabilitation, are also an integral part of the management of Chronic Obstructive Pulmonary Disease (COPD). They focus on improving the physical and psychological well-being of patients by prioritizing exercise training, nutritional guidance, education, and psychosocial interventions. The multidisciplinary character of pulmonary rehabilitation aims not only to enhance the physical capacity but also to treat comorbid diseases that are frequently observed in COPD patients, such as depression and anxiety. Evidence shows that patients with mental comorbidities are more symptomatic and have increased hospitalization rates, highlighting the importance of incorporating mental health support into pulmonary rehabilitation interventions. While pharmacological treatment is valuable, the overall nature of non-pharmacological treatment is essential for improving the quality of life of COPD patients and achieving long-term benefits (Rahi et al., 2023). Organized exercise training is one of the most critical aspects of pulmonary rehabilitation, having been shown to significantly enhance exercise capacity and alleviate the symptoms of dyspnea. Through tailored exercise regimens aimed at each patient's functional capacity, the programs not only strengthen lung function but also have a positive impact on muscle endurance and strength. Education is also a key element of pulmonary rehabilitation. Patients are provided with knowledge regarding the management of their disease, early warning signs of decompensation, and making lifestyle modifications that can enhance their health outcomes. This educational aspect instills a sense of control and self-management, particularly in patients with difficulty in the problematic aspects of COPD (Macleod et al., 2021). Therefore, the inclusion of exercise and education in the pulmonary rehabilitation program is crucial for maximizing health gain. Aside from physical training and education, pulmonary rehabilitation also involves total psychological support. The association between COPD and psychiatric disorders like depression and anxiety has been noted, where studies have indicated poorer health status and increased use of healthcare in patients with such comorbidity. Addressing these issues within the scope of pulmonary rehabilitation can lead to significant improvement in patients' mental well-being, along with disease management. Non-drug interventions like cognitive behavioral therapy can be incorporated within rehabilitation interventions to assist patients in coping with the psychological distress of COPD. The multidimensional nature of these interventions not only alleviates respiratory symptoms but also enhances emotional resilience, ultimately leading to a more comprehensive management of chronic obstructive pulmonary disease (Rahi et al., 2023).

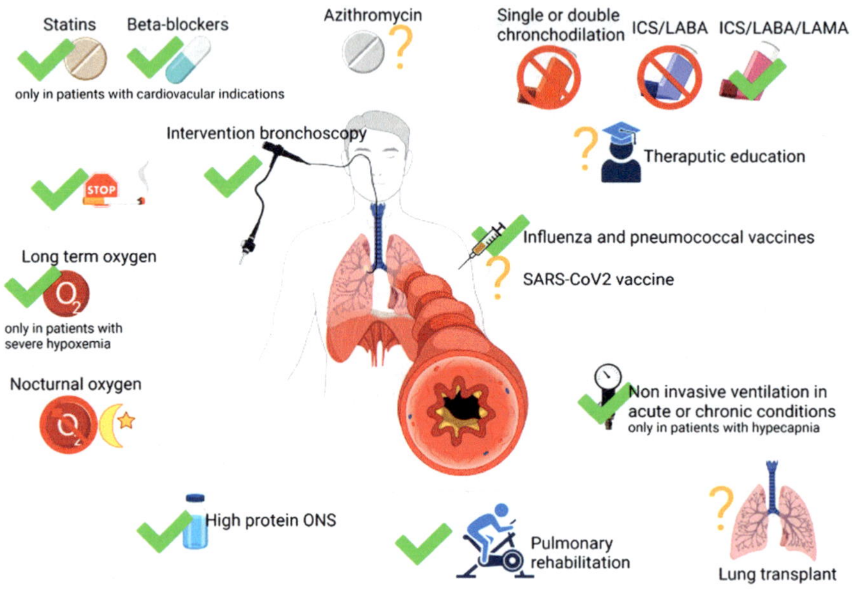

Figure 11.10. Non-pharmacological interventions.

Source: https://ars.els-cdn.com/content/image/1-s2.0-S2590041223000478-gr1.jpg

11.4.3. Surgical Options (Lung Volume Reduction Surgery, Transplantation)

The management of Chronic Obstructive Pulmonary Diseases (COPD) generally consists of surgical interventions, including lung volume reduction surgery (LVRS) and lung transplantation, as primary interventions for severe cases. LVRS is applied only to patients with emphysema, a form of COPD characterized by the destruction of alveoli, leading to defective lung function and breathlessness. LVRS aims to remove involved segments of lung in an effort to enhance the overall mechanics of the respiratory unit, thereby enhancing airflow and allowing for more efficient gas exchange in preserved lung tissue. This procedure, which can be performed using multiple methods such as video-assisted thoracoscopic surgery (VATS), has been effective, particularly for patients who are appropriately selected and for whom standard medical therapies are not successful (Mulryan et al., 2024). Research has revealed that LVRS could be a cost-effective option for treating severe emphysema, and different surgical methods yield varying costs and results. A cost comparison of LVRS from research illustrates VATS-LVRS as the most economical at a mean of €12,896 per patient, and its comparison with bronchoscopic endobronchial valve implantation and robotic LVRS is demonstrated (Mulryan et al., 2024). The financial impact of these surgical procedures is critical to health systems, as they weigh resource allocation against delivering the best patient care. Because LVRS can have a profoundly impactful effect on quality of life, particularly for individuals with severe COPD, its cost implications contribute to informed policy and clinical decisions regarding the provision and utilization of these procedures. Transplantation remains another focal surgery for patients with advanced end-stage COPD, particularly for those whose lung function is severely compromised despite other therapy. Lung transplantation generally provides a second life opportunity for patients with incapacitating symptoms, enabling them to return to normal everyday activities that might otherwise be impossible. However, candidacy for the procedure must be thoroughly evaluated since hazards of transplantation, like rejection and postoperative complications, make multidisciplinary management a necessity. Decision-making should balance the advantages on one side with the risks involved, demanding careful patient selection and adjuvant therapy for an optimal outcome (Opanasenko et al., 2023). Finally, LVRS and lung transplantation are essential procedures in the spectrum of surgical procedures in treating COPD, proving the need for innovation in improving the prognosis and life quality in patients.

Test Your Knowledge

1. What are the pharmacological treatments?
2. What are the non-pharmacological interventions?

11.5. Management of COPD

Learning Outcome

1. Importance of lifestyle changes (smoking cessation, exercise)
2. Role of patient education and self-management
3. Monitoring and follow-up care

Effective management of Chronic Obstructive Pulmonary Disease (COPD) requires a multifaceted approach tailored to the specific circumstances of each patient. At the heart of this is determining the severity of the disease, which will inform the treatment. Spirometry is the tool that clinicians utilize to measure lung function, on the basis of which COPD can be staged. This stratification enables healthcare providers to select appropriate pharmaceutical treatments, such as bronchodilators and corticosteroids, which are crucial for symptom control and the prevention of exacerbations. The individualization of treatment regimens not only improves patient care but also facilitates improved compliance with therapy, underlining the importance of ongoing monitoring and patient education as fundamental components of optimal COPD management. Interventions that engage patients in their own care can significantly enhance quality of life and reduce the burden of this chronic disease. Recent advances in pharmacotherapy highlight the evolving nature of COPD management. With ongoing R&D activity with inhalation treatments, including combination inhalers and long-acting medications, patients can now enjoy more effective and better-tolerated therapies that treat symptoms and improve lung function. These advances highlight the importance of staying current with clinical recommendations, as they continually evolve in response to new evidence. The Global Initiative for Chronic Obstructive Lung Disease (GOLD) periodically updates its reports to address this need, providing clinicians with comprehensive information on the latest therapeutic strategies. New treatment strategies take into account individual patient choice and individual health profiles, such that not only evidence-based but also individualized management strategies are implemented, which is critical to optimize treatment outcomes and patient satisfaction. Beyond pharmacological strategies, non-pharmacological interventions play a crucial role in the overall management of COPD. These interventions also include smoking cessation programs, pulmonary rehabilitation, and lifestyle modifications to enhance overall physical function and respiratory health. Smoking cessation is the most significant intervention for the prevention of worsening of COPD, with proven benefit in morbidity and mortality. Pulmonary rehabilitation programs also enhance exercise tolerance and alleviate symptoms, underscoring the importance of an active patient role in managing their condition. As COPD is a chronic disease, mental health management and the practice of supportive care routines are just as vital. By investigating the implementation of holistic treatment models, medical caregivers can better equip patients to cope with the complexity of living with COPD, leading to improved health outcomes and a better overall quality of life.

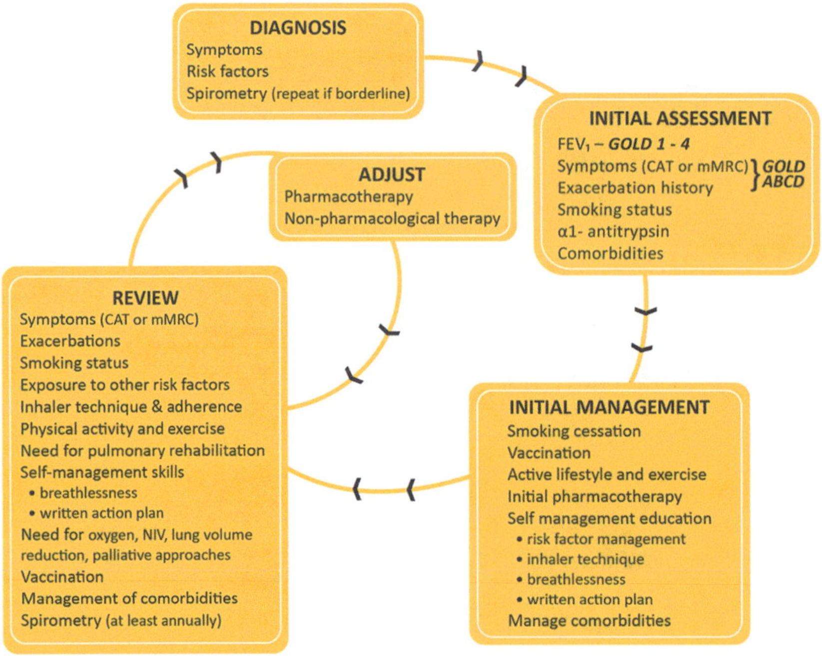

Figure 11.11. Management of COPD.

Source: https://cdn.sanity.io/images/7uf7fwhe/production/a48fde6d14cbe51d1e7e74fb3a6a041da736f4b3-960x840.png

11.5.1. Importance of Lifestyle Changes (Smoking Cessation, Exercise)

Chronic Obstructive Pulmonary Disease (COPD) is a significant health and quality-of-life threat, and thus needs to be managed. Of all the interventions, modifying lifestyle through smoking cessation and increased physical activity is the most important among the essential interventions. The major etiologic factor for COPD is smoking, and smoking cessation can slow disease progression considerably and improve pulmonary function. Studies consistently show that former smokers enjoy better health than the smoking population. Additionally, smoking cessation not only makes the progression of the disease worsen further, but also renders pharmacological treatment more effective. Hence, control of smoking behavior is most crucial in COPD management strategy, since the advantages do not just end at symptom relief but also involve long-term stabilization of the disease and improved overall well-being. Apart from quitting smoking, physical exercise plays an integral part in the treatment of COPD. Exercise enhances the function of respiratory muscles, enhances exercise tolerance, and reduces symptoms of dyspnea. Tailored exercise programs enhance patients' functional status and quality of life to a significant level. Evidence has shown that COPD patients who undergo proper exercise programs experience less breathlessness with exertion and can cope better with the disease's limitations. Physical activity also provides COPD patients with a sense of independence and empowerment, so they actively contribute to taking care of themselves. By integrating exercise into their practice, patients can reap appreciable benefits, making it an essential component of COPD's holistic management. More than individual health outcomes, the significance of lifestyle change applies to public health as well. Large-scale lifestyle interventions, such as cessation of smoking and exercise, can decrease the medical burden of COPD. Pre-existing ESC guidelines, implementation of these strategies is among the improvements of patient outcomes and prevention of hospitalization for the exacerbation of COPD (Visseren et al., 2021). It is recommended that healthcare providers incorporate these lifestyle changes into care plans, enabling patients to maintain long-term improvements in their health. Aside from that, public or community interventions to improve awareness regarding smoking risks and exercise may lead to decreased prevalence of COPD. Lastly, by endorsing lifestyle modification, the medical community can be a significant force in enhancing the quality of life for COPD patients, while also addressing broader population health concerns (Lyon et al., 2022).

11.5.2. Role of Patient Education and Self-Management

Effective patient education, then, is key to the management of Chronic Obstructive Pulmonary Disease (COPD) with substantial influence on an individual's ability to engage in self-management. With enhanced knowledge regarding the disease and its impact, educational programs can help patients recognize their symptoms, comply with proper medication, and understand the need for lifestyle modification. Evidently, participation in structured self-management programs significantly improves the quality of life, functional status, and mental well-being of patients. For instance, a randomized controlled trial found that patients receiving self-management-focused education revealed statistically significant improvements on selected patient-reported outcomes, for instance, depression and anxiety levels, relative to usual care (Tsaousi et al., 2024). This highlights the need for comprehensive educational interventions to be integrated into the care continuum for patients with COPD. The relevance of individually tailored educational interventions is based on their ability to address specific knowledge deficits and adapt to a range of disease severity. Evidence demonstrates that individuals with a history of exacerbations have increased levels of awareness of critical domains, such as symptom identification and when to refer to healthcare providers. These results suggest a linear association between the severity of disease and the effectiveness of educational interventions in enhancing vital self-management skills. Specifically, knowledge about exacerbation recognition improved notably in patients with moderate-to-severe COPD, highlighting the need for education to be responsive and relevant to the patient's own experience (Fischer et al., 2024).

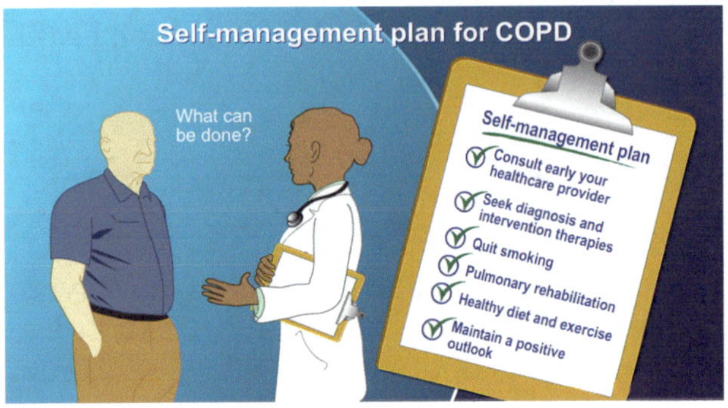

Figure 11.12. Self-management plan for COPD.

Source: https://www.animatedCOPDpatient.com/en-COPD/content.ashx?file=COPD01/slides/m1_slide_12.jpg

Therefore, medical professionals must prioritize the development of patient-specific learning materials that appeal to patients' needs, aiming to promote autonomy in managing their condition. Multidimensionality in patient education encompasses not only the provision of information but also the development of self-management skills, enabling patients to take proactive action in their health management. This approach includes educating patients in skills such as controlled breathing exercises, the proper use of inhalers, and drug regimens. Furthermore, there is a need for an environment of supportive healthcare in which patients feel comfortable exchanging information about their disease care. Effective communication between patients and health providers is also necessary, as it enables patients to report matters of concern and fear regarding their condition. Lastly, as evidenced by other studies, enhancing patient education and empowering self-management has been shown to induce greater health outcomes, reduced healthcare utilization, and increased patient satisfaction, providing a rationale for an interprofessional model of healthcare in COPD practice (Tsaousi et al., 2024).

11.5.3. Monitoring and Follow-Up Care

Optimal follow-up treatment and monitoring are the most significant aspects in the management of Chronic Obstructive Pulmonary Disease (COPD). Monitoring enables doctors to detect changes in a patient's condition at an early stage, thereby facilitating the provision of timely interventions. Follow-up visits should be based on regular assessments of lung function through spirometry, as well as the observation of symptoms such as dyspnea and cough. These tests facilitate individualized treatment regimens as well as the identification of complications that may occur. Moreover, the use of patient-reported outcome measures can enhance the understanding of a patient's functional status and quality of life, thus enabling the development of personalized care plans. The use of prescribed follow-up care regimens not only optimizes therapeutic benefit but also enhances patient engagement, resulting in active management of their condition by the patients. Pharmacotherapy titration according to follow-up evaluation is necessary to optimize treatment in COPD patients. Patients will, as time passes, develop exacerbations of their condition that will necessitate a re-assessment of their drug therapy. According to clinical guidelines, the management of COPD exacerbations can include the initiation or intensification of pharmacotherapy, such as bronchodilators and corticosteroids, based on the severity of the exacerbation. Infection with bacteria is typically tracked to guide prescribing behavior, under which the clinician must be judicious in the use of antibiotics. For instance, in the case of acute exacerbations involving bacterial infections, recommendations postulate the truncation of antibiotic therapy to five days if specific clinical presentations are observed (Rachael A Lee et al., 2021). This move aims to limit the overuse of antibiotics while addressing antimicrobial resistance issues, and to ensure effective treatment of COPD exacerbations. In addition to medication therapy, follow-up care must include education and support interventions for patients with COPD. Smoking cessation and pulmonary rehabilitation are key to long-term disease management through lifestyle changes. Monitoring these non-pharmacological therapies on a regular basis helps assess their efficacy and adherence, resulting in improved overall health. Healthcare professionals may also utilize telemedicine as part of follow-up treatment, particularly for patients with mobility issues or those residing in remote areas. Telemedicine consultations can be suitable for continued contact and proper, timely adjustment of the care regimen. Through the incorporation of an integrated approach that combines both clinical evaluation and patient education, health professionals can maximize the treatment of COPD and substantially improve patients' quality of life.

Test Your Knowledge

1. What is the role of patient education and self-management?
2. What is monitoring and follow-up care?

11.6. Impact of COPD On Quality of Life

Learning Outcome

1. Physical limitations and daily activities
2. Psychological effects and mental health considerations
3. Economic burden and healthcare costs

The effect of chronic obstructive pulmonary disease (COPD) on quality of life cannot be stressed enough, as it certainly alters the various facets of daily living in individuals affected by the same. Many patients with COPD experience restrictions in physical activities, and this can lead to physical inactivity. The reduction in mobility, coupled with the chronic breathlessness that is characteristic of the condition, results in an intense sense of frustration and powerlessness. Therefore, most patients report a decline in their emotional well-being, and they end up becoming anxious and depressed as they grapple with the limitations that accompany their illness. Apart from undermining their interpersonal relations, this emotional burden even disrupts social activity, as they feel lonelier. Studies have established that the quality of life of undiagnosed COPD patients is quite diminished, as such patients experience more difficulty with their health status compared to those diagnosed with COPD (Gerstein et al., 2023). Moreover, the impact of COPD extends to occupational domains, e.g., job productivity and employment in the workplace. Most patients experience symptoms that are detrimental to their ability to perform at their previous work level, resulting in increased absenteeism and impaired professional performance. The economic impact is considerable since loss of work productivity not only results in individual financial costs but also maximizes the cost to healthcare systems regarding attempting to meet the increased demand for medical care and treatment. Chronic worsening, the hallmark that is common to COPD, adds only to the scenario by promoting hospitalizations that can disrupt the work schedule of a patient and add to financial burdens further (Hurst et al., 2020). Since the workforce cannot balance health needs with work needs, the quality of life is compromised, leading to a vicious cycle of worsening symptoms and escalating socioeconomic demands. The interplay of physical restriction and emotional health is indicative of the multifaceted impact of COPD on quality of life. Since the mere task of breathing is so strenuous, subjects will learn to live with the different self that could be void of prior interests or passions. The psychosocial impact of chronic disease is enormous and may lead to hopelessness as patients accept the reality of permanent disability. Coping with these demands requires a collaborative approach incorporating medical management, psychological counseling, and community interventions, which enhance social support. This holistic method not only addresses the physiological aspects of COPD but also acknowledges the psychosocial and emotional effects the disease has on patients. By understanding these interacting variables, we can begin developing more suitable intervention programs that aim to improve the overall quality of life for individuals with COPD (Gerstein et al., 2023).

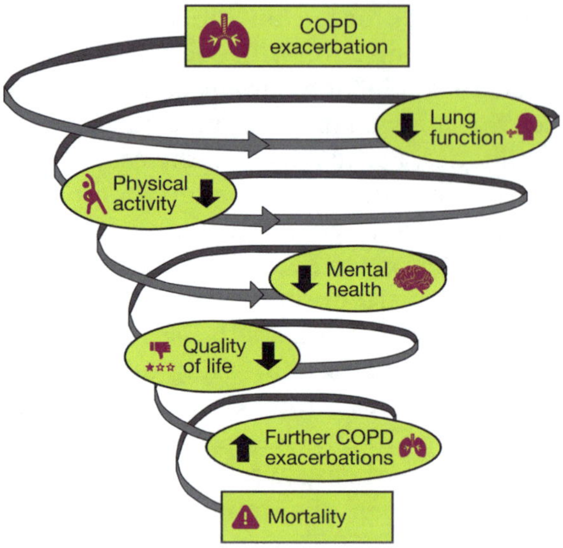

Figure 11.13. Impact of COPD on quality of life.

Source: https://www.ejinme.com/cms/10.1016/j.ejim.2019.12.014/asset/bcbaac53-ce05-4889-a4c3-fd8730ac7df3/main.assets/gr2_lrg.jpg

11.6.1. Physical Limitations and Daily Activities

Physical disability in COPD patients has a significant influence on the performance of activities of daily living. The debut and recurrent manifestation of COPD, such as dyspnea and fatigue, is likely to limit patients from achieving activities that were previously tolerable for them. Thereafter, patients risk experiencing reduced engagement in social, recreational, and occupational activities, and thus lose some aspects of their quality of life. Moreover, the chronic state of such physical impairments initiates a cycle of decreased physical activity, aggravation of respiratory signs and symptoms, and further debilitation. This dynamic interaction between limited physical capacity and daily tasking justifies the importance of understanding how COPD not only affects lung function but also affects the quality of life of people with COPD. Activities of Daily Living (ADL), such as fundamental needs like bathing, dressing, and cooking, are typically significantly compromised by COPD. The patients report greater challenge in these everyday functions, which can instill dependency and frustration. Tools such as the London Chest Activity Daily Living (LCADL) scale provide feedback about the patients' self-estimated capability to manage ADL in the framework of their respiratory illness. A decrease in their ability to execute everyday tasks can cumulate a feeling of isolation and powerlessness, further exacerbating mental illness issues such as those around chronic disease. By identifying the specific activities that are problematic, healthcare professionals can structure interventions that enable patients to regain autonomy and improve their quality of life (Karande et al., 2024). Pulmonary rehabilitation is now a well-established cornerstone treatment for enhancing the daily functioning of patients with COPD. Studies indicate that standardized rehabilitation programs not only enhance physical capacity and symptom reduction but also improve overall quality of life. For instance, while recording the positive outcomes of such therapy, a recent study found significant score improvement in LCADL, lung function, and exercise capacity after an 8-week duration pulmonary rehabilitation program. Patients also reported an enhanced ability to carry out domestic work and physical activity, demonstrating the groundbreaking potential of dedicated therapy on their lifestyle. Hence, overcoming physical constraints through systematic intervention not only aligns with the management of the physiological function of COPD but also involves the engagement of patients in purposeful activities, affirming the hypothesis that more enhanced lung health is directly related to an improved daily experience (Karande et al., 2024).

11.6.2. Psychological Effects and Mental Health Considerations

The psychological effect of chronic obstructive pulmonary disease (COPD) extends beyond the disease's physical manifestations, significantly affecting the mental health of the individual. Depression and anxiety are common comorbidities that develop due to the inevitable fear of deterioration and limitation on physical activity. Being unable to engage in previously enjoyable activities may result in social withdrawal, culminating in a vicious cycle of hopelessness and poor quality of life. Also, the uncertainty of disease progression is a problem that patients can struggle with, which may leave them even more helpless. Addressing these psychological issues is essential, not just because they complicate daily functioning, but also because they impair effective control of the disease itself. Thus, healthcare providers must take the initiative in the assessment of mental health status and integrating psychological care into the overall treatment plan for COPD patients. Effective coping strategies and mental health care are essential to manage the psychological load of COPD. Cognitive-behavioral therapy (CBT) has proven effective in equipping patients with coping skills to reinterpret thoughts, reducing depression and anxiety symptoms. Support groups can also offer significant social support, encouraging feelings of belonging among individuals who share similar issues. Such social interaction can reduce feelings of loneliness and enhance coping mechanisms. Furthermore, physicians must start treating the patient's mental health problem early in therapy. By utilizing a combined psychological and physical approach from the beginning, physicians can anticipate improved compliance with therapy and better outcomes. Thus, both clinical and psychological care must be considered as two sides of a comprehensive COPD care package. Lastly, the broader social ramifications of the psychological impact of COPD cannot be overlooked. Caregiving families typically have a heavy emotional burden, which in turn adds to increased risk factors for their own mental health conditions, like caregiver burnout and depression. This was particularly the case with the COVID-19 pandemic, which intensified feelings of stress and anxiety in patients and caregivers alike. With the value of unpaid caregiving estimated at $339.5 billion in 2022, the financial burdens of mental illness percolate outward from the individual to affect health care systems and society broadly. Solutions to these domains require policy shifts in healthcare at the systemic level, as well as increased resources for mental health care. Through the availability of such programs for caregivers and the integration of mental health care into COPD treatment models, it is possible to ease some of the severe psychological effects endured by individuals with this chronic condition, as well as those who take care of them.

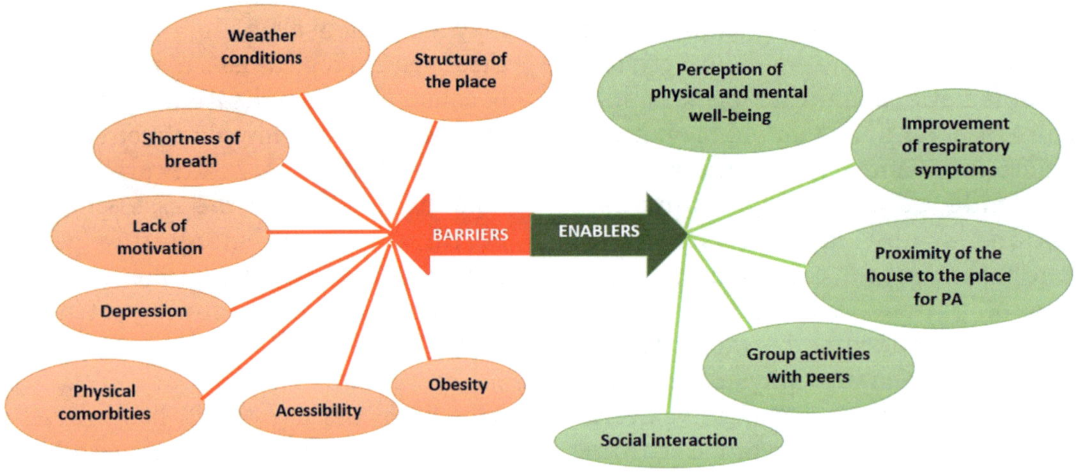

Figure 11.14. Psychological effects and mental health considerations of COPD.

Source: https://media.springernature.com/lw685/springer-static/image/art%3A10.1038%2Fs41533-024-00386-7/MediaObjects/41533_2024_386_Fig3_HTML.png

11.6.3. Economic Burden and Healthcare Costs

Chronic Obstructive Pulmonary Disease (COPD) is a substantial economic burden, significantly affecting not only health systems but also the productivity of society. Prevalence of COPD, coupled with its multi-modal treatment requirements, has led to escalating healthcare expenditure across the board. Exacerbating patients are hospitalized, which not only drives direct medical costs through acute services but also manifests in longer-term fiscal effects through ongoing drug needs and rehabilitation services. The cumulative impact of these expenses also underscores a compelling need for strategic healthcare policy initiatives that would seek to contain and minimize the cost of COPD, such that resources are efficiently channeled towards maximizing patient outcomes. Moreover, an analysis of the economic impacts of COPD is critical in emphasizing the importance of preventive measures for reducing disease rates and control costs in the long term, since such measures can lead to astronomical savings by the health care system as well as patients. The economic impact of COPD extends beyond direct healthcare expenditures, having significant effects on workforce productivity and the economy as a whole. Illness absenteeism and diminished work capacity can result in high business loss to employers and become a factor in decreased national economic output. The trend is particularly alarming since the number of elderly persons at risk of COPD continues to grow. Air pollution has also exacerbated the severity of diseases, adding to the burden of illnesses and increasing healthcare costs associated with respiratory ailments, including COPD. As noted in recent research, regional differences are significant about air pollution and related healthcare expenses linked to respiratory disease, indicating that more polluted states face disproportionate economic issues due to health factors. Understanding these economic factors is crucial in designing specific public policies, not just addressing the problem of air quality but also reducing the healthcare economic burden of chronic illnesses like COPD (Ahmed et al., 2025). Investing in preventive healthcare and early interventions can go a long way in reducing the economic costs of COPD. Widespread smoking cessation programs, environmental management, and public education can potentially lower the number of exacerbations of COPD and hospitalizations. Furthermore, effective management of chronic obstructive pulmonary disease through patient-tailored treatment strategies can lower the rate of acute exacerbations, which contribute to higher costs. Recent analysis has shown that states with extensive public health initiatives experienced reduced healthcare spending, as well as improved health outcomes for patients with COPD. By prioritizing prevention and improving air quality, policymakers can not only mitigate the healthcare costs associated with COPD but also reduce the economic costs resulting from decreased workforce productivity. Lastly, addressing the economic strain of COPD requires a multidisciplinary approach that involves healthcare professionals, policymakers, and society as a whole, thus necessitating the consideration of both the health and economic implications of this pressing healthcare issue (Alexander et al., 2025).

Test Your Knowledge

1. What are the physical limitations?
2. What are the psychological effects and mental health considerations?

SUMMARY

The management of Chronic Obstructive Pulmonary Diseases (COPD) is demanding, particularly in maintaining patient adherence to therapeutics. The success in applying inhaled corticosteroids and long-acting β2 agonists (ICS/LABA) demonstrates what can be accomplished in optimizing patient outcomes. However, a retrospective cohort study revealed that non-adherence continues to be a problem because only a small percentage of patients maintained their medication regimen as prescribed after one year of treatment initiation (Czira et al., 2024). The findings reveal that while primary treatment may prove beneficial, long-term success hinges on continued participation and adherence by patients, again advocating for improved methods in patient education and support. Furthermore, socioeconomic status bears directly upon COPD patient compliance rates. It has been demonstrated that there is poorer compliance among patients from lower socioeconomic backgrounds, and this correlates with poorer health outcomes. These results have essential implications insofar as they make a case for healthcare providers to tailor care based on patients' socioeconomic status (Basnet et al., 2024). Through understanding of such dynamics, treatment can be designed not only to cure medical disease but also to address socioeconomic problems faced by patients, potentially to achieve long-term health care better. At the end of the day, addressing COPD's complexity involves a multifaceted approach that includes pharmacologic therapy, patient education, and awareness of socioeconomic factors. The studies reviewed reveal significant discrepancies in intervention efficacy and adherence, underscoring the urgent need for systematic change in how healthcare systems manage COPD. Patient involvement in individualized treatment plans and support mechanisms can lead to better rates of adherence, lower exacerbations, and overall quality of life. This holistic response is crucial in confronting the chronic character of COPD and improving the health of individuals with this disabling condition.

The controversy surrounding COPD has raised a few significant aspects crucial in determining the cause and effects of the disease. One considerable aspect is maternal health in the development of COPD among children. It has been conclusively proven that mothers who smoke during pregnancy increase the risk of COPD among children. Specifically, findings from a Mendelian randomization analysis revealed a very high odds ratio, illustrating that maternal smoking at birth enhances the risk of COPD in children (IVW, $OR=35.13$; $p<0.001$). Additionally, after adjusting for maternal illnesses, the association remained very strong, reinforcing the influence of maternal behaviors and environmental exposures in early life and their long-term impacts on respiratory outcomes (Jian et al., 2025). Alongside maternal factors, the interaction of COPD with autoimmune diseases must be considered. There is evidence from studies that a causal relationship may exist between COPD and several autoimmune diseases, and this reveals a network of comorbidities that complicates COPD management. While the original Mendelian analysis was unable to create a causative correlation of importance between COPD and autoimmune diseases, reverse Mendelian randomization identified relevant correlations of magnitude between rheumatoid arthritis and osteoarthritis as risk factors for the onset of COPD. Exactly, the odds ratio indicates a high risk, with an OR of 377.313 for rheumatoid arthritis, necessitating a combined clinical approach to manage COPD patients (Yu et al., 2024). Implications of such findings are multi-pronged, including the necessity of a complete awareness of the determinants of COPD. This includes not only maternal and genetic determinants but also the influence of concomitant autoimmune conditions. Clinicians need to be aware of such correlations to enhance patient care and implement early interventions. Moreover, population-level prevention measures to reduce maternal smoking may have long-term effects on the respiratory health of generations to come. In any case, the salient features highlighted create a complex interdependence of environmental, genetic, and autoimmune factors in the etiopathogenesis of COPD, which requires an interdepartmental approach to research as well as treatment.

KEY TERMS FROM THIS CHAPTER

- Chronic bronchitis
- Airflow limitation
- Alpha-1 antitrypsin deficiency
- Mucus hypersecretion
- Alveolar destruction
- Barrel chest
- Chronic cough
- Pulmonary hypertension
- Exacerbations
- FEV1/FVC ratio
- Emphysema
- Smoking
- Chronic inflammation
- Bronchial wall thickening
- Air trapping
- Dyspnea
- Sputum production
- Cor pulmonale
- Spirometry
- Bronchodilators

CRITICAL THINKING QUESTIONS

1. Which of the following conditions is the most common cause of COPD?

a. Tuberculosis

b. Smoking

c. Occupational exposure to asbestos

d. Allergic reactions

2. COPD is characterized by which of the following pathophysiological changes?

a. Reversible airway obstruction

b. Irreversible airflow limitation

c. Alveolar over-inflation only

d. Predominantly restrictive lung defect

3. Which spirometry finding is typical of COPD?

a. Increased FEV_1/FVC ratio

b. Decreased FEV_1 and decreased $FEV_1/$ FVC ratio

c. Normal FEV_1 with decreased FVC

d. Increased total lung capacity with increased FEV_1

4. Which type of COPD is characterized by "pink puffers"?

a. Chronic bronchitis

b. Emphysema

c. Asthma

d. Bronchiectasis

5. Which of the following is a typical clinical feature of chronic bronchitis?

a. Dyspnea without cough

b. Chronic productive cough for at least 3 months in 2 consecutive years

c. Acute onset of chest pain

d. Weight loss and cachexia

Short Answer Questions

1. What are the two main conditions classified under COPD?
2. What is the primary risk factor for developing COPD?
3. Describe the characteristic airflow limitation seen in COPD.
4. What is the significance of the FEV1/FVC ratio in diagnosing COPD?
5. Name two common symptoms of COPD.

Answer to Critical Thinking Questions

1. (b) 2. (b) 3. (b) 4. (b) 5. (b)

REFERENCES

1. Azaman, N. M., Ghafar, N. A., Azhar, A., Fauzi, A. A., Ismail, H. A., Idrus, S. S. S., Mokhjar, S. S., & Hamid, F. A. (2018). Investigation of concrete floor vibration using Heel-Drop test. *Journal of Physics Conference Series, 995*, 012027. https://doi.org/10.1088/1742-6596/995/1/012027
2. Ahmed, K. M., Salih, A. M., Raoof, B. K., Ahmed, T. N., Mohammed, B. A., Yaqub, K. Q., Ali, R. A., et al. (2025). Economic burden of air pollution and healthcare costs for respiratory diseases in the United States of America. *International Journal of Scientific Research and Modern Technology*. https://www.semanticscholar.org/paper/9dc9c7ac7774b2870530b513ce0a4001b9a92e3c (accessed on 16th June 2025).
3. Alexander, B. D., Bresnik, M., Anupindi, R., Pizzicato, L., DeKoven, M., Lovelace, B., Coleman, C. I., et al. (2025). P-1010. Clinical and economic burden of changing initial antifungal regimens in invasive aspergillosis: A hospital perspective. *Open Forum Infectious Diseases, 12.* https://www.semanticscholar.org/paper/09142a38398de9f9340cc195609a5717138281b4 (accessed on 16th June 2025).
4. Alzheimer's Association. (2023). 2023 Alzheimer's disease facts and figures. *Alzheimer's & Dementia, 19*, 1598–1695. https://doi.org/10.1002/alz.13016 (accessed on 16th June 2025).
5. Amaducci, S., Bacci, E., Baldacci, S., Bartoli, et al. (2018). Inhalation therapy in the next decade: Determinants of adherence to treatment in asthma and COPD. https://core.ac.uk/download/152415584.pdf (accessed on 16th June 2025).
6. Ban, W., & Rhee, C. (2022). Role of nuclear factor erythroid 2–related factor 2 in chronic obstructive pulmonary disease. *Tuberculosis and Respiratory Diseases, 85*, 221–226. https://www.semanticscholar.org/paper/0b2c8cfbe7a9bdcbd982937bccefdd7c90ba45a8 (accessed on 16th June 2025).
7. Basnet, S., Vijaya, Y., Durga, S., Yadav, K., Adhikari, S., & Sijina, K. S. (2024). Effects of socioeconomic and clinical factors on treatment adherence in patients with chronic obstructive pulmonary diseases patient: Focus on inhalation therapy. *Asian Journal of Pharmaceutical and Clinical Research*. https://www.semanticscholar.org/paper/63cf08f666dd0607276bc59a82125f99f92f2a8a (accessed on 16th June 2025).
8. Bobowicz, M., Jassem, E., & Jassem-Bobowicz, J. M. (2009). Advanced chronic obstructive pulmonary disease (COPD). https://core.ac.uk/download/268447669.pdf (accessed on 16th June 2025).
9. Cacciottolo, J. (2013). Lung health and outdoor air pollution: A review. https://core.ac.uk/download/83019957.pdf (accessed on 16th June 2025).
10. Choi, J. Y., Song, J., & Rhee, C. (2022). Chronic obstructive pulmonary disease combined with interstitial lung disease. *Tuberculosis and Respiratory Diseases, 85*, 122–136. https://www.semanticscholar.org/paper/137c20cbe478c7676f655fded1c7986130d24f48 (accessed on 16th June 2025).
11. Chukmaitov, A., Deng, Y., Lin, S. Y., et al. (2020). Multi-morbidities are not a driving factor for an increase of COPD-related 30-day readmission risk. https://core.ac.uk/download/323474274.pdf (accessed on 16th June 2025).
12. Conti, V., De Marchis, L., Graziani, C., et al. (2016). Blood and sputum biomarkers in COPD and asthma: A review. https://core.ac.uk/download/159268735.pdf (accessed on 16th June 2025).

13. Czira, A., Banks, V., Requena, G., Wood, R., Tritton, T., Wild, R., Compton, C., et al. (2024). Treatment pathways, economic burden and clinical outcomes in new users of inhaled corticosteroid/long-acting B2-agonist dual therapy with chronic obstructive pulmonary disease in a primary care setting in England: A retrospective cohort study. *BMJ Open, 14.* https://www.semanticscholar.org/paper/d5a6645594ff48bc58f8c7dfdaaf473a67a87c01 (accessed on 16th June 2025).

14. Dos Santos, N. C., Camelier, A., Menezes, A. K., Cavalcanti de Almeida, V. D., Maciel, R. B. T., & Camelier, F. W. R. (2024). Effects of the use of beta-blockers on chronic obstructive pulmonary disease associated with cardiovascular comorbidities: Systematic review and meta-analysis. *Tuberculosis and Respiratory Diseases, 87*, 261–281. https://www.semanticscholar.org/paper/15cee4b0f85d64bf5f3d341bfba19cb3846cb615 (accessed on 16th June 2025).

15. Fischer, C., Siakavara, M., Alter, P., Vogelmeier, C., Speicher, T., Pott, H., Watz, H., et al. (2024). Association of patients' knowledge on the disease and its management with indicators of disease severity and individual characteristics in patients with chronic obstructive pulmonary disease (COPD): Results from COSYCONET 2. *Patient Preference and Adherence, 18*, 2383–2393. https://www.semanticscholar.org/paper/21c3c9b5734783433a1bedfb471bb42a108c1f9b (accessed on 16th June 2025).

16. Gerstein, E., Bierbrier, J., Whitmore, G. À., Vandemheen, K. L., Bergeron, C., Boulet, L. P., Côté, A., et al. (2023). Impact of undiagnosed chronic obstructive pulmonary disease and asthma on symptoms, quality of life, healthcare use, and work productivity. *American Journal of Respiratory and Critical Care Medicine, 208*, 1271–1282. https://doi.org/10.1164/rccm.202307-1264oc (accessed on 16th June 2025).

17. Gogou, E., Kotsiou, O. S., Siachpazidou, D., Pinaka, M., Varsamas, C., Bardaka, F., Gerogianni, I., et al. (2021). Underestimation of respiratory symptoms by smokers: A thorn in chronic obstructive pulmonary disease diagnosis. *npj Primary Care Respiratory Medicine, 31.* https://doi.org/10.1038/s41533-021-00226-y (accessed on 16th June 2025).

18. Gordon, M., Gangemi, A., Sandwith, E., Kumaran, M., & Kueppers, F. (2025). Vascular pathology in alpha 1 antitrypsin deficient chronic obstructive pulmonary disease and emphysema patients: Case reports. *The Application of Clinical Genetics, 18*, 1–7. https://www.semanticscholar.org/paper/437d2be6a1a3154aa007004439b55e2709dd49d9 (accessed on 16th June 2025).

19. Hagan, G. W., Jones, P. W., Onishi, K., Yoshimoto, K., et al. (2014). Prevalence of airflow limitation in outpatients with cardiovascular diseases in Japan. https://core.ac.uk/download/29469357.pdf (accessed on 16th June 2025).

20. Halpin, D., Criner, G. J., Papi, A., Singh, D., Anzueto, A., Martínez, F. J., Agustí, A. A., et al. (2020). Global initiative for the diagnosis, management, and prevention of chronic obstructive lung disease. The 2020 GOLD Science Committee Report on COVID-19 and chronic obstructive pulmonary disease. *American Journal of Respiratory and Critical Care Medicine, 203*, 24–36. https://doi.org/10.1164/rccm.202009-3533so (accessed on 16th June 2025).

21. Hanania, N. A., & Celli, B. (2024). Phosphodiesterase inhibition as a therapeutic strategy for chronic obstructive pulmonary disease: Where we have been and what lies ahead. *Chronic Obstructive Pulmonary Diseases.* https://www.semanticscholar.org/paper/3eb301ce8ce61c43793b8953973446ca5e6ed93d (accessed on 16th June 2025).

22. Hurst, J. R., Skolnik, N., Hansen, G. J., Anzueto, A., Donaldson, G. C., Dransfield, M. T., & Varghese, P. (2020). Understanding the impact of chronic obstructive pulmonary disease exacerbations on patient health and quality of life. *European Journal of Internal Medicine, 73*, 1–6. https://doi.org/10.1016/j.ejim.2019.12.014 (accessed on 16th June 2025).

23. International Meetings and Science (IMsci). (2024). Heterogeneity of inflammatory processes and pathways driving chronic obstructive pulmonary disease pathology. *EMJ Respiratory*. https://www.semanticscholar.org/paper/4c22d485501061b5e5e3d4700baf20f3bb8aa0c8 (accessed on 16th June 2025).

24. Ismailov, I., Kalmatov, R., Abdurakhmanov, B., Mirza, A. M., & Chaurasia, J. K. (2024). Role of reactive oxygen species in the pathogenesis of bronchial asthma and obstructive pulmonary diseases: Systematic review. *Advancements in Life Sciences*. https://www.semanticscholar.org/paper/12db5d56d2173e630f851f6a91a0351f01494b25 (accessed on 16th June 2025).

25. James, S. L., Abate, D., Abate, K. H., Abay, S. M., Abbafati, C., Abbasi, N., Abbastabar, H., et al. (2018). Global, regional, and national incidence, prevalence, and years lived with disability for 354 diseases and injuries for 195 countries and territories, 1990–2017: A systematic analysis for the Global Burden of Disease Study 2017. *The Lancet, 392*, 1789–1858. https://doi.org/10.1016/s0140-6736(18)32279-7 (accessed on 16th June 2025).

26. Jian, Q., Huo, H., Mu, F., & Wang, F. (2025). Maternal smoking around birth as a risk factor for offspring chronic obstructive pulmonary disease: Evidence from Mendelian randomization. *Tobacco Induced Diseases, 23*. https://www.semanticscholar.org/paper/0f4a3afcba124d4c9cfe1cd31142b9616b378133 (accessed on 16th June 2025).

27. Jörres, R. A., Kellberger, J., Kotschy-Lang, N., Nowak, D., et al. (2012). Long-term efficacy of pulmonary rehabilitation in patients with occupational respiratory diseases. https://core.ac.uk/download/16432253.pdf (accessed on 16th June 2025).

28. Karande, B., Gosavi, N., & Godse, A. (2024). Impact of pulmonary rehabilitation on lung functions and quality of life in chronic respiratory disease patients. *IP Indian Journal of Immunology and Respiratory Medicine.* https://www.semanticscholar.org/paper/403e5d0c4db27c81d18335c1d91fd3507d12649f (accessed on 16th June 2025).

29. Kim, W. I., Pak, S. W., Lee, S. J., Park, S. H., Lim, J. O., Kim, D. I., Shin, I., et al. (2024). Copper oxide nanoparticles exacerbate chronic obstructive pulmonary disease by activating the TXNIP-NLRP3 signaling pathway. *Particle and Fibre Toxicology, 21*. https://www.semanticscholar.org/paper/c3558232f5099ecf1d0ea519b9076b90b2338bcf (accessed on 16th June 2025).

30. Kita, K., Gawinowska, M., Chełmińska, M., & Niedoszytko, M. (2024). The role of exhaled breath condensate in chronic inflammatory and neoplastic diseases of the respiratory tract. *International Journal of Molecular Sciences, 25*. https://www.semanticscholar.org/paper/394b20d0941057f155a8b8dda402f377fc7816e6 (accessed on 16th June 2025).

31. Kwok, W. C., Tam, T. C. C., Sing, C., Chan, E. W., & Cheung, C. L. (2024). Validation of diagnostic coding for chronic obstructive pulmonary disease in an electronic health record system in Hong Kong. *Hong Kong Medical Journal = Xianggang Yi Xue Za Zhi*. https://www.semanticscholar.org/paper/58563b2b40c79039b8563452a72100b859c1e846 (accessed on 16th June 2025).

32. Lee, R. A., Centor, R. M., Humphrey, L. L., Jokela, J. A., Andrews, R., & Qaseem, A. (2021). Appropriate use of short-course antibiotics in common infections: Best practice advice from

the American College of Physicians. *Annals of Internal Medicine, 174*, 822–827. https://doi.org/10.7326/m20-7355 (accessed on 16th June 2025).

33. Lu, R., Xu, K., Qin, Y., Shao, X., Yan, M., Liao, Y., Wang, B., et al. (2022). Network pharmacology and experimental validation to reveal effects and mechanisms of icariin combined with nobiletin against chronic obstructive pulmonary diseases. *Evidence-Based Complementary and Alternative Medicine: eCAM, 2022*. https://www.semanticscholar.org/paper/df3632044b28a3d76919039668fde4d668739b95 (accessed on 16th June 2025).

34. Lyon, A. R., López-Fernández, T., Couch, L. S., Asteggiano, R., Aznar, M. C., Bergler-Klein, J., Boriani, G., et al. (2022). 2022 ESC Guidelines on cardio-oncology developed in collaboration with the European Hematology Association (EHA), the European Society for Therapeutic Radiology and Oncology (ESTRO) and the International Cardio-Oncology Society (IC-OS). *European Heart Journal, 43*, 4229–4361. https://doi.org/10.1093/eurheartj/ehac244 (accessed on 16th June 2025).

35. Macleod, M., Papi, A., Contoli, M., Beghè, B., Celli, B. R., Wedzicha, J. A., & Fabbri, L. M. (2021). Chronic obstructive pulmonary disease exacerbation fundamentals: Diagnosis, treatment, prevention and disease impact. *Respirology, 26*, 532–551. https://doi.org/10.1111/resp.14041 (accessed on 16th June 2025).

36. Marks, G. (2025). Monitoring pulmonary rehabilitation and long-term oxygen therapy for people with chronic obstructive pulmonary disease (COPD). https://core.ac.uk/download/pdf/30675577.pdf (accessed on 16th June 2025).

37. Mazzone, P. J., & Lam, L. (2022). Evaluating the patient with a pulmonary nodule. *JAMA, 327*, 264–264. https://doi.org/10.1001/jama.2021.24287 (accessed on 16th June 2025).

38. Monsó, E., & Reidl, J. (2015). Glucocorticoids and antibiotics, how do they get together? https://core.ac.uk/download/328839801.pdf (accessed on 16th June 2025).

39. Mulryan, K., Sorensen, J., Waller, D., & Redmond, K. (2024). Lung volume reduction surgery: A micro-costing analysis from a national tertiary referral center. *European Journal of Cardio-Thoracic Surgery: Official Journal of the European Association for Cardio-Thoracic Surgery*. https://www.semanticscholar.org/paper/b37e64c9d5f38cee74882babfde073b3b18bee44 (accessed on 16th June 2025).

40. Opanasenko, M., Konik, B., Tereshkovych, O., Stepaniuk, A. M., Levanda, L., Bychkovskyi, V., Shalagay, S., et al. (2023). Lung volume reduction surgery (clinical cases). *Tuberculosis, Lung Diseases, HIV Infection*. https://www.semanticscholar.org/paper/6df5e87b9ff73a3d5edc605bb39b672876dd4d21 (accessed on 16th June 2025).

41. Rahi, M. S., Thilagar, B., Balaji, S., Prabhakaran, S. Y., Mudgal, M., Rajoo, S., Yella, P. R., et al. (2023). The impact of anxiety and depression in chronic obstructive pulmonary disease. *Advances in Respiratory Medicine, 91*, 123–134. https://doi.org/10.3390/arm91020011 (accessed on 16th June 2025).

42. Rutkowski, S. (2021). Management challenges in chronic obstructive pulmonary disease in the COVID-19 pandemic: Telehealth and virtual reality. *Journal of Clinical Medicine, 10*, 1261–1261. https://doi.org/10.3390/jcm10061261 (accessed on 16th June 2025).

43. Sepúlveda-Loyola, W., Osadnik, C., Phu, S., Morita, A. A., Duque, G., & Probst, V. S. (2020). Diagnosis, prevalence, and clinical impact of sarcopenia in COPD: A systematic review and meta-analysis. *Journal of Cachexia Sarcopenia and Muscle, 11*, 1164–1176. https://doi.org/10.1002/jcsm.12600 (accessed on 16th June 2025).

44. Sönnerfors, P., Jacobson, P., Andersson, A., Behndig, A., Bjermer, L., Blomberg, A., Blomqvist, H., et al. (2024). The challenges of recruiting never-smokers with chronic obstructive pulmonary disease from the large population-based Swedish CArdiopulmonary bioImage study (SCAPIS) cohort. *European Clinical Respiratory Journal, 11*. https://www.semanticscholar.org/paper/2082d634b7c5a324ba69a1e9d121cf53cd9af3eb (accessed on 16th June 2025).

45. Terry, P., & Dhand, R. (2020). Inhalation therapy for stable COPD: 20 years of GOLD reports. *Advances in Therapy, 37*, 1812–1828. https://doi.org/10.1007/s12325-020-01289-y (accessed on 16th June 2025).

46. Tsaousi, F., Bouloukaki, I., Christodoulakis, A., Ierodiakonou, D., Tzanakis, N., & Tsiligianni, I. (2024). A chronic obstructive pulmonary disease self-management intervention for improving patient-reported outcomes in primary care in Greece. *Medicina, 60*. https://www.semanticscholar.org/paper/d2bcda979240c69702c461b30203d1f247624a17 (accessed on 16th June 2025).

47. Vahanian, A., Beyersdorf, F., Praz, F., Milojevic, M., Baldus, S., Bauersachs, J., Capodanno, D., et al. (2021). 2021 ESC/EACTS Guidelines for the management of valvular heart disease. *European Heart Journal, 43*, 561–632. https://doi.org/10.1093/eurheartj/ehab395 (accessed on 16th June 2025).

48. van der Leest, S., & Duiverman, M. L. (2018). High-intensity non-invasive ventilation in stable hypercapnic COPD: Evidence of efficacy and practical advice. *Respirology, 24*, 318–328. https://doi.org/10.1111/resp.13450 (accessed on 16th June 2025).

49. Visseren, F. L. J., Mach, F., Smulders, Y. M., Carballo, D., Koskinas, K. C., Bäck, M., Bénétos, A., et al. (2021). 2021 ESC Guidelines on cardiovascular disease prevention in clinical practice. *European Heart Journal, 42*, 3227–3337. https://doi.org/10.1093/eurheartj/ehab484 (accessed on 16th June 2025).

50. Volkow, N. D. (2020). Collision of the COVID-19 and addiction epidemics. *Annals of Internal Medicine, 173*, 61–62. https://doi.org/10.7326/m20-1212 (accessed on 16th June 2025).

51. Wang, H., Ge, C., Zhang, Z., Geng, Z., & Zhang, L. (2024). Effects of physical activity and sedentary behavior on serum vitamin D in patients with chronic obstructive pulmonary disease. *Advances in Clinical and Experimental Medicine: Official Organ Wroclaw Medical University*. https://www.semanticscholar.org/paper/9c94145fedaae922b44778dc1d2563f00fb3b3f6 (accessed on 16th June 2025).

52. Wang, Q., Su, W., Liu, J., & Zhao, D. (2023). Advances in the investigation of the role of autophagy in the etiology of chronic obstructive pulmonary disease: A review. *Medicine, 102*. https://www.semanticscholar.org/paper/579b1c74e251b237904fc6acd8a7fe18b0394418 (accessed on 16th June 2025).

53. Xie, M., Liu, X., Cao, X., Guo, M., & Li, X. (2020). Trends in prevalence and incidence of chronic respiratory diseases from 1990 to 2017. *Respiratory Research, 21*. https://www.semanticscholar.org/paper/ea17a3fb19a9e13d8cada0d81d4a29d97622e35d (accessed on 16th June 2025).

54. Yu, X., Cheng, X., Lv, L., Wang, N., Li, M., Ji, W., Liu, T., et al. (2024). The association between chronic obstructive pulmonary disease and autoimmune diseases: A bidirectional Mendelian randomization study. *Frontiers in Medicine, 11*. https://www.semanticscholar.org/paper/6b0e7d899ef56d65c4a893641f92fbf4a8641ad6 (accessed on 16th June 2025).

55. Zeppenfeld, K., Tfelt-Hansen, J., Riva, M., Winkel, B. G., Behr, E. R., Blom, N. A., Charron, P., et al. (2022). 2022 ESC Guidelines for the management of patients with ventricular arrhythmias and the prevention of sudden cardiac death. *European Heart Journal, 43*, 3997–4126. https://doi.org/10.1093/eurheartj/ehac262 (accessed on 16th June 2025).

56. Zhang, J., Sun, K., Jagadeesh, A., Falakaflaki, P., Kayayan, E., Tao, G., Haghighat Ghahfarokhi, M., et al. (2024). The potential and pitfalls of using a large language model such as ChatGPT, GPT-4, or LLaMA as a clinical assistant. *Journal of the American Medical Informatics Association: JAMIA*. https://www.semanticscholar.org/paper/d750928ede2438b495d482dc8cb4f2be7bafcf62 (accessed on 16th June 2025).

57. Zöller, D., Haverkamp, C., Makoudjou, A., Sofack, G., Kiefer, S., Gebele, D., Pfaffenlehner, M., et al. (2024). Alpha-1-antitrypsin-deficiency is associated with lower cardiovascular risk: An approach based on federated learning. *Respiratory Research, 25.* https://www.semanticscholar.org/paper/f183623c9921265e61db7e532be71f4444052933 (accessed on 16th June 2025).

RESPIRATORY FAILURE

12

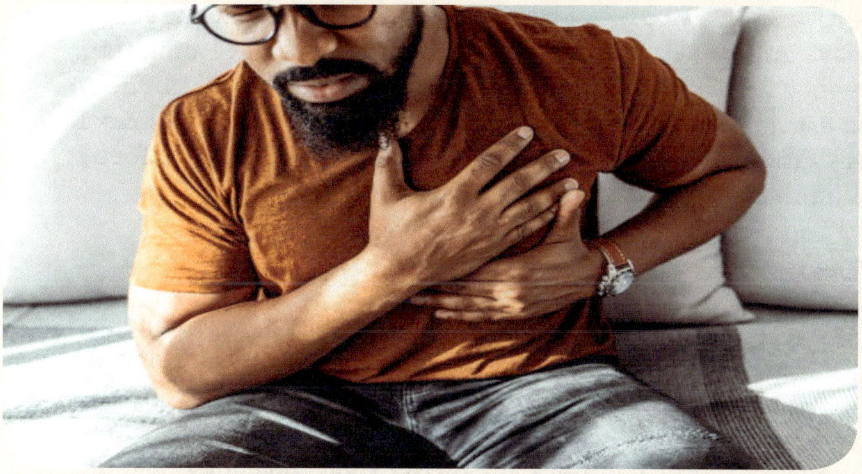

LEARNING OBJECTIVES

After studying this chapter, you will be able to:

1. Explain the types of respiratory failure
2. List the causes of respiratory failure
3. Describe symptoms and diagnosis
4. Understand the treatment options
5. Focus on the complications associated with respiratory failure
6. Explore the prevention strategies

Introduction

The topic of respiratory failure is a severe public health problem with the presentation of failure of the respiratory system to maintain sufficient gas exchange. The condition results from a range of etiologies that can be acute or chronic and cause hypoxemia or hypercapnia. Interdependence between the cardiovascular and respiratory systems in a critical manner elucidates the complexity of respiratory failure, where diseases such as pneumonia, chronic obstructive pulmonary disease (COPD), and acute respiratory distress syndrome (ARDS) have the capacity to lead to serious complications. Healthcare practitioners need to understand the etiopathogenesis, clinical presentations, and management of respiratory failure. A strategy that is advanced enough to consider both the physiological change and the overall health condition of the patients is at the core of managing and treating this life-threatening condition successfully, highlighting the need for early intervention and diagnosis in improving patient outcomes.

The pathophysiology responsible for respiratory failure can be broadly classified into two types: type I respiratory failure, characterized by hypoxemia but not hypercapnia, and type II respiratory failure, which is accompanied by both hypoxemia and hypercapnia. Such a classification helps clinicians to organize the therapeutic strategy. For instance, pneumonia typically presents with type I respiratory failure due to impaired gas exchange in the alveoli. In contrast, conditions like COPD would typically present with type II respiratory failure as a consequence of compromised airway and alveolar obstruction. Identification of the specific type and cause of respiratory failure is crucial to initiate targeted treatment, which may range from supplemental oxygen and mechanical ventilation to pharmacological interventions. As the science of respiratory therapies advances, there is an urgent need to compare the efficacy of traditional and new treatments in treating respiratory failure. Current studies have revealed the far-reaching impact of extrinsic influences, such as cosmetic procedures, on respiratory health, revealing unexpected complications. For example, a case report highlighted a case involving a young woman who developed acute respiratory distress syndrome following silicone injections, suggesting the risk associated with unregulated medical treatments. Cases underline the importance of medical professionals being constantly vigilant about such procedure complications. Health care professionals can be trained to diagnose and manage complications like silicone embolism syndrome through ongoing education in risks associated with cosmetic treatment. In light of the broadened etiology of respiratory failures, it is necessary to raise awareness and improve training in detecting potential adverse effects due to unconventional medical practices, which would further underscore the necessity of an integrated approach to respiratory health.

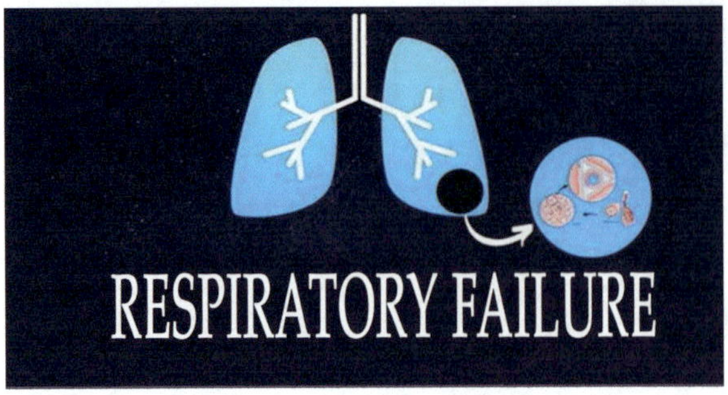

Figure 12.1. Respiratory failure.

Source: https://external-content.duckduckgo.com/iu/?u=https%3A%2F%2Ftse1.mm.bing.net%2Fth%3Fid%3DOIP.pNCsYiwTk7ub9E3WeMyn4QHaFI%26r%3D 0%26pid%3DApi&f=1&ipt=344681dbd48f9203ff6763d5ac352f6eb19a853f988c253106b6d42c9f7d6e48

Definition of Respiratory Failure

The concept of respiratory failure is fundamental to the pathophysiology of both acute and chronic respiratory illnesses. It gives an explanation of the breakdown of the respiratory system to maintain satisfactory gas exchange, leading to profound hypoxemia or hypercapnia. In the clinical context, respiratory failure is classified clinically into two broad categories: acute respiratory failure and chronic respiratory failure. Acute respiratory failure is rapid in onset and can be caused by numerous conditions, such as pneumonia, sepsis, or aspiration, that disrupt normal lung function. Chronic respiratory failure is slow to develop and is typically associated with underlying pulmonary conditions such as COPD or restrictive lung diseases. The distinction between these categories is essential not only for diagnosis but also for determining the appropriate management strategies for infected patients. Respiratory failure is defined to encompass not only the blood gas physiological values but also the clinical implications of inadequate respiratory function. Diagnosis typically involves several clinical markers, such as arterial blood gas PaO_2 and $PaCO_2$ levels. The presence of such abnormalities indicates impaired gas exchange, resulting in systemic effects on oxygenation and the removal of carbon dioxide. Also, the Acute Respiratory Distress Syndrome (ARDS) is a typical example of cases where the diagnostic criteria for respiratory failure are met, necessitating immediate and intensive assessment as well as management. With increasing research, complex definitions based on clinical evidence and some pathophysiological notions are emerging, emphasizing the complexity in managing respiratory failure, particularly under critical conditions, for which custom-made care protocols are needed to ensure lung function preservation and improved outcomes. In addition to being aware of the physiological conditions associated with respiratory failure, one should also consider various etiologies that can lead to hospitalizations affecting the respiratory system. An algorithmic classification is usually employed by hospitals for such events to standardize clinical trials and outcomes. have an accurate definition of respiratory failure, as causative conditions with similar presentations may differ. As seen in idiopathic airflow pulmonary fibrosis (IPF)-associated research, it is essential to identify infections or precipitating events as an exacerbation since shown (Behr et al., 2024). This not only aids in the treatment of the acute event, but also determines patients' longitudinal care plan that they may need to prevent subsequent complications. Ultimately, a definitive and robust definition of respiratory failure serves both clinical practice and research equally well, enhancing the ease with which medical practitioners can address this vital aspect of respiratory well-being.

Importance of Understanding Respiratory Failure

A clear understanding of respiratory failure is not only essential for managing patients immediately, but also for public health. Respiratory failure, or the inability of the respiratory system to sustain adequate gas exchange, can be caused by conditions such as chronic obstructive pulmonary disease (COPD), pneumonia, or acute lung injury. In these complex cases, prompt intervention and early treatment are crucial to avert complications resulting from severe respiratory failure. For example, elderly patients with acute liver failure have a high risk of opportunistic infections, which can complicate the treatment and worsen the prognosis of respiratory function. The interconnection of liver function and respiratory status advocates the exercise of caution in monitoring and managing comorbidity and demonstrates that a holistic approach to patient care is essential in improving prognosis and quality of life, as evidenced by the case noted in Wu et al. (2024). Sensitivity to underlying respiratory failure mechanisms facilitates evidence-based establishment of effective treatment and preventive measures.

The complexity of respiratory distress can frequently necessitate an interdisciplinary approach for optimal management. In a child, like in the case of the three-year-old boy with recurrent respiratory distress, it could be challenging but important to distinguish between several likely causes, such as genetic disorders or gastroesophageal reflux disease (GERD). Respiratory failure in a child can lead to significant developmental delay, since prolonged illness may blunt physical and mental growth. Therefore, active care and regular follow-up are imperative to address physical health requirements as well as developmental milestones, highlighting the need for healthcare providers to remain current on the multifaceted presentation of respiratory conditions.

As expounded in Daidone et al., (2024), the information guarantees improved patient outcomes and the efficacy of treatment plans. Apart from special instances, the understanding of respiratory failure can be applied to the broader context of healthcare systems and resource usage as well. Effective management of respiratory failure plays a crucial role in reducing healthcare costs associated with prolonged hospitalization and intensive care unit admission. By investing in education and awareness about the condition, healthcare professionals can maximize preventative treatment strategies, ultimately yielding improved patient outcomes in general. Public health interventions, such as vaccination, smoking cessation, and effective public health policies, can have far-reaching implications in reducing the incidence of respiratory failure-causing diseases. Untreated respiratory disease can have crushing social costs, which highlights the necessity of considering respiratory failure as a clinical entity but also as a matter of public health for which there is a need for multilateral involvement between healthcare providers and policymakers.

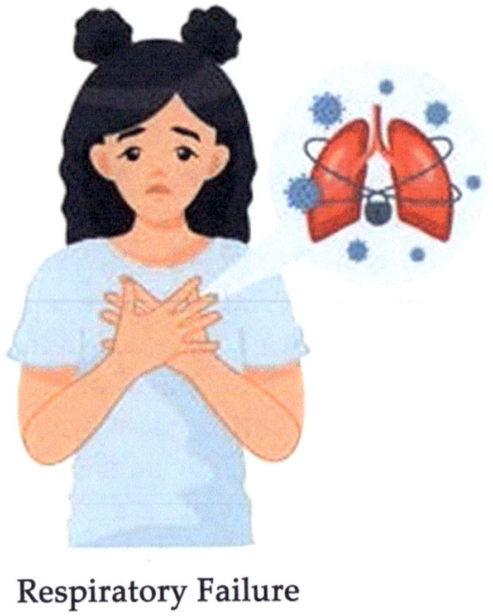

Figure 12.2. Woman Respiratory Failure Pneumonia Shortness Breath.

Source: https://www.shutterstock.com/image-vector/woman-respiratory-failure-pneumonia-shortness-260nw-2049737762.jpg

12.1. Types of Respiratory Failure

Learning Outcome

1. Acute Respiratory Failure
2. Chronic Respiratory Failure
3. Hypoxemic vs. Hypercapnic Respiratory Failure

Respiratory failure is generally classified into two broad categories based on the underlying pathophysiological mechanisms of gas exchange abnormality: hypoxemic and hypercapnic respiratory failure. Hypoxemic respiratory failure, or type I, occurs when there is inadequate oxygenation of the blood with normal ventilation. The syndrome is commonly associated with diseases that compromise the ability of the lungs to oxygenate the blood, such as pneumonia, pulmonary edema, and acute respiratory distress syndrome (ARDS). In all these cases, arterial blood gas analysis typically reveals a low arterial oxygen tension (PaO_2) with normal or low carbon dioxide tensions ($PaCO_2$). It is vital to identify the characteristics of these two forms because therapeutic options vary significantly, influencing patient outcomes and guiding clinical interventions to manage respiratory failure effectively. Hypercapnic respiratory failure, also known as type II respiratory failure, is characterized by elevated levels of carbon dioxide resulting from inadequate ventilation, as opposed to a problem with oxygenation. This type is typically seen in such disorders as chronic obstructive pulmonary disease (COPD), asthma, central nervous depression, or neuromuscular disease that diminish the respiratory muscles' efficiency to increase lung capacity appropriately. Hypercapnic respiratory failure most typically occurs in patients with increased $PaCO_2$ accompanied by a decrease in pH, indicating respiratory acidosis. The management of hypercapnic respiratory failure involves the use of therapies that improve ventilation, either through non-invasive positive pressure ventilation or intubation in severe cases. Both types of respiratory failure are characterized by distinct presentations, enabling healthcare providers to tailor their approach and improve clinical outcomes to a significant degree. In addition to the two main types of respiratory failure, mixed respiratory failure is also possible, where both hypercapnia and hypoxemia occur together. This type of presentation makes clinical management more complicated and is seen in the most critically ill patients with severe lung disease or chronic illness exacerbations. Mixed respiratory failure must be carefully diagnosed through thorough patient history and lab work to diagnose underlying causes accurately. Delicate coordination of treatment is necessary to effectively treat both deficit oxygenation and ventilation. Understanding the subtleties involved in the categories of respiratory failure better equips practitioners to provide optimized care and initiate proper therapies, which ultimately leads to an improvement in prognosis and patient quality of life during such life-threatening health issues.

12.1.1. Acute Respiratory Failure

Acute respiratory failure (ARF) is a critical clinical syndrome characterized by an inability of the respiratory system to facilitate adequate gas exchange and thus produce hypoxemia and/or hypercapnia. ARF can emerge suddenly, and prompt medical intervention is essential to avoid a catastrophic outcome. Several etiologies cause ARF, including pneumonia, exacerbation of chronic obstructive pulmonary disease (COPD), pulmonary embolism, and acute respiratory distress syndrome (ARDS). Pathophysiologic mechanisms responsible for ARF typically involve ventilatory dysfunction, diffusing capacities, or shunting. Clinicians should have an understanding of these mechanisms in order to effectively diagnose and manage ARF, as timely intervention can significantly improve patient outcomes. Healthcare providers are responsible, when caring for ARF, to apply a mix of clinical knowledge and technological advances to provide adequate care and avoid potentially lethal scenarios. The management of acute respiratory failure requires a structured approach with an emphasis on rapid evaluation and treatment. High-flow nasal oxygen therapy (HFNOT) has also proven to be an effective strategy in managing acute hypoxemic respiratory failure, as it can lead to improvements in oxygenation without the need for invasive ventilation. Evidence suggests that it tends to identify its superiority over standard oxygen therapy, ultimately curtailing the progression of treatment needs in most cases. Noninvasive ventilation (NIV) is also a key intervention, particularly in patients with respiratory acidosis and COPD exacerbations. Moreover, for patients with respiratory failure caused by a reversible etiology, extracorporeal membrane oxygenation (ECMO) provides a life-sustaining intervention when other therapeutic means have been exhausted. These new treatments underscore the development of treatment strategies tailored to the needs of ARF patients, with a focus on the importance of early treatment in enhancing overall outcomes. In addition to the urgency of clinical intervention, the long-term consequences of acute respiratory failure are a significant concern, particularly about prognosis and quality of life. ARF patients often go on to develop chronic complications, such as impaired pulmonary function and increased healthcare utilization, down the road in their clinical course. Such research considerations, as the need for nutritional support and pulmonary rehabilitation, have become part of complete care in this context. Specifically, data have shown that nutritional deficiency will additionally exacerbate the severity of respiratory disease, and hence the need for personalized nutritional care in these patients' management strategies is underlined. To the extent that the pathophysiology of respiratory failure is increasingly understood, especially in diseases such as idiopathic pleuroparenchymal fibroelastosis (iPPFE), the ARF dilemma becomes even more urgent. Improving prognosis models and treatment remains the primary goal of ongoing research, ultimately aimed at optimizing patient outcomes and facilitating recovery from this complex disorder (Ishii et al., 2025; Gruszka et al., 2025).

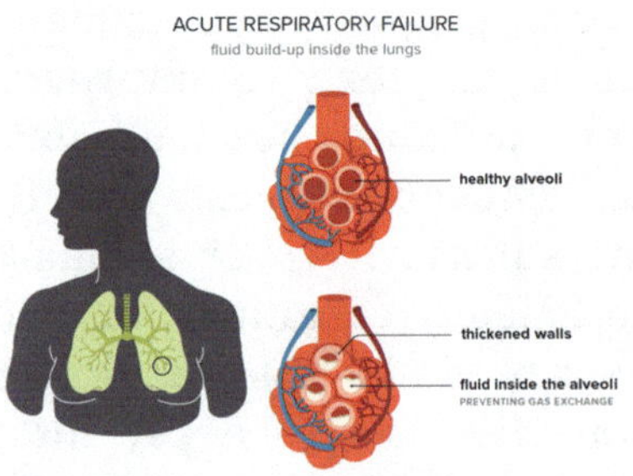

Figure 12.3. Acute respiratory failure.

Source: https://i0.wp.com/post.medicalnewstoday.com/wp-content/uploads/sites/3/2022/04/acute-respiratory-failure-1296x1061-body-1024x841.png?w=1155&h=2265

12.1.2. Chronic Respiratory Failure

When dealing with chronic respiratory failure, the key feature to be considered is the relationship between the physiologic processes and the diseases involved. Chronic respiratory failure is often caused by diseases such as COPD, interstitial lung disease, and cystic fibrosis, which are linked to progressive lung impairment. These diseases result in ineffective gas exchange, leading to elevated levels of carbon dioxide in the blood and reduced levels of oxygen, a syndrome known as hypoxemia. Patients with these chronic conditions not only bear the physiological weight of respiratory failure but also the psychosocial burdens, which can significantly compromise their quality of life. The interplay of these factors necessitates holistic management strategies that are specifically tailored to meet both medical and supportive care needs, as respiratory failure requires a multifaceted approach to ensure proper treatment (Boland et al., 2013).

The psychosocial consequences of chronic respiratory failure cannot be overemphasized. Dyspnea, fatigue, and pain are debilitating symptoms experienced by most patients that severely impede daily activities and social functioning. The psychological impact is distressing, which may lead to isolation and despair. Palliative care has now become a fundamental aspect of treating chronic respiratory failure, with an emphasis not only on symptom relief but also on enhancing patients' overall well-being. Recommendations are currently to include palliative care for all those with life-prolonging chronic lung disease, irrespective of prognosis. This integrated approach is designed not only to alleviate physical suffering but also psychological distress related to chronic respiratory failure, hence offering patients a broader care model (Boland et al., 2013). Further, breaking down barriers for successful palliative care in chronic respiratory failure is crucial to improving patient outcomes. Despite growing recognition of the role of comprehensive care, specialist palliative care is not available to most patients with non-malignant lung diseases. Research suggests that effective communication between respiratory and palliative care teams can result in improved symptom control and more comprehensive support mechanisms for patients and their families. Subsequent research should focus on defining optimal models of care delivery that encompass both pharmacotherapy and non-pharmacotherapy interventions, and that address care gaps. Through an evolving understanding of chronic respiratory failure, maximizing care techniques will play a key role in mitigating the impact of this disabling disease, fostering a more enabling environment for individuals affected by it (Boland et al., 2013).

12.1.3. Hypoxemic Vs. Hypercapnic Respiratory Failure

Understanding the distinction between hypoxemic and hypercapnic respiratory failure is paramount for effective clinical management. Hypoxemic respiratory failure is characterized by insufficient oxygen in the blood, typically attributed to causes such as pneumonia, pulmonary edema, or acute respiratory distress syndrome (ARDS). The arterial oxygen levels fall, while carbon dioxide (CO_2) may be normal or slightly elevated. The primary therapy for hypoxemic failure is typically the administration of supplemental oxygen or other interventions, such as high-flow nasal oxygen (HFNO). Present evidence suggests that HFNO is a viable treatment option for acute hypoxemic respiratory failure caused by COVID-19, although it does not definitively affect mortality, but rather hospital length of stay, thereby impacting patient management strategies (Sjauw et al., 2025). In contrast, hypercapnic respiratory failure is caused by inadequate ventilation, leading to the accumulation of CO_2 in the blood. It often happens with patients who have chronic obstructive pulmonary disease (COPD), which leads to alveolar hypoventilation. Arterial blood gas examination during hypercapnic failure reveals elevated levels of CO_2 and associated potential oxygen deficiencies. Treatment primarily involves noninvasive ventilation (NIV), which aids in regulating ventilation and gas exchange. Some forms of NIV, including average volume-assured pressure support (AVAPS) and fixed pressure support, have been studied for effectiveness in chronic hypercapnic respiratory failure. Data show that while both modes are effective in controlling CO_2, neither has a measurable benefit in clinical outcomes (Evans et al., 2024). The strategies for managing hypoxemic and hypercapnic respiratory failure reflect the relevant underlying pathophysiological mechanisms, which necessitate personalized therapies. Healthcare providers must distinguish between the two forms of respiratory failure to optimize treatment protocols and patient outcomes. For instance, the inability of patients with hypoxemic failure to be adequately oxygenated may justify more aggressive treatment, including the use of mechanical ventilation for severe failure. Patients with hypercapnic failure require a focus on optimizing ventilation to reverse CO_2 retention. Lastly, being familiar with regulatory mechanisms and patient-specific factors is crucial in formulating effective treatment plans for managing respiratory failure.

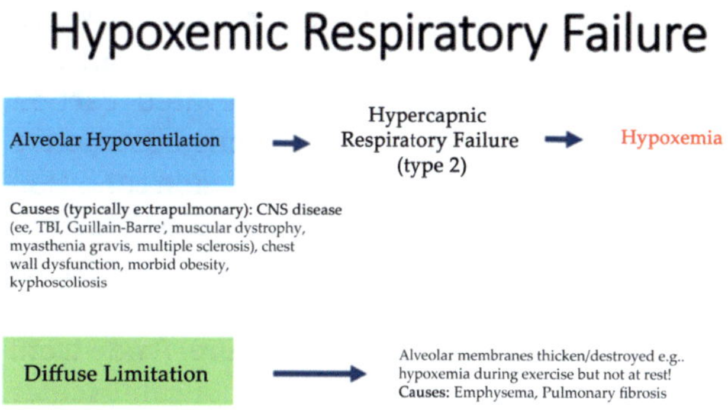

Figure 12.4. Hypoxemic respiratory failure.

Source: https://external-content.duckduckgo.com/iu/?u=https%3A%2F%2Fo.quizlet.com%2FOQ7B0KcvCHp3c1aNFJBWew.png&f=1&nofb=1&ipt=4b121cbb5e126d029995cb4a26832fca610514dadbe3a19eb204cf09ad68d57a

Test Your Knowledge

1. What is acute respiratory failure?
2. What is chronic respiratory failure?

12.2. Causes of Respiratory Failure

Learning Outcome

1. Obstructive Lung Diseases
2. Restrictive Lung Diseases
3. Central Nervous System Disorders

The pathogenesis of respiratory failure is complex and can be broadly categorized into two types: hypoxemic and hypercapnic. Hypoxemic respiratory failure occurs when the lungs are unable to supply sufficient oxygen to the blood, often as a result of causes such as pneumonia, acute respiratory distress syndrome (ARDS), or pulmonary embolism. For example, pneumonia can lead to inflammation and fluid accumulation within the alveoli, impairing gas exchange and resulting in decreased blood oxygen levels. Hypercapnic respiratory failure occurs when the body is unable to effectively eliminate carbon dioxide, resulting in elevated carbon dioxide levels in the blood. Chronic obstructive pulmonary disease (COPD) is a common condition that belongs to this class of respiratory failure, with airway blockade denying the passage of carbon dioxide, which can lead to respiratory acidosis and ultimately organ failure. Aside from infections and chronic diseases, neuromuscular disorders are significant causes of respiratory failure. COPD and myasthenia gravis disrupt the neural pathways that control breathing. These diseases can weaken the diaphragm and intercostal muscles, causing patients to experience insufficient breathing. Due to this, patients develop hypoventilation, resulting in gas exchange insufficiency and carbon dioxide accumulation. Central nervous system origin reasons, such as stroke or traumatic brain injury, have the ability to provoke respiratory failure due to the interference with the brain's respiratory centers. The implications of these conditions extend beyond mere respiratory distress because chronic respiratory failure may result in severe complications, including acute lung injury and multi-organ failure, highlighting the imperative need for early management and diagnosis. In addition, the onset of diseases like SARS-CoV-2 has introduced a new dimension of respiratory failure etiology by inducing acute respiratory symptoms and complications that could result in rapid deterioration. COVID-19 can cause severe pneumonia and acute lung injury, leading to hypoxemic respiratory failure, which may need vigorous respiratory support such as mechanical ventilation.

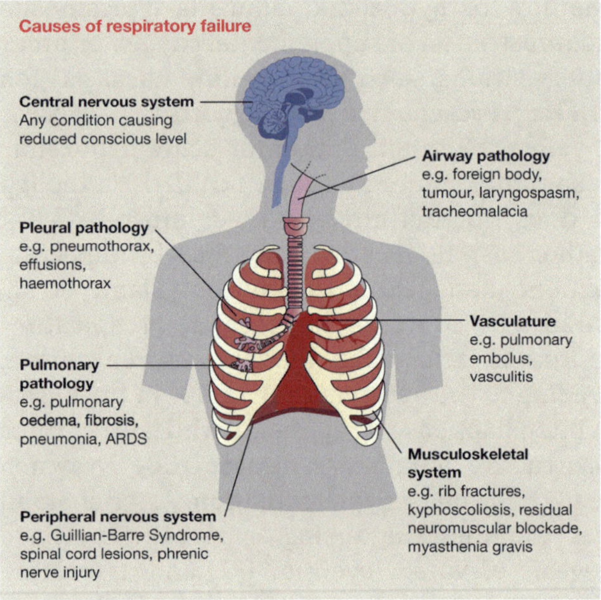

Figure 12.5. The causes of respiratory failure.

Source: https://www.surgeryjournal.co.uk/cms/10.1016/j.mpsur.2024.07.007/asset/aae5beab-f693-40d4-8510-f5a0da20bbae/main.assets/gr1_lrg.jpg

There is also a finding that COVID-19 is complicated by thromboembolic events, such as pulmonary embolism, which further aggravates the clinical profile and impairs respiratory function by blocking pulmonary arteries. Studies have found that in COVID-19, the interplay between inflammation and coagulation has a profound effect on respiratory mechanics.

Finally, an understanding of the multifactorial etiology of respiratory failure, including the influence of viral infections and complications arising from them, is critical for designing effective therapy regimens and optimizing patient outcomes (Wichmann D, 2020; Chopra et al., 2020).

12.2.1. Obstructive Lung Diseases

Obstructive lung disorders, with restriction of airflow, are a leading cause of respiratory failure, an acute illness in which the respiratory apparatus cannot provide satisfactory gas exchange. Chronic airway narrowing and inflammation characterize asthma, chronic obstructive pulmonary disease (COPD), and bronchiectasis as prototypic members of this category. These diseases increase airway resistance, making it difficult for air to flow during exhalation and trapping air inside the lungs. These physiological changes can be a causative agent of acute respiratory failure, where oxygen levels become critically low and carbon dioxide levels become high, leading to hypercapnia. Understanding the pathophysiology of these obstructive diseases is key since early intervention and treatment are essential in avoiding exacerbations that can lead to respiratory failure (Panetti et al., 2024).

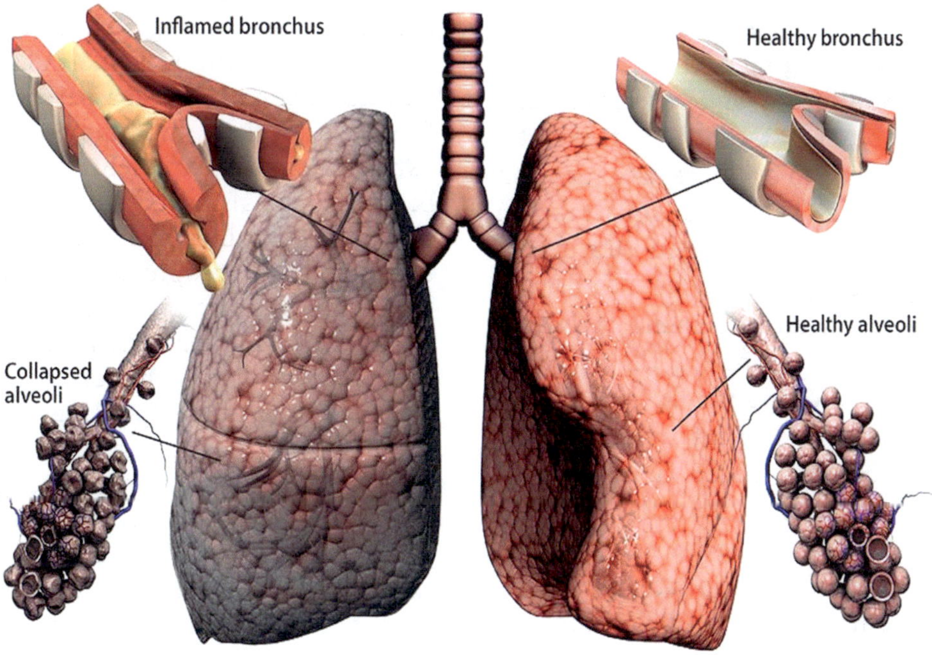

Figure 12.6. Obstructive lung diseases.

Source: https://external-content.duckduckgo.com/iu/?u=https%3A%2F%2Fimages.fineartamerica.com%2Fimages-medium-large-5%2Fchronic-obstructive-pulmonary-disease-gunilla-elamscience-photo-library.jpg&f=1&nofb=1&ipt=382a166548e7329368e4639245c102b71f806332d716d71bd4cd26171dae27ff

The relationship between obstructive lung diseases and respiratory failure also highlights the importance of patient management therapy aimed at controlling inflammation and bronchoconstriction. In conditions like asthma, acute worsening due to rapid and uncontrolled narrowing of the airways can be life-threatening and needs immediate intervention with treatment strategies such as bronchodilators and corticosteroids. In COPD, the chronic nature of the illness can lead to constant recurrence of respiratory failure that must be controlled both pharmacologically and with lifestyle interventions to enhance patients' respiratory function. Furthermore, improvements in pulmonary rehabilitation have been encouraging in improving exercise tolerance and quality of life in such patients. With the rising prevalence of obstructive lung diseases globally, health care systems cannot help but change by using preventive measures and early intervention programs to manage the associated risks of respiratory failure (Narala et al., 2024). Furthermore, the role of pulmonary function tests and imaging techniques in the diagnosis and monitoring of obstructive lung diseases cannot be overstated. The diagnostic tests enable clinicians to evaluate lung function thoroughly, provide critical information regarding airflow limitation, and the extent of lung injury. Lastly, the development of biomarkers and artificial intelligence presents new opportunities for improving the accuracy of diagnoses and therapeutic interventions. For example, biomarkers of inflammation and oxidative stress can aid in the customization of therapy based on individual patient characteristics, particularly in the management of exacerbations that may precipitate respiratory failure. As research continues to uncover the multifaceted mechanisms involved in obstructive lung diseases, future approaches must incorporate a multidisciplinary approach, including prevention, early diagnosis, and novel treatments (Panetti et al., 2024).

12.2.2. Restrictive Lung Diseases

Restrictive lung diseases represent a significant category of pulmonary diseases characterized by a compromised lung capacity to expand, resulting in abnormal pulmonary gas exchange function. It leads to naturally impairing the structural function of the lung tissue or respiratory mechanics, which causes reduced lung volumes such as total lung capacity and vital capacity. Since gas exchange is impaired, patients may develop dyspnea and fatigue symptoms that add to exacerbated respiratory failure. Conditions such as interstitial lung disease, neuromuscular disease, and obesity hypoventilation syndrome are reflective of restrictive lung diseases that add significantly to the risk of acute respiratory failure, particularly following exposure to environmental or physiological stresses, such as noted in clinical case reports among children (Panetti et al., 2024). Diagnosis and management of restrictive lung disease are crucial in preventing respiratory failure and promoting patient outcomes. Clinicians employ a combination of clinical assessment, pulmonary function testing, and imaging modalities to estimate the extent of lung damage. Arterial blood gas analysis is a particularly valuable diagnostic tool by which clinicians can quantify the extent of respiratory compromise and formulate specific interventions. For instance, in the treatment of restrictive respiratory failure due to pneumonia, novel therapies such as phosphatidylcholine liposomes have been found useful in restoring respiratory function through the optimization of gas exchange parameters and increasing metabolic activity in compromised patients (Rozova et al., 2023). Notably, early intervention greatly improves the prognosis of patients with the sinister presentations of restrictive lung diseases. Furthermore, the connection between restrictive lung disease and respiratory failure emphasizes the importance of a multidisciplinary treatment plan. In addition to pharmacological therapy, supportive care, including pulmonary rehabilitation and respiratory therapy, can significantly enhance lung function and quality of life in affected individuals. Patient-education techniques, including the recognition of exacerbation symptoms and the application of lifestyle modifications to minimize risk, are also central to practical management algorithms. As a result of the complex pathophysiology in restrictive lung disease, ongoing research is needed to develop novel therapeutic interventions and diagnostic strategies that would bridge the care gaps. The integration of newer diagnostic modalities, such as artificial intelligence and biomarker testing, has the potential to bring about paradigm-shifting changes in the diagnosis and management of the nuances of restrictive lung disease and related risks of respiratory failure (Rozova et al., 2023; Panetti et al., 2024).

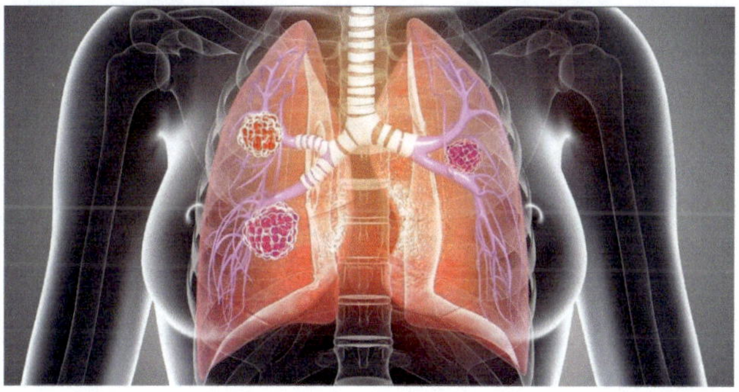

Figure 12.7. Restrictive lung diseases.

Source: https://lunginstitute.com/wp-content/uploads/2022/07/Restrictive-Lung-Disease.jpg

12.2.3. Central Nervous System Disorders

The relationship between diseases of the Central Nervous System (CNS) and respiratory failure is multifaceted, accentuating the significance of neurological health in maintaining respiratory function. CNS disorders such as stroke, traumatic brain damage, and neurodegenerative disease can cause significant impairments in the adaptive capacity of the brain for the control of breathing effort. The brainstem, holding vital respiratory centers, may be compromised by these conditions, leading to ineffective ventilation and oxygenation. In the case of severe brain injury, for example, the function of the brainstem may be compromised, resulting in hypoventilation or apneic attacks, which can lead to respiratory failure. Furthermore, the degree of respiratory failure in CNS disease patients is often a management problem, necessitating advanced interventions such as mechanical ventilation and even extracorporeal support systems to sustain life amidst critical respiratory incapacitation. Moreover, the interaction between CNS disease and respiratory failure emphasizes the importance of overall management strategies. Autonomic nervous system dysregulation affecting respiratory pattern and drive is common in CNS disease patients. Dysregulation of the autonomic nervous system can lead to respiratory complications such as aspiration pneumonia or atelectasis, further exacerbating the neurological condition of the patients as well as treatment results. The rising incidence of cases of respiratory failure that are associated with CNS disorders requires that attending doctors employ multidisciplinary strategies in actively monitoring and managing such patients. The employment of newer techniques, such as extracorporeal membrane oxygenation (ECMO), has gained increased use over the past few years and offers a viable lifeline to patients with CNS injuries or diseases who have severe respiratory failure. This approach reflects the novel background of treatment options available in critically ill patients with increasing understanding of interdependency between neurological and respiratory dysfunction (Lorusso et al., 2021).

Ultimately, recent research highlights the significant implications for COVID-19-related CNS complications, which can lead to rising rates of respiratory failure. Various research illustrates the neurological manifestations of SARS-CoV-2 infection, including encephalitis, acute cerebrovascular accidents, and ongoing neurocognitive impairments. These reports indicate that COVID-19 is not only respiratory in consequences but also has profound CNS impacts that potentially predispose the subjects towards respiratory issues. Given that CNS disease develops as a result of infectious processes, it alerts us to be cautious in monitoring those suspected of having neurological complications from COVID-19. Further, the results of post-mortem examination reflect pathophysiological mechanisms like thromboinflammation, consistent with coagulopathy data that can worsen both CNS and respiratory outcomes in severely infected individuals (Wichmann D, 2020). To this end, gaining knowledge of these interactions is integral to improving management strategies against both CNS disorders and their respiratory complications in the background of ongoing health challenges.

Test Your Knowledge

1. What are the obstructive lung diseases?
2. What are the central nervous system disorders?

12.3. Symptoms and Diagnosis

Learning Outcome

1. Common Symptoms of Respiratory Failure
2. Diagnostic Tests and Procedures
3. Importance of Early Diagnosis

Diagnosis of respiratory failure symptoms is critical in guiding the on-time diagnosis and treatment. The presentation may include shortness of breath, tachypnea, and a sense of suffocation that can aggravate depending on concomitant conditions. Notably, the symptoms are exacerbated in COPD patients such that the symptoms of acute respiratory infection, including COVID-19, are camouflaged. This overlap is often problematic to diagnose, as the recognition of chronic symptomatology and acute change is rendered challenging. Proper classification of respiratory symptoms is required by healthcare providers, as per guidelines from the Global Initiative for Chronic Obstructive Lung Disease, to provide appropriate management, especially in periods with heightened prevalence of respiratory illness. Additionally, careful symptom evaluation guides the decision to order further diagnostic tests, ultimately leading to effective treatment (Halpin et al., 2020).

Respiratory failure diagnostic approaches must be methodical and thorough, often relying on the incorporation of clinical assessment, radiographic imaging, and laboratory studies. The initial diagnosis is made through a complete patient history and physical examination, aiming to identify the causes of respiratory distress. Arterial blood gas (ABG) measurement is a key diagnostic tool, as it measures oxygen and carbon dioxide concentrations in blood, thereby revealing respiratory alkalosis or acidosis. Imaging modalities, such as chest X-rays or computed tomography scans, may also be used to diagnose lung pathology. During the COVID-19 pandemic, diagnosis has become more complex due to the novel symptoms and their overlap with established respiratory illnesses. The early identification of

SARS-CoV-2 through polymerase chain reaction (PCR) testing may impact management plans, especially in cases of coinfection or exacerbation (Wiersinga et al., 2020). In addition to routine diagnostic regimens, integration of telemedicine has transformed symptom assessment and management of patients with respiratory failure. It is feasible to identify deteriorating respiratory symptoms at an early stage through remote consultations, thereby facilitating timely management. Interestingly, in the ongoing COVID-19 pandemic, this practice has gained immense importance, as many patients suffering from respiratory diseases would hesitate to report for conventional face-to-face encounters for fear of exposure. Furthermore, monitoring technology has also advanced to provide healthcare practitioners with real-time data concerning patients' oxygen saturation levels and breathing patterns. Such developments supplement traditional methods of diagnosis and allow for more personalized modes of healthcare. Lastly, the diversified approach to diagnosing symptoms of respiratory failure emphasizes the importance of a comprehensive knowledge base on respiratory health, especially considering the increasing global respiratory challenges (Halpin et al., 2020; Wiersinga et al., 2020).

12.3.1. Common Symptoms of Respiratory Failure

The clinical presentation of respiratory failure encompasses a multitude of symptoms that signify the primary failure of the respiratory system to facilitate adequate gas exchange. The two most common symptoms in patients with respiratory failure are tachypnea and dyspnea. Shortness of breath, or dyspnea, can be caused by decreased oxygenation or increased carbon dioxide pressure in the blood. It can be complained of by patients as a feeling of being choked or an increase in effort to breathe, thereby causing discomfort. It is particularly emphasized in acute settings as a sign where patients exhibit a modified respiratory pattern that is rapid, shallow, or tachypneic. This is a normal reaction to hypoxemia, a resulting condition that needs immediate evaluation and treatment for enhancing respiratory function and preventing further deterioration of the patient's condition. Cyanosis, blue discoloration of the skin and mucous membranes, is another dramatic respiratory failure sign. This body sign characterizes severe hypoxemia because it is substantiated by elevated levels of deoxygenated hemoglobin in the blood. Cyanosis appears in patients near the lips, fingers, or other peripheral areas and serves as a visible signal for caregivers to consider supplemental oxygen or intervention therapy. The finding of cyanosis is concerning, as it highlights the degree of respiratory compromise and necessitates prompt clinical intervention. Altered mental status may also be present in cases of respiratory failure, where decreased oxygenation affects cerebral function. Patients can manifest in confusion, lethargy, or agitation, suggesting possible respiratory distress. This cognitive impairment underscores the need to find and cure the etiology of respiratory failure in a quest to re-establish adequate oxygen delivery to essential organs and prevent fatal complications. Without any doubt, respiratory failure can also be manifested by other systemic symptoms like exhaustion and exercise intolerance. Patients will tend to present with undue malaise and reduced exercise tolerance due to their compromised respiratory mechanism. Fatigue is a prevalent by-product of the chronically elevated cost of breathing, which perpetuates a cycle of decreased activity and worsening symptoms. The emotional impact of chronic respiratory failure should not be downplayed either, with despair or apprehension being frequent companions to the perception of breathlessness. Such psychosocial issues make patients' burdens more challenging, and a multidisciplinary approach is necessary. Treating the physical and emotional aspects of respiratory failure is critical to improving the quality of patients' lives overall and to achieving the best results from recovery, a concept picked up in recent studies into post-COVID-19 readjustments in health and the multi-faceted character of recovery from severe respiratory treatment (Wichmann, 2020; Chopra et al., 2020).

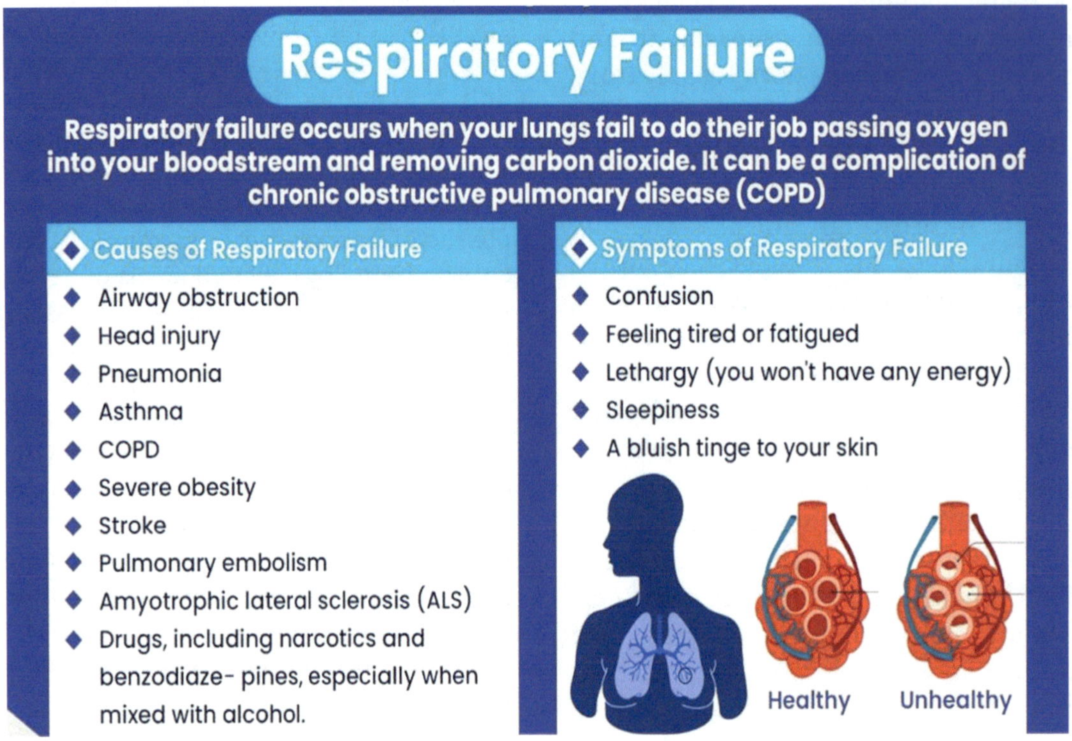

Figure 12.8. Symptoms of respiratory failure.

Source: https://www.sparshdiagnostica.com/wp-content/uploads/2025/01/Respiratory-Failure-1024x1024.jpeg

12.3.2. Diagnostic Tests and Procedures

Diagnostic testing for respiratory failure is crucial for determining the etiology and tailoring treatment plans to individual needs. Arterial blood gas (ABG) analysis, which measures efficiency of gas exchange, and imaging tests such as chest X-ray and computed tomography (CT) scans are frequently employed diagnostic tests. ABGs provide valuable information about the levels of oxygen and carbon dioxide in the blood, which healthcare providers can use to determine the type of respiratory failure—either hypoxemic or hypercapnic. Imaging modalities enable the visualization of lung structure and the detection of pathological processes, such as pneumonia, pulmonary edema, or other obstructive conditions. Systematic diagnostic strategies are critical in risk populations, such as patients with hematological malignancies, in whom the pathophysiologic complexity of respiratory failure can complicate both prognosis and management (Azoulay et al., 2016).

In conjunction with standard diagnostic tools, advanced techniques play a crucial role in elucidating the cause of respiratory failure. Bronchoscopy, often coupled with bronchoalveolar lavage (BAL), enables direct visualization of the airways, allowing for the sampling of respiratory secretions for microbiological analysis. It is particularly worthwhile in cases of suspected pneumonia or opportunistic infection, where prompt diagnosis can have a significant impact on prognosis. The efficacy of these processes, as in the case of critically ill patients, has been attributed to the identification of specific pathogens that contribute heavily to treatment and mortality rates (Azoulay et al., 2016).

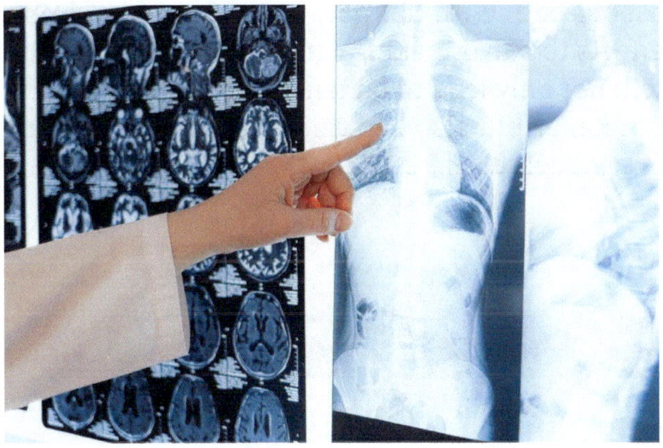

Figure 12.9. Diagnostic tests and procedures for respiratory failure.

Source: https://coughpro.com/wp-content/uploads/2022/09/diagnostic-tests-.jpg

Furthermore, viral infections, such as severe acute respiratory syndrome (SARS), necessitate timely diagnostic methods to identify pathogens, and thus the timeliness of response in respiratory emergencies. The integration of different diagnostic tests and procedures forms a core framework for effective management of respiratory failure. The correlation of clinical assessments with focused investigation enables medical practitioners to construct a multiplicity of understanding about the patient's condition. Identifying the etiology in undetermined cases of respiratory failure is necessary because certain factors are correlated with increased mortality, hence the need for detailed investigation (Azoulay et al., 2016). Finally, a systematized diagnostic process not only enhances results in individual patients but also improves overall management plans for critical care settings. With the ongoing advancement of technology and medical intelligence, diagnostic tests will become increasingly complex, further refining our understanding and treatment of respiratory failure.

12.3.3. Importance of Early Diagnosis

The importance of early diagnosis of respiratory failure cannot be overstated, as it directly impacts the patient's prognosis and treatment course. Early detection of the etiology of respiratory worsening enables timely interventions, thereby reducing the incidence of complications. Apart from making immediate therapeutic interventions such as oxygen therapy and mechanical ventilation possible, early diagnosis also provides a window for the use of specific etiologic treatments for respiratory failure. For instance, in the case of genetic diseases like severe combined immunodeficiency (SCID), early screening of newborns can significantly enhance survival rates. Especially, those treatments initiated before 3.5 months of age lead to an increase in the survival rate to 94%, while for later-diagnosed persons, there is a lower percentage of survival. Consequently, the incorporation of systematic screening programs into clinical procedures can notably improve patient outcomes for respiratory failure conditions (Hernadez et al., 2025). In clinical practice within hospitals, undiagnosed or misdiagnosed respiratory disease typically results in late responses to treatment, hence worsening the patients' condition and raising mortality rates. For example, pulmonary tumor embolism predisposes patients to progressive respiratory failure, but its non-specific presentation tends to complicate diagnosis. Standard imaging procedures, such as computed tomography angiography and echocardiography, are likely to result in poor specificity; thus, such categorical diagnoses are typically made post-mortem. This. It illustrates how a failure in early diagnosis not only hinders timely care but also proves to be fatal. A high index of suspicion for malignancy complications should be maintained among clinicians for patients with unexplained respiratory symptoms to facilitate timely intervention and diagnosis. This highlights the pressing need for diagnostic innovation to aid in the detection of diseases most likely to lead to respiratory failure (Ščerbakovs et al., 2025). In addition, the linkage between timely diagnosis and successful treatment extends beyond immediate clinical results to involve ramifications in overall public health. Increasing cases of respiratory disease and associated morbidity necessitate anticipatory disease detection and management action. By encouraging interventions such as augmented training among nursing personnel and patient education regarding the symptomatology of respiratory distress, health systems can significantly reduce early diagnosis rates. Furthermore, by employing technology, including machine learning and telemedicine, risk patients could be identified sooner. Early diagnosis and correct diagnosis can be a critical preventive measure against acute respiratory failure and may also reduce healthcare expenditure associated with longer hospital stays. Joint efforts towards making early diagnosis a priority will not only lead to enhanced individual patient outcomes but also healthier populations overall (Hernadez et al., 2025).

Test Your Knowledge

1. What are the common symptoms of respiratory failure
2. What are the diagnostic tests and procedures?

12.4. Treatment Options

Learning Outcome

1. Oxygen Therapy
2. Mechanical Ventilation
3. Pharmacological Interventions

The treatment of respiratory failure is multidisciplinary, with treatment provided based on the etiology, severity, and patient-specific factors. Supportive care provides the foundation for treating respiratory failure, stabilizing the patient's condition and ensuring adequate oxygenation. This may include supplemental oxygenation, non-invasive ventilation (NIV), and in cases of extreme severity, intubation followed by mechanical ventilation. The aim is to afford sufficient gas exchange without causing further complications secondary to substandard oxygenation or hypercapnia. Newer therapeutic strategies, especially in the context of infectious conditions like COVID-19, emphasize the importance of such maneuvers. Indeed, effective antiviral therapies and immunization are still in the pipeline as mainstay elements in the prophylactic management of respiratory failure from viral infection (Habas et al., 2020). Besides supportive therapy, drug treatment has a significant role to play in the management of respiratory failure. The use of corticosteroids has gained significance, particularly for patients who have acute respiratory distress syndrome (ARDS) caused by infections such as COVID-19. The medication aims to reduce inflammation within the lungs, thereby improving general pulmonary function. Studies have shown that the prompt use of corticosteroids can significantly reduce the mortality rate in more severe conditions (Li et al., 2020). Moreover, adding bronchodilators can enhance airway obstruction and ventilation in individuals with chronic obstructive pulmonary disease or asthma. As studies continue to unfold, identifying the most appropriate dosages and treatment regimens remains the top priority to achieve the utmost therapeutic advantages in the treatment of respiratory failure. Convalescent plasma therapy is another new-fangled treatment option that has been studied in COVID-19-infected patients with respiratory comorbidities. It involves the administration of plasma from survivors of the virus with the expectation that the neutralizing antibodies contained within it would be of value to the immune system in active infections. Some hope has been noted in early reports, particularly in those with severe respiratory manifestations, although definitive evidence of its efficacy has not yet been demonstrated. For instance, whereas convalescent plasma therapy was associated with a substantial improvement in some clinical parameters, statistical significance was not established in larger demographic analyses (Li et al., 2020). Therefore, further studies are needed, and future clinical trials should focus on optimizing criteria for patient selection and identifying specific populations that would derive the maximum benefit from this novel therapeutic approach.

12.4.1. Oxygen Therapy

The administration of oxygen therapy in the treatment of respiratory failure is essential, particularly in individuals with chronic obstructive pulmonary disease (COPD) and other hypoxemic conditions. Oxygen therapy helps alleviate the signs and symptoms of hypoxia by increasing tissue oxygenation, thereby preserving vital bodily functions. Clinical practice guidelines recognize the importance of integrating both pharmacologic and non-pharmacologic treatments in an attempt to enhance improved quality of life and survival in the patient. For patients with COPD, long-term oxygen therapy (LTOT) is used in those who exhibit persistently low blood oxygen levels. Not only does the therapy increase oxygen saturation, but it has also been correlated with reduced hospital readmissions and mortality, proving the effectiveness of the therapy in chronic disease conditions (Marks G). Oxygen therapy is also evolving with advancements in technology that increase patient compliance and results. The existence of portable oxygen concentrators (POCs) enables patients to maintain mobility during oxygen therapy. Intelligent portable oxygen concentrators (iPOCs) are technologies that adjust oxygen flow automatically in line with patients' physical activity levels as monitored in real-time. Such equipment ensures that the patient receives the correct oxygen amount based on their level of activity, thereby enhancing compliance with guideline therapy. iPOCs' performance has been demonstrated, with superior accuracy in oxygen adjustments and improved general oxygenation compared to standard models (Do Lña et al., 2020). The advancements not only demonstrate improved health results but also significantly enhance the quality of life of individuals with chronic respiratory diseases. Although oxygen therapy has certain benefits, it is applied unevenly across the population. Evidence indicates that many eligible patients are not being treated with LTOT, sometimes due to a lack of awareness or healthcare system restrictions (Marks G). Monitoring access to and uptake of oxygen therapy is critical for identifying gaps and informing appropriate interventions. Improved data on the use of therapy can highlight barriers and help inform strategic planning to enhance its delivery. Addressing these disparities is central to the bigger picture of the treatment of respiratory failure, eventually resulting in patients being treated with comprehensive care that also includes timely and appropriate oxygen therapy as part of a general multi-faceted treatment for chronic respiratory disease. Not only does this overall process contribute to individual patient care improvement, but it also contributes to decreasing the overall issue of respiratory disease in healthcare systems.

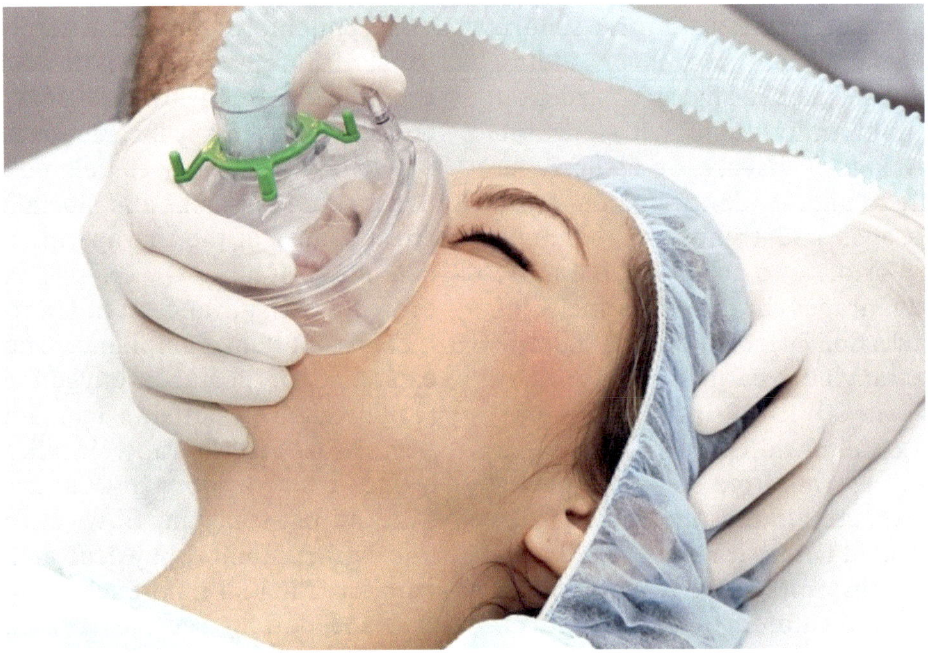

Figure 12.10. Oxygen therapy.

Source: https://www.safestroke.eu/wp-content/uploads/2017/02/oxygen-mask.jpg

12.4.2. Mechanical Ventilation

Mechanical ventilation is a valuable intervention for patients with respiratory failure, particularly when spontaneous breathing is inadequate to meet the body's metabolic needs. Mechanical ventilation involves the delivery of controlled breaths with the help of a ventilator, which delivers sufficient oxygenation and elimination of carbon dioxide. In situations involving acute respiratory distress syndrome (ARDS), potentially caused by reasons such as pneumonia and sepsis, mechanical ventilation assumes significance. The ventilatory approach—i.e., assist-control vs. pressure support ventilation—has a significant impact on clinical outcomes and must be tailored based on patient-specific factors. Detailed familiarity with the patient's underlying pathology informs the choice of ventilatory mode and settings, highlighting the importance of an integrated mechanical ventilation strategy in critically ill patients, in particular those with sepsis-related respiratory failure and septic shock (Evans et al., 2021). The physiological impact of mechanical ventilation is complex and demands close observation and titration. When mechanical ventilation is applied, the provider must balance tidal volumes, rates, and pressures to provide adequate ventilation while preventing ventilator-induced lung injury (VILI). Low tidal volume strategies are encouraged in patients with ARDS through research, which has shown that using low tidal volumes (approximately 6 mL/kg of predicted body weight) can prevent alveolar overdistension, with the goal of preserving lung function in the long term. In addition, using optimal positive end-expiratory pressure (PEEP) has improved oxygenation without the threat of repeated alveolar opening and closure. Such measures are of utmost importance in averting mechanical ventilation complications, emphasizing vigilance during informed decision-making and ongoing monitoring of patient response during the management of ongoing respiratory failure (Naicker et al., 2020). Severe respiratory failure may also require resorting to advanced ventilation techniques, such as high-frequency oscillatory ventilation or extracorporeal membrane oxygenation (ECMO). These therapies, while more invasive, can be life-saving in refractory hypoxemia or hypercapnia in nonresponding patients. Particularly in sepsis-induced ARDS, where the lung function is acutely damaged, such therapy can provide temporary respiratory support while the underlying pathology has a chance to recover. Research within critical care settings continues to examine the optimization of mechanical ventilation, with nuances for different patient populations, such as those presenting with respiratory disease due to COVID-19, which have emerged with their unique set of challenges and demands in mechanical ventilation practices. This assists healthcare practitioners in making life-and-death decisions on the management of respiratory failure (Naicker et al., 2020).

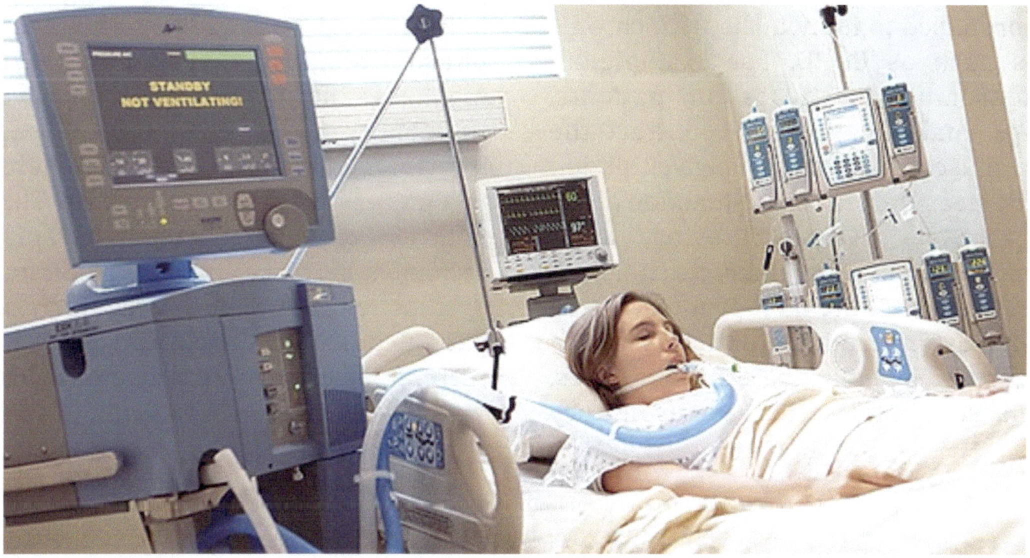

Figure 12.11. Mechanical ventilation.

Source: https://static.wixstatic.com/media/101914_c8af3edb378f4462a44273fa4535d3e3~mv2.png/v1/fill/w_568,h_304,al_c,q_85,usm_0.66_1.00_0.01,enc_avif,quality_auto/101914_c8af3edb378f4462a44273fa4535d3e3~mv2.png

12.4.3. Pharmacological Interventions

Pharmacologic intervention is a crucial component in the treatment of respiratory failure, particularly in reversing the underlying pathophysiologic processes that contribute to this life-threatening condition. The use of bronchodilators, corticosteroids, and other respiratory agents is aimed at maintaining airway patency, reducing inflammation, and preserving gas exchange. Beta-agonists such as albuterol are examples, with the latter exerting its action on bronchial smooth muscle to cause vasodilation and consequent relief of bronchospasm. Furthermore, corticosteroids like prednisone are commonly applied to suppress inflammatory processes in the lungs, which can be exacerbated in conditions such as acute respiratory distress syndrome (ARDS). By properly acting on these processes, pharmacological intervention can successfully alleviate symptoms and improve overall respiratory capacity in infected individuals. In addition to bronchodilators and corticosteroids, respiratory failure can also be addressed through the incorporation of pharmacologic interventions that augment respiratory muscle function. These interventions may include medications that enhance the strength and endurance of respiratory muscles, which are often compromised in individuals with chronic conditions such as COPD. For example, in certain neuromuscular drugs for patients, these drugs enable patients to contract the respiratory muscles, thus improving ventilation successfully. Measurement of the function of the respiratory muscle becomes necessary under such circumstances because it directs clinicians on the effectiveness of the therapy intervention and triggers customized interventions that can be adjusted based on individuals' specific needs. In addition, combining , such as respiratory muscle training, can yield improved results for patients undergoing pharmacological treatment. This approach is consistent with current advances in clinical practice. Further, newer pharmacologic treatments such as adaptive servo-ventilation (ASV) are showing promise for the treatment of central sleep apnea (CSA) associated with respiratory failure, particularly among patients with heart failure. ASV is a new positive airway pressure therapy that is synchronized to a patient's breathing patterns, therefore providing individualized ventilation support. Although recent meta-analysis findings indicate that ASV has no significant effect on critical cardiac parameters, such as left ventricular ejection fraction, it still provides potential benefits for certain subgroups of heart failure (Aleid et al., 2024). This ever-evolving pharmacological therapeutic environment highlights the need for ongoing investigation to identify the optimal patient populations for treatment with these new therapies and to optimize treatment protocols. Through the addition of new pharmacotherapies, which increment the management of respiratory muscle dysfunction, the aim is ultimately to improve patient outcomes in various presentations of respiratory failure (Poddighe et al., 2024).

Test Your Knowledge

1. What is oxygen therapy?
2. What is mechanical ventilation?

12.5. Complications Associated With Respiratory Failure

Learning Outcome

1. Cardiovascular Complications
2. Infections and Sepsis
3. Long-term Pulmonary Damage

Complications related to respiratory failure are of utmost significance, contributing to morbidity and mortality in the involved populations. Ventilator-associated pneumonia (VAP) in mechanically ventilated patients is a significant problem. VAP is not only a common complication but is also a major cause of more extended hospital stays and increased healthcare costs. It is most often caused by situations such as airway colonization and the compromised immune response due to systemic illness. Furthermore, patients of respiratory failure can experience prolonged ventilation therapy, which puts them at greater risk of developing complications such as diaphragm dysfunction and critical illness myopathy, making it even harder to recover.

Management of such complications is essential, as they not only lead to poorer clinical outcomes but also necessitate a more complex and resource-intensive approach to patient care. A second significant complication arises from the use of lung rest strategies during treatment, particularly in neonates undergoing extracorporeal membrane oxygenation (ECMO). Choice of ventilator settings plays a vital role in determining respiratory failure outcomes. For example, conventional mechanical ventilation has been associated with higher rates of supportive care and potentially prolongs the duration of ECMO, as indicated by evidence that various levels of positive end-expiratory pressure affect the overall treatment time (Aghai et al., 2017). This practice deviation from ventilator standard can lead to unexpected delays before weaning patients from ventilation, increasing hospital length of stay, and aggravating the risk of other complications such as pulmonary hypertension or lung injury. Thus, optimizing ventilatory management emerges as pivotal in minimizing these resultant risks, ultimately decreasing patient harm. Moreover, the general prognosis of complications of respiratory failure may affect patient management and operative outcomes, particularly in patients with underlying conditions. For instance, those with neuromuscular diseases undergoing surgery are at high risk of complications of respiratory failure. In a study of complications associated with neuromuscular scoliosis, a significant proportion of patients experienced adverse events that negatively impacted their treatment course and outcomes (Calderaro et al., 2017). These findings emphasize the importance of thorough preoperative assessments and effective measures to prevent complications. By understanding the interaction between surgical risks and respiratory failure, clinicians are able to predict better and manage complications and offer an improved, proactive regimen of care to vulnerable populations.

12.5.1. Cardiovascular Complications

COVID-19 has revealed profound cardiovascular complications that may occur to augment respiratory failure, bringing into focus their complex interrelation. The interrelation between pulmonary infections like COVID-19 and cardiovascular wellbeing is complex; acute respiratory distress syndrome (ARDS) presents in severe diseases, leading to a cascade of cardiovascular stress. Research indicates that approximately 42% of COVID-19 pneumonia patients subsequently develop ARDS, an acute hypoxemic respiratory failure, and are often complicated by underlying cardiovascular disease, such as hypertension and myocardial injury. The presence of such comorbidities renders it difficult to clinically manage respiratory failure since the patient is at increased risk of morbidity and mortality and needs intense monitoring and personalized therapeutic interventions (Gibson et al., 2020). In critically ill patients, the cardiac effects of respiratory failure are adverse, usually in the form of myocardial dysfunction. Release of cardiac biomarkers such as troponins during COVID-19 has been correlated with higher mortality rates by virtue of myocardial injury and consequent complications such as cardiogenic shock and decreased vascular tone, inducing hypotension. This damage to the myocardium can complicate respiratory failure management options because, as well as placing an added burden on the heart, it depletes the reserve capacity needed to cope with hypoxia secondary to compromised pulmonary function. Clinicians are thus increasingly required to address both respiratory and cardiac stewardship in a multifaceted approach to patient management (Lorenzo et al., 2020). In view of the urgency of confluence of respiration and cardiovascular functions in patients with COVID-19 and ARDS, a coordinated plan of management becomes the need of the hour. Early identification of cardiovascular complications is crucial in order to improve outcomes in affected groups. Interventions may include the provision of supportive therapies like fluid resuscitation, the use of vasopressors, and close monitoring of cardiac function through echocardiography. Furthermore, understanding the unique presentations of ARDS, including those associated with COVID-19, such as inflammatory mechanisms leading to multiorgan pulmonary and cardiovascular injury, informs the development of changing treatment protocols with the overall aim of reducing the incidence of respiratory failure. Through this double aim, not only is resolution from acute respiratory distress encouraged but also the high cardiovascular risk imposed by chronic hypoxemia is reduced (Gibson et al., 2020).

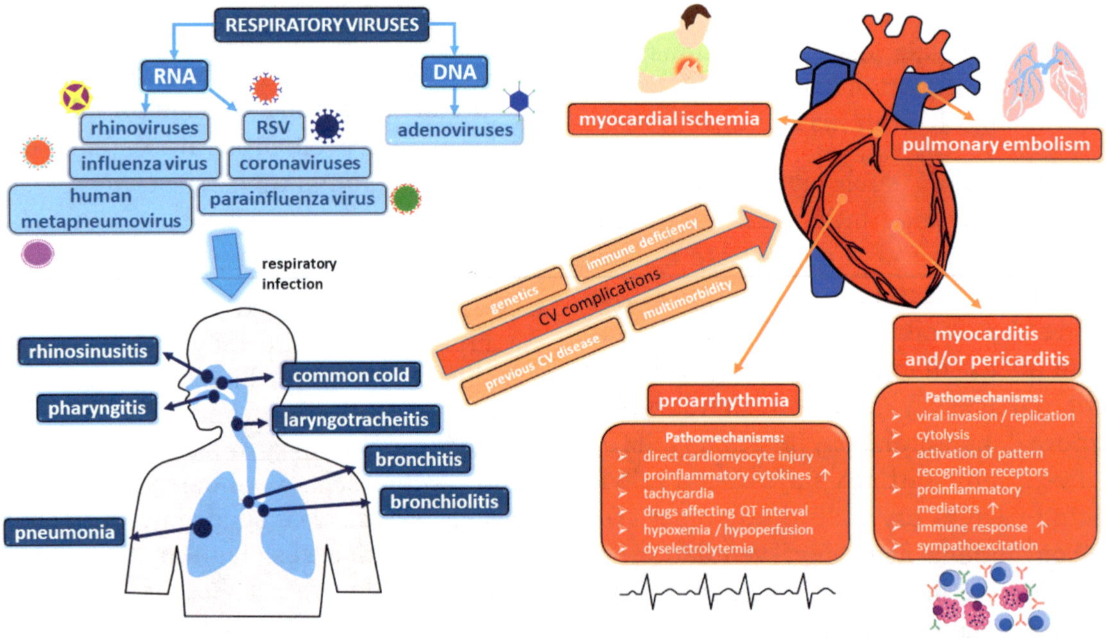

Figure 12.12. Cardiovascular complications with respiratory failure.

Source: https://www.mdpi.com/biomedicines/biomedicines-11-00071/article_deploy/html/images/biomedicines-11-00071-g001.png

12.5.2. Infections and Sepsis

The association between infection and sepsis is central to the pathophysiology of respiratory failure. Sepsis ensues when the host response to infection results in catastrophic organ dysfunction, typically in conjunction with acute respiratory distress syndrome (ARDS). The Surviving Sepsis Campaign promotes early recognition and treatment of sepsis, with guidelines that recommend the early use of antimicrobial therapy within one hour of recognizing sepsis. Such early treatment will significantly enhance patient outcomes, thereby reducing the risk of developing severe respiratory complications, such as ARDS. In addition, the severity of sepsis-associated respiratory failure is a sign of a deranged immune response, which may cause injury to the lungs and disrupt normal respiratory dynamics, ultimately leading to gas exchange derangements and oxygenation failures required for patient survival (Evans et al., 2021). The pathophysiology mechanisms of sepsis are multifactorial and include both direct and indirect effects on lung function. For instance, the induction of toll-like receptor 4 (TLR4) by pathogen-associated molecular patterns may trigger an inflammatory cascade, resulting in increased vascular permeability and pulmonary edema. This highly effective inflammatory process, although required to neutralize infection, can inadvertently result in extreme tissue damage that causes respiratory failure. In addition, the relationship between sepsis and dysregulation of surfactant production in the lungs has the potential to exacerbate the course of ARDS since functional surfactant loss compromises lung mechanics and gas exchange. Understanding the intricate interactions between infection, TLR4 signaling, and lung function has the potential to shed light on the targets of therapy for reversing the progression of respiratory failure in septic patients (Aboudounya et al., 2021). The clinical management of sepsis-related respiratory failure involves a comprehensive and multidisciplinary approach. The treatment protocols can include supportive care measures such as mechanical ventilation and fluid resuscitation, in combination with the administration of broad-spectrum antibiotics to combat the responsible infection.

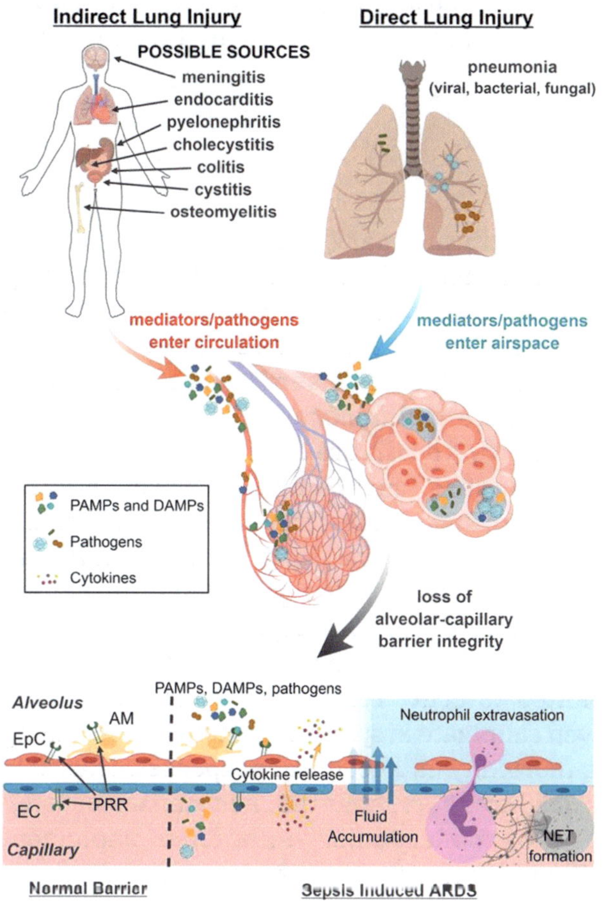

Figure 12.13. Infections and sepsis with respiratory failure.

Source: https://df6sxcketz7bb.cloudfront.net/manuscripts/124000/124061/medium/jci.insight.124061.f1.jpg

New recommendations suggest the use of balanced crystalloids instead of normal saline for fluid resuscitation to minimize the deleterious effects of hyperchloremic metabolic acidosis. Furthermore, corticosteroids are also used to modulate the hyperinflammatory response in septic patients. Equally vital is addressing the long-term condition of the survivors, who tend to have persistent respiratory dysfunction and other organ dysfunction. Developing follow-up programs that assess and support patient recovery following sepsis can enhance their functional status and quality of life, highlighting the need for ongoing care in this high-risk patient group (Evans et al., 2021).

12.5.3. Long-Term Pulmonary Damage

Chronic pulmonary damage is a serious consequence of most chronic respiratory disorders that tend to cause severe health complications that tend to exacerbate respiratory failure. Disorders such as chronic obstructive pulmonary disease (COPD) and pulmonary fibrosis are extensively documented to impair lung function over time progressively. The disorders cause structural and functional changes within the lung tissue, leading to inefficient gas exchange, which ultimately culminates in chronic respiratory insufficiency. The effect of this chronic impairment is not limited to acute respiratory symptoms; it can even culminate in systemic complications, adding to morbidity and healthcare expenses. Thus, it is crucial to understand the mechanisms of long-term pulmonary injury in order to implement efficient therapeutic interventions aimed at countering its development and addressing the consequences of respiratory failure. Furthermore, the chronic pulmonary damage is generally made worse by environmental hazards and lifestyle causes, such as smoking, pollution, and occupational hazards. Chronic exposure to these risk factors typically accelerates or triggers deterioration in lung function, leading to the development of irreversible injury-based diseases. Of specific note is the role of recurrent pulmonary embolism (PE), which has the potential to cause chronic thromboembolic pulmonary hypertension. This condition not only affects pulmonary status but can also cause right ventricular failure and have a significant impact on overall cardiovascular status. Accurate risk stratification and management are key in handling such complications. It has been observed in literature that early interventions improve outcomes in individuals at risk. Thus the use of multidisciplinary approaches to handling the burden of long-term pulmonary insult becomes all the more pertinent (Bellis et al., 2018). The impact of chronic pulmonary damage is extensive, necessitating increased concern and earlier intervention strategies in the healthcare system. Respiratory failure from chronic lung illness is common among patients who often have a poorer quality of life with ongoing symptoms of dyspnea and fatigue. This case highlights the importance of prompt diagnosis and treatment, which can lead to lifestyle modifications, medication, and, in severe cases, surgery. Available lung health improvement measures, such as anti-smoking campaigns and environmental regulations, are important in the prevention of chronic pulmonary injury. Through prevention and management, the healthcare community can significantly improve outcomes among those at risk of respiratory failure, thereby reducing both the clinical and socioeconomic burden of these chronic conditions (Zibrak et al., 2014).

Test Your Knowledge

1. What are the cardiovascular complications?
2. What is long-term pulmonary damage?

12.6. Prevention Strategies

Learning Outcome

1. Smoking Cessation Programs
2. Vaccination and Infection Control
3. Management of Chronic Respiratory Conditions

Effective prevention strategies are necessary to manage the onset of respiratory failure, particularly in the case of pneumonia, the leading cause of this fatal disorder. Primary prevention strategies aim to reduce the chance of pneumonia by taking measures such as immunization, quitting smoking, and managing comorbidities. Vaccines, for example, against pneumococcus and influenza, are highly effective in reducing the rates of pneumonia in susceptible groups, such as the elderly and patients with chronic respiratory conditions. Further, encouraging quitting smoking can have long-term implications because smoking itself is a significant risk factor for the development of respiratory infections. By focusing on such preventive interventions, healthcare providers can significantly reduce the cases of respiratory failure due to pneumonia, ultimately saving lives and lowering healthcare expenses associated with acute care procedures (Moon et al., 2025). Secondary prevention interventions are equally important in the early recognition and treatment of pneumonia, aiming to prevent progression to acute respiratory failure. This includes the use of risk assessment methods, such as the Pneumonia Severity Index (PSI), and the utilization of specific biomarkers, including procalcitonin and C-reactive protein. These methods enable early diagnosis and allow clinicians to implement proper antibiotic therapy without unnecessary delay, improving patient outcomes. New technologies such as machine learning algorithms for real-time stratification of pneumonia patients also supplement traditional assessment methods. By enhancing the speed and precision of pneumonia diagnosis, secondary prevention interventions contribute significantly to reducing the number of patients who develop respiratory failure, highlighting the importance of continued investment in detection and intervention strategies (Moon et al., 2025). Tertiary prevention interventions, targeted at maximizing the care for patients who are already experiencing respiratory failure, are critical in preventing complications and improving recovery outcomes. This intervention phase involves the use of noninvasive respiratory assistance and lung-protective ventilatory strategies, along with bundled care, in intubated patients. Novel treatments, such as diaphragm pacing, have also been making headlines recently, particularly in ROHHAD syndrome, where regular mechanical ventilation may not be the optimal approach. This method has been shown to have the potential to improve respiratory function and minimize dependency on invasive ventilation strategies. Implementing these tertiary prevention procedures will significantly reduce the impact of respiratory failure and enhance the patient's quality of care, underscoring the need for multidimensional input in addressing this life-threatening condition.

12.6.1. Smoking Cessation Programs

Smoking cessation programs play a vital role in addressing the public health crisis associated with respiratory failure, particularly in view of the extensively documented implications of lung function resulting from smoking. The increasing prevalence of chronic respiratory diseases, such as COPD and lung cancer, underscores the necessity for such programs. Evidence indicates that successful smoking cessation programs can dramatically decrease the prevalence of respiratory failure, consequently enhancing general patient outcomes. They tend to utilize a multicomponent approach, including behavioral assistance, pharmacological intervention, and social support, in an effort to assist individuals with cigarette smoking cessation. Addressing both the physical and psychological components of addiction, smoking cessation programs have the potential to result in sustained abstinence. This multi-faceted approach is imperative as it not only caters to the immediate need of quitting but also equips the subjects with coping strategies for maintaining a smoke-free lifestyle, impacting respiratory health directly, and reducing the prevalence of respiratory diseases. The incorporation of technology advancements in smoking cessation programs has revolutionized the way assistance is being provided to subjects who wish to quit smoking. Digital health technologies, such as cell phone applications and internet forums, have become increasingly popular and effective. These websites often provide personalized guidance, support, and access to a like-minded community, all making quitting easier than ever. Recent research has shown that app users achieve higher quit rates than those using conventional methods alone, demonstrating a desire to keep up with newer technology. Also, these interventions can be adjusted to fit individual lifestyles, making them as effective as possible. As smartphones are becoming a focus of daily routines, integrating technology with smoking cessation may be an essential step in curbing smoking and subsequently tobacco-related respiratory failure incidences, as highlighted in recent healthcare-related literature. The impact of smoking cessation programs extends beyond individual health; it also yields additional community and economic benefits. By decreasing the number of smokers, these programs have the ability to counteract the financial strain on healthcare systems typically associated with smoking disease treatment, such as respiratory failure. Moreover, healthier populations are responsible for increased productivity and decreased absenteeism, which fosters a healthy economy. Population-based programs with an educational and preventive focus create environments that support healthier lifestyle choices. One such example is public health campaigns, commonly initiated in addition to cessation strategies, to inform citizens about the hazards of smoking and the available aids to stop smoking. Lastly, incorporating smoking cessation measures into broader public health programs is crucial to avert the high incidences of respiratory failure and improve the quality of life for hundreds of thousands of patients.

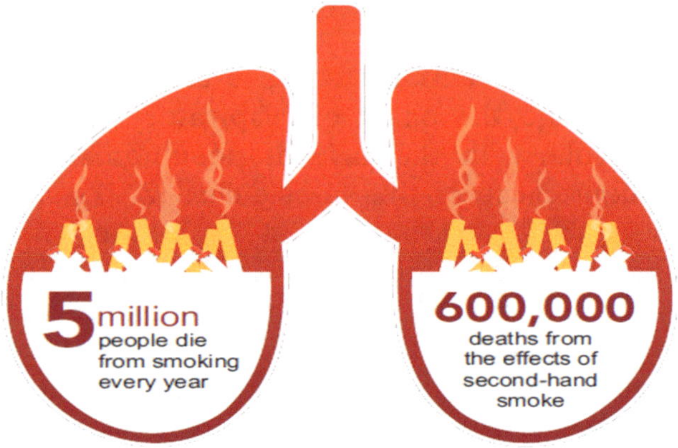

Figure 12.14. Smoking cessation programs.

Source: https://www.sgh.com.sg/patient-care/specialties-services/Respiratory-and-Critical-Care-Medicine/PublishingImages/pages/smoking-cessation-clinic/Lung-smoking-cessation.png

12.6.2. Vaccination and Infection Control

Vaccination plays a crucial role in preventing infections, particularly for respiratory diseases that can lead to respiratory failure. Vaccines immunize the body to fight and respond against some pathogens, which can reduce the incidence of infections such as pneumonia, influenza, and COVID-19, all of which can significantly impact respiratory function. Through prevention of these infections, vaccines significantly reduce respiratory failure complications, particularly among high-risk populations, including the elderly and those with underlying conditions. The existence of vaccines for various respiratory pathogens has been integral to curbing morbidity and mortality rates as well as improving overall respiratory health outcomes. Hence, vaccination promotion, along with public health measures, becomes a pressing need of the hour to reduce the number of severe respiratory infections that can lead to respiratory failure and necessitate intensive medical interventions. In addition to vaccination, strict infection control measures must be implemented to prevent respiratory infections and their subsequent impact on respiratory function. Optimal infection control strategies encompass a range of interventions, including regular hand hygiene, wearing personal protective equipment, and isolating infected individuals. These measures of intervention are most relevant within healthcare settings, where risk of transmission is increased. As an illustration, in cases of respiratory infections like the COVID-19 pandemic, strict infection control strategies have had to be adopted to protect healthcare providers and vulnerable patients. The concurrent implementation of vaccination and infection control strategies forms the foundation for a comprehensive program to manage respiratory infections, ultimately preventing respiratory failure in susceptible populations. All such overall approaches are critical, particularly in high-prevalence regions, where community-based interventions have the potential to reduce rates of transmission as well as complications risks substantially. The emergence of novel respiratory viruses, such as severe acute respiratory syndrome coronavirus 2 (SARS-CoV-2), underscores the ongoing need for effective vaccination and infection control measures. The pandemic of COVID-19 illustrated the noteworthy impact of viral infections on respiratory health, with high rates of respiratory failure and associated mortality, especially in unvaccinated groups (Hui et al., 2022). COVID-19 vaccination has proved to be one of the most powerful tools in controlling this virus and preventing the severe consequences of the disease, reaffirming the need for mass campaigns promoting vaccine coverage. In addition, the rapid evolution of diagnostic and treatment protocols to contend with COVID-19 underscores the dynamic nature of infection control in practice. As we continue to fight new respiratory infections, continuous research and public health interventions will be vital to ensuring that vaccination remains the foundation of infection prevention and respiratory healthcare, thereby reducing the burden of respiratory failure in the population (Yadav, 2024).

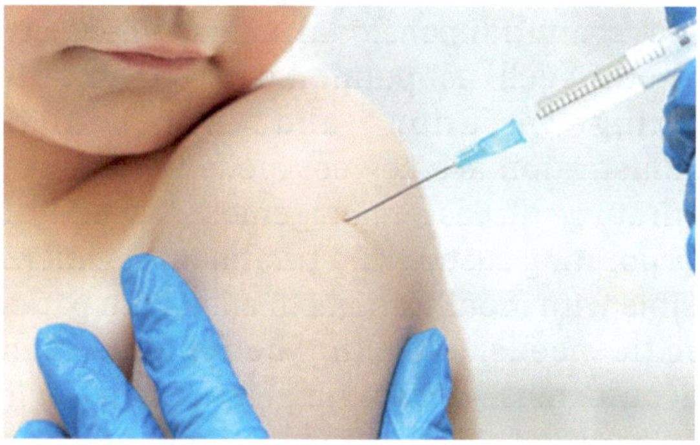

Figure 12.15. Vaccination and infection control for respiratory failure.

Source: https://www.kauveryhospital.com/wp-content/uploads/2023/12/88-3.jpg

12.6.3. Management of Chronic Respiratory Conditions

Management of chronic respiratory diseases, most notably chronic obstructive pulmonary disease (COPD) and obstructive sleep apnea (OSA), is essential in averting respiratory failure. The two pathologies are capable of occurring concurrently, and this leads to a condition called overlap syndrome (OS) that immensely complicates therapeutic management. Hypoxemia and hypercapnia and its sequelae often confront OS patients with profound implications of higher hospitalization rates as well as an elevated mortality rate. Effective management requires an integrated approach, including active screening and regular monitoring of nocturnal hypoxia. By addressing the complexities of managing both COPD and OSA, healthcare providers can intervene more effectively for the individual, such as non-invasive ventilation, which is crucial in OS patients, particularly in the management of acute exacerbations. Apart from this, reductionist orientations in the mitigation of clinical practices can enhance outcomes and improve the quality of life for patients with such chronic diseases worldwide (Sun et al., 2025). For knowing the role of chronic respiratory disorders, the healthcare professionals must follow a multidimensional management style. Methods such as pulmonary rehabilitation, smoking cessation, and bronchodilator administration are key components of chronic respiratory disease management. In addition, incorporating customized treatment regimens is feasible with modifications to align with patient-specific needs, enabling better compliance and outcomes. Continuing education on the importance of self-management and adherence to prescribed therapies has a significant impact on patients' quality of life. Interventions promptly in patients presenting with acute exacerbations of respiratory distress due to chronic disease are essential to prevent the progression to respiratory failure. Such interdisciplinary management ensures that all aspects of a patient's chronic disease are addressed, leading to improved outcomes (Sun et al., 2025). Over the last few years, the growing awareness of the effects of substances such as e-cigarettes and their potential to aggravate chronic respiratory disease has mounted. The emergence of e-cigarette or vaping product use-associated lung injury (EVALI) demonstrates that there is a requirement for caution in respiratory care. Patients presenting with symptoms characteristic of chronic respiratory disease may actually have EVALI, and it becomes challenging for traditional management practices to be efficacious. Challenges in diagnosing and treating EVALI emphasize the importance of ongoing education and research on the impact of vaping on lung function. Treatment of EVALI is often successful with corticosteroids and supportive care, particularly in patients with acute respiratory distress syndrome (ARDS). Therefore, it is essential to have complete knowledge of the latest trends in respiratory health, such as the impact of vaping, in order to effectively treat chronic respiratory diseases and prevent severe consequences, including respiratory failure.

Test Your Knowledge

1. Illustrate the smoking cessation programs.
2. How are chronic respiratory conditions managed?

SUMMARY

This respiratory failure analysis embodies the severity and complexity of conditions among such patients. New evidence suggests a heavy burden associated with respiratory failure, particularly in groups with co-existing comorbidities. Research indicates that patients being ambulanced, in a state of having a hard time breathing, fall into categories like pneumonia, cardiac failure, and chronic obstructive pulmonary disease (COPD) (Archer et al., 2016). An awareness of this complexity is essential, as healthcare systems must adjust their services to accommodate the diverse needs of a patient group. An appreciation of the epidemiology of respiratory failure gives an understanding of focused interventions that can enhance outcomes for these patients, ultimately to establish better healthcare provision and more effective resource allocation within emergency medicine. Furthermore, advances in modalities of respiratory support have been pivotal in the care of acute and chronic respiratory failure. Non-invasive interventions, such as high-flow nasal therapy (HFNT), have increasingly gained popularity and are currently used extensively in clinical practice, enhancing patient outcomes and comfort (Cortegiani et al., 2019). This advancement reflects the ongoing evolution in treatment modalities to provide adequate respiratory support. By administering warmed and humidified oxygen with higher flow rates, HFNT addresses both the oxygenation and ventilation needs of patients suffering from respiratory distress. Further studies in this area are needed to standardize treatment and assess the long-term effects of novel therapies, ensuring they effectively meet clinical needs. In general, care for respiratory failure is a critical healthcare area that requires a multidimensional approach to treatment for patients. Respiratory distress is a vulnerable population of patients who are not only suffering from respiratory distress but also other health conditions, which make management complex. With the evolution of knowledge about respiratory failure, clinical responses will also need to follow variable patient populations. Care systems will need to incorporate information related to the epidemiology of respiratory distress and emerging therapies, such as HFNT. These results collectively will maximize outcome measurement, enhance patient care, and enable a more robust response to the ongoing threats of respiratory failure in medicine.

Respiratory failure is significant in clinical practice and public health. It is primarily characterized by the respiratory system's inability to perform adequate gas exchange, resulting in hypoxemia or hypercapnia. Specific causes of respiratory failure include chronic obstructive pulmonary disease (COPD), pneumonia, and acute respiratory distress syndrome (ARDS). All of these conditions demonstrate mechanisms by which underlying pathophysiological processes lead to departure from normal respiratory function. Treatment varies across the board, underscoring the importance of taking an individualized approach with each patient's unique clinical picture. For instance, therapy can range from supplemental oxygenation to invasive mechanical ventilation, underlining the urgency of early diagnosis and treatment. As expounded in the literature, the role of systematic reviews in chronic respiratory conditions cannot be overstated, particularly in improving knowledge and guiding best patient care (Page et al., 2021). The history of respiratory failure can be either acute or chronic in nature and demands special clinical knowledge to improve patient outcomes. Acute respiratory failure evolves speedily and typically requires immediate intervention, whereas chronic respiratory failure evolves over decades and necessitates careful management of comorbid conditions. Several studies emphasize the importance of early detection of these conditions to prevent the onset of respiratory failure. The integration of newer therapeutic modalities, including pharmacological advancements, is a significant factor in improving survival rates and enhancing the quality of life for patients. As stated, the antitumor activity exhibited by pembrolizumab and axitinib in patients with advanced renal cell carcinoma serves to remind us of how emerging treatments are capable of revolutionizing treatment paradigms (Brian I. Rini et al., 2019). Continued research in the field of respiratory medicine is necessary to understand the evolving pathogenesis and treatment paradigms underlying respiratory failure. Aside from the initial management of respiratory failure, longer-term interventions must also be considered to enhance recovery and avoid recurrence. Conditioning and pulmonary rehabilitation programs have been shown to be valuable adjuncts to management. These programs emphasize the importance of exercise and learning and are designed to give patients greater control of their illness. Additionally, the use of telemedicine and remote monitoring equipment facilitates continuous patient engagement, thus enabling timely intervention when deterioration ensues. The ongoing focus on capacity development through systematic reviews underscores the need for amalgamation and synthesis of evidence-based practice, potentially spread widely to healthcare practitioners (Page et al., 2021). Lastly, the intricate treatment strategy for respiratory failure is a convergence of clinical expertise, research ingenuity, and commitment towards improving patient outcomes in respiratory medicine.

KEY TERMS FROM THIS CHAPTER

- Hypoxemia
- Type 1 respiratory failure
- PaO2
- Ventilation-perfusion mismatch
- Dead space ventilation
- Mechanical ventilation
- Oxygen therapy
- Work of breathing
- Fatigue
- Pulmonary edema
- Hypercapnia
- Type 2 respiratory failure
- PaCO2
- Shunt
- Acidosis
- Non-invasive ventilation (NIV)
- Acute Respiratory Distress Syndrome (ARDS)
- Dyspnea
- Respiratory muscle failure
- Hyperventilation

CRITICAL THINKING QUESTIONS

1. **Respiratory failure is defined by which of the following?**
   a. $PaO_2 < 60$ mmHg with or without $PaCO_2 > 50$ mmHg
   b. $PaO_2 > 80$ mmHg and $PaCO_2 < 40$ mmHg
   c. $PaCO_2 < 35$ mmHg only
   d. Normal blood gases with respiratory distress
2. **Type 1 respiratory failure is primarily characterized by:**
   a. Hypoxemia with normal or low $PaCO_2$
   b. Hypercapnia without hypoxemia
   c. Normal oxygenation with hypercapnia
   d. Neither hypoxemia nor hypercapnia
3. **Which of the following conditions is most likely to cause type 2 respiratory failure?**
   a. Pulmonary embolism
   b. Acute respiratory distress syndrome (ARDS)
   c. Chronic obstructive pulmonary disease (COPD) exacerbation
   d. Pulmonary edema
4. **What is the most appropriate initial treatment for type 1 respiratory failure?**
   a. Mechanical ventilation without oxygen
   b. Supplemental oxygen therapy
   c. Diuretics
   d. Bronchodilators only
5. **Which of the following is a potential complication of respiratory failure?**
   a. Pulmonary hypertension
   b. Diabetes mellitus
   c. Cerebral edema
   d. Renal calculi

Short Answer Questions

1. Define respiratory failure.
2. What are the two main types of respiratory failure?
3. What is the primary cause of type 1 (hypoxemic) respiratory failure?
4. Which blood gas parameter is used to diagnose respiratory failure?
5. Name three common causes of type 2 (hypercapnic) respiratory failure.

Answer to Critical Thinking Questions

1. (a) 2. (a) 3. (c) 4. (b) 5. (a)

REFERENCES

1. Aboudounya, M. M. & Heads, R. J. (2021). COVID-19 and Toll-Like Receptor 4 (TLR4): SARS-CoV-2 may bind and activate TLR4 to increase ACE2 expression, facilitating entry and causing hyperinflammation. *Mediators of Inflammation, 2021*, 1–18. https://doi.org/10.1155/2021/8874339 (accessed on 16th June 2025).
2. Alapati, D., Aghai, Z. H., Hossain, M. J., Dirnberger, D. R., Ogino, M. T., & Shaffer, T. H. (2017). Lung rest during extracorporeal membrane oxygenation for Neonatal Respiratory Failure—Practice Variations and Outcomes. *Pediatric Critical Care Medicine, 18*(7), 667–674. https://doi.org/10.1097/pcc.0000000000001171Aleid, A. M., Alqerafi, A., Alhejaili, I. S., Alsaedi, M. N., Almutairi, D. M. A., Al Shankiti, H. A. M., Almaslamani, N. W., et al. (2024). Assessing the efficacy of adaptive servo-ventilation in heart failure patients: A systematic review. *Journal of Advanced Trends in Medical Research*. https://www.semanticscholar.org/paper/e631f562f70d9e991c4ab0f3006cec6d0c224a63 (accessed on 16th June 2025).
3. Archer, P., Asha, S. E., Bryant, M., et al. (2016). Epidemiology, prehospital care and outcomes of patients arriving by ambulance with dyspnea: An observational study. https://core.ac.uk/download/196603319.pdf (accessed on 16th June 2025).
4. Azoulay, E., Benoit, D., Bruneel, F., et al. (2016). Increased mortality in hematological malignancy patients with acute respiratory failure from undetermined etiology: A Groupe de Recherche en Réanimation Respiratoire en Onco-Hématologique (Grrr-OH) study. https://core.ac.uk/download/84044246.pdf (accessed on 16th June 2025).
5. Behr, J., Brown, K. K., Ford, P., et al. (2024). An adjudication algorithm for respiratory-related hospitalisation in idiopathic pulmonary fibrosis. https://core.ac.uk/download/610638336.pdf (accessed on 16th June 2025).
6. Bhagani, S., Gillespie, S. H., & Hawkey, P. M. (2003). Severe acute respiratory syndrome (SARS): Breathtaking progress. https://core.ac.uk/download/1669004.pdf (accessed on 16th June 2025).
7. Boland, J., Martin, J., Ross, J. R., et al. (2013). Palliative care for people with non-malignant lung disease: Summary of current evidence and future direction. https://core.ac.uk/download/151156967.pdf (accessed on 16th June 2025).
8. Calderaro, C., Di Sanzo, V., Ferretti, A., et al. (2017). Rate of complications due to neuromuscular scoliosis spine surgery in a 30-years consecutive series. https://core.ac.uk/download/98337785.pdf (accessed on 16th June 2025).
9. Chopra, V., Flanders, S. A., O'Malley, M., Malani, A. N. & Prescott, H. C. (2020). Sixty-day outcomes among patients hospitalized with COVID-19. *Annals of Internal Medicine, 174*, 576–578. https://doi.org/10.7326/m20-5661 (accessed on 16th June 2025).
10. Cortegiani, A., Gregoretti, C., & Spoletini, G. (2019). Physio pathological rationale of using high-flow nasal therapy in the acute and chronic setting: A narrative review. https://core.ac.uk/download/224993362.pdf (accessed on 16th June 2025).
11. Daidone, C., & Carper, S. (2024). Differential diagnosis and interdisciplinary workup of a pediatric patient with an unknown immune condition: Chronic respiratory distress secondary to viral illness and developmental consequences. *Cureus, 16*. https://www.semanticscholar.org/paper/9ef2f4b50379d210db7e522cb26162d6de177f8e (accessed on 16th June 2025).

12. Davies, M. J., D'Alessio, D. A., Fradkin, J., Kernan, W. N., Mathieu, C., Mingrone, G., Rossing, P., et al. (2018). Management of hyperglycemia in type 2 diabetes, 2018. A consensus report by the American Diabetes Association (ADA) and the European Association for the Study of Diabetes (EASD). *Diabetes Care, 41*, 2669–2701. https://doi.org/10.2337/dci18-0033 (accessed on 16th June 2025).

13. De Bellis, A., D'Abramo, M., Frati, G., et al. (2018). Surgical embolectomy for acute massive pulmonary embolism: State of the art. https://core.ac.uk/download/188822613.pdf (accessed on 16th June 2025).

14. De Lorenzo, A., & da Cruz Lamas, C. (2020). COVID-19 and the cardiovascular system. *Heart Vessels and Transplantation, 4*, 37–37. https://doi.org/10.24969/hvt.2020.197 (accessed on 16th June 2025).

15. Doña, L., Jiménez, A. L., Muñoz, A., Zara, P., Morillo, P. S., et al. (2020). Automated home oxygen delivery for patients with COPD and respiratory failure: A new approach. https://core.ac.uk/download/322903467.pdf (accessed on 16th June 2025).

16. Evans, A., Alam, A., & Nugent, K. (2024). Average volume-assured pressure support versus fixed pressure support in chronic hypercapnic respiratory failure: A systematic review and meta-analysis. *The Southwest Respiratory and Critical Care Chronicles*. https://www.semanticscholar.org/paper/e7df8e1315cf2dcbaadbe31a18f2701958fad1a0 (accessed on 16th June 2025).

17. Evans, L., Rhodes, A., Alhazzani, W., Antonelli, M., Coopersmith, C. M., French, C., Machado, F. R., et al. (2021). Executive summary: Surviving sepsis campaign: International guidelines for the management of sepsis and septic shock 2021. *Critical Care Medicine, 49*, 1974–1982. https://doi.org/10.1097/ccm.0000000000005357 (accessed on 16th June 2025).

18. Evans, L., Rhodes, A., Alhazzani, W., Antonelli, M., Coopersmith, C. M., French, C., Machado, F. R., et al. (2021). Surviving sepsis campaign: International guidelines for management of sepsis and septic shock 2021. *Critical Care Medicine, 49*, e1063–e1143. https://doi.org/10.1097/ccm.0000000000005337 (accessed on 16th June 2025).

19. Gibson, P. G., Qin, L. & Puah, S. H. (2020). COVID-19 acute respiratory distress syndrome (ARDS): Clinical features and differences from typical pre-COVID-19 ARDS. *The Medical Journal of Australia, 213*, 54–54. https://doi.org/10.5694/mja2.50674 (accessed on 16th June 2025).

20. Gruszka, S., Wolff, A., Bryła, K., Szewczyk, M., Udziela-Gil, H., Lewandowska, D., Rosińska-Lewandoska, D., et al. (2025). Modern approach to the treatment of acute respiratory failure–from nasal cannula to ECMO. *Journal of Education, Health and Sport*. https://www.semanticscholar.org/paper/a1bd62f56ac7b6261d38e70da12ded7631426880 (accessed on 16th June 2025).

21. Gustafsson, U., Scott, M. J., Hübner, M., Nygren, J., Demartines, N., Francis, N., Rockall, T., et al. (2018). Guidelines for perioperative care in elective colorectal surgery: Enhanced Recovery After Surgery (ERAS®) Society recommendations: 2018. *World Journal of Surgery, 43*, 659–695. https://doi.org/10.1007/s00268-018-4844-y (accessed on 16th June 2025).

22. Habas, K., Nganwuchu, C., Shahzad, F., Gopalan, R. C., Haque, M., Rahman, S., Majumder, M. A. A., et al. (2020). Resolution of coronavirus disease 2019 (COVID-19). *Expert Review of Anti-infective Therapy, 18*, 1201–1211. https://doi.org/10.1080/14787210.2020.1797487 (accessed on 16th June 2025).

23. Halpin, D., Criner, G. J., Papi, A., Singh, D., Anzueto, A., Martínez, F. J., Agustí, A. A., et al. (2020). Global Initiative for the Diagnosis, Management, and Prevention of Chronic Obstructive Lung Disease. The 2020 GOLD Science Committee Report on COVID-19 and Chronic Obstructive Pulmonary Disease. *American Journal of Respiratory and Critical Care Medicine, 203*, 24–36. https://doi.org/10.1164/rccm.202009-3533so (accessed on 16th June 2025).

24. Hernadez, O., Bartlett, V., Browne, S., Corey, K., Gass, D., McCall, C., Molinari, L., et al. (2025). Baby's First Test: Importance of the newborn screen in the diagnosis of SCID. *Journal of Human Immunity*. https://www.semanticscholar.org/paper/0a9445da23b7e52205473cf346c894220a608f01 (accessed on 16th June 2025).

25. Hui, D., & Zumla, A. (2022). Advances in the epidemiology, clinical features, diagnosis, clinical management and prevention of coronavirus disease 2019. *Current Opinion in Pulmonary Medicine, 28*, 166–173. https://www.semanticscholar.org/paper/e5c811f32f07888544165288427d60fe4eed1667 (accessed on 16th June 2025).

26. Ishii, H., Kinoshita, Y., Hamada, N., Fujita, M. & Kushima, H. (2025). Idiopathic pleuroparenchymal fibroelastosis: Diagnosis and management. *Expert Review of Respiratory Medicine*. https://www.semanticscholar.org/paper/6650f84fb5c17935a0054dcaa71b2905d9e16215 (accessed on 16th June 2025).

27. Johnson, L. M., Pulskamp, T. G. & Berlau, D. J. (2025). The latest developments in synthetic approaches to Duchenne muscular dystrophy. *Expert Review of Neurotherapeutics, 25*, 311–321. https://www.semanticscholar.org/paper/4683ba1c517640eeff243f98e813b3ab3351f47d (accessed on 16th June 2025).

28. Li, L., Zhang, W., Hu, Y., Tong, X., Zheng, S., Yang, J., Kong, Y., et al. (2020). Effect of convalescent plasma therapy on time to clinical improvement in patients with severe and life-threatening COVID-19. *JAMA, 324*, 460–460. https://doi.org/10.1001/jama.2020.10044 (accessed on 16th June 2025).

29. Lin, C., & Robison, J. (2024). Silicone embolism syndrome causing altered mental status and respiratory failure after an unlicensed gluteal silicone injection: A case report. *Clinical Practice and Cases in Emergency Medicine, 8*, 151–154. https://www.semanticscholar.org/paper/080b1757033095612bf91a8e77dd240392190ee0 (accessed on 16th June 2025).

30. Lorusso, R., Shekar, K., MacLaren, G., Schmidt, M., Pellegrino, V., Meyns, B., Haft, J. W., et al. (2021). ELSO interim guidelines for Veno arterial extracorporeal membrane oxygenation in adult cardiac patients. *ASAIO Journal, 67*, 827–844. https://doi.org/10.1097/mat.0000000000001510 (accessed on 16th June 2025).

31. Marks, G. (2025). Monitoring pulmonary rehabilitation and long-term oxygen therapy for people with chronic obstructive pulmonary disease (COPD). https://core.ac.uk/download/pdf/30675577.pdf (accessed on 16th June 2025).

32. Moon, J. Y., El Labban, M., Gajic, O. & Odeyemi, Y. (2025). Strategies for preventing and reducing the impact of acute respiratory failure from pneumonia. *Expert Review of Respiratory Medicine, 19*, 205–221. https://www.semanticscholar.org/paper/4837bac6cd99d07df7a1a1161350cb1601f08d0d (accessed on 16th June 2025).

33. Naicker, S., Yang, C. W., Hwang, S. J., Liu, B. C., Chen, J. & Jha, V. (2020). The novel coronavirus 2019 epidemic and kidneys. *Kidney International, 97*, 824–828. https://doi.org/10.1016/j.kint.2020.03.001 (accessed on 16th June 2025).

34. Narala, V. R., Narala, S. R., Subramani, P. A., Panati, K. & Kolliputi, N. (2024). Role of mitochondria in inflammatory lung diseases. *Frontiers in Pharmacology, 15*. https://www.semanticscholar.org/paper/8076ef884b74e727b7440607b0d0e00b7c2e52a2 (accessed on 16th June 2025).

35. Page, M. J., Moher, D., Bossuyt, P. M., Boutron, I., Hoffmann, T., Mulrow, C. D., Shamseer, L., et al. (2021). PRISMA 2020 explanation and elaboration: Updated guidance and exemplars for reporting systematic reviews. *BMJ*. https://doi.org/10.1136/bmj.n160 (accessed on 16th June 2025).

36. Panetti, B., Bucci, I., Di Ludovico, A., Pellegrino, G., Di Filippo, P., Di Pillo, S., Chiarelli, F., et al. (2024). Acute respiratory failure in children: A clinical update on diagnosis. *Children, 11*. https://www.semanticscholar.org/paper/ccdbd2cee5910ae21d415e52282ffeb8ecfb46af (accessed on 16th June 2025).

37. Poddighe, D., Van Hollebeke, M., Rodrigues, A., Hermans, G., Testelmans, D., Kalkanis, A., Clerckx, B., et al. (2024). Respiratory muscle dysfunction in acute and chronic respiratory failure: How to diagnose and how to treat? *European Respiratory Review, 33*. https://www.semanticscholar.org/paper/d20197fae395b0d617d8936f79809b52fc21682f (accessed on 16th June 2025).

38. Prokopev, G. G., Abidova, M. M., Postnikova, E. V., Shorina, M., Mihajlova, A. D., Zhilina, S. S., Sulejmanov, A. B., et al. (2025). Diagnostic criteria and effective treatment strategies for respiratory failure in children with ROHHAD-syndrome. *Rossiyskiy Vestnik Perinatologii i Pediatrii (Russian Bulletin of Perinatology and Pediatrics)*. https://www.semanticscholar.org/paper/bd4a83904353c8282904027427d162de04fb67de (accessed on 16th June 2025).

39. Rini, B. I., Plimack, E. R., Stus, V. P., Gafanov, R., Hawkins, R. D., Nosov, D., Pouliot, F., et al. (2019). Pembrolizumab plus axitinib versus sunitinib for advanced renal-cell carcinoma. *New England Journal of Medicine, 380*, 1116–1127. https://doi.org/10.1056/nejmoa1816714 (accessed on 16th June 2025).

40. Rozova, K. & Shapovalova, A. S. (2023). Clinical effectiveness of phospholipids in patients with restrictive respiratory failure due to lung tissue inflammation. *Tuberculosis, Lung Diseases, HIV Infection*. https://www.semanticscholar.org/paper/c0f964afc610f04f92788f3f75f860a7416ad976 (accessed on 16th June 2025).

41. Ščerbakovs, K., Mihejeva, V., Dubencovs, S., Stunda, E. & Zentina, D. (2025). Pulmonary tumor embolism from gastric adenocarcinoma causing respiratory and cardiac failure may not be identified on standard ante-mortem imaging. *European Journal of Case Reports in Internal Medicine, 12*. https://www.semanticscholar.org/paper/28a69e3d573d0859a2d2df9c023e303dbda01dc9 (accessed on 16th June 2025).

42. Sjauw, D. J. T., Hessels, L. M., Duiverman, M., Elshof, J., Janssen, M. L., Türk, Y., Heunks, L., et al. (2025). High-flow nasal oxygen vs. conventional oxygen therapy in patients with COVID-19 related acute hypoxemic respiratory failure and a do not intubate order: A multicenter cohort study. *Respiratory Research, 26*. https://www.semanticscholar.org/paper/31d1b28289e92550b2ffa16e71486e7272a68b89 (accessed on 16th June 2025).

43. Sun, W. & Chen, Y. H. (2025). [Impact and management of comorbidities in patients with chronic obstructive pulmonary disease and obstructive sleep apnea]. *Zhonghua Jie He He Hu Xi Za Zhi = Chinese Journal of Tuberculosis and Respiratory Diseases, 48(4)*, 392–395. https://www.semanticscholar.org/paper/f950d1ea44ee4fc59a8f14c3727cc2eb1606ef77 (accessed

on 16th June 2025).

44. Suzuki, Y. & Kuriyama, A. (2024). Prolonged suppressive antibiotic therapy for inferior vena cava filter infection following emphysematous pyelonephritis and cystitis: A case report. *Annals of Medicine and Surgery, 86*, 2176–2180. https://www.semanticscholar.org/paper/da5a86336f812839bc4d94cdac3ed47ae6df87a3 (accessed on 16th June 2025).

45. Urlapu, K., Venkatram, S., Soliman, M., Ronderos, D. & Diaz-fuentes, G. (2023). Acute respiratory failure due to vaping-induced lung injury: A case report and management review. *International Journal of Innovative Research in Medical Science*. https://www.semanticscholar.org/paper/281abf074bf227f421937dd774a89f5bb9f689fd (accessed on 16th June 2025).

46. Wichmann, D. (2020). Autopsy findings and venous thromboembolism in patients with COVID-19. *Annals of Internal Medicine, 173*, 1030–1030. https://doi.org/10.7326/l20-1206 (accessed on 16th June 2025).

47. Wiersinga, W. J., Rhodes, A., Cheng, A. C., Peacock, S. J. & Prescott, H. C. (2020). Pathophysiology, transmission, diagnosis, and treatment of coronavirus disease 2019 (COVID-19). *JAMA, 324*, 782–782. https://doi.org/10.1001/jama.2020.12839 (accessed on 16th June 2025).

48. Wu, J., Yu, J., Li, H., Wang, Y. & Xu, R. (2024). Fatal invasive Aspergillus infection in an elderly patient with hepatitis E: A case report and literature review. *Medicine, 103*. https://www.semanticscholar.org/paper/ea2be8392234ebef0f171fe26526457bd35520c2 (accessed on 16th June 2025).

49. Yadav, S. (2024). Understanding the complexities of post-tuberculosis lung disease: Implications for global health. *IP Indian Journal of Immunology and Respiratory Medicine*. https://www.semanticscholar.org/paper/515136dc61c8694f1897a39a01f54605d11d8450 (accessed on 16th June 2025).

50. Zibrak, D., & Price, D. (2014). Interstitial lung disease: Raising the index of suspicion in primary care. https://core.ac.uk/download/25497515.pdf (accessed on 16th June 2025).

INDEX

A

Abnormal lung sounds 12, 28
Acid-fast bacilli (AFB) 253, 288, 289
Acid-fast bacilli (AFB) staining 289
Acidosis 428
Acute pneumonia 29
Acute Respiratory Distress Syndrome (ARDS) 428
Acute respiratory failure 18, 97, 107, 109, 186, 217, 295, 304, 307, 317, 324, 400, 403, 405, 407, 408, 414, 423, 430, 431, 432
Adaptive respiratory function 58
Adenoid hypertrophy (AH) 49
Airborne ultrasound surface motion camera (AUSMC) 22
Airborne ultrasound surface motion cameras (AUSMC) 9
Airflow limitation 391
Air-fluid level 215
Air trapping 391
Airway hyperresponsiveness 355
Airway obstruction 19, 27, 73, 128, 141, 163, 210, 216, 328, 334, 336, 337, 340, 350, 355, 374, 375, 376, 392, 415
Airway resistance 49, 71, 79, 84, 85, 86, 94, 118, 407
Allergens 100, 101, 140, 355
Allergic bronchopulmonary aspergillosis (ABPA) 322
Alpha-1 antitrypsin deficiency 391
Alveolar destruction 356, 391
Alveolar epithelium 44, 119, 147, 181
Alveolar macrophages 124, 133, 134, 143, 144
Alveolar stage 70
Alveolar surface tension 56, 81
Alveolar ventilation 104
Anaerobic bacteria 215
Anesthesiology planning 3
Angiotensin-converting enzyme 2 (ACE2) 46
Antifungal therapy 309, 322
Antimicrobial peptides 143
Antimicrobial susceptibility testing 288
Arrhythmia 15
Arterial blood gas (ABG) 18
Arterial blood gas (ABG) analysis 165, 178, 412
Aspergillosis 294, 297, 322, 323
Aspiration pneumonia 192, 203, 215
Asthma 20, 26, 34, 147, 151, 177, 179, 182, 220, 289, 327, 329, 330, 331, 332, 334, 338, 341, 343, 346, 347, 350, 351, 352, 354, 355, 357, 359, 360, 392
Auscultation 1, 3, 4, 8, 9, 10, 11, 12, 13, 14, 18, 22, 23, 25, 26, 27, 28, 30, 31, 32, 155, 339

B

Barrel chest 391
Bilateral wheezing 27
Blastomycosis 322, 323
Bradypnea 14

Branching morphogenesis 70
Breathing process 80
Breathlessness 15
Bronchi 2, 3, 4, 5, 6, 7, 40, 41, 43, 44, 45, 46, 47, 49, 50, 70, 78, 79, 112, 113, 114, 115, 116, 132, 185, 195, 200, 209, 210, 216
Bronchial breath sounds 31
Bronchial hyperreactivity 27, 62
Bronchial tree 70
Bronchial wall thickening 215, 391
Bronchiectasis 185, 188, 189, 209, 210, 214, 215, 217, 268, 288, 322, 392
Bronchoconstriction 355
Bronchodilators 355, 378, 391, 429
Broncho-obstructive syndrome 13, 14
Bronchopneumonia 215
Bronchopulmonary dysplasia 42
Bronchoscopy 169, 170, 178, 179, 206, 207, 208, 412
Bronchovesicular breath sounds 12
Bronchus-associated lymphoid tissue (BALT) 143

C

Canalicular stage 70
Capnography 178
Carbon dioxide expulsion 5, 65
Cardiac disease 15, 17
Cardiovascular system 3, 76, 101, 431
Cavitary lesion 216
Cellular metabolism 77, 87, 93
Cellular respiration 81, 90
Cellular signaling mechanisms 43
Chemoreceptors 104, 144
Chest expansion 31
Chest pain 13, 16, 17
Chest physiotherapy 215
Chest tightness 334, 337, 355
Chest ultrasound 178
Chest X-ray 21, 178, 179, 198, 200, 253, 323
Chronic bronchitis 179, 364, 391, 392
Chronic cough 288, 391
Chronic irritation 13
Chronic lower respiratory disease 78, 109
Chronic mouth breathing 49
Chronic obstructive pulmonary disease (COPD) 12, 14, 24, 26, 27, 28, 29, 32, 70, 77, 88, 97, 99, 101, 106, 121, 131, 142, 151, 153, 161, 162, 163, 167, 174, 177, 195, 205, 298, 329, 369, 371, 376, 385, 387, 393, 394, 396, 399, 401, 402, 403, 405, 406, 407, 415, 422, 425, 427, 429, 432
Chronic Obstructive Pulmonary Disease (COPD) 27, 42, 79, 85, 95, 196, 363, 364, 365, 366, 367, 370, 373, 374, 375, 377, 378, 379, 381, 383, 384, 388
Chronic productive cough 215, 392
Ciliated pseudostratified columnar cells 50
Clinical assessments 6, 12, 159, 413
Clinical management 14, 97, 196, 207, 219, 230, 263, 283, 329, 403, 405, 421, 432
Clinician-patient relationship 2
Clubbing 31
Coccidioidomycosis 297, 322, 323
Community-acquired pneumonia (CAP) 186, 190, 191, 215
Computed tomography (CT) 18, 20, 160, 177, 186, 207, 211, 304, 305, 372, 412
Congenital anomalies 60, 61, 62
Congestive heart failure 15, 23
Continuous positive airway pressure (CPAP) 83
Continuum poroelastic model 83
Cor pulmonale 391
Cough reflex 143
Crackles 23, 31, 32
Cryptococcosis 322, 323
Cyanosis 13, 31, 411
Cylindrical bronchiectasis 215
Cytokines 355

D

D-dimer testing 16
Dead space ventilation 428
Diagnostic accuracy 1, 2, 16, 21, 25, 149, 152, 154, 156, 157, 159, 164, 166, 169, 171, 173, 175, 178, 195, 248, 272, 273, 305, 318, 368, 372
Diagnostic process 3, 14, 25, 152, 155, 158, 167, 177, 273, 372, 413
Diffusing capacity for carbon monoxide (DLCO) 178, 179

Diffusion 88, 104, 161, 162, 163
Directly Observed Therapy (DOT) 238
Ductus arteriosus 57
Dyspnea 13, 14, 15, 16, 18, 26, 27, 98, 151, 154, 186, 198, 200, 207, 261, 272, 299, 302, 312, 313, 315, 316, 335, 337, 355, 370, 371, 376, 379, 383, 384, 386, 391, 392, 404, 408, 411, 422, 428, 430

E

Early fetal development 45
Embryogenesis 39, 41, 52, 55, 58, 61, 69
Embryonic development 39, 42, 43, 46, 52, 53, 68, 71
Embryonic stage 70
Emphysema 179, 391, 392
Empyema 215
Environmental reservoirs 288
Eosinophilia 322
Eosinophils 253, 355, 356
Epithelial cells 4, 44, 48, 49, 58, 69, 73, 78, 116, 117, 119, 126, 128, 129, 130, 131, 133, 134, 135, 136, 137, 142, 144, 145, 180, 301
Epithelial-mesenchymal interactions 40
Eustachian tubes 48
Exacerbations 371, 391
exercise pulmonary hypertension (exPH) 75
Exhaled nitric oxide test 178
Exhaustive assessment 8
Expiratory reserve volume 104
Extrapulmonary diseases 16

F

Fetal growth 43, 53
Forced expiratory volume (FEV) 79
Forced Expiratory Volume in one second (FEV1) 18, 161
Forced vital capacity (FVC) 28, 95, 162, 340
Forced Vital Capacity (FVC) 18, 161
Functional residual capacity 104
Fungal spores 322

G

Gas exchange 2, 3, 4, 5, 6, 15, 41, 43, 44, 47, 48, 49, 50, 51, 53, 54, 56, 57, 58, 59, 60, 64, 65, 66, 67, 68, 69, 75, 77, 78, 79, 80, 81, 84, 85, 86, 87, 88, 89, 90, 91, 94, 95, 97, 99, 101, 103, 113, 114, 115, 116, 119, 128, 144, 161, 162, 163, 167, 168, 185, 186, 364, 380, 399, 400, 401, 402, 403, 404, 405, 406, 407, 408, 411, 412, 414, 417, 421, 422, 427
Gastroesophageal reflux disease 27, 329, 340, 349, 401
Gene signals 55
Genetic integrity 46
Genetic variation 46
Goblet cells 70, 143, 144
Granulomatous inflammation 322

H

Healthy pregnancy 42
Hemoglobin 89, 104
Hemoptysis 215, 216
Histamine release 143
Histoplasmosis 297, 322, 323
Holistic patient-oriented care 2
Hospital-acquired pneumonia (HAP) 192, 215
Hydatid cyst 322
Hypercapnia 3, 399, 400, 403, 407, 414, 417, 425, 427, 428, 429
Hyperresonance 31, 32
Hyperventilation 428
Hypoxemia 3, 8, 13, 23, 399, 400, 403, 404, 411, 417, 420, 425, 427, 428, 429
Hypoxic drive 104
Hypoxic environments 57, 80

I

IgA antibodies 143
IgE-mediated hypersensitivity 355
Immunocompromised host 288, 322
Inflammation 110, 121, 125, 355, 430
Inflammatory response 143
Inhaled corticosteroids 342, 355, 378
Inspection 8, 10, 31, 32, 154
Inspiratory muscle fatigue 6
Inspiratory reserve volume 104, 105
Intercostal muscles 4, 6, 7, 8, 78, 80, 81, 82, 84, 103, 406

Intercostal muscles contract 4, 6, 84
Intercostal retractions 31
Interstitial pneumonia 215
Intrapulmonary pressure 81, 85
Intrathoracic pressure 81, 83, 84, 85, 88
Intrathoracic pressure dynamics 81

L

Larynx 2, 3, 4, 5, 7, 41, 48, 77, 78, 114, 115, 116
Lobar pneumonia 32, 215
Löffler's syndrome 322
Lower respiratory tract 4, 7, 8, 41, 47, 48, 49, 50, 72, 79, 116, 119, 186, 220, 325
Lung abscess 188, 201, 215, 217, 219, 220
Lung anatomy 42, 44, 157, 200, 305, 372
Lung biopsy 178
Lung branching morphogenesis 43
Lung bud 70
Lung cancer 16, 72, 140, 150, 151, 154, 157, 165, 169, 171, 173, 176, 196, 201, 219, 371, 423
Lung carcinoma 14, 171
Lung compliance 57, 83, 84, 85, 86, 90, 97
Lung development 40, 43, 46, 53, 54, 55, 59, 60, 61, 63, 66, 71
Lung function 1, 15, 18, 19, 21, 26, 28, 30, 37, 40, 45, 52, 55, 56, 58, 59, 76, 77, 80, 83, 95, 97, 98, 99, 100, 103, 105, 109, 121, 134, 141, 154, 155, 162, 163, 164, 165, 168, 188, 193, 195, 196, 203, 213, 293, 294, 310, 322, 328, 331, 334, 335, 336, 338, 340, 342, 344, 346, 350, 354, 367, 368, 369, 370, 372, 373, 374, 375, 376, 377, 378, 379, 380, 381, 382, 384, 386, 387, 400, 401, 408, 417, 421, 422, 423, 426
Lung homeostasis 54, 331
Lung maturation 43, 60
Lung maturity 42
Lung parenchyma 18, 23, 63, 83, 186, 190, 201, 202, 204, 208, 214
Lung tissue 5, 8, 22, 29, 43, 54, 61, 81, 83, 85, 115, 134, 152, 169, 179, 185, 186, 187, 202, 206, 211, 213, 300, 301, 302, 303, 311, 366, 375, 380, 408, 422, 433
Lymphoid tissue 143

M

Macrolide antibiotics 288
Magnetic Resonance Imaging (MRI) 157, 159, 178
Mantoux test 178, 253
Mast cells 355
Maternal health 42
Maternal microbiome 62
Maternal microplastic exposure 62
Maturation 45, 54
Mechanical ventilation 107, 416, 417, 428, 429
Mechanomyography 82, 107
Mental distress 15
Mesenchymal tissue 44
Microbiota 40, 41, 47, 56, 59, 63, 70, 72, 112, 113, 124, 125, 126, 145, 146, 180, 256, 314, 321
Microbiota-gut-brain axis 40, 47, 56, 70, 72
Microcirculatory sufficiency 90
Micro-computed tomography (micro-CT) 81
Minute ventilation 104
Molecular movement 77
Morphogenesis 41
Mucociliary clearance 143
Mucus hypersecretion 355, 391
Mucus-secreting glands 48
Mucus secretion 86
Mu-opioid receptors (MORs) 93
Muscle activity 82
Mycobacterium abscessus 262, 263, 267, 282, 288
Mycobacterium avium complex (MAC) 263, 273, 280, 288, 289
Mycobacterium kansasii 288
Mycobacterium tuberculosis 167, 223, 224, 225, 227, 228, 230, 231, 233, 235, 236, 244, 246, 249, 251, 254, 256, 257, 258, 259, 260, 262, 265, 272, 289, 291

N

Nasal cavity 2, 4, 7, 47, 48, 50, 78, 115, 116
Nasal congestion 7
Nasal hairs 119, 143
Necrotizing pneumonia 215
Neonatal breathing 57
Neonatal circulation 57
Neonatal life 39, 57, 74
Neonatal respiration 45, 56, 57, 58
Neonatal respiratory distress syndrome (NRDS) 58

Neuromechanical coupling 81, 109
Nodular infiltrates 288
Non-invasive ventilation (NIV) 428
Nonproductive cough 14, 189
Nontuberculous mycobacteria (NTM) 261, 263, 266, 288
Normal respiratory pathophysiology 79

O

Opioid-induced respiratory depression (OIRD) 93
Opportunistic infection 288
Oxidative burst 143
Oxygenate tissues 2
Oxygen therapy 415, 416, 428
Oxygen transport 80, 87, 89, 90, 91
Oxyhemoglobin dissociation curve 104

P

Paenibacillus odorifer 54, 72
Palpation 1, 3, 8, 10, 11, 12, 13, 22, 28, 29, 30, 31, 32, 154, 155
Paragonimiasis 322
Paranasal sinuses 48
Parasitic lung infiltrates 322
Partial pressure of carbon dioxide 104
Partial pressure of oxygen 104
Pathogenesis mechanisms 64, 267
Pathological dysfunction 1
Patient care 1, 10, 11, 15, 17, 23, 24, 42, 61, 152, 159, 165, 168, 172, 174, 195, 197, 274, 283, 286, 296, 300, 316, 322, 343, 381, 390, 401, 416, 419, 427
Patient education 2, 8, 19, 27, 162, 275, 285, 340, 348, 381, 383, 384, 385, 390, 414
Patient history 2, 3, 16, 22, 24, 25, 34, 152, 153, 154, 159, 188, 279, 299, 304, 306, 367, 403, 410
Peak expiratory flow rate (PEFR) 19, 27, 178, 355
Peak flow meter 18, 20
Peak flow metering 19
Pectus excavatum 31
Percussion 1, 3, 14, 18, 28, 30, 31, 32
Perfusion 104
Phagocytosis 143
Pharynx 2, 3, 4, 7, 41, 47, 48, 77, 78, 115, 116, 119, 120, 128, 129, 131, 134, 142, 187
Physical examination 1, 2, 4, 26, 30, 152, 154, 155, 338, 339
Pleural effusion 8, 11, 14, 20, 28, 30, 32, 154, 179, 207, 216, 265
Pleural fluid analysis 178
Pleuritic disorders 16
Pneumocystis jirovecii pneumonia (PJP) 322
Pneumonia 26, 28, 186, 189, 190, 191, 192, 198, 200, 402, 423
Polysomnography 178
Postnatal condition 57
Postnatal growth 52, 54
Postnatal life 54
Postpartum lung growth 40
Prenatal exposure 60, 63, 64
Preterm birth 53
Primary ciliary dyskinesia 45, 60
Pseudoglandular stage 49, 70
Pulmonary airways 44
Pulmonary capillaries 3, 51, 67, 90
Pulmonary development 58
Pulmonary disease 5, 12, 14, 21, 24, 26, 27, 28, 29, 32, 42, 46, 63, 64, 70, 77, 81, 83, 88, 95, 97, 99, 101, 106, 121, 131, 142, 151, 153, 154, 160, 161, 162, 163, 167, 174, 177, 186, 188, 192, 195, 205, 212, 220, 254, 259, 261, 263, 265, 266, 267, 276, 285, 289, 290, 291, 293, 297, 298, 303, 311, 329, 360, 363, 364, 369, 370, 371, 376, 380, 385, 387, 389, 393, 394, 395, 396, 397, 399, 401, 402, 403, 405, 406, 407, 415, 422, 425, 427, 429, 432, 433
Pulmonary edema 32, 356, 428, 429
Pulmonary embolism 16, 35, 88, 159, 179, 403, 406, 422, 431
Pulmonary etiology 15
Pulmonary function tests 5, 19, 149, 152, 154, 158, 356, 408
Pulmonary function tests (PFTs) 161, 178
Pulmonary hemodynamics 76
Pulmonary hypertension 391, 429
Pulmonary physiology 85, 103
Pulmonary surfactant 57, 71, 104

Pulmonary vasculature development 46
Pulse oximetry 18, 178
Pus formation 215

R

Reflex bronchoconstriction 143
Residual volume 97, 104, 105, 179
Respiratory ailment 26
Respiratory airway 41
Respiratory anatomy 1, 5, 55, 68
Respiratory apparatus 47, 51, 65, 81, 115, 119, 140, 407
Respiratory development 39, 42, 43, 45, 46, 53, 54, 55, 56, 59, 60, 61, 63, 70
Respiratory disease care 14
Respiratory distress 3, 7, 10, 13, 14, 15, 22, 23, 24, 25, 27, 28, 30, 34, 36, 41, 45, 50, 53, 58, 60, 61, 85, 92, 97, 98, 103, 124, 133, 143, 154, 167, 170, 186, 199, 207, 214, 266, 308, 310, 321, 329, 368, 399, 400, 401, 402, 403, 405, 406, 410, 411, 414, 415, 416, 418, 419, 420, 421, 426, 427, 429, 430, 431
Respiratory diverticulum 41, 43, 44
Respiratory embryogenesis 44
Respiratory epithelium 53, 69, 70, 143
Respiratory health 2, 3, 10, 12, 19, 20, 22, 40, 41, 44, 46, 47, 48, 49, 51, 52, 53, 54, 55, 56, 57, 58, 59, 60, 61, 62, 63, 64, 65, 69, 70, 76, 77, 78, 79, 81, 88, 91, 95, 96, 97, 99, 103, 111, 114, 115, 116, 120, 122, 126, 128, 131, 134, 136, 137, 138, 141, 162, 186, 188, 193, 294, 307, 314, 328, 335, 336, 343, 348, 350, 368, 369, 382, 391, 400, 411, 424, 425, 426
Respiratory health care 2
Respiratory illnesses 6, 10, 16, 18, 26, 43, 64, 86, 99, 121, 153, 195, 198, 200, 214, 295, 303, 313, 329, 333, 338, 363, 370, 377, 400, 410
Respiratory mechanism 5, 411
Respiratory muscle failure 428
Respiratory pathology 3, 22, 26, 77, 178, 293, 295, 321
Respiratory physiology 1, 20, 65, 67, 76, 77, 78, 79, 81, 84, 85, 86, 87, 88, 89, 90, 91, 92, 93, 94, 95, 96, 97, 99, 100, 101, 102, 103, 104, 137
Respiratory rate 3, 8, 13, 23, 27, 28, 31, 56, 91, 93, 104, 118, 328
Respiratory system 1, 2, 3, 4, 5, 6, 7, 8, 10, 11, 12, 13, 14, 16, 17, 18, 19, 20, 21, 22, 23, 30, 32, 33, 34, 39, 41, 42, 43, 44, 46, 47, 48, 49, 51, 52, 53, 54, 55, 56, 57, 58, 61, 62, 63, 64, 65, 66, 67, 68, 69, 70, 71, 73, 74, 75, 76, 77, 78, 79, 80, 81, 82, 83, 84, 94, 95, 97, 101, 103, 105, 108, 111, 112, 113, 114, 115, 117, 118, 119, 120, 121, 122, 123, 124, 125, 128, 129, 130, 131, 133, 134, 135, 137, 139, 140, 142, 143, 185, 190, 205, 269, 293, 294, 302, 334, 360, 399, 400, 401, 403, 411
Respiratory therapy 8, 22, 31, 308, 408
Respiratory tract 2, 3, 7, 8, 11, 12, 39, 40, 41, 42, 43, 44, 45, 46, 47, 48, 49, 50, 52, 53, 54, 55, 56, 57, 58, 59, 60, 61, 62, 63, 64, 65, 67, 68, 69, 70, 71, 72, 73, 101, 112, 113, 116, 117, 118, 119, 120, 121, 123, 124, 126, 128, 135, 140, 143, 144, 146, 169, 181, 193, 300, 313, 321, 336, 339, 367, 368, 374, 375, 376, 395
Respiratory tree 45, 192
Reynolds-Averaged Navier-Stokes equations 84
Rib cage 6
Risk assessment 3, 369, 423

S

Saccular (cystic) bronchiectasis 215
Saccular development 49
Saccular stage 70
Schistosomiasis 322
Serological tests 322
Shortness of breath 13, 15, 334, 335, 411
Skin and soft tissue infection 288
Spirometry 18, 19, 161, 162, 178, 340, 355, 381, 391
Sputum analysis 165, 167, 178
Sputum culture 166, 200, 253, 288
Sputum production 14, 154, 188, 206, 210, 215, 269, 370, 372, 391
Status asthmaticus 355
Strongyloidiasis 322
Submucosal glands 50, 129, 147, 182
Surfactant production 70, 144
Surfactant proteins 143
Systemic disturbances 1
Systemic resistance 86
Systemic treatment 16

T

Tachycardia 16
Tachypnea 7, 13, 14, 410, 411
Tactile fremitus 31, 32
Teratogenic developmental disorders 44
Thoracentesis 178, 179
Thoracic cavity 4, 6, 34, 80, 81, 82, 83, 84, 177
Thoracic radiography 3, 33
Thoracic resonance 14
Thoracic volume 4, 6, 81, 82
Tidal volume 95, 96, 104, 105
Tissue elasticity 11, 83
Total lung capacity 95, 104, 179
Trachea 2, 3, 4, 5, 7, 22, 32, 40, 41, 43, 44, 45, 46, 47, 48, 49, 50, 56, 71, 78, 79, 113, 114, 115, 116
Tracheal deviation 31
Tracheoesophageal fistula 45, 61
Tracheoesophageal septum 70
Transdiaphragmatic pressure measurement 82
Treatment regimens 191, 288
Tuberculin test 178
Tuberculosis (TB) 223, 224, 226, 231, 239
Type 1 respiratory failure 428, 429
Type 2 respiratory failure 428
Type II pneumocytes 70, 144
Type I pneumocytes 70, 144

U

Ultrasound elastography 11
Upper airway 78, 94, 108
Upper respiratory tract 7, 47, 48, 49, 51, 115, 116, 144

V

Vaccine development 78, 246, 247, 248, 284
Varicose bronchiectasis 215
Ventilation 3, 81, 103, 104, 178, 179, 414, 416, 428
Ventral respiratory column (VRC) 92
Vesicular breath sounds 31
Viral infection 14, 306, 371, 414
Visual assessment 8, 10, 13
Visual examination 10
Visual inspections 8
Vital capacity 96, 104, 105

W

Wheezes 31, 155